SPORTS INJURIES
The Unthwarted Epidemic

Second Edition

Edited by

Paul F. Vinger
Earl F. Hoerner

PSG PUBLISHING COMPANY, INC.
LITTLETON, MASSACHUSETTS

Library of Congress Cataloging in Publication Data
Main entry under title:

Sports injuries.

Includes bibliographies and index.
1. Sports—Accidents and injuries. 2. Sports—Accidents and injuries—Prevention.
I. Vinger, Paul F. II. Hoerner, Earl F. [DNLM: 1. Athletic Injuries. 2. Sports
medicine. QT 260 S7702]
RD97.S73 1985 363.1′4 85-3703
ISBN 0-88416-498-5

Published by:
PSG PUBLISHING COMPANY, INC.
545 Great Road
Littleton, Massachusetts 01460

First Edition 1981
Second Edition 1986

Printed in the United States of America.

International Standard Book Number: 0-88416-498-5

Library of Congress Catalog Card Number: 85-3703

Last digit is the print number: 9 8 7 6 5 4 3 2

Contributors

Marlene J. Adrian, PhD
Director, Biomechanics Research Laboratory
University of Illinois at Urbana-Champaign
Urbana, Illinois

Judith D. Bentkover, PhD
Visiting Lecturer of Health Policy and Management
Harvard School of Public Health
Christopher Walker Fellow
Kennedy School of Government
Harvard University
Cambridge, Massachusetts

Carl S. Blyth, PhD
Professor and Chairman
Department of Physical Education
University of North Carolina
Chapel Hill, North Carolina
Chairman, American Football Coaches Association Committee on Football Injuries and Fatalities

Victoria R. Brown, MS
Human Factor Analyst
Directorate for Hazard Identification and Analysis
US Consumer Product Safety Commission
Washington, DC

Dennis Burns, MFA
President, Pro-tec, Inc.
Bellevue, Washington

Robert C. Cantu, MD
Chief of Neurosurgical Service
Chairman, Department of Surgery
Director of Medical Education
Director, Service of Sports Medicine
Emerson Hospital
Concord, Massachusetts

Cosmo R. Castaldi, DDS
Chairman, American Society for Testing and Materials, Hockey Committee
Professor and Chairman
Department of Pediatric Dentistry
University of Connecticut
Farmington, Connecticut

C. Frazier Damron, PeD
Professor and Director
Safety Studies Program
Department of Curriculum and Instruction
School of Education
University of Wisconsin
Madison, Wisconsin

Steven J. Danish, PhD
Professor and Chair of Psychology
Virginia Commonwealth University
Richmond, Virginia

Deborah L. Feltz, PhD
Assistant Professor
Youth Sports Institute
Michigan State University
East Lansing, Michigan

Steven T. Gaunya, RPT
Mt. Vernon Rehabilitation Center
Alexandria, Virginia

Daniel Hanley, MD
College Physician
Bowdoin College
Brunswick, Maine
Physician for US Olympic Teams 1960–1968
Medical Commission International Olympic Committee

Christine E. Haycock, MD
Associate Professor of Surgery
College of Medicine and Dentistry
New Jersey Medical School
Newark, New Jersey
Member, AMA Committee on Medical Aspects of Sports

John S. Hayward, PhD
Professor, Department of Biology
University of Victoria
Victoria, British Columbia
Canada

Joseph M. Healey, Jr, JD
Assistant Professor
Community Medicine and Health Care
University of Connecticut School of Medicine
Farmington, Connecticut

Voigt R. Hodgson, PhD
Professor, Department of Neurosurgery
School of Medicine
Wayne State University
Detroit, Michigan

Earl F. Hoerner, MD, MPH
Professor of Orthopedic Rehabilitation
University of Connecticut
School of Medicine
Farmington, Connecticut
Director, Human and Sport
Performance Laboratory
University of Connecticut
Storrs, Connecticut

Thomas E. Hoerner, MD
Orthopedic Surgeon
Team Physician
Merrimack College
North Andover, Massachusetts

Edward S. Horton, MD
Clinical Research Center
Medical Center Hospital of Vermont
Burlington, Vermont

William F. Hulse
Senior Research Consultant
American Society of Testing
and Materials
Philadelphia, Pennsylvania

Ralph Kylloe, EdD
President, Kylloe and Associates
Littleton, Massachusetts
Former Visiting Assistant Professor
Purdue University

Sheldon Langer, DPM, FACFO
President, The Langer Biomechanics
Group
Deer Park, New York

Merrill G. Liteplo, MD
Clinical Instructor in Dermatology
Harvard Medical School
Boston, Massachusetts

Edward M. Milner
Manager, Products Technology
Recreational Products
Monsanto Company
St. Louis, Missouri

Ashby C. Moncure, MD
Assistant Clinical Professor
Harvard Medical School
Boston, Massachusetts
Physician for Boston Bruins

Chauncey A. Morehouse, PhD
Professor of Physical Education
Pennsylvania State University
University Park, Pennsylvania

Frederick O. Mueller, PhD
Professor of Physical Education
University of North Carolina
Chapel Hill, North Carolina

John J. Murray, MD
Clinical Associate Professor
of Pediatrics
College of Medicine
University of Vermont
Burlington, Vermont
Medical Officer, Cross-country venue
XIII Winter Olympic Games
Lake Placid, New York

Arthur M. Pappas, MD
Professor of Orthopedics
University of Massachusetts
School of Medicine
Worcester, Massachusetts
Medical Director
Boston Red Sox

E. C. Percy, MD
Associate Professor of Orthopedics
College of Medicine
The University of Arizona
Health Sciences Center
Tucson, Arizona

John W. Powell, PhD, AT, C
Instructor in Health Education
Pennsylvania State University
University Park, Pennsylvania

Arnold E. Reif, DSc
Research Professor of Pathology
Boston University School of Medicine
Boston, Massachusetts

Francis X. Rockett, MD
Clinical Instructor, Surgery
Harvard Medical School
Boston, Massachusetts
Physician for Harvard University
Football Team

Allan J. Ryan, MD
Editor-in-Chief
The Physician and Sportsmedicine
Minneapolis, Minnesota

Jennifer L. Shaw, BS
Research Assistant
University of Connecticut
School of Medicine
Farmington, Connecticut

Arthur J. Siegel, MD
Medical Director
Hahnemann Hospital
Brighton, Massachusetts

Harriet G. Tolpin, PhD
Associate Professor of Economics
Simmons College
Boston, Massachusetts

Hal Trumble
Executive Director
Amateur Hockey Association
of the United States
Colorado Springs, Colorado

Paul F. Vinger, MD
Emerson Hospital
Concord, Massachusetts
Assistant Clinical Professor
in Ophthalmology
Harvard Medical School
Boston, Massachusetts
Chairman, Eye Safety Committee
American Society of Testing and Materials

James P. Webb, RN
Former Olympic contender

Earle W. Wilkins, Jr, MD
Associate Professor of Surgery
Harvard Medical School
Boston, Massachusetts
Physician for the Boston Bruins

Kent S. Wilson, MD
Assistant Clinical Professor
Department of Otolaryngology
University of Minnesota
Minneapolis, Minnesota

Contents

Foreword

Injuries are a part of sport, as they are of all our activities of daily living. In sport the difference is that there is a better opportunity to prevent injuries, and in organized sports activities to identify them more promptly, provide appropriate emergency and definitive management, and help to prevent reinjury by effective rehabilitation and proper advice regarding the return to practice and competition. The tremendous universal interest in sports medicine today among people in all walks of life who are involved in many different types of physical activities has supported developments and improvements in all of these aspects of prevention and management of sports injuries so that they are currently more effective than ever.

Injury prevention begins with the physical evaluation of athletes before entering their sports seasons. Today we know better the particular hazards of each sport, are able to identify the physical deficiencies or defects that increase the chances of injuries when those who have them are exposed to such hazards, and are enjoying more and better examinations of young athletes. There appears to be a tendency, even for individual recreational athletes, to seek such preparticipation evaluation.

An important factor in preventing sports injuries is the physical conditioning of the athlete. Strength, coordination, flexibility and power are being more seriously considered in the training of athletes today and we have developed better techniques and equipment to help us.

In all sports where protective equipment is required on or off the athlete, we have better products available as the result of new materials and improved designs. Greater attention has been given as well to protecting other athletes from the impact of such protective equipment on them.

When injuries occur, recent advances in understanding the biomechanics involved and knowledge of tissue resistance to stress have made it possible to make accurate diagnoses more rapidly. This has been facilitated by the introduction of such sophisticated devices as the arthroscope, computerized automated tomography and radioisotope bone scanning.

Surgical management of sports injuries has benefitted from long-term evaluation of the results of specific reparative techniques such as repair and replacement of the anterior cruciate ligament and follow-up of the results of both surgical and nonsurgical treatment of other conditions such as shoulder separation. The development of more reliable surgical techniques and more efficient surgical instruments has rendered surgical management in many circumstances a more conservative approach than nonsurgical methods.

Finally, the rehabilitation of the injured athlete has become more effective through recognition of the desirability of restoring early range of movement as soon as consistent with appropriate tissue healing time and through other measures taken to preserve muscle strength and prevent atrophy during the treatment process. Correct timing of the return to sports practice and competition helps to reduce recurrent injury and shortens temporary disability.

Allan J. Ryan, MD

Foreword

SECTION I
Monitoring Sports Injuries

CHAPTER 1
Injury Surveillance Systems for Sports

C. Frazier Damron, PeD
Earl F. Hoerner, MD
Jennifer L. Shaw, BS

Many persons who engage in physical activities do so neither well nor wisely. To enjoy them one has to be free from injury and illness. Yet disabilities in sports stem primarily from accidental causes. The athlete who spends months or years in strenuous conditioning programs may lose the results of that effort in a matter of seconds. An injury to a key member of a team may destroy a chance for victory.

The benefits of a sport depend upon efforts to prevent and control injuries. Yet the recent growth of sports equipment and facilities and the number of participants has far outstripped the controls designed to make play safe yet enjoyable. When injuries are measured in days and years of lost time and productivity, it is evident that sports accidents are a major safety problem.

Until recently, reports on recreational sports lacked reliable injury data. Since most participation has been on an individual and unorganized basis, there generally has been no central reporting of accidents. Although an increasing number of national and private organizations are now routinely reporting accidental injuries, even in organized athletics and in physical education, completion and analysis of accident and medical reports have been resisted by both participants and sports leaders.

Major breakthroughs in the scientific analysis and interpretation of the causes of sports injuries are anticipated as the result of studies by individual physicians and teams composed of physicians, trainers, coaches, and athletic doctors. Much of this valuable medical research has been conducted by the American Medical Association Committee on the Medical Aspects of Sports. The Association has *Standard Nomenclature of Athletic Injuries.*

An effective accident data system depends upon the collection and effective analysis of valid and reliable data and material evidence. If utilized properly, such a system can eliminate most potential accident hazards and minimize the consequences of those that do occur.

ACCIDENTS AND INJURIES DEFINED

Accident

The control of accidental injuries is complicated by the many definitions of *accident.* In sports, an accident is an unplanned event capable of resulting in loss of time, property damage, injury, disablement, or even death. To complicate matters further, the term *accident* is defined by every agency that accumulates such data for measurement purposes. Sports fans may refer to an event as an accident while a player or coach may consider it an injury. Identifying an event as an accident is predicated upon the causal factors in that

---

Adapted from: C.F. Damron. *Accident Surveillance System for Sports.* Sports Safety Series, Monograph No. 2. Washington, DC: American Alliance for Health, Physical Education and Recreation, 1977.

setting, the possibilities of prevention or control, and the seriousness of the harm.

Injury

All injury is damage. Two types of injuries are defined in the safety field: *restricted-activity injuries*, and *disabling injuries* confining the victim to bed.

Half of an estimated 50 million sports injuries require only brief medical attention with no restrictions of the person's usual activity. One injury in five confines a person to bed. According to the National Health Survey, a "bed-disabling injury" is one that confines a person to bed for more than half of the daylight hours on the day of an accident or on a following day. The National Safety Council defines a disabling injury as an injury that prevents a person from performing his usual activities for a full day beyond the day of the injury.

Each data system defines its terms slightly differently, but the parameters of a reportable injury always include the requirement for medical attention and a resulting restriction of participation. In the near future, it seems likely that sports injuries will be more accurately defined as to the quantitative limits of damage to person and property. The public is currently demanding improved product reliability to increase safety in the air, in automobiles and at work. Should they make similar demands for greater safety in sports, professionals in the field must be prepared.

NEED FOR A DATA SYSTEM

An effective system produces appropriate evidence about human and environmental variables for each accident episode, as well as variables having to do with products used. Such a system also promotes needed corrective measures and follow-up evaluation. The development of an effective system involves several processes:

1. Expedient uniform recording on standard forms of all near-miss incidents to indicate potentially hazardous situations or conditions,
2. Expedient uniform recording on standard forms of all accidents,
3. Prompt and thorough investigation of both near-miss and actual accidents,
4. A process for summarizing and analyzing accident data,
5. Conclusions and recommendations for corrective actions,
6. An accountable scheme for assessing and monitoring corrective measures.

The "state of the art" of accident data systems for surveillance of sports accidents leaves much to be desired. None of the systems at local, state, or national levels, maintains a balanced focus. However, even though they vary widely in scope, purpose, and procedures, there are common threads of emphasis. For example, practically all the systems are designed to focus upon after-the-incident events. Priority attention is focused upon injuries requiring medical attention, and which result in observable restricted activity or specific lost time from a particular sports activity.

Limitations of this nature significantly reduce the capabilities for obtaining a complete accounting of all accidents. These episodes, no matter how minor, need to be studied carefully even if no personal injury occurred, because each is an indication that something needs corrective attention. Clues to guide remedial actions are needed, to prevent recurrence of behaviors or conditions that could have more serious consequences. The data base provided by such systems is the only objective means for obtaining the evidence to implement corrective measures and appraise their effectiveness. Furthermore, effective systems are needed to account for particular features such as:

1. Unique risks and potential hazards associated with each sport activity,
2. Competitive behaviors common to all sports, including the desire or need to take risks,
3. Personal variables of participants such as their interest, motivation, skill, maturity, and knowledge,
4. Societal influences that affect behavior and performance of participants and their leaders,
5. Inadequate and overcrowded sport areas and facilities,
6. Discrepancies and failures of sports products and especially personal protective supplies, devices, and clothing,
7. Laxity of officials in enforcing the rules and regulations designed to safeguard participants.

A few sports such as football, hockey, and skiing have benefited from specialized systems yielding limited evidence used in controlling several accident-producing hazards. However, the list of sports that need more valid and reliable data to guide prevention and control is long.

A similar need exists in the sports, whose participants range from hundreds to millions. Their numbers continue to increase dramatically, as does the accident toll. These sports include snowmobiling, skin and scuba diving, water skiing, sky gliding and parachuting, backpacking, and a host of others.

PUBLIC INVOLVEMENT IN ACCIDENTS

Recreation and sports provide people with increasing opportunities for adventure, excitement, status, and enjoyment. Over 90% of Americans engage in at least one of more than 75 outdoor athletic and recreational sports activities. The current explosion in recreational sports is unprecedented; people have more time and money to spend in this rapidly expanding area.

Of the 200 million people in the United States over 110 million swim annually. Fifty million use boats, 40 million fish, and the same number use fire weapons with 20 million of them hunting annually. About 30 million persons camp each year, 35 million bowl, 4 million ski, 15 million water ski, and 3 million fish through the ice in 10 states.

It is estimated that over $25 billion are spent annually on recreational sports. It is difficult to estimate how costly sports accidents are to our people in terms of injuries and damage to equipment.

In the United States millions of people engage in sports annually, with only a few fatal injuries. Few realize that a sports death may be caused by factors usually not considered as related to obvious risk. For example, nearly 20% of all deaths of athletes are caused by heatstroke.

INHERENT RISKS

In sports, participants seek exciting, vigorous, challenging, and emotionally satisfying activities. This is the joy of the game. To such players the question of risk is of secondary importance. Many athletes minimize the danger. They accept the demands of vigorous contact sports and expect a number of hard blows in achieving optimal physical performance. Some seek the fun of sports even though they are physically and emotionally unprepared for it. To do so increases the likelihood of injury.

Calculating the Risks

An athlete runs a 50-50 chance of receiving an injury.[3] About 90% of all sports-related injuries are contusions and minor muscle pulls. They may not be accidental but inherent to the sport. The remaining 10% are more serious. They require appropriate therapeutic measures and should be assessed as to their accidental or nonaccidental nature.

About 20% of the one million youngsters who play football sustain an injury to knee, shoulder, or ankle each year. Fifty thousand nonprofessional players require surgery on the knee. There are also frequent microtraumatic lesions that become apparent in later life and cause arthritic impairments. About 25 to 30 persons die of football-related impairments annually. This fatality rate affects 1 of every 25,000 varsity players, or 1 per 3 million hours of exposure. What does society trade off for these injuries and deaths?

In Clarke's study on sport risks, comparisons are made of the hazards of football, power boating, auto and horse racing, and activities included in daily living. Football has the lowest death rate of all the activities investigated. Clarke contends, "What constitutes undue risk from participation in sports remains intuitive" and "...the more sound a research program, the more the undue-risk question can be put on an individual basis." An assessment of risks must include fatality and injury rates. There must also be reports on pathologic studies of individuals who have evidence of microtraumatic lesions that become apparent and debilitating in later life.

Certain risks taken by players become evident only after careful medical study of the adverse results of sports activity. A boxer who had demonstrated superior ability nonetheless died from the first blow on his head. A basketball player who bumped his head against the chest of an opponent also died because he too, had a very thin skull. These are examples of anomalies that are determined after injury and can seldom be detected prior to participation in a vigorous sport. What is needed is to determine which conditions can be detected prior to serious injury and to exercise appropriate measures to protect athletes from harm. For example, many swimmers are saved from drowning through effective community safety programs. To curb deaths and injuries in sports requires many environmental and human controls that reflect a full understanding of the dangers.

Contact and Noncontact Sports

Athletic activities are generally categorized as contact or noncontact sports. Injuries sustained in contact sports are generally considered to be the result of stress, competition, and collisions that are expected parts of the game, and not of accidental origin. The injured player may contend an accident caused his impairment or he may admit that he exceeded his performance capabilities.

When the hazards of an activity are known, the probability of injury is curtailed. Therefore players must understand the control of hazards. This responsibility rests fully on sports administrators. Even experienced players need continued excellent coaching, strong drives for maintaining and increasing skilled performance, and a community that does not make unreasonable demands of its athletes.

It is apparent that risks are exceedingly hard to quantify. Data to assess them are lacking. A basic philosophy of safety in sports has not as yet spread in our society. With a wider acceptance of safety concepts, information will become increasingly available on risks.

THE DEMOGRAPHICS OF SPORTS ACCIDENT SYSTEMS INCLUDING SPORTS ACCIDENT DATA

National data on sports accidents are now being collected by various agencies whose reports provide information on trends associated with sports hazards. Until recently, *Accident Facts*, an annual publication of the National Safety Council, reported school sports accidents; now annual issues abstract information on significant injuries within cities, states, or community areas. Many local organizations contribute their recurrent accident experience. Agencies within schools and colleges usually contribute information to state and national agencies.

There is not a complete accident data system that encompasses all educational institutions in a particular state. However, a few states have some type of system in operation. The state educational agency usually initiates accident data systems for use by elementary and secondary schools. The State Board of Health or some other state agency also provides this service. Certainly effective statewide systems can enhance surveillance of sports accidents.

Still, national or state sports accident information may not meet the needs of local agencies seeking to control hazards that are unique to their communities.

BASIC CONSIDERATIONS FOR ACCIDENT DATA SYSTEMS

The Organizational Process

The priority a sports accident data system should receive, and the need for an organized approach, was aptly given by Schwank (personal communication, 1975):

> Reporting, collecting and analyzing data on sports injuries, the first of four themes for the congress, is properly listed first, for we must base our actions regarding safety in sports upon valid and reliable data. I would not take off for a backpacking trip through one of our beautiful wilderness areas in Montana without a topographical map. Neither should we, without significantly reliable data, campaign for changes in football rules, attempt to set standards for protective sports equipment or make complaints or recommendations to the Consumer Product Commission, the Football Rules Committee, or any other such commission or committee. Without the map, without the data, one must surely wander, get lost, or at least encounter problems that he should have been able to avoid.

Communications

An organized communication network is critical to the development of an effective system. Someone must conceive, formulate, and transmit system information to receivers. An effective communication network is the only means to coordinate all the varied efforts of those interested in and associated with system development.

Established principles provide guidance in designing and implementing a system communication plan. In topical outline form these are:

1. Determine objectives
   - Increase awareness
   - Change attitudes
   - Achieve acceptance
   - Obtain support
2. Analyze the receivers (audiences)
   - Agency administrators and staff
   - Heads of departments, divisions, areas
   - Participants
   - Parents
   - Representatives of community and state agencies
   - News media
3. Select appropriate techniques for reaching each audience
   - Clarify system definitions
   - Obtain receiver involvement
   - Utilize social action (which emphasizes shared values and objectives)
4. Evaluate the effectiveness of the communications process
   - Through a systematic access scheme
   - Informal questionnaires
   - Person-to-person interviews
   - Analyze responses (related to system and communications objectives)
   - Make appropriate changes

As system technology and procedures become more sophisticated, a comprehensive, multipurpose information network for sports accident data should develop.

Goals

The goals of an effective sports data system are primarily to provide factual evidence to protect and defend the integrity of sports activities. An effective system should have three corollary purposes: 1) to provide reliable statistical data from which effective measures can be formulated to prevent or minimize the consequences of accidents that do occur, 2) to provide guidance toward enhancing the enjoyment of sports while at the same time imposing restraints that protect the welfare of all participants, and 3) to provide information for developing and improving the total safety program. The first purpose should receive the primary emphasis simply because the other two cannot be accomplished until it is well on the way toward successful attainment. A uniform terminology is needed, that will be acceptable to users. Persons with responsible roles in the system must understand each term and its appropriate use in operational applications. When all terms and definitions are uniformly stated, accident data from a wide variety of sources can be compared. Without such standardization valid comparisons are not possible.

Authority

The legal authority of a sports data system is vested in the chief administrator or board of the parent agency, be it a school, university, or other public or private institution. The person who is assigned and accepts the responsibility should be certain that it is officially designated by the legal authority, preferably in writing. The nature, scope, and duties should be prescribed, understood, and agreed upon by both parties.

Policies

Policy statements need to be clearly written, following the decision-making process that sets the direction for the system. Policies are effective to the extent that the system's leaders and workers have contributed to the policy statements and understand the meanings and values associated with each. Examples of some general policies are:

1. All departments, divisions, or systems in which any sports activity is conducted will participate in the uniform accident data system.

2. A qualified person will be assigned the responsibility of coordinating and monitoring the total accident data system for sports.

3. The system will be conducted according to established uniform policies and procedures for reporting, investigation, analysis, summarization, dissemination, and follow-up evaluations.

4. Complete details will be recorded on all sports accidents and near-accidents that may be potentially dangerous.

An example of specific policy is: The person immediately responsible for the sports activity shall notify the proper authorities when a serious accident occurs.

Budgeting

Budgeting is extremely important to the development and operation of an effective data system. Effectively coping with this challenge requires the system's leaders to understand thoroughly the financial conditions, sources of income, and the outcome desired by the parent agency. Budgets should be based on justifiable needs without guesses or assumptions.

Personnel

Qualified leadership is required to organize, manage, and maintain an effective sports accident data system. Fundamental knowledge of the basic components of the system and how each relates to the other is a basic need.

A persistent personnel problem is the recruitment and selection of supportive staff and on-line workers to assist the system administrator. One of the more powerful means of obtaining supportive assistance is through group actions by means of formalized or ad hoc committees, special study or task force groups. These groups should include balanced representation among system users and supporters. When possible, the core members of the group should include a physician, dentist, nurse, parent, athletic trainer, athletic director, coach, safety coordinator, physical education teacher, administrator, custodian, facilities manager, and student or participant.

Education

The organizational efficiency of a system will depend upon the education provided for leaders and workers alike. The range of educational needs begins during the planning stage, extends through the operational phase, and continues on through the improvement and refinement phases. New personnel will need an orientation to the system and experienced personnel will need refresher and reinforcement learning opportunities.

Evaluation

Evaluation of a data system is the process of determining the effectiveness of the system. It can be a problem for agency administrators and the system leaders. The end product of the system often has not been defined well enough to permit anyone to determine the extent to which the system is "successful." Also, the total system may operate in an informational vacuum. Some data are unused because they are irrelevant; other data receive no response by system leaders or workers because they are not considered data.

These types of problems can only be uncovered and remedied by an evaluation. It is an important process not to be overlooked.

Reporting Definitions

Reporting is the foundation of an effective accident data system. It must be prompt and accurate and must cover accidents and near-accidents on appropriate forms.

In planning or refining the reporting process, it is important that key administrators, staff, and participants be encouraged to provide their ideas, suggestions, or criticisms.

It is fundamental that terms and definitions be understood by all personnel. Examples of fundamental terms for reporting sports accidents have been identified and defined by Silverwood, who pointed out that "reporting processes are not identical for all purposes and there are differences in reporting practices among high school, college, and agency programs because of the variations in organizational responsibilities to the participant." His terms and definitions are as follows:

Participant. An individual permitted by a school or agency to take part in one of its sponsored activities.

Accident, sponsor jurisdiction. An accident that occurs on the property established by the sponsor to serve the practice or competition of participants and during the period that participation is sponsor-sanctioned.

Accident, nonschool jurisdiction. An accident that occurs outside the jurisdiction of the sponsor.

Accident, reportable. A sponsor-jurisdiction accident that results in an injury to a participant. Customarily, a reportable accident occurs when the injury requires first aid or medical treatment. Under this reporting plan, often no differentiation is made between "reportable" and "recordable" accidents.

Accident, recordable. A sponsor-jurisdiction accident that results in injury to a participant and deprives (or would deprive) him of medically approved complete participation in that activity on the day following injury.

These examples illustrate the critical role of definitions in reporting. Additional examples from other sources emphasize the need for clarity and specificity of a definition.

Injury An injury is defined as one which occurred as a result of participation in an organized football program at the high school level, for which medical treatment was received, or which resulted in restriction of [a student's] usual activity, for one day beyond the day of injury.

Reportable injury A reportable injury is one that requires the injured to desist from the activity, absent himself for a period of time and require either first aid or medical attention. An injury to the hand, neck, or spine must be reported, regardless of how slight it appears to be.

Disability injury This is any injury that results in death, permanent total or partial disability, or temporary total disability that occurred in the course of employment.

Nondisabling injury Any injury is called disabling if it requires medical treatment including first aid, but does not result in death, permanent impairment, or temporary total disability.

Recordable accident A recordable accident is any accident that results in a) severe pupil injury which causes the loss of one-half day or more of school time, or b) nonschool time, and/or c) a school jurisdictional accident which causes any property damage.

School jurisdiction accidents Such accidents occur on school property, during school-sponsored activities conducted off school property, or to students walking to and from school property.

Students are defined as children, youth, or adults who are officially enrolled or involved in any school-sponsored classes or activities. Included are classes or other activities at any educational level or special programs, eg, recreation, clubs, special education, Headstart, and the like.

Additional terminology related to the reporting process is provided in *Standard Nomenclature of Athletic Injuries* published by the American Medical Association.

Reporting Forms

In determining the appropriate reporting forms, the content and format should be carefully selected and designed in accord with the goals and definitions established for the system. If all sports accidents, including near-miss types, are to be reported, a form for that purpose will include items considerably different than in a system that requires reports of only medically treated injuries. In addition, form items may be needed to fulfill other needs such as insurance claims, legal requirements, or athletic conference regulations. In states where liability for sports accidents exists, an item should be included on the form for witnesses and administrators to sign.

There is an essential body of basic information that is prerequisite to the summarization and analysis of sports accident data. If additional data for a particular purpose such as research or insurance are needed, other forms can be devised. A basic requirement is that they be simple enough to be completed easily in a minimum amount of time. There is a basic minimum of information needed on an accident report form. Silverwood lists the essential descriptive components as follows:

1. Time-place-activity identification
2. Participant identification
3. Participant complaint
4. Description of the accident
5. Mechanism of injury
6. Medical diagnosis and disposition
7. Nature and day of medical clearance for return to a conditioning program
8. Day of medical clearance for return to complete participation.

It should be recognized that data from these minimum report form items can produce only gross information for use in determining and implementing corrective actions. However, they can produce general evidence of problem areas and accident patterns that can be used by decision-makers to direct further inquiry or implement corrective actions.

Reporting Procedures

The most vital aspect of the reporting process is that it be complete, accurate, and uniform. Deficiencies and inaccuracies can lead to faulty summaries and erroneous conclusions. The solution to this problem lies primarily in the education the reporters receive about the mechanics and standards of accurate reporting.

The process for routing a completed report form needs to be established and included with the instructions for the use of the form. Examples of recipients are the coordinator designee for the sports accident data system, the general coordinator or director of the total safety program, the administrative head of the program unit in which the accident occurs, the agency administrator or his designee, the insurance carrier, the attending physician, and other approriate personnel as needed.

Investigation

The purpose of investigating sports accidents is to obtain the best possible information about causative factors so that appropriate countermeasures may be devised to prevent similar occurrences. This process, effectively carried out, may lead to discovery of new or unnoticed hazards that need correction. In addition, the scheme can provide clues for improving other elements of data system functions.

Ideally all accidents need investigation. Priority should be given to the incidents that are most numerous, or to those involving situations or conditions with high risk potential. This may involve "near-miss" episodes as well as "minor" accidents. For instance, if mouthguards become faulty by warping or cracking, it will become known through an effective reporting process whether there is a near-miss or actual injury. Equipment failures should be investigated whether or not an injury occurs.

Routine investigations in which a nondisabling injury occurs can usually be done by system personnel. Whoever is assigned this role needs to understand the goal and values of the investigation process. Every investigation is conducted for two reasons: to find out how to prevent recurrence and thus protect the welfare of other participants, and to obtain facts needed for insurance claims. Fixing blame or establishing liability are not factors to be considered. He or she should also have at least general understanding of the nature of sports activities, including specific knowledge of the human variables, and also those pertaining to products and environment: for example, the rules of the sport, standards for court, field, and equipment, and the contributing causes commonly associated with sports activities.

Effective conduct of an investigation begins at the time each accident occurs and should proceed in all appropriate directions. The more delay involved, the greater the difficulty in obtaining all related facts, information, and objects associated with the accident. Memory reliability of the injured victim and witnesses decreases rapidly as time passes. Therefore, priority must be given to an immediate appraisal of the accident scene. Prompt investigations cannot be initiated or managed properly unless systematically planned in advance of need.

The facts collected from an investigation will provide evidence of the "what" and "how" aspects of the accident. Determining the "why" will depend upon an analysis of the facts. Every accident has features that include a number of possible contributing causes. These can involve personal protective equipment, environmental elements, and the behavioral actions associated with the sport activity. Each of these areas should receive the open-minded attention of the investigation. To come to a conclusion that the accident was fortuitous—"just one of those accidents which couldn't be prevented"—is less than superficial. To limit the analysis merely to personal negligence is another valueless conclusion. When negligence is involved there is an underlying reason.

The findings and recommendations resulting from an accident investigation should be discussed with decision-making personnel in the agency and with leaders of the accident data system. Prompt implementation of corrective measures depends primarily upon how well this is done.

All too often, the corrective measures recommended and decided upon are not implemented. The main reason is the failure to establish controls which insure that compliance will be checked and monitored. It is the responsibility of agency administration to establish such controls.

DATA SUMMARIZATION

The summarizing of sports accident data is relatively easy when planned in a systematic manner. The focus should be upon format that allows pertinent tabulations of raw data and summarization of total figures. The basic objectives to consider are:

1. Determine what accident data are most needed or desired by the sponsoring agency. Questions to guide deliberations are: to what extent does age, weight, and sex influence accident experience? What is the frequency and severity of injuries for each sport activity? What is the accident experience for each department, division, or school? What locations account for the most accidents? What environmental or equipment factors are involved in the accidents? What situations and behaviors are contributing to the accidents? What do patterns and trends of accident experience indicate? What is the cost of accidents to the agency, insurance company, and participants?

2. Decide how often summarized data are desired. It is a basic tenet that the expediency of decision-making and corrective actions is in proportion to the availability of data summaries for analysis and interpretation. For agencies sponsoring sports activities, unless under a legal mandate such as professional sports, the frequency of summary reporting is a local decision. The agency can maintain the autonomy of its system completely or it can elect to participate in a system developed by an athletic or sports conference to which it belongs.

3. Make certain that all accident report data are in accord with the definition of a recordable accident before recording the information on summary charts. Recordable accidents for jurisdictional and nonjurisdictional accidents are to be included depending on the objectives established for the system.

Manual Summarization

If the manual technique is to be employed for tabulating and summarizing the data, certain principles should be considered. These are:

1. The design for the summary chart or charts should be patterned according to the arrangement of the items on the report forms.

2. The size, shape, and format of the main chart or charts should be designed to accommodate the volume of reports, number of sports activities, and number of participants involved.

3. The person transferring the data from the accident report form to the summary chart should be thoroughly familiar with reporting terminology and codes so that the information is interpreted and classified accurately.

The possible combinations of summary charts are numerous. If each item on a report is valid, each can be summarized. It is strategic, however, to select the more critical items, such as lost time, hazardous behaviors, faulty equipment, and sex. Equal attention also needs to be given to the summaries, which by further breakdown are likely to produce clues for further summarization, and so on. Known or suspected accident problem areas are a priority clue in these decisions.

Machine Processing Summarization

Another technique for summarizing data is by means of machine data processing. This computerized process can tabulate, sort, summarize, and print out all pertinent information. This permits accident data to be accumulated constantly, deposited at a central place, and kept ready for rapid retrieval. The main value in using the computerized data processing technique is that accident information can easily be made available without cost in staff time for clerical chores. Data can be summarized in a variety of ways, with little effort, in a few minutes.

A critical aspect in establishing an effective summarization process for sports accident reports is for data processing and sports personnel to develop an initial understanding of the nature of each other's work. This sets the stage for cooperative efforts that are necessary for later development of the analysis stage. Two points are emphasized that relate to this computerized technique for summarizing data:

1. An accident report form will be needed that contains information to be coded. It will be easier to code if the information items are arranged in the order required for computer card layout.

2. An accident reporting code will be needed so that each item for which information is desired will have a code that can be key-punched onto a punched card.

The staff will also need to know what data are needed, how often the reports are desired, and what use is to be made of them. These are the same decisions that have to be made for manual processing.

Data Analysis

Analysis basically involves the summarized total of raw data and the calculation of injury frequency and severity rates. "Frequency" is the measure of actual accidental injury experience by showing how often injury occurs. "Severity" indicates the rate at which participation time is being lost. Figuring these rates takes into account several variables such as number of participants involved, the number of participant days or hours, and the seriousness of injury consequences. Analysis processes are not identical for all purposes, and agencies vary in such practices because responsibilities to clientele and participants differ. However, most analysis approaches follow similar patterns.

Key terms and definitions pertinent to understanding analysis that have been developed by Silverwood for use in sports systems are quoted as follows:

Frequency rate This is the ratio of the number of recorded accidents to exposure, and is expressed in terms of participation-hours. It can be determined by the following equation:

$$\frac{\text{Number of recorded injuries} \times 1{,}000{,}000}{\text{Exposure (No. persons} \times \text{No. hours)}} = \text{Injury frequency rate.}$$

This formula is applicable for overall injury rates for a total data system, a specific system for sports only, and even for special investigations. The injury per participant-hour (or man-hour) presents a more realistic portrayal than injury per days of sports accident experience.

In adapting the equation for the particular sport of skiing, injury rates could be presented in terms of number of injuries per thousand man skier days, basing the population on the number of days lift tickets are issued (L.R. Young, unpublished data, 1974).

Severity rate Severity rate makes use of severity days, defined as total lost days charged for injuries resulting in disability (impaired performance in that activity). Lost days include days of disability following the end of the sports season.

An equation for computing severity rate relates lost time to exposure.

$$\frac{\text{No. severity days} \times 100{,}000}{\text{Exposure (No. persons} \times \text{No. school days)}} = \text{Severity rate.}$$

With this formula, arbitrary lengths of absence from participation are chargeable to accidents that result in death or permanent disability. In sports where disability is more significant in terms of participant performance capabilities, definitions need to be carefully scrutinized to assure that the severity rate accurately reflects the injury situation.

Since the unit of exposure may need to be equally applicable to the overall situation and the specific sports activities, hours of participation might be substituted for school days in the preceding formula. In doing so, it may be advisable to change the 100,000 index to 1,000,000 to arrive at a workable formula.

Average lost time charged Besides frequency and severity rate, a third measure of accident experience is the average participation days charged per disability injury. This is a seldom-used measure, which can reveal the seriousness of injuries on the average. It may also reveal sports accident conditions or situations not readily apparent from a review of frequency or severity rates alone. Thus, it has potential for making possible a more complete evaluation of injury experience.

In determining the relationship between the total days charged and the total number of disabling injuries, the average days lost from participation may be calculated by either of the following formulas:

$$\text{Av days lost (from participation)} = \frac{\text{Total days (of season)}}{\text{Total disabling injuries (per season)}}$$

or

$$\text{Av days lost (from participation)} = \frac{\text{Severity rate}}{\text{Frequency rate}}$$

Even though nondisabling sports injuries are not usually included in computing frequency and severity rates, records should be kept of them and scrutinized regularly. The records should show, for example, the frequency of occurrence, the organizational unit in which the injuries occurred, the types of injuries, and the relationships to disabling injuries. Computing their frequency rate can be done in the same manner as the disabling injury frequency rate, by multiplying the number of participant cases requiring medical (or first aid) attention by 1,000,000 and dividing the product by the participant-hours of exposure.

Accident Analysis

It is essential that the record of each injury include at least one item in each of the following categories:

1. Nature of injury, ie, principal physical characteristics.
2. Part of body affected.
3. Source of injury, ie, the identification of the object, substance, exposure, or bodily motion that directly produced the injury.
4. Accident type, ie, the event that directly resulted in injury.
5. Hazardous conditions.
6. Agency of accident, ie, the identification of the object, substance, or premises in or about which the hazardous condition existed.
7. Unsafe act, ie, violation of commonly accepted safe procedure or practice

which directly contributed to the occurrence of the accident.

After injury rates have been used to identify the sports activity in which injuries occur most frequently, an analysis of individual cases will provide the information necessary to determine needed corrective measures. Further analysis in terms of hazardous condition, agency of the accident, and unsafe acts should be based upon accident investigation reports.

Data Comparison and Interpretation

At the appropriate time during analysis, a comparison of current frequency and severity rates with those of previous years is helpful in discerning trends toward or deviations from normal accident experience. Such comparisons can be tricky unless uniform definitions and procedures have been used in the system. Exceptional caution should be used in comparing rates with the state or national average. In most cases data from different systems are not compatible for comparison. Furthermore, because sports statistics from national sources are of necessity based upon accident summaries that are derived from incomplete data, national rates tend to be appreciably lower than those of an agency that obtains reports on all recordable accidents.

For accident data to be valid and reliable, they must be collected and treated in a uniform manner. In the absence of uniform definitions, valid comparisons of sports accident data from different sources is not possible. While basic interpretive guidelines can be provided by precisely stated definitions, objectives, and policies, there are always interpretive decisions to be made which fall outside the realm of these factors. Final judgment of exceptions must be made by local system decision-makers and applied uniformly on a continuous basis throughout the total system.

NATIONAL SYSTEMS INCLUDING SPORTS ACCIDENT DATA

The National Electronic Injury Surveillance System (NEISS)

NEISS is a national accident data system designed to determine the nature and scope of product injuries to consumers. The system is administered through the US Consumer Product Safety Commission, a regulatory agency of the federal government. It has rule-making authority and its policies are set by five commissioners, who are nominated by the President, confirmed by the Senate, and serve fixed terms. The agency's mission is to reduce the risk of injury among consumers while using consumer products, including those used in competitive and recreational sports. A consumer product is defined as any article manufactured for sale to, or for intended use by, consumers in or around the home, at school, or in recreation.

The Commission has a variety of ways to deal with hazardous products depending on the severity of the risk each represents. It has authority to ban or seize "imminently hazardous products." If the risk is neither immediate nor severe but still considered "unreasonable," mandatory standards can be promulgated that will reduce the injury risk. Where the risk is less, the Commission may rely on voluntary standards and voluntary compliance.

Manufacturers, distributors, and retailers must report to the Commission any defective sport product that does or could present a substantial hazard to a consumer. The Commission may then order the defective product to be recalled, repaired, replaced, or repurchased by the manufacturer. Also the Commission has authority for conducting research to determine cause and prevention of product-related injuries, and it has extensive information-gathering authority, including access to company records, relating to safety aspects of a product.

A vital part of the information-collecting process is NEISS. According to the Commission, this system for surveillance and investigation of product-related injuries is presently the most important tool in the field of product safety. It is the only statistically valid, nationwide system for continuous monitoring of consumer product-related injuries. This system has two particular advantages.

First, the system is national in scope. Since NEISS is based on a representative sample of hospital emergency rooms throughout the country, we can for the first time make statistically valid projections to the United States population of the number and types of injuries seen in hospital emergency rooms. Now 119 hospitals are participating in the NEISS program, comprising a representative sample of about 5000 emergency rooms in the continental United States. Statistically valid projections of all data categories can, therefore, be made for any given reporting period.

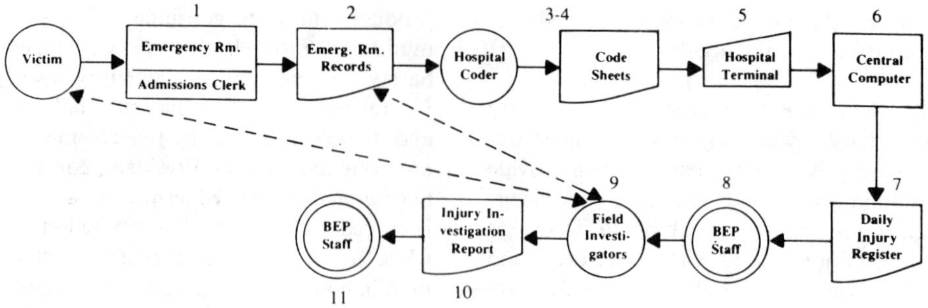

Figure 1-1 Path of an injury through the NEISS system.

A second advantage of NEISS is that data on all emergency room patients having product-related injuries are transmitted electronically from each reporting source to a central computer in Washington, DC, every 24 hours. This type of reporting insures that the data are current. It further provides a mechanism for the rapid analysis of information which, in turn, can be the basis for initiating a field investigation.

Injuries as defined in this program are instances of trauma requiring competent medical care or resulting in at least one day of restricted activity. The data include injuries related to products used in the household, in recreational activities, and in institutional environments.

Surveillance, as made possible through this program, will provide an unprecedented capability for monitoring injury patterns, as well as for isolating specific aspects of the injury problem. Further, an assessment of the effectiveness of remedial programs will be possible through this same hospital network.

The hospital surveillance program is the first major segment of a total injury data effort. Plans are also being made for utilizing death certificates on a national basis for obtaining product injury information.

To illustrate more specifically the NEISS concept as it relates to sports safety, Figure 1-1 provides a schematic diagram of the NEISS process.

Sports Injury Data

The nature and extent of sports injury data available through NEISS are valuable particularly to professionals dedicated to the improvement of sports safety programs.

With these data, estimated frequencies can be determined which will indicate the number of cases reported to hospital emergency rooms nationwide that are associated with a specific product or activity. Summaries can then be compiled to show age groups and accident types.

In addition, a matrix report can be constructed for the product description showing the relative distribution of diagnoses and body parts injured. The matrix model can be adapted to any product-related injury study.

Another NEISS capability allows totals to be summarized for each product and activity, and listed according to frequency of reports. For example, Figure 1-2 shows selected items with the highest frequency rank under the category of Sports and Recreational Equipment.

The Commission has an organized informational and educational campaign in the form of the *NEISS News* which is the primary means of routine distribution of NEISS data. This is a monthly periodical that usually contains short articles on product safety and specific data on more than 100 products or combinations of products. It is supplemented by periodic news releases on, for example, "Consumer Product Safety Commission Offers Football Safety Tips."

Contributions of NEISS to Sports Product Standard

The role of the Commission in the development of standards for sports and other products is primarily of a mandatory nature as prescribed in the Consumer Product Safety Act. The Act, however, provides unique provisions that allow the public first opportunity in standard developments. If there are no offers from the public, if a public effort is unsuccessful, or if a public offer comes from a single agency, then the Commission is allowed to write a standard.

The initial phase of the process is a determination by the Commission that a consumer product is

Product #	Product Description	f	S
P1200	**SPORTS AND RECREATIONAL EQUIPMENT**		
1202	Bicycle and Bicycle Equipment	17,411	33
1211	Football, Activity and Related Equipment	12,591	22
1205	Basketball, Activity and Related Equipment	9,492	16
1204	Baseball, Activity and Related Equipment	8,983	23
1265	Sports Ball, not specified	3,207	18
1241	Swings	2,788	30
1216	Snow Skiing and Associated Equipment	1,887	20
1214	Hockey Equipment	1,640	27
1210	Fishing Equipment	1,569	26
1231	Swimming Pools and Associated Equipment, not including Above-Ground Pools	1,415	79
1245	Ice Skates	1,164	21
1266	Volleybll	1,161	15
1244	Playground Climbing Apparatus	1,094	30
1242	Slides	1,010	34
1263	Mini-Bikes	1,003	34
1267	Soccer	1,000	22
1219	Tennis and Badminton Equipment	918	19
1270	Wrestling — Organized Activity and Related Equipment	756	25
1272	Gymnastics and Associated Equipment	749	22
1212	Golf Equipment except Golf Carts	704	31
1200	Sports and Recreational Equipment	636	25
1233	Trampolines	551	20
1203	Boats, Motors and Accessories for Recreational Use	502	48
1218	Snowmobiles	480	44
1206	Bowling, Activity and Related Equipment	474	16
1237	Gas, Air and Spring Operated Guns	452	38
1262	Swimming Pools, Above-Ground	432	59
1217	Sleds	424	33
1201	Playground Equipment not elsewhere classified	414	26
1209	Exercise Equipment	408	36
1264	Water Skiing and Associated Equipment	359	24
1273	Toboggans	321	34
1268	Track and Field Activities, and Related Equipment	300	23
1230	Camping Trailers, other than Mobile Homes	264	28
1236	Unlicensed Motor Scooters and Go-Karts	248	23
1243	See Saws	226	26

Figure 1-2 NEISS frequency rank of injuries related to sports and recreational equipment, July 1972 through June 1973.

an "unreasonable" risk. Since the law does not prescribe precise definitions or rules for distinguishing between reasonable and unreasonable risks, the Commission makes such a judgment based on several factors, as follows:

1. The number and severity of the accidents involving the product,
2. The contributing role of the product in the accidents,
3. Whether the hazards the product presents can be eliminated by technically feasible actions,
4. What expense would be involved in required modifications,
5. Whether the risk to the user of the product is assumed knowingly or unknowingly, voluntarily or involuntarily,
6. The uniqueness of the function the product serves,
7. Public exposure to the product.

The use of NEISS surveillance and investigative data is encouraged by the Commission particularly for product performance assessments and modifications and consumer education programs. Examples of agencies or disciplines, which can beneficially use NEISS findings in planning and implementing injury control programs, are manufacturers, education, medicine, and safety and health councils. Additional information concerning NEISS and the operations of the Commission can be obtained by writing to: US Consumer Product Safety Commission, Washington, DC 20207.

The National Center for Health Statistics (NCHS)

This Center is a component of the Public Health Service, US Department of Health, Education and Welfare. The Center's mission is to develop and maintain systems capable of providing reliable, general purpose, national, descriptive health statistics on a continuing basis and to publish these statistics for use by the health industry and related industries, both public and private. The Center's concept of health statistics includes injuries, and injury data are collected and reported regularly. Occasionally special reports on the subject are released. But this general information and data are of little practical value to the sports world. The Center does not collect data on sports injuries or accidents but only the place of injury such as recreation areas.

Occupational Safety and Health System

A system for recording work-related injuries and illnesses, including those occurring in professional sports, was established by the Occupational Safety and Health Act (OSHA) of 1970. Amateur sports injuries or illnesses are not included because no employment relationship exists. The act provides for a rigorous, accurate set of statistics to bolster standard setting and compliance activities. The OSHA directs the Secretary of Labor, in consultation with the Secretary of Health, Education and Welfare, to "develop and maintain an effective program of collection, compilation, and analysis of occupational safety and health statistics." The Secretary of Labor has assigned to the Bureau of Labor Statistics the responsibility for this program. In many states, a statistical grant agency cooperates with the Bureau in administering the record-keeping program. The date of July 1, 1971, marked the beginning for records keeping and reporting under the Act.

Some of the record-keeping regulations have been difficult to apply to professional sports. In certain cases, such as professional football, assistance was requested in applying the record-keeping requirements to the unique situations involved. As a result a letter of guidance was prepared by the Bureau of Labor Statistics and sent to individual teams of both the National and American Football Leagues. One area of guidance in the letter clarifies the concept of lost workdays that presents a difficult problem for professional teams. For example, if a player spends time from a practice session treating a bruised ankle in a whirlpool bath, does it count as a "lost workday"? If a player's ability to participate in a practice session is doubtful, the management must decide whether or not the player could participate, in his current condition, in a game situation. If he could, there would not be a case; if he could not, it would be recorded as a lost workday of restricted activity.

In conclusion, it should be pointed out that this relatively new system has the potential for contributing significantly to improvements in accident data system developments. With vigorous implementation it could no doubt expedite the identification of corrective measures needed to control injuries and other losses in professional sports and those sponsored by employers covered by the Act. There is, however, no plan to publish accident data information about individual or professional sports as a whole.

Additional information and materials concerning this system are available on request from the regional offices of the Bureau of Labor Statistics, or the Office of Occupational Safety and Health Statistics, Washington, DC.

The National Safety Council System

Accident reporting guidelines and materials designed for use in educational institutions have been provided by the National Safety Council for many years. The system can be used as prescribed or adopted for local developments.

Elementary and Secondary Schools The forms developed for elementary and secondary schools include: a standard student accident report form, monthly student accident summary forms (for boys and girls), and annual student accident summary forms (for boys and girls).

The Standard Student Accident Report is used for recording the details of student accidents and injuries. As can be noted in Figure 1-3 the form is applicable for all accidents, including those that occur in sports.

Detailed instructions are provided to guide recorders in completing it. The need for precise recording of precise information is emphasized.

A code sheet gives a breakdown of general and specific classifications of accident details. Selected general coding classifications are provided as part of the system and are applicable to sport accidents. Every school system should require a report of some kind, so that school authorities know of all accidents that occur in activities or events sponsored under school jurisdiction. Preventive and control measures can be formulated only when the details are precisely known. This information also provides some protection for school personnel should liability become an issue.

The purpose of distinguishing between types and severity of accidents is twofold: first, to provide the school with information relative to all school jurisdiction accidents and with non-school jurisdiction accidents causing injury to pupils, and second, to provide a standard method with a common base in order to compare and analyze accident and injury data within a school system, or with other school systems, or with national statistics. The terms used to distinguish these purposes are reportable (any accident for which a report is filled out) and recordable (any accident to be included in standardized statistical treatment of the data).

An investigation of all recordable accidents is suggested. The investigation reports are submitted on the standard student accident report forms and sent to the safety program administrator or coordinator.

The Student Accident Summary forms (for boys and girls) are used for preparing monthly summaries of recordable accidents as reported on the Standard Student Accident forms. They summarize important information and facts to be observed and used primarily for decision-making.

(check one)
School Jurisdictional
Non School Jurisdictional

RECOMMENDED
STANDARD STUDENT ACCIDENT REPORT
(See instructions on reverse side)

(check one)
Recordable ☐
Reportable Only ☐

School District:
City, State:

General

1 Name | 2 Address

3 School | 4 Sex Male ☐ Female ☐ | 5 Age | 6 Grade/Special Program

7 Time Accident Occurred
Date | Day of Week | Exact Time | AM / PM

Injury

8 Nature of Injury

9 Part of Body Injured

10 Degree of Injury (check one)
Death | Permanent | Temporary (lost time) | Non Disabling (no lost time)

11 Days Lost
From School | From Activities Other Than School | Total

12 Cause of Injury

Accident

13 Accident Jurisdiction (check one)
School: Grounds | Building | To and From | Other Activities Not on School Property
Non School: Home | Other

14 Location of Accident (be specific) | 15 Activity of Person (be specific)

16 Status of Activity | 17 Supervision (if yes, give title & name of supervisor) Yes ☐ No ☐

18 Agency Involved | 19 Unsafe Act

20 Unsafe Mechanical/Physical Condition | 21 Unsafe Personal Factor

22 Corrective Action Taken or Recommended

23 Property Damage
School $ | Non School $ | Total $

24 Description (Give a word picture of the accident, explaining who, what, when, why and how)

Signature

25 Date of Report | 26 Report Prepared by (signature & title)

27 Principal's Signature

This form is recommended for securing data for accident prevention and safety education. School districts may reproduce this form adding space for optional data. Reference: Student Accident Reporting Guidebook, National Safety Council, 425 N. Michigan Avenue, Chicago, Illinois 60611 1966 34 pages

Figure 1-3 The National Safety Council's recommended standard student accident report form.

These summaries are of proved diagnostic value in determining status and trends of accident occurrence. Also, evidence of critical safety problems can be identified and action taken on a regular short-term basis.

Machine data processing should be given a top priority in analyzing and summarizing data if the volume of reports warrants it. The amount and type of data which can be obtained by this means is practically unlimited and the tasks can be completed in minutes. This machine process can provide source materials not normally available from the manual processing method because of staff and time limitations.

The following example illustrates this system's capabilities for identifying and monitoring sports accident problems.

The safety coordinator in a large school system was reviewing the monthly summary chart. He noted that a disproportionately high number of accidents were occurring in team sports under school jurisdiction. This became evident from the tabulations recorded for the chart item "activity, by classification of accident." The highest incidence was in varsity football. He then summarized the football accidents by: status of the activity, nature of injury and parts of the body injured, agency involved, unsafe physical condition, unsafe act, and unsafe personal factor.

In investigating further he found that most of the incidents were broken teeth and mouth damage and that no mouth guards were being used. The problem was discussed with the safety coordinator, coaching staff, physical education teachers, and school administrators. The local dental association assisted in developing corrective measures. An experimental mouthpiece was developed that could be fitted individually for each football player. Funding was approved to purchase mouth guards for participants, and all players were required to wear them. During the next football season no tooth damage was reported.

The Annual Student Summary forms are used for annual consolidation of all recordable accidents reported for the year. ("Reportable-only" accidents are not included in the monthly or annual summaries.) These data then provide the essential information for calculating the accident frequency rate and the average severity rate by grade level. These rates are valuable for a variety of comparative purposes, especially for direct comparisons with overall rates.

The frequency rates relate the number of accidents or injuries to exposure factors. A definitive measure for sports accidents is frequency rates calculated on the basis of "participant (student) hours" rather than "student days." The "participant hour" figure is harder to estimate, but it gives more valid evidence of accident experience. For example, it accounts for the hourly "time a participant spends in a particular sport activity" in relation to the number of injuries in each category. Results are expressed in terms of one million student hours. (See "Data Analysis.")

The system administrator can compute injury frequency rates on a monthly, semester, or annual basis for all sports in the school system. This can be done for one school, by grades, or by activities. He can compare rates on the same basis and determine where improvements are needed. A comparison of annual (or other time periods) frequency rates with previous years is possible for all sports or selected sports in a single or several schools.

Severity indicates the seriousness of injuries for totals of accidents or for specific areas or activities. In addition, results can be compared year by year to determine negative or positive results. Severity information can be obtained either generally, that is, the total accident experience of a school or school system; or specifically, as the total accident experience of an activity or activities. The severity rate is illustrated with frequency rate, in "Data Analysis." The concept is similar to that for figuring frequency rates.

Institutions of higher learning A general accident data system designed for institutions of higher learning has also been available during recent years from the National Safety Council. However, the Council's activities in this area will be discontinued when the current supply of materials is expended. This means there will no longer be a national resource organization to assist higher education personnel in establishing and maintaining general systems. This fact plus the paucity of significant system literature reduces the likelihood of effective general systems being developed in most of these institutions. With the exception of the few that maintain a system designed for local use, the outlook is bleak for improved accountability in reducing accident experience among student populations, in sports and otherwise.

SCHOOL AND COLLEGE ACCIDENTS AND INJURIES

Secondary Schools

Information on the number of participants in secondary school sports is available from the National Federation of State High School Athletic Associations. The ten most popular high school sports as determined by participation are listed here:

	No. of Schools	No. of Partici-pants
Football—11 Man	13,959	853,537
Basketball	20,227	676,559
Track and Field (Outdoor)	16,836	623,139
Baseball	13,002	360,157
Wrestling	6870	226,681
Cross-country Skiing	7818	144,488
Golf	8650	93,841
Tennis	6221	83,717
Swimming	3229	83,286
Volleyball	3519	63,144

Some ratios of injuries and accidents to the total number of participants have been calculated for various sports. Current studies list sports as having a high, middle, or low hazard rate. With improved research designs, it will be possible to identify more clearly which sports have a high incidence of danger and which do not. Even within a sport it will be possible to determine which activity is more hazardous than others (such as an offensive or defensive position in football), and how the hazard may relate to equipment used or not used.

Sports-related accidents in the secondary schools of New York State that were studied by Pechar fell into two categories: those related to personal factors (ie, physical and mental-emotional factors) and those related to administrative factors. Pechar states that 62% of the accidents were caused by personal factors and 38% by administrative factors. Physical factors included fatigue and muscular weakness. Mental-emotional factors causing accidents were ranked in this order: disregarding instructions, taking unnecessary chances, and acting before thinking.

A study of accidents in 207 public junior high schools by Dissinger reveals that three-fifths of the 1626 accidents occurred in physical education or closely related activities. Boys were involved in accidents in basketball, football, softball, and baseball. Girls met with accidents primarily in basketball and volleyball.

Junior high school football produced one injury for every 10 participants in one season at a school in Fort Lauderdale, Florida. Two-thirds of the injuries were sustained at practice, the rest during games.

College Accidents

A study conducted by the American College Health Association on 22 college and university campuses showed that 207,000 full-time students reported 14,487 injuries of which 1247 were disabling. Victims of nearly three-fourths of the injuries were men. One out of eight men and 1 of 12 women were injured. Eight percent of the injuries were disabling beyond the day of the accident.

In a study on college physical education accidents Florio and Stafford found that nearly 60% of the injuries occurred in the gymnasium and not on outdoor facilities. They recorded that the most hazardous sports were touch football, ice skating, and personal defense. The highest accident rate occurred in team and contact sports.

SELECTED ACCIDENT DATA SYSTEMS FOR SPORTS

National Collegiate Athletics Association Injury Surveillance System

The National Collegiate Athletic Association (NCAA) implemented a Football Injury Surveillance System in 1982 that promises to provide extremely useful data regarding major injury trends in secondary schools and colleges. In 1983, the system was expanded to encompass the sports of women's volleyball, wrestling, women's gymnastics, baseball, men's lacrosse and women's lacrosse. Eventually, it will cover all NCAA sponsored sports.

According to Zemper, Research Coordinator for the system, when fully implemented, it will be collecting data from approximately a 10% sample of all NCAA member institutions participating in each specific sport. The statistically valid, stratified sampling will be distributed by NCAA division and geographical region of the country and should allow projection of the data to the entire set of participating schools.

The NCAA Committee on Competitive Safeguards and Medical Aspects of Sports will use the data to evaluate and revise recommended policies for the guidance of member institutions in developing sound and safe athletic programs.

A reportable injury in the NCAA system is any injury which meets three broad-based criteria: first, that it occurred as a result of participation in an organized sport practice or contest; second that the injury required medical attention; and third, that the injury resulted in restriction of the athlete's participation for one or more days beyond the day of injury.

Athletic trainers at NCAA institutions in the sampling regularly complete and submit two clear and simple types of forms. They are paid an honorarium for reporting for their sport each season. Their accuracy, efficiency and promptness are imperative to maintaining the system's integrity.

The hallmark of the NCAA forms for data collection is their simplicity. The NCAA has basic data on each participating institution and completing the Injury Surveillance System forms consists primarily of circling code numbers corresponding to the conditions of an injury on one of two standard forms. An IBM System 34 computer stores the data and reports it as injury rate per 1,000 athlete-exposures. An athlete-exposure is defined as "one athlete participating in one practice or contest, where she or he is exposed to the possibility of athletic injury".

A weekly exposure form is completed and mailed by each trainer each week whether or not any reportable injuries have occurred. It records the number of practices and contests and average number of participants for the week. If applicable, questions about artificial versus natural surfaces are also answered.

The second type of form deals specifically with individual injuries. Anonymity is emphasized for the athletes, but the form thoroughly investigates all possible criteria which could have contributed to the injury.

The Football Individual Injury Surveillance Form differs somewhat from the general form used for other sports so it can include questions about types of injuries and conditions unique to football. For other sports, a standard form is filled out which investigates common concerns, then several questions relating specifically to each sport are also answered.

Parameters investigated include weather and temperature conditions, type of injury, part of body injured and equipment being utilized at time of injury as well as situational factors. These include position of the player on the field, type of contact with another player if another player was involved in the injury, and time during the match when injury occurred.

If the Safeguards Committee is particularly concerned about the safe use of a piece of equipment or the quality of different designs of equipment, the form is modified to incorporate these concerns. For example, questions regarding the use of knee braces in football and possible correlates with injuries to those wearing them or those who are hurt by the impact of another player's knee brace were recently added to the football form.

The NCAA System is especially important since the only other sport injury data system, the National Athletic Injury Reporting System, stopped collecting data for high school and college level athletic programs in June, 1983. Although some interesting trends seem to have been identified from the first few years of data collection, Zemper cautions against drawing any conclusions based on such short-term data. Long-term studies will reveal the broad patterns and determine risk factors much more accurately than could be revealed from looking at the data from only one or two seasons. Data from the NCAA system could eventually eliminate most potential accident hazards and minimize the consequences of those accidents that do occur. Only through accurate analysis can needs be identified and safeguards implemented which will give the participants the best protection possible, the protection they deserve.

National Athletic Injury Reporting System (NAIRS)

NAIRS was a surveillance system "conceived out of the reality that existing sports injury data were incomplete, obsolete, or fallacious." It was a practical means for obtaining and interpreting continuous information on the incidence and associated circumstances of athletic injuries or illnesses (to male and female). It also had great potential for operations on a national scale.

A principal investigator is responsible for data interpretation and review of research-related access requests. A coordinator is responsible for the data collection process, including the training and monitoring of recorders in close cooperation with the National Athletic Trainers Association.

Significant Aspects of the System

NAIRS was designed specifically for varsity sports for which detailed weekly information is needed. However, the system permitted sponsors of any organized sport activity to participate with inexpensive modifications. Therefore, factors that significantly influence the frequency and severity of athletic injuries and illness can be monitored in a variety of settings. A major contribution of the system was the establishment of baseline data or endemic levels of occurrence of injury or illness among athletes. From these data, patterns of prevalent factors that influence incidence can be observed. Assessments can then be made as to whether a shift in frequency has occurred. The resulting evidence can be used to guide decisions regarding corrective measures. In addition, the reference data bank kept current by the system was a valuable asset to the conduct of in-depth investigation.

The system could service any organized athletic sport, for male, female, or coed groups in school, college, university, or agency. Surveillance capabilities for physical education, intramurals, and recreation programs could be accommodated.

Reporting and Data Collection

NAIRS input organization is planned for a low-cost operation. It is not dependent on the use of highly trained investigators or medical record libraries or records. For this reason certified NATA (National Athletic Trainers Association) trainers are key persons in the data collection and reporting processes. Duties and responsibilities of key personnel are as follows:

NAIRS Coordinator Athletic trainer who supervises the data collection process and the training of system personnel.

District Coordinator Athletic trainer in each of 10 geographical districts who supervises NAIRS interests.

Cluster Coordinators Trainers who supervise the use of NAIRS in a particular locality.

Recorder One who fills out NAIRS forms for a given institution.

Athletic Director The person who oversees the intervention of NAIRS and monitors the protocol for interpreting NAIRS requirements and periodic results.

NAIRS Terminology

Fundamental to the operation of the system are basic definitions which help the recorder complete the forms accurately. The definitions are specified for recording potentially significant injuries and are purposely designed to avoid analysis of nuisance injuries. The key definition prescribes the disabling character of any injury. Any injury or illness that keeps the athlete from participation on the performance day (practice or game) following the day of onset is reportable. Selected definitions developed for the system are as follows:

Athlete (participant) A student is a participant if he or she maintains candidacy for varsity competition by subscribing to the institution's eligibility rules, procedures, and schedule.

Participation (return to participation) An athlete is participating if he or she has health supervisory clearance or coach permission for engaging in activities generally expected of the athlete's varsity teammates.

Practice (participation-day) Only those coach-directed sessions that include physical activity are recordable practices.

Reportable injury or illness Injuries and illnesses meeting any of the following definitions are reportable:

1. Brain concussion. Any brain concussion is reportable if the athlete must be held for observation before return to play is permitted.
2. Dental injury. Any dental injury is reportable if it should receive professional attention.
3. Any injury or illness causing cessation of an athlete's customary participation throughout the participation-day following day of onset is reportable.
4. Any injury or illness that requires substantive professional attention before the athlete's return to participation is permitted is reportable.

These definitions are meant to separate the nuisance injuries which warrant little attention and do not materially affect performance, from the health problems that have potential or demonstrated significance.

THE SIGNIFICANCE OF DATA SYSTEM DEVELOPMENT

The development and implementation of an effective accident data system for sports is significant to many. One of the more important benefits accrues to the agency which sponsors the sport.

The management indicates its interest and concern for the safety, health, and social welfare of those actively involved in the sports program it sponsors. Such efforts influence the morale and performance within the agency, thus increasing the efficiency of the accident data system and resulting often in substantial savings. Data from the system may also be used to protect against public criticism and legal entanglements.

The emotional or psychological climate may alter the accident rate. Some communities are very sports-minded and make unusual demands on players and coaches (the violence that erupts at some international soccer contests is legendary and regrettable). Other communities that may not care to support sports programs seek to jettison contests and recreational programs because of injuries, rivalries, disputed responsibilities or other problems that arise. Often their assessment is illogical; they decide to outlaw contests in lieu of finding a satisfactory solution that retains the values of sports.

Parents or guardians of participants will have a primary interest in an effective data system, the preventive aspects that could eliminate the "unreasonable" risks involved in the sports activity in which their family members participate. However, when an injury does occur, parents or guardians are also benefited by knowing what to anticipate in severity of damage and extent of recovery. Emotional suffering is reduced and often the financial burden as well.

National conferences on accident prevention in physical education, athletics and recreation, published as *Sports Safety*, volumes 1-6, contain recommendations of safety specialists from many disciplines and sources. While intended primarily for school personnel, they are also useful to other agencies and sports governing bodies. They stress that to reduce sports accidents and prevent their recurrence, all accidents must be investigated, causes determined and corrective action taken. This necessitates effective reporting and investigation to provide information for administrative guidance, program development and evaluation, legal analysis and improvement of equipment.

The participants, of course, are the persons most directly benefited by an accident data system. A majority of them are not keenly aware of the injury risks involved. They lack precise knowledge of the hazards in sports activities. They tend to believe that an accident can not happen to them. They make a gross assumption that their sponsoring agency and its supervisory or instructional personnel will automatically assure that all hazards are eliminated or reasonably controlled. They deserve the best protection possible.

SUGGESTED READINGS

Accident Facts. Chicago: National Safety Council. 1968.

Accident Facts. Chicago: National Safety Council, 1969.

Bettinghaus, E.P., and Miller, G.R. *Keeping the Public Informed: Accent on Accountability.* Denver: Department of Education, 1973.

Borich, G.D. (Ed.) *Evaluating Educational Programs and Products.* Englewood Cliffs, NJ: Educational Technology Publications, 1974.

Borozne, Morehouse, and Pechar. *Sports Safety Monographs 1-6.* Washington, DC: American School and Community Safety Association (AAHPER), 1971.

Byrd, O.E. *Health.* Philadelphia: W.B. Saunders, 1971, p. 69.

Clark, G. A little less mayhem on a Sunday afternoon. *Job Safety and Health* 3:10-17, 1975.

Clarke, K.S. Calculated risk of sports fatalities. *JAMA.* 197:894-896, 1966.

Clarke, K.S. *NAIRS I, Recorder's Handbook, 1975-1976.* University Park, Pa: Pennsylvania State University, 1975.

Dissinger, J.K. Accidents in junior high school physical education programs. *Res Q.* 37:495, 1966.

Dzenowagis, J.G. Injuries in men's physical education and intramural sports. *Safety Monographs for Colleges and Universities #14.* Chicago: National Safety Council, 1962.

Eastman, R. *The School Budget Cycle: A Continuing Process.* Winneconne, Wis: Wisconsin Association of School Boards, 1967.

Esch, A.F. The national electronic injury surveillance system (NEISS). *The Medical Aspects of Sports.* Proceedings of the 15th National Conference. Chicago: American Medical Association, 1974.

Fisher, L.B. The organization of campus safety programs. *Safety Monographs for Colleges and Universities #9.* Chicago: National Safety Council, 1959.

Florio, A.E., and Stafford, G.T. *Safety Education,* 3rd Ed. New York: McGraw-Hill, 1969.

Gottman, J.M., and Clasen, R.W. *Evaluation in Education: A Practitioner's Guide.* Itasca, Ill: Peacock Publishers, 1971.

Hall, H. Rehabilitating the injured knee, ankle or shoulder. *Patient Care* 2:68, 1968.

Health News. *Medical News.* August, 1969, p. ii.

Lippincott, H. How to get the values of university accident prevention. *Safety Monographs for Colleges and Universities #9.* Chicago: National Safety Council, 1959.

The Mission and Policies of the National Center for Health Statistics. Washington, DC: US Department of Health, Education and Welfare.

Monthly Labor Review. Reprint 2794. Washington, DC: US Department of Labor, 1974, pp. 14–19.

Morgan, H. How Louisiana has used the guidebook to develop its student accident reporting system. *National Safety Congress Transactions: School and College Safety* 23:40–43, 1967.

NAIRS. University Park, Pa: Pennsylvania State University.

National athlete injury reporting system. Editorial. *Safety Forum* 1:2, 1974.

Occupational Safety and Health Statistics: Concepts and Methods. Report 438. Washington, DC: US Department of Labor, 1975.

Pechar, S.F. A study of the nature, frequency, and related personal and administrative factors of physical education accidents among boys in the junior and senior high schools in New York state. EdD Dissertation, New York University, 1961.

Practical Safety Communications. Macon, Ga: International Safety Academy, 1971.

Robinson, R.I. *NCAA Football Head and Neck Injuries in Eastern Colleges.* Cortland, NY: State University of New York at Cortland.

School Safety Policies with Emphasis on Physical Education, Athletics, and Recreation. Washington, DC: American Association for Health, Physical Education, and Recreation, 1968, pp. 27–28.

Seaton, D.C. et al. *Administration and Supervision of Safety Education.* New York: Macmillan, 1969.

Seaton, D.C., Stack, H.J., and Loft, B.I. *Administration and Supervision of Safety Education.* New York: Macmillan, 1969, p. 228.

Silverwood, G.P. Accident investigation and reporting. Edited by C.P. Yost. In *Sports Safety.* Washington, DC: American Association for Health, Physical Education, and Recreation, 1970.

Standard Nomenclature of Athletic Injuries. Chicago: American Medical Association, 1966.

Standard Nomenclature of Athletic Injuries. Chicago: American Medical Association, 1966.

Student Accident Reporting Guidebook. Chicago: The National Safety Council, 1966.

Using Injury Statistics. Bulletin 255. Washington, DC: US Department of Labor, 1963.

US Consumer Product Safety Commission. NEISS: an overview. *NEISS News* 3:1–8, 1975.

US Consumer Product Safety Commission. National electronic injury surveillance system. *NEISS News* 1:2, 1973.

Weinstein, Twerski, Piehler, et al. *Products Liability and the Reasonably Safe Product.* New York: John Wiley & Sons, 1978.

Zemper E.D. NCAA injury surveillance system. Paper presented at the 1984 Olympic Scientific Congress, Eugene, Oregon, July 1984.

CHAPTER 2
Government's Role in Data-Gathering

Victoria R. Brown, MS

Millions of people participate daily in organized sports and many others participate on a recreational basis. Data sources indicate that thousands are injured and require medical attention while engaging in these activities. Many of these injuries are needless. Many arise from taking unreasonable risks.

Sports participation is growing at the community and recreational level and for women at the high school and college level. It is growing in individual or lifetime sports such as tennis, skiing, and jogging. Despite this trend, little is known about the risks involved. It is probably fair to say that sports injury rates are higher where no controls are enforced. Younger children, because of their limited experience, are not likely to exercise judgment as to the inherent risks in a sport. In analyzing the injury data on all sports injuries it is necessary to determine the risks, eliminate those that are unreasonable, and control those that are predictable.

Frequently, injury data are analyzed only when serious accidents occur. But the frequency and chronic nature of other less serious injuries may be of equal or more meaning, especially as they affect youth during the developmental years. It is necessary to understand the developmental limitations of the individuals involved and the physiologic, psychologic, and biomechanical factors before assessing reasonable or unreasonable risks of injuries.

CONSUMER PRODUCT SAFETY COMMISSION

Many organizations are involved in sports safety and sports injury investigation. The Consumer Product Safety Commission (CPSC) is one of the federal agencies. The Consumer Product Safety Commission is an independent federal regulatory agency with the primary goal of protecting consumers against unreasonable risk of injury from hazardous products. Through the Consumer Product Safety Act (CPSA) of 1972, the Commission was granted broad authority to issue and enforce safety standards on more than 10,000 consumer products that may present an unreasonable risk of injury.

The Act defines the term consumer product as "...any article, or component part thereof, produced or distributed for sale to a consumer for use in or around a permanent or temporary household or residence, a school, in recreation, or otherwise; or for the personal use, consumption or enjoyment of a consumer in or around a permanent or temporary household or residence, a school, in recreation, or otherwise,..."[1]

As stated in the Law, the purposes of the CPSA are:

1. To protect the public against unreasonable risks of injury associated with consumer products,
2. To assist consumers in evaluating the comparative safety of products,
3. To develop uniform safety standards for consumer products and to minimize conflicting state and local regulations,
4. To promote research and investigations into the causes and prevention of product-related deaths, illnesses, and injuries.

Under the section on product safety information and research, the Act further states that:

> The Commission shall ...(1) maintain an injury information clearinghouse to collect, investigate, analyze, and disseminate injury data, and information, relating to the causes and prevention of death, injury, and illness associated with consumer products, and (2) conduct such continuing studies and investigations of deaths, injuries, diseases, other health impairments, and economic losses resulting from accidents involving consumer products as it deems necessary.[1]

National Electronic Injury Surveillance System (NEISS)

In order to fulfill these responsibilities the Commission maintains an injury surveillance system that daily monitors statistically selected hospital emergency rooms nationwide for injuries associated with consumer products. This system, known as NEISS (National Electronic Injury Surveillance System) was discussed in Chapter 1. It has shown that a significant number of injuries reported from emergency rooms have been associated with sports. In 1983, of an estimated 10.3 million injuries associated with consumer products approximately 2.7 million were related to sports and recreational activities (Table 2-1).[2]

Injury cases reported through NEISS indicate that a product is involved in, but does not necessarily cause, an accident. Selective follow-up investigations determine the precise circumstances surrounding the injuries.

NEISS serves as the major vehicle for describing the magnitude of sports injuries. To the extent that the data are valid they provide a basis for comparing relative incidence and types of sport injuries. At face value the problem appears extreme. Sports-associated injuries represent over 25% of all injuries reported by NEISS.

As with any injury surveillance system, there are some inherent limitations in NEISS. For example, NEISS data, as a measure of sports product-associated injuries, are affected by the following considerations:

Table 2-1
NEISS Report of Injuries Related to Sports and Recreational Equipment, 1983

	Estimate	Percent of injuries to 5-14 year age group	Number of cases reported
Bicycles or accessories	571,196	60.5	11,488
Baseball, N.O.S.	216,335	29.4	4011
Baseball, organized	165,845	29.2	2699
Baseball, informal	95,610	33.1	2004
Basketball, N.O.S.	235,328	20.4	4945
Basketball, organized	112,674	29.6	2052
Basketball, informal	113,676	22.6	2135
Football, N.O.S.	186,830	38.9	3853
Football, organized	129,419	36.9	2305
Football, informal	108,635	43.1	2061
Soccer, N.O.S.	51,840	44.3	1108
Soccer, organized	33,052	20.4	677
Soccer, informal	23,764	51.1	436
Volleyball, N.O.S.	43,502	19.5	865
Volleyball, organized	22,893	28.7	364
Volleyball, informal	16,768	17.0	267
Trampolines	11,995	56.7	215
Gymnastics, N.O.S.	19,160	61.9	395
Gymnastics, organized	25,443	62.9	410
Gymnastics, informal	7848	67.9	143
Wrestling	56,481	32.5	1016
Weightlifting	42,662	15.3	912
Swings and swing sets	77,507	56.5	1561
Slides, playground	40,006	48.7	779
Monkey bars	45,619	77.6	975
Track and field	65,007	21.6	1240
Ice hockey	26,928	24.9	398
Water skiing	29,619	5.9	402
Snow skiing	42,938	23.7	557
Golf	18,377	24.6	313
Skateboards	16,836	56.5	414
Squash, racquetball and paddle ball	36,002	3.6	730
Tennis	29,524	15.6	557
Swimming pool, N.O.S.	43,492	44.2	890

1. A large number of such injuries are treated by private physicians.
2. In the absence of relevant exposure data it is difficult to establish sports injury rate.
3. Prior to October 1978 NEISS reporting made no distinction between injuries incurred in organized and unorganized sports activities.

CPSC PROGRAM TEAMS

There are six program teams within the CPSC, one of which addresses injuries associated with sports and recreational products or activities. The team is comprised of a staff with disciplines in epidemiology, human factors, economics, engineering, information and education, and law enforcement and compliance.

Because of the product-specific orientation of the Consumer Product Safety Act, attempts have been made to devise regulatory strategies that separate product-related from activity-related injury. It was found, however, that product and activity cannot be separated.

The Commission examines the complete sports environment, including products, playing fields, climatic conditions, rule formulation, and participant interaction. This includes interaction with the related industries and rule-making bodies of organized sports.

At present, mandatory product regulation does not appear to provide the desired results. It is difficult to isolate specific causes of sports injuries in general. It is even more difficult to determine that a sports product was at fault because of mechanical failure or poor design. Therefore, remedial efforts become quite controversial. The issue becomes: if cause-effect relationship between a sports injury and a product can not be identified, how can any preventative measure be implemented? Furthermore, if a remedial strategy is initiated (through information and voluntary standards support) aimed at reducing an identified risk, how does one determine the efficacy of the action taken? In other words, for *x* amount of dollars and staff time how many sports-associated deaths, fractures, or concussions can reasonably be eliminated? Currently, the answer to this question is only speculative.

Petitions

There are several ways by which the sports and recreation team may take action with regard to a sports product. The two primary channels are petition, and voluntary standards activity.

The Commission may be petitioned by any concerned individuals to initiate corrective actions on a product they feel is hazardous.[3] After a petition is accepted the Commission has 120 days to evaluate available engineering and economic data along with data on injuries. Then they make a decision whether to grant, deny, or defer the petitioner. The Commission has been petitioned twice to set mandatory safety standards on synthetic turf, and on football helmets and shoes. Petitions regarding synthetic turf were denied twice. The Commission considered the data submitted insufficient to support a finding that a consumer product safety rule was necessary.

A petition on football helmets and shoes was submitted on the basis that they presented an unreasonable risk of injury. Action on it was deferred until late in 1979, when it was reevaluated and denied.

Additional products evaluated are: bicycles, swimming pool slides, skateboards, minibikes.

Voluntary Standards

It is generally believed that the most effective handling of sports and recreation products is by voluntary standards. Organizations have developed these on products used in the following sports: football, hockey, gymnastics, fencing, wrestling, and baseball; and on the following products: golf carts, snowmobiles, swimming pools, spas, trampolines, snow ski bindings, mouth guards and eye protectors.

The Commission generally views development of voluntary standards as supportive. They provide data as requested, or through staff review and comments on proposed standards.

In fiscal year 1985, the Commission will be addressing baseball-related injuries associated with children 5 to 14 years of age. A special study conducted in 1983 identified 85,000 organized baseball–related emergency room treated injuries to children 5 to 14 years of age. During the years 1973 to 1983, 51 baseball-related deaths involving victims 5 to 14 years of age were reported to CPSC. The majority of fatal injuries reported were victims struck by a baseball or softball (35 of 51 deaths). In at least 20 of these cases, the death was a result of being struck in the chest with a ball.[6,7]

Under a contract to be completed by May 1985, the CPSC will try to 1) identify the mechanism(s) of death which occurs as a result of chest impact from a baseball or softball, 2) determine if an injury threshold tolerance can be established, and 3) identify current test methods or establish new ones designed to measure the impact attenuation characteristics of chest protectors.

Information and Education

The Commission's information and education program provides the framework for cooperation with industry and the total community of consumers. Informational and educational programs have been developed in all media to promote increased awareness of product safety among consumers. The potential for injury in sports activities and the need for wearing protective equipment are emphasized. Since some of the safety problems associated with athletic and sports products are user- or use-related, emphasis is directed toward rule-making organizations, athletic coaches, and sports directors.

INJURY DATA COLLECTION—WHY AND WHO?

The time-honored "assumption of risk" in sports is too often touted as a basis for accepting injuries. The debate continues over what risks are reasonable or unreasonable. It is unreasonable, however, for a high school football player to die or to be paralyzed because of an improperly fitted, maintained, or designed helmet. It seems also unreasonable that ice hockey players can needlessly loose their eyesight or sustain fractured facial bones because they do not wear face masks. While readily available on the market, masks are not required by all hockey rules committees.

However, the magnitude and extent of sports-associated injuries, which are less identifiable, point to the need for better sports injury data. Lack of funds and time, and scarcity of qualified investigators have compounded the problems involved in establishing a universally acceptable data collection system.

Hayes[4] contends that:

> Many of the risks taken are unnecessary and could be reduced without changing the nature of the activity. What is required is a scientific approach to the problem involving many disciplines. If we are to understand the phenomenon of sport, the manner must be conducive to the collection of data and subjected to statistical analysis and inference.

Clarke[5] states:

> Decision-makers in sports face both conflicting revelations of the nature and extent of health and safety problems in sports, and conflicting recommended solutions to these problems. Further, they face this with little research data to verify or refute respective contentions.

Development and utilization of an effective surveillance system will assist in identifying the number and severity of sports injuries and their effects upon the participants.

While the primary goal of such information should be prevention of injuries, its immediate use will be in the courtroom. Millions of dollars are tied up in litigations concerning football helmets alone. The manufacturers of gymnastic equipment also face court action. This has led to the formation of the United States Gymnastics Association to certify instructors who teach gymnastics and activity by the NCAA Subcommittee on Medical Aspects of Sports warning athletes of the risks of injury in selected sports.

The National Athletic Injury Reporting System (NAIRS), also discussed in Chapter 1, has been encouraged and utilized by CPSC as an alternate data base for decision-making. NAIRS attempts to determine the degree to which a product may or may not be involved in an injury incident. CPSC utilized data provided by NAIRS for responses to the petitions involving synthetic turf and football helmets.

The data collection system must be sensitive enough to reflect the specific injured body part, the specific nature of play (ie, organized vs unorganized), and the human factors involved. Prior to its redesign in 1978–1979, NEISS did not provide the necessary detail to meet the program needs. The inclusion of the nature of play and of body joints injured on the surveillance reports has strengthened their contribution. However, because of the nature and complexity of sports injuries it is clear that more detailed data on them are needed. However, even with additional detail, it will be difficult to identify causal factors for injuries.

The Issue

There are many reasons why injury records should be maintained. A few are:

1. To determine more realistically the level of assumed risk in a given sports activity,
2. To determine areas where follow-up or specific research may be needed,
3. To support the development of voluntary standards for protective equipment by manufacturers,
4. To measure the social costs of the sports health injury problem.

The real question is: in the absence of a uniform and universally accepted sports injury data collection system what can be done?

Special-interest or independent groups could attempt to establish a system. The government could act as an independent vehicle without the bias that may prevail in self-governing sports organizations. It could communicate with key individuals and organizations and serve as a repository and disseminator of information.

Funding could be alleviated if a government body were established. Very often sports organizations either do not have the monies needed to support large-scale data collection or they give other areas higher priority.

The content of this paper reflects the views of the author, and does not necessarily reflect the views of the U.S. Consumer Product Safety Commission, nor does the mention of trade names, commercial products, or organizations imply endorsement by the Commission.

REFERENCES

1. *U.S. Consumer Product Safety Commission Annual Report, October 1979.* Compilation of Laws Administered by CPSC, April, 1979. Washington, DC: The Commission, 1979.

2. Tabulation of data from the National Electronic Injury Surveillance System, January 1, 1977, through December 31, 1978. Washington, DC: US Consumer Product Safety Commission, 1979.

3. US General Services Administration. *Code of Federal Regulations,* 16. Washington, DC: National Archives and Records Service, 1979.

4. Hayes, D. Risk factors in sport. *Human Factors* 16:454–458, 1974.

5. Clarke, K.S. Premises and pitfalls of athletic injury surveillance. *J Sports Med.* 3:292–295, 1975.

6. Overview of sports related injuries to persons 5–14 years of age. U.S. Consumer Product Safety Commission, Directorate for Epidemiology, December 1981.

7. Baseball and softball related injuries to children 5–14 years of age. U.S. Consumer Product Safety Commission, Directorate for Epidemiology, June 1984.

CHAPTER 3
Pros and Cons of Data-Gathering Mechanisms

John W. Powell, PhD, AT, C

For the past sixty years athletic programs in educational institutions throughout the United States have been expanding rapidly. As the participation in sports widened and the variety and intensity of the activities increased, the injuries that occurred gained the attention of agencies responsible for the administration of high school and college athletic programs. Thus the field of sports safety, including injury prevention, emergency procedures, and follow-up care, moved to the head of the list of administrative concerns.

BACKGROUND

As the literature regarding sports injuries is examined, several recurrent shortcomings can be observed.

1. Much of the information was generated from studies using very small populations, ie, one year for a few teams or several teams for one or two years.
2. Several studies did not clearly establish a definition for an injury. Each project may have had slightly different definitions thus affecting the overall interpretation and the comparability of the findings.
3. Seldom did the individuals asked to record data have knowledge of the variables to be recorded prior to the injury. Without this knowledge, end-of-season questionnaires had to be completed with existing records. Sometimes intuition and recall were mixed with real data in order to complete the recording requirements for the studies undertaken.
4. Although most studies agreed that within athletic programs, sprains, strains, and contusions were the most common types of injury, rarely was the relative severity of these injuries discussed. There was little consistency in either medical or research definitions of injury severity in the primary records kept.

The ability to interpret findings of the existing studies is limited. Systematic data collection, consistent and widely accepted definitions of injury, and overall participant exposures to a sport are necessary in order to enhance the utility of the recorded data. Simply reporting injury frequency does not provide enough data for decision-making. Injury frequencies must be standardized to a given population or total sport exposure, and the resulting rates of injury must be monitored over successive years. Long-term rates will provide the most useful data regarding the injuries either for a single program or for the same sport in many institutions.

A landmark project utilized many of the positive features necessary to interpret sports injury data accurately. This investigation collected specific data from several high school programs in North Carolina. Systematic definitions and recorder-monitoring procedures were established. The data gathered in the study are useful in evaluating the football programs in North Carolina. But the carry-over value to other states is limited compared to what could have been done by a similar effort on a national scale.

Based on the design of the Blythe and Mueller study of North Carolina high schools, and the basic research techniques used in the field of epidemiology, a surveillance system was developed that could collect data for a variety of institutions and sports: the National Athletic Injury/Illness Reporting System (NAIRS). Thanks to interdisciplinary collaboration of a variety of sports professionals, the NAIRS system was able to accumulate injury data for eight years from over 30 different sports and over 200 colleges and high schools nationwide. Within the system the number of schools reporting for each sport varies from year to year while the consistency of the overall injury patterns were maintained. The capability of the NAIRS system was well established when the opportunity to continue collecting data was terminated due to a lack of financial support. The eight years of data collected from 1975–1982 will stand as a reference for several years. Future attempts at monitoring risk patterns in sports will be able to identify with and profit from the experiences of this project.

USING SURVEILLANCE DATA

The most beneficial way for an individual institution to avail itself of surveillance data is to be a contributor to the data base. This commitment makes it possible for the institution to evaluate changes occurring within its own programs. It can also use the data from the entire base to study current injury patterns for each sport recorded. The opportunity to do this on a year-to-year basis can provide rules committees with good evidence on which to base future decisions on sports safety.

Questions posed to the NAIRS data base were in budget planning, equipment utilization, and risk decisions on health insurance programs for the athletic department. On a larger scale, information was used to assess the impact of rules changes on the risks of participation. Particular styles of play or conditioning programs were studied as to their impact on injury rates. An individual also could compare personal experiences to a broader base than one locale. The ideal use of the data base was to complement the local experience by producing a base line from national data.

The ability to collect data systematically for any organized sport was built into the NAIRS concept of surveillance recording. The sport codes were developed and the computer could handle large amounts of input. An individual recorder was limited in ad hoc inquiry to questions based on variables which were recorded. If data from sports with small numbers of participating schools were used, the analysis was restricted somewhat. The larger subsets of data provided a wide variety of potential for interpretation. The full utilization of the accumulated data depends on the skill of the user to interpret the number and incorporate them into a foundation for decision making.

Data Collection for Unorganized Sports

The ability to collect and interpret data from less organized sports such as jogging, hang gliding, or mountain climbing poses unusual problems. While data collection in these areas is not impossible, it is very difficult and demands cooperation among a variety of disciplines.

The foundation for the collection of data from organized sports is based on the concept of on-site recording by a trained observer. The recorder for the NAIRS data was the certified athletic trainer or the agent at the member institution. An individual recorder was responsible for an entire team for a season, and makes note of personal and sport-related variables, exposure numbers, and the circumstances that exist at the time of each injury. In unorganized sports the difficulty in recording injuries stems from the absence of such a control. These athletes usually participate on their own schedules. No immediate care is generally available for any injuries that occur and the individual usually only presents himself to a primary health care facility if his injury limits his normal activity. The primary care center thus becomes the point of entry for these people into an injury recording system. The NAIRS system was able to modify its original computer software to accomodate to the needs of these primary health care centers.

In order to establish a system of injury data collection for the unorganized sports, the practitioner must have consistent access to the site where athletes with these injuries appear for treatment. Recording in clinics and hospitals as well as physicians' offices could provide local officials with valuable information. This could be used for the development of community education programs for fitness, programs for training emergency care personnel, and for the overall benefit of the weekend athlete. By knowing the injury patterns for a given program useful information could be developed to assist in preventing injuries to its participants. Any decisions made regarding sports safety within the community could be easily evaluated from the before and after pictures available from a continuous data base.

The key to the development of data collection for unorganized sports depends on the interest of sports professionals and the cooperation of the local medical community. The physician, clinic, and hospital staff must be systematically coordinated through a central location. There must be reasonable agreement on what is to be recorded, by whom, and in which health care units. Group cooperation and flexibility must be continuing parts of the process.

DATA DISPLAY

An important aspect of any system of data collection is the procedure used to interpret the findings. In general, interpretation should be confined to the framework of the question that generated the data. If data were sought from game-related conditions, then interpretation and display should be confined to only those conditions. Some questions may apply only to practice conditions and other questions may combine both game and practice conditions. Caution must be exercised to see that the findings are not extended beyond the questions unless the former are offered specifically as opinions or interpretations of the researcher.

NAIRS Definitions

The foundation of a strong surveillance data base lies in the quality of the specific definition for injury, severity and exposure. For example, the NAIRS established a *reportable* injury as one that limits athletic participation for at least the day after the day of onset. Within the NAIRS framework a MINOR injury is one that limits the athlete's participation for seven days or less. An injury is MODERATE if participation is limited for more than 7 but less than 21 days. The term MAJOR refers to time-loss from participation of more than 21 days.

The NAIRS category of severe injury includes those injuries which have long-term societal implications such as death, quadriplegia, or amputation. In addition, injuries are assigned to one of two groups: *reportable* injuries include all occurrences reported to NAIRS, and *significant* injuries are those that limit participation for more than seven days.

There are several methods of interpreting frequency data. Absolute frequencies, percentages, and rates are the most common. Absolute frequencies and percentages are weakened by their dependency on the population size. Rate calculations are more useful because of the standardized denominators such as 100 participants or 1000 athlete exposures.

Within the NAIRS system both denominators are used under specific conditions. Rates are generally calculated by dividing the number of injuries by the number of participants or athletic-exposure. An athlete-exposure (AE) is defined as an opportunity to be injured. If 50 athletes have 50 practice sessions and 7 games, the total athlete-exposure is found by multiplying athletes × practices and athletes × games and summing the two. In this case, the total athlete exposure equals 2850 $[50^2 + (50 \times 7)]$. NAIRS college football accumulated over 1.5 million athlete-exposures in the four years 1975 to 1979 using this definition.

Incidence Rates for College Football

Overall football injuries for the 1975, 1976, and 1977 football seasons are shown in Table 3-1.

To illustrate the use of case rates generated by NAIRS, a small data set for the first three seasons are used and displayed in Table 3-1. Inherent in the question of risk is the concept of "chances for injury." The numbers in the table seem to indicate over 90 cases/100 athletes. Included in these rates are individuals who sustained more than one injury. To clarify the issue, add to Table 3-1 the content of Table 3-2. The total injured athletes/100 athletes reflects the number of persons injured at least once but not twice per 100 athletes. From

Table 3-1
Overall Football Injuries
1975–1977 (NAIRS Data)

	1975	1976	1977
Total cases/100 athletes	97.7	93.2	91.5
Significant cases/100 athletes	26.2	24.8	24.6

Table 3-2
Numbers of Teams and Numbers of Atlhktes Injured
1975–1977 (NAIRS Data)

	1975	1976	1977
Number of programs	42	37	69
Number of athletes	3738	3330	6348
Total injuries/100 athletes	97.7	93.2	91.5
Significant injuries/100 athletes	26.2	24.8	24.6
Total injured athletes/ 100 athletes	55.1	58.2	52.4
Significantly injured athletes/ 100 athletes	24.7	22.1	24.0

these data it appears that slightly more than 50% of a 100 man squad will sustain some type of injury. Since the significant injury/100 athletes and the significant injured athlete/100 athletes are similar, this probably indicates that if an athlete receives one significant injury, he probably will not receive a recorded one. The addition of the number of teams per season and athletes per season adds perspective to the overall impact of the data.

To complete the picture Table 3-3 adds to Table 3-2 the consideration of injuries per 1000 athlete-exposures (AE) as defined earlier.

Although the rates per 1000 athlete-exposures seem to indicate a downward trend for injury over the three years, these small differences may be random errors or sampling errors due to the size of the data base.

Table 3-3
Injuries per 1000 AE
1975–1977 (NAIRS Data)

	1975	1976	1977
Number of programs	42	37	69
Number of athletes	3738	3330	6348
Total injuries/100 athletes	97.7	93.2	91.5
Significant injuries/100 athletes	26.2	24.8	24.6
Total injured athletes/100 athletes	55.1	58.2	52.4
Significantly injured athletes/ 100 athletes	24.7	22.1	24.0
Total injuries/1000 AE	11.8	11.3	10.9
Significant injuries/1000 AE	3.2	3.0	2.9

When comparing rates per 1000 athlete-exposures among various sports, special consideration should be given to the nature of the sport and the relative impact similar injuries would have for each of two athletes in their respective sports. Table 3-4 displays selected rates per 1000 athlete-exposures for the 1975–1977 recording years.

The differences observed between men's and women's experiences are probably real and the search for the human factors that influence these rates may provide the key as to the reasons for them.

DATA INTERPRETATION

The complete consideration of the human factors, the nature of the game, and the facilities used in association with the game all interact to produce a sequence of events that lead to injury. As each area is analyzed, the complexity of the interpretation increases.

Cause and Effect

Sports enthusiasts continually attempt to attach the concept of cause and effect to the numbers of injuries that they observe or experience. The use of large data base such as that gathered by NAIRS, addresses the cause-effect concept in a systematic way. To do this the following two points must be held firmly in mind: 1) if a causal relationship exists between variables, the epidemiologic surveillance

Table 3-4
Significant Injury Rates per 1000 Athlete (Women's Sports Labeled F) Exposures, 1975–1977

	Number of College teams surveyed			Total injury rate/1000 AE			Significant injury rate/1000 AE		
	1975	*1976*	*1977*	*1975*	*1976*	*1977*	*1975*	*1976*	*1977*
Wrestling	15	15	29	11.6	11.3	7.7	4.4	4.6	3.3
Football	42	37	69	11.8	11.3	10.9	3.2	3.0	2.9
Basketball	30	22	41	7.2	7.5	6.7	1.8	2.1	1.5
Basketball (F)	21	13	10	7.1	10.0	8.3	2.1	3.1	2.1
Field hockey	14	15	18	4.4	5.3	5.6	0.7	1.0	0.9
Ice hockey	9	6	10	11.4	13.6	9.1	2.4	2.9	2.3
Soccer	15	11	14	8.6	10.8	8.3	2.0	2.5	2.0
Baseball	12	12	16	1.1	2.1	1.6	0.5	0.3	0.6
Volleyball (F)	12	12	25	2.4	4.4	4.8	1.0	1.0	1.0
Softball (F)	10	8	11	2.1	1.9	2.3	0.7	0.6	0.6

will show the association, but 2) an association demonstrated by surveillance data does not necessarily mean that the relationship is causal. In order to imply causality to a described association, tests must be applied and systematic reevaluation carried out as more data are generated. The greater the exposure for the longer period of time, the more readily the question of causality can be addressed.

Several points should be noted:

1. Large-scale surveillance is required if the risk of sports participation is to be quantified accurately.
2. Large-scale recording can be accomplished but requires interdisciplinary cooperation among persons and agencies involved in sports administration.
3. Once data have been generated, extreme caution and meticulous analysis must be carried out before any statement of causality can be established.
4. In view of the statement of causality the data can be analyzed to provide decision-makers a sound base from which to choose relevant courses of action.

Acceptable Risk

The judgment of how much risk is acceptable for the participants in sports will always be a function of personal and collective values. To be able to base that judgment on systematically collected data that quantify risks will provide sports with better decisions on safety and increased benefits for the participants. Therefore, surveillance of athletic injuries must be continued and expanded. The emphasis for programs such as NAIRS must come from sports governance agencies and must be implemented in individual programs. Schools and clinics have the manpower. The task is to bring the system and the manpower together on a nationwide basis.

SUGGESTED READINGS

Alles, W.F., Powell, J.W., Buckley, W.E., and Hunt, E.E. The national athletic injury/illness reporting system 3-year findings of high school and college football injuries. *J Orthopaedic Sports Physical Ther.* 1(2):1979.

Blyth, C.S., and Mueller, F.O. An epidemiologic study of high school football injuries in North Carolina, 1968–1972. Final report. US Consumer Product Safety Commission, Washington, DC: US Government Printing Office, 1972.

Clarke, K.S. Premises and pitfalls of athletic injury surveillance. *J Sports Med.* 3(6):1975.

Clarke, K.S., Miller, and Sayers J. Sports injury data collection and interpretation. *Interscholastic Athletic Administration.* 1(3):1975.

Clark, K.S., and Miller, S.J. The national athletic injury/illness reporting system (NAIRS). *Proceedings—Second National Conference on Sports Safety.* Chicago: American School and Community Safety Association. October 1976.

NAIRS Staff. An epidemiological examination of the association of selected products with related injuries in football 1975-1977. *Report to the U.S. Consumer Product Safety Commission.* March 1979.

Powell, J.W. Research in athletic training—NAIRS model. *Proceedings of NATA Professional Education Conference.* Nashville, Tenn. 1978, pp. 15–24.

CHAPTER 4
Proposals for Improvement

Edward M. Milner

The majority of recent sports injury studies have addressed specific issues or problems. This approach has limited their utility and frequently led to misinterpretation, especially if several years have passed between data collection and review. An ongoing system for sports injury study is needed that will accomplish these ends:

1. Serve the needs of the various groups who seek to reduce the frequency and severity of sports injuries,
2. Permit analysis of trends as well as single season data,
3. Allow valid comparisons between different levels and styles of play, both during the same season and across several years,
4. Make data interpretation as direct and precise as possible.

PRESENT STUDIES AND THEIR USERS

The following are some needs of audiences to be served by sports injury data systems.

Rules makers need to know which sports activities are associated with the highest injury frequencies and severities.

Coaches and players need to know the risk of injury associated with various techniques of practice and play.

Administrators need to know the status of their programs and equipment relative to other organizations at the same levels of participation.

Manufacturers of sports equipment need to evaluate the performance of their products against the overall market in order to determine needed changes or the results of product modifications. They also face the exposure of the ongoing "sue syndrome" in the field of product liability, and need data to defend themselves when they are doing a good job.

The public needs an unbiased and rational appraisal of the risks associated with various sports, especially those supported with public funds, as well as the benefits that are derived from those programs.

Insurers need to have a basis on which to establish properly the costs of insurance coverage.

Most sports injury studies made in recent years have dealt with one or several of these needs, but there has been no single program addressed to all of them. Some of the best known studies are reviewed here.

The *National Electronic Injury Surveillance System* (NEISS)[1] of the US Consumer Product Safety Commission uses data from the emergency rooms of selected hospitals. However, this may not represent the injuries of organized team sports, many of which are not processed through emergency rooms. The hospitals were selected on a general population basis rather than on a sports participation basis. Some sports, such as skiing, are probably undersampled, since the system includes relatively few hospitals in regions where skiing is a major activity.

Studies made for special interest groups such as the National Football League make no attempt (quite properly) to relate their findings to injuries at other levels of play such as among colleges or high schools.

The excellent work done by The *National Athletic Injury/Illness Reporting System (NAIRS)*[2] has been hampered by a lack of long-term funding, as well as by limited sampling at the high school level, and by dependence on the motivation and accuracy of volunteer participants.

The *North Carolina High School Study*[3] did a superb job within high school football near the University of North Carolina, showing the advantages of using a small number of highly trained investigators, establishing baseline data, and impressing various experimental conditions on portions of the study population. But such attention to detail was costly and would be difficult to operate on a nationwide basis, and the study is now over 10 years old.

The majority of organized sports programs in the United States are related to our educational systems (with the notable exceptions of programs such as Little League baseball, Pop Warner football, and amateur hockey). It seems logical to go to the organizations coordinating school-related sports to set up administration of a comprehensive, ongoing program of injury data collection and analysis. The number of sports administrative bodies is small: the National Collegiate Athletic Association, the National Alliance for Intercollegiate Athletics, the National Junior College Athletic Association, the National Federation of State High School Associations, and the American Alliance for Health, Physical Education, Recreation, and Dance. These, plus the associations of a few states not affiliated with one of the above groups, cover almost all school-related sports activities in the United States. Most of these groups are already communicating through their Joint Commission on Competitive Safeguards and Medical Aspects of Sports. They are joined by professional support groups such as the National Athletic Trainers Association and the American College Health Association.

An adequate system of injury study should build on the foundations already laid by the NAIRS and North Carolina groups.

NAIRS software is designed to permit compatible data entry at different levels of study and reporting detail. It uses sport-related terminology specific to many different sports. It has been "debugged" to the degree that data can be edited for content and consistency before entry and can be retrieved promptly as needed for study.[2]

The North Carolina group provided careful on-site auditing of the input data for accuracy and completeness through the use of a controlled sample population and a small group of professional investigators.[3] These practices should be included in the ongoing system for at least a portion of the participating teams, establishing a continuing baseline of audited data against which comparisons can be made.

SUGGESTED GUIDELINES

Under the leadership of a group such as the Joint Commission on Competitive Safeguards and Medical Aspects of Sports, it should be possible to set up a system along the following lines.

Administration

The national sports injury study programs should be administered within systems already in place. They can be coordinated under the auspices of the Joint Commission on Competitive Safeguards and Medical Aspects of Sports.

Sampling

Sampling and data input should include a controlled sample group for each sport and level of play. There should also be provisions for voluntary data input from concerned individual schools, teams, and conferences.

For controlled samples, a statistically valid group of teams should be selected for each level of play in the sports studied. They will serve as the controlled sample population. Various areas of the country should be represented to account for regional differences in climate, and in style and intensity of play. Data collection from the control group of teams should be carried out by paid investigators and closely audited by the program administrators. Admittedly this approach is expensive, but it represents the best chance to assure consistency, accuracy, and completeness of the data.

Voluntary samples will be made up of those schools (or teams or conferences) desiring to participate in the injury surveillance program to improve the safety of their own programs. When allowed to do so on a voluntary basis, they will pay their own expenses for data collection and reporting, using a compatible but somewhat simpler format similar to the NAIRS II System. The individual team or organization can compare its own results with those of the "control" teams for its own level of play as well as with the averages for all participants. The data from voluntary participants would be stored separately from that for the control sample. It could be pooled with the controlled sample data where statistically appropriate to increase the precision of various estimates.

Data Access

Summaries of the data related to overall sport participation—in both games and practice sessions—should be routinely published for the use of rules makers, sports administrators, and coaches. Where appropriate, internal data should be available to qualified researchers, but with safeguards to protect the privacy of the institutions and players involved.

Access to equipment-related data by equipment manufacturers is an important need if design and quality improvements are to continue. This access should be on a self-supporting basis for participating manufacturers, perhaps through an associate membership or as a "patron." To avoid misuse of competitive information, the data for a given manufacturer's products should be made available only to the individual supplier. Data for all suppliers would be averaged and reported by style or design categories (for example, shoes by the number and arrangement of cleats, or helmets by padding and suspension features). This would permit a supplier to compare the results for his products by style and category with overall industry results. He could not make comparisons against individual competing suppliers' products.

At the central data-processing facility, knowledgeable professionals should watch the data as they come in from all sources, both controlled and voluntary, and should be available for consultation. Problems of terminology and diagnosis can be avoided by consistency checks as the data are received, as has been done by NAIRS.

These consulting editors would be charged with maintaining the confidentiality of the individuals and organizations supplying the raw data.

AUDIT SYSTEM

No surveillance system is better than the quality of its input data. Accordingly, provisions must be made for continual audit as the data are generated. Some balance must be reached between the geographic locations of the control teams and their accessibility for auditor visits. This can be done by the use of regional clusters of control teams. This would permit a small number of well-qualified auditors to visit each control team several times during each season and check the accuracy of its data. They would review diagnoses and the length of time injured players were not available for sports participation. They could also determine the circumstances of injuries.

Similarly, each participating team should receive routine summaries of its own injury records for comparison with sportwide averages. Participants should not have data that can be identified as coming from other teams or individuals. *Rigorous protection of the privacy of individuals, teams, and manufacturers is ethically essential, and is critical to the continuation of voluntary participation in a valid sports injury data system.*

The audit provisions become a combination of the audit features of both the North Carolina High School Study, with its use of on-site auditors, and the NAIRS provision for content editing and central consultation.

FUNDING

In recent years the majority of injury study and prevention programs have sought and generally received funding from governmental sources. Such funding is seldom adequate, and is not assured from year to year. Some of the provisos of governmental funding acts tend to force inefficient if not counterproductive recording measures. How much better for sports injury studies if their funding is provided from within the sports world itself, with participation from all levels of sports and athletics.

Each year professional sports activities depend on amateur and educationally centered sports for their players and many of their coaches, as well as for their audiences who generate gate and television receipts. These are excellent reasons why professional sports should contribute regularly and generously to programs that will help make all sports safer.

College football and basketball are "big business," but are already loaded with the burden of supporting nonrevenue sports and intramurals. Nevertheless, there is good reason to believe that a better knowledge of sports injury causes and frequencies will help reduce the cost of sports injuries not to mention their effects on the lives of injured athletes. A modest per capita tax or contribution, dedicated to reduction of injuries, from each institution sponsoring organized sports programs is appropriate as well as good business.

Most manufacturers of sports equipment are relatively small organizations, although many are business entities within large corporations. The manufacturers of athletic equipment have already contributed to such projects as the development of improved football helmet standards, through the National Operating Committee for Standards in

Athletic Equipment (NOCSAE). They also helped support the early stages of the NAIRS effort. This support should be continued and increased, but the reduction of sports injury severity and frequency is the responsibility of all the groups involved.

One of the principal virtues of sports participation is its teaching of teamwork through individual responsibility and effort. The same virtue should be practiced in the support of an adequate program of sports injury surveillance and study, to the end that those who participate may do so more safely.

REFERENCES

1. US Consumer Product Safety Commission. Fact Sheet. *News Briefing Papers.* Sept. 28, 1973.

2. Clarke, K.S. Final Report, *Development of the National Injury/Illness Reporting System.* Washington, DC: US Consumer Product Safety Commission, 1976.

3. Blyth, C.S., and Mueller, F.O. An epidemiological study of high school football injuries in North Carolina 1968–1972. Washington, DC: US Consumer Product Safety Commission, 1974.

SECTION II
Socioeconomic Considerations

CHAPTER 5
The Economic Costs of Sports Injuries

Harriet G. Tolpin, PhD
Judith D. Bentkover, PhD

When Doctors Tolpin and Bentkover were asked to write a chapter on economic aspects of sports injuries, they chose to focus on the economic costs associated with such injuries. It became quite clear early in their research efforts that providing actual estimates of economic costs of even a single type of injury was precluded by the lack of data necessary to derive such estimates.

Although the economic cost of sports injuries has not been subjected to formal analysis prior to this effort, the economic cost of illness has been a research issue that has received substantial attention over the last two decades. In this chapter, the authors examine the state-of-the-art cost of illness methodology and develop a conceptual and analytical framework for the estimation of the economic cost of sports injuries.

As the authors demonstrate, this framework provides a basis for rational discussion and decision-making regarding the use of protective devices in sports. However, the dearth of appropriate data is the binding constraint that impedes the estimation of the economic cost of sports injuries. The authors underscore the exhortations of several of the other authors in this book and call for the development and maintenance of a consistent, reliable data base. Such an information system would facilitate future research in this area.

The Editors

A PUBLIC POLICY PERSPECTIVE

In 1982 U.S. national health expenditures were $322.4 billion, a sum that will account for 10.5% of total expenditures for all goods and services in the economy that year. It is now widely accepted that the resources available to meet health care needs are limited. Thus rational allocation of those resources must proceed with careful analysis of the costs and benefits of alternative health practices. Estimation of economic cost of specific diseases and injuries is of great interest to both public and private sector decision-makers who allocate funds, since rational allocation depends on such information.

Already, conscious decisions are being made. National health planning guidelines require that hospitals ration beds. Federal reimbursement policies implicitly assign priorities that govern the use of health care goods and services. The availability of physicians and the rapidity of technologic advancement affect many decisions. These include which health care services will be produced and the means by which and to whom they will be delivered.

In order to formulate public health policy, current information on both the efficacy of alternative medical interventions and their associated cost and benefits must be evaluated by decision-makers. Only then can incentives to adopt a set of cost-effective health practices be formulated.

The reason for studying the costs of sports-related injuries is that treatment of many such injuries requires a substantial number of resources. Also, a significant number of these injuries can be prevented. Although protective equipment is widely available, its use is often rebuffed by players. Masks, helmets, and similar gear are associated with inconvenience and stigma. In this situation, a comprehensive cost analysis can serve as an important aid in the decisions relating to the allocation of resources directed toward the prevention of these injuries.

THE CONCEPT OF ECONOMIC COST

An economist defines the cost of a good or service as the benefits foregone from other goods and services that cannot be produced because the resources have been used to produce the particular good in question. Thus economic cost is often termed opportunity cost in the sense that resources used in one way mean the sacrifice of those opportunities that would be available if resources were used another way. "Economic cost of sports injuries" refers to the opportunity cost that society incurs by diverting resources from alternative uses in order to diagnose and treat injuries associated with sports. The computation of the economic cost of sports injuries is based on estimates of the value of those diverted resources.

Economic costs of injuries are of two types: direct and indirect. Direct costs are those expenditures paid for by the patient, the patient's family, and third party reimbursement agencies. In particular, these expenditures result from the explicit outlay of resources necessary to diagnose and treat the injury under consideration. Direct costs of sports injuries thus include the costs of emergency room and/or hospital treatment, physicians, dentists, and other professional services, drugs, medical supplies, physical therapy, rehabilitation services, and follow-up care. From a societal perspective, direct costs also include expenditures for 1) research and personnel training oriented towards detection, treatment, and prevention; and 2) expenditures for related facilities and equipment.

Indirect costs are not directly associated with the treatment of an injury but are incurred as a result of the injury. These costs result primarily from reduced productivity and increased morbidity or mortality. The notion here is that there is a cost in terms of foregone output of those individuals suffering from premature death or disability as the result of a sports injury. Foregone production results in reduced consumption by the patient and his family and affects the rest of society in reduced tax revenues and increased needs for public assistance.

SOCIETAL AND SOCIAL COSTS

Two other types of costs also need to be considered in cost-of-injury estimates: societal and social.

Societal Costs

Those costs that must be taken into account when considering cost of injury from the societal perspective include insurance administration costs, and legal and court costs.

From the societal perspective it is appropriate to identify insurance administration costs incurred by agencies covering selected medical events associated with injury.

The legal and court costs are associated with adverse side effects of treatment or product liability. They consume resources that could be channeled into alternative uses. To estimate them one must know the likelihood of an injured person pursuing litigation. For cases settled in court, the overall costs are dependent upon the value of the time spent by lawyers and judges on the case, the contribution made by legal support services, and an appropriate proportion of variable court overhead expenses.

Since legal costs are borne by the individual as well as by society, exclusion of these costs will result in a slight underestimate of the total private economic costs.

Social Costs

The term social costs refers to psychosocial deteriorations that result from illness or injury. The concept of social cost recognizes, for example, that mortality influences the family and its life cycle, that morbidity may affect duration of marriages, and that significant associations exist among morbidity, economic dependence, and social isolation. Many injuries may bring about personal catastrophies that are not quantitatively estimated. Victims may suffer loss of a body part or speech, disfigurement, disability, impending death, pain, and depression. This person, as well as those around him or her, may be forced into a changed environment: economic dependence, social isolation, loss of career and education opportunities, and relocation of living quarters. Such changes are likely to induce anxiety and resentment, reduce self-esteem, and precipitate emotional problems. Mental illness may develop and family conflict and/or suicide may be the result. Disrupted development and delinquency may occur among children.

Marital instability has associated with it economic costs (eg, lawyer and court fees, alimony, child support) as well as psychosocial costs. Long-term emotional damage to family members may necessitate expenditures for counseling and therapy services. Child neglect and even abuse may be a consequence of psychosocial deteriorations resulting from disability and/or reduced quality of life associated with illness or injury.

As with direct and indirect costs, the first step in incorporating social costs into cost-of-injury estimates requires their identification and enumeration. Although this identification step is relatively straightforward in the case of direct and indirect costs—that is, expert medical opinion can supply this type of information—identification of social costs is a much more difficult undertaking. Since expert medical opinion generally encompasses a biomedical model of disease, psychosocial aspects of disease states are often not considered, particularly in terms of their effects on family members.

QUANTIFICATION OF ECONOMIC COSTS

In order to quantify the economic costs of a specific sports injury it is necessary to identify diagnosis, treatment, and follow-up requirements. Figure 5-1 illustrates some of the possible variations in the course of treatment and in the residual impairment status; it also delineates resource needs for each phase of treatment.

To identify precisely the resources required (for example, the number of physician visits, dosage of specific drugs), expert medical opinion must be relied upon. A detailed description of needs can then be developed for each type of sports injury. Of course, the part of the body affected, severity of the injury, and the age and physical status of the injured individual are all considered in this process.

There are two ways to calculate direct costs: 1) estimates of unit costs of health care goods and services can be multiplied by the number of goods and services required; or 2) aggregate total expenditures (eg, hospital expenditures, physicians' services) can be distributed by diagnosis using utilization and cost estimates from various sources.

Although indirect costs include several components, only a few items can be quantified. Morbidity and mortality account for the largest component of indirect costs. They are commonly measured in terms of the value of foregone output that sports injury patients would have produced if they had not incurred their injuries. (Another way to assess value is the "willingness-to-pay" method, discussed in Limitations Imposed by Data.) Again, medical judgment relating to level of post-discharge disability and life expectancy are important considerations in valuation.

The major societal costs—insurance administration, legal, and court costs—must be estimated on the basis of available data and some relatively arbitrary assumptions such as the percentage of total insurance administration costs attributable to claims involving sports injuries.

Although the measurement of societal costs may be conceptually straightforward, in practice, because of significant data limitations, these costs are either not included in cost-of-injury estimates or they are assumed to be some fixed proportion of expenditures in another direct cost category. To the extent that societal estimates are omitted, total economic costs will be underestimated. However, the inclusion of arbitrary estimates of societal cost may not be a preferable alternative.

Quantification of social costs is currently the focus of much methodologic discussion. It is in this area that the state-of-the-art is least developed. Some promising first steps have been taken in quantifying quality-of-life considerations through functional status indexes. For example, the intensity and duration of pain can be inferred from the amount of pain-killing drugs required. But relatively little has been done in terms of developing indicators of psychosocial distress and enumerating its consequences. Costs of psychotherapy and psychiatric care are, at this point, all that are available.

Areas of controversy remain with respect to direct and indirect costs. The problems in these areas center more around quantification than around identification and enumeration. In the area of social costs, however, significant work needs to be done on identification and enumeration before addressing problems of inadequacy and non-comparability of data.

In order to compute the economic cost of one patient's sports injury, it is necessary to combine the available estimates of all of the above costs. To arrive at the economic cost of all instances of a particular type of sports injury, it is necessary to multiply estimates of its incidence by the economic cost of one such injury. Finally, to compute the total costs of sports injuries, it is necessary to aggregate incidence estimates and economic cost estimates.

Within this basic methodological framework the economic costs of sports injuries to individuals and to society can be computed. It is possible to estimate the costs of sports injuries by age, sex, specific parts of the body, and severity levels.

Prior to our presenting examples of the application of this methodology, however, it is necessary to discuss two additional steps that are involved in the quantification of economic costs.

First, in order to coordinate all calculations and thereby ensure relevant combinations of cost and incidence, it is necessary arbitrarily to choose a base year. Once this year is designated, all costs must be based on prevailing price levels in that year, and incidence rates must correspond to population in that year.

Second, in order to avoid the overvaluation of costs occurring in future years, economic costs extending over a period of years must be converted to a present value in the base year by using an appropriate discount rate. Although there is widespread agreement on the necessity to discount

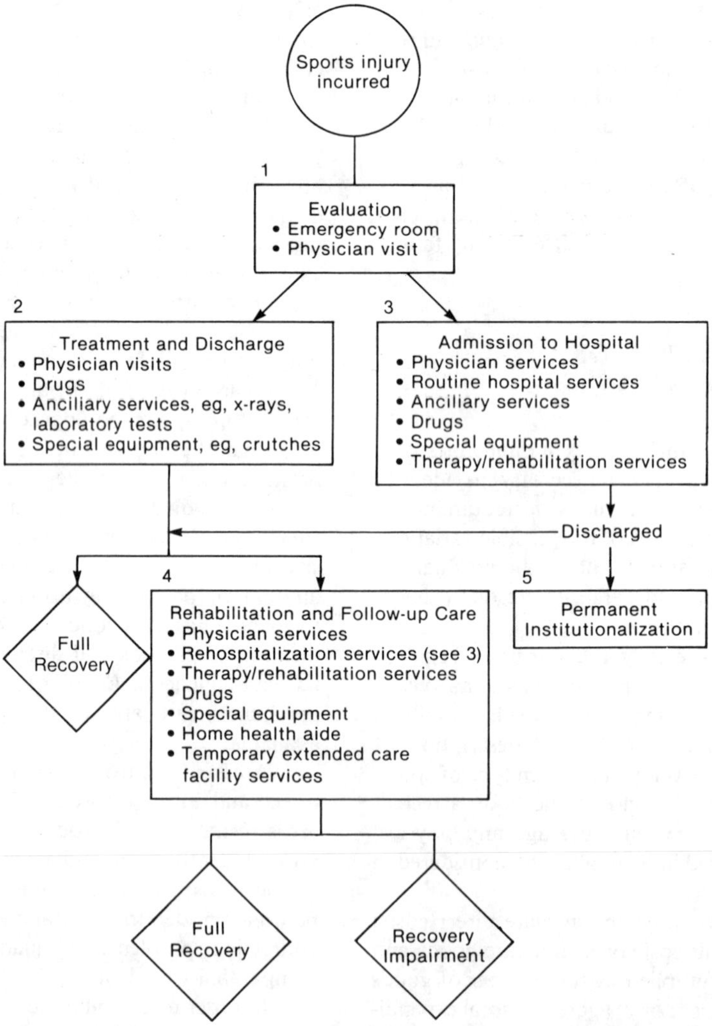

Figure 5-1 Treatment and resource requirements of a sports-injury patient.

future costs, there is no corresponding level of agreement on the level at which the discount rate should be set.

Some economists have argued that the discount rate used in public decision-making should reflect the opportunity cost of public capital in other ventures, including investment alternatives in the private sector. This policy implies that a relatively high discount rate, ie, one close to the market rate interest in the private sector, be employed. Other economists suggest that a lower rate of interest, which is more representative of a social rate of time preference, be employed. This lower rate would give more weight to costs occurring in the future and presumably would give more recognition to the welfare of future generations bearing these costs.

ECONOMIC COST OF A SINGLE SPORTS INJURY: TWO ILLUSTRATIVE CASES

Case 1: Ice Hockey Injury

A 25-year-old man was hit in the eye with a stick while playing ice hockey. The injury ultimately necessitated a corneal transplant after which the player's vision was fully restored and recovery was complete.

The necessary steps in the evaluation and treatment of this injury were identified to include the following (Resource requirements were obtained from Paul Vinger, MD):

1. Immediately following the injury the player went directly to a hospital emergency room where the injury was diagnosed as a severe corneal abrasion. The eye was patched and the patient was told to see an ophthalmologist the next day.
2. The patient saw the ophthalmologist, was given a complete eye examination, and told to return for follow-up.
3. In ensuing weeks the severe abrasion turned into a recurrent erosion and four further follow-up visits were required.
4. On the fourth visit, a soft "bandage" contact lens was prescribed.
5. Three additional follow-up visits ensued. The erosion treatment was not effective and the patient developed a corneal ulcer.
6. The patient was hospitalized for six days of intravenous treatment for the ulcer.
7. Following discharge, the patient was seen another four times by the ophthalmologist for observation and treatment.
8. The ulcer healed with a dense scar, significantly impairing the patient's vision. The patient elected to undergo a corneal transplant requiring five days of hospitalization.
9. The transplant was successful and treatment ended after four additional visits following hospital discharge.

In order to calculate the direct costs associated with this sequence of events, the resources utilized in each of the treatment steps must be identified and valued. This information appears in Table 5-1.

Case 1 estimates the total cost of an injury that leaves no permanent disability, has a relatively short course of treatment, and does not result in

Table 5-1
Economic Cost of an Ice Hocky Injury: Severe Corneal Abrasion in a 25-year-old Man

Direct Costs*	
Emergency room visit	$ 52
Complete exam by ophthalmologist	36
Four follow-up visits at $21	84
"Soft bandage" contact lens	180
Three follow-up visits at $21	63
Six days' hospitalization at $263 per day	1570
MD cost	156
Four follow-up visits at $21	84
Corneal transplant	
Five days' hospitalization at $262 per day	1308
Surgical fees	1248
Assistant fee	250
Anesthetist fee	260
Four follow-up visits at $21	84
Total direct costs	$5375
Indirect Costs (Work days lost at $68.30 per day)†	
MD visits, 15 visits at ½ day each	513
Corneal ulcer treatment, 10 days	683
Corneal transplant, 21 days	1435
Insurance administration costs‡	210
Total indirect costs	$2841
Total Economic Costs	$8216

*These costs are based on actual unit costs inflated to fiscal year 1980. Detailed calculations are available from the authors upon request.

†Earnings data are based on Arthur D. Little, Inc. estimates prepared for the National Center for Health Services Research, Office of the Assistant Secretary for Health Research, Statistics, and Technology, Public Health Service U.S. Department of Health, Education, and Welfare pursuant to Contract No. 233-78-3013.

‡Insurance administration costs are assumed to be equivalent to 3.9% of total direct cost expenditures.

significant morbidity. Thus the direct costs associated with the injury comprise the bulk of the total injury costs. Indirect costs are relatively small, and no costs are incurred beyond the year in which the injury was sustained. Case 2 presents cost estimates of a spinal cord injury sustained while playing football. This injury does result in permanent disability, significant morbidity and costs, both direct and indirect, which are incurred over the lifetime of the injured player. Direct and indirect costs are substantial and recurring.

Case 2: Football Injury

A 20-year-old man playing wide receiver in a football game was running a crossing pattern over the middle. The quarterback threw a pass and the receiver was tackled in midair with a high hit by a player coming from the opposite direction. The wide receiver fell to the ground and was motionless. He was taken by ambulance to the nearest hospital emergency room under spinal cord precautions and was diagnosed as having a fracture of the sixth cervical vertebra with spinal cord involvement. This injury left the player a permanently impaired quadriplegic who was never able to resume gainful employment.

The diagnostic, therapeutic, and rehabilitative treatment necessitated by this injury are assumed to be as follows:[1]

1. The patient was transported by ambulance to the emergency room and received emergency treatment.
2. He was admitted to a general hospital for the acute care phase of his treatment and then transferred to a spinal cord injury center for subacute care and rehabilitation (235 days).
3. The patient was discharged and returned to his home. One-time home modifications (eg, ramps, widening of doors, bathroom modifications) were made.
4. The purchase of certain medical equipment and appliances such as a wheelchair and an electric hospital bed was required.
5. The patient enrolled in an active vocational rehabilitation program six months after hospital discharge. It consisted of a complete and detailed vocational evaluation and training, and work adjustment.

For the remainder of his life, certain additional resources were required by the patient.

6. Although the patient did not need to be institutionalized following hospital discharge, he did require continuing assistance and received attendant care at home (approximately six hours per day).
7. Each year he was readmitted to the hospital for both routine checkups and treatment of common complications such as decubitus ulcers and urinary tract infections (15 days per year of rehospitalization).
8. The nature of the injury necessitated the use of drugs and medical supplies, particularly those associated with bowel and bladder control programs.
9. The nature of the injury also necessitated special expenditures for such items as transportation, laundry, bedding, clothing, and nonmedical appliances.

Resource requirements and estimates of the costs of this particular injury appear in Table 5-2. In this table two discount rates have been specified:

Table 5-2
Economic Cost of a Football Injury
Severe Spinal Cord Injury (in $FY 1980)

	6%	10%
Direct Costs*		
Initial Costs	$101,858	$101,764
Emergency assistance		
- Ambulance @ $75		
- Emergency room treatment Services @ $437		
Initial hospitalization		
- 235 days @378 = $88,830		
Home modifications @ $9946		
Vocational rehabilitation†	2570	2476
Annual Costs	228,442	166,343
Medical equipment and appliances $554/yr		
Attendant care costs 6 hr/day @ $5.10/hr for 350 days = $10,710/yr		
Rehospitalization 15 days/yr @ $378/day = $5670/yr		
Drugs and medical services $1126/yr		
Miscellaneous service and supplies $895/yr		
Total Direct Costs	$330,300	$268,107
Indirect Costs		
Foregone earnings‡	394,740	233,306
Insurance administrative costs§	12,882	10,456
Total Indirect Costs	407,622	234,762
Total Economic Costs	737,922	511,869

*These costs are based on actual unit costs inflated to $FY 1980. Detailed calculations are available from the authors upon request.
†A one-time cost assigned to the year following the onset of injury.
‡Earnings data are based on Arthur D. Little, Inc., estimates prepared for DHEW, NCHSR pursuant to Contract 233-78-3013.
§Insurance administration costs are assumed to be equivalent to 3.9% of total direct cost expenditures.

10% and 6%. Ten percent is a close approximation to the present opportunity cost of public capital, if that capital were invested in the private sector. Six percent, on the other hand, is a more intermediate value that more closely approximates the social discount rate. Using each of these rates, the present value of future costs can be determined with reference to a base year, such as fiscal year 1980.

Aggregate Cost of Sports Injuries

In order to estimate the aggregate economic cost to the nation of sports injuries for a given year, it is necessary to 1) estimate the economic cost of injury associated with a given sport for all individuals injured while engaged in that sport for the given year, and 2) aggregate these cost estimates across all sports. The task of aggregating costs across sports is straightforward. However, the task of estimating the cost of injuries associated with a given sport cannot be completed at the present time because of unavailability of necessary data.

In this section we present the conceptual and methodologic issues involved in estimating the expected economic costs of injuries associated with a given sport. Data requirements necessary for such an estimation effort are then discussed.

In order to estimate direct and indirect costs of all injuries associated with a sport, one needs an estimate of the number of injuries in that sport in a given year. These figures must again be classified according to age and sex of the injured persons, and the type and severity of injury. For example, indirect costs attributable to productivity losses, if valued according to a human capital approach, will tend to be higher for men than for women and for persons in high income-generating years than for either the very young or the very old. Direct costs will vary with type and severity of injury since resource requirements involved in treatment will vary similarly. Indirect costs will be related to the type and severity of injury since morbidity and mortality are also affected by these dimensions of injury.

One must also know resource requirements for treating an injury of given type and severity for an individual of a particular sex and age. These are multiplied by per unit costs in calculating direct costs of the injuries. In some cases direct costs are recurring; that is, certain expenditures must be made beyond the year in which the injury occurs. Appropriately discounted, they must be multiplied by survival probabilities. For example, direct costs to be incurred two years from date of injury must be multiplied by the probability that the injured individual will be alive two years after the injury occurs. Survival probabilities, in turn, depend on the age and sex of the person injured, the type of injury, and its severity.

In order to estimate indirect costs, estimates of morbidity and mortality for the injured population are required. The most common way of converting these estimates into indirect cost figures is to use expected lifetime earnings tables which are available by sex and age groups.

To summarize, in order to calculate the direct and indirect costs of injuries associated with a given sport incurred in a particular time period, the following information is required:

1. incidence of injury by age and sex
2. type of injury incurred
3. severity of injury
4. resources required in the diagnosis and treatment, and per unit costs of such resources
5. morbidity and mortality estimates associated with each type of injury.

This list points out the necessity for a consistent, reliable sports injury reporting system as a prerequisite to estimating the economic costs of sports injuries.

LIMITATIONS IMPOSED BY DATA AND THE STATE-OF-THE-ART

As has just been shown, the implementation of the economic cost of injury methodology is dependent upon substantial data requirements. One of the most serious problems in assessing the societal impact of sport-related injuries is inadequacy of data on their extent, incidence, type, and severity.

Data Limitations

Although a variety of systems do exist for the gathering and reporting of information related to sports injuries, none of these data collection systems was designed to provide national data representative of total injuries associated with a particular sport. Data that do exist either represent injuries associated with organized sports or injuries associated with unsupervised, unorganized sports activities. Much of the data, having been collected for specific purposes, are not in a form amenable to the categorizations necessary for calculations of economic costs. A convincing case is presented in Chapters 1, 2, and 3 for the development of a standardized, consistent, and reliable injury reporting system. Such a reporting system could be structured in such a way that incidence data with data describing the injured person (age and sex) and the person's injury (by type and severity) would provide the raw data necessary to begin to estimate economic costs.

Although clinical literature contains a wealth of information concerning the nature of sports injuries and available treatment regimens, relatively little data are available concerning the corresponding health care resources consumed in the treatment process, their associated costs, and the duration and degree of disability associated with the injuries. What data sources are available are discussed below.

In terms of disease or illness-specific data, standard codes for classifying diseases, disabilities and causes of death are provided by the International Classification of Diseases (ICD). The ICD codes are used in vital statistics, in health services research and health status surveys, in indexing admitting and discharge diagnoses in hospital records, and in designating clinical problems associated with claims for inpatient and outpatient care under public and private reimbursement programs. Hence, ICD codes provide a means of obtaining information concerning injury-specific health care resource needs and associated costs. Gaining access to meaningful disease-specific data for estimating costs of injury is difficult, however, because much of it is dispersed among many sources and contained in huge computer files of hospital discharge abstracts and claims files. Often constraints of time and money (and at times access) preclude using such data.

Far more data are available concerning a patient's resource needs during the acute illness, especially one requiring hospitalization, then concerning the longer term needs of those with a lengthy outpatient recovery and rehabilitation phase or a chronic, recurring condition. One possible approach to filling this data gap involves the careful documentation of activities of patients over an extended period of time through an audit trail of patient records for various types of inpatient and outpatient care. Alternatively, since many hospitals use abstracting services for both bills and medical records, pairing two records for patients with a given injury could provide data concerning hospital stays and associated charges and even potentially for repeat hospital stays. The feasibility of approaches such as these would have been established and the considerable costs involved weighed against the benefits provided by the acquisition of additional data.

Estimates of indirect costs such as foregone earnings or of a stream of future direct costs extending over lifetime require the use of vital statistics data. Life expectancies by age groups are computed by the Bureau of Vital Statistics of the National Center for Health Statistics based on actual mortality experience at one point in time. In cases of serious injuries or those resulting in permanent physical or mental disabilities, life expectancy data are required for the calculation of foregone earnings and future health care costs. There are at present no work experience or earnings data for disabled populations, and although life expectancies for any disabled and chronically ill individuals are undoubtedly shorter than those for the normal population, hard data are lacking. Clearly, the issue of long-term disabling injuries and their costs need future consideration.

In general, estimated health care service needs —whether derived from actual data or from estimates provided by expert medical opinion—are multiplied by unit costs for services in order to arrive at a total cost. Although this seems to be a straightforward process, consistent, national cost data for the whole range of acute care, rehabilitative, outpatient, and long-term care services are not available. Often costs (or charges) from one area or one hospital are used, with the result that totals cannot be generalized to the country as a whole.

In sum, data limitations present significant problems in cost-of-injury analyses. For sports-related injuries, data problems are particularly serious because consistent and reliable injury incidence data are not available. In conjunction with an injury reporting system, a mechanism for gathering information regarding health care resource utilization associated with the treatment of injuries needs to be developed. One possible mechanism might involve the recording of resource utilization data for selected samples of injured persons. The type of information that would be useful in generating cost estimates as well as a sample form for recording such information appears in Figure 5-2.

Methodological Issues

It is also important to point out that the methodology discussed is subject to the limitations imposed by the state-of-the-art.

Figure 5-2 Patient Profile Data Collection Form

	Year of Injury*	Future Years* (Specify period)
Direct Cost Element		
Emergency assistance prior to hospitalization, emergency transportation to hospital and medical treatment on arrival at hospital		
Initial short-term acute hospitalization		
Routine and ancillary services		
Physical rehabilitation		
Special equipment		
Long-term care		
Physical rehabilitation		
Rehospitalization		
Physician services		
Pharmaceuticals		
Supplies and special medical devices		
Home care		
Home modifications		
Indirect Cost Element		
Days lost from work		
Disability status for remainder of life		

*Indicates specific type of sources used, number of units (eg, two outpatient specialists visits) and per unit cost if available.

First, in terms of quantification of indirect costs, the basic difficulty with estimating losses due to premature death and/or disability is the problem of valuing human life. Various methods have been suggested for valuation of human life including implicit values of society and individuals, value statements explicit in the political and judicial process, explicit value statements by individuals ("willingness to pay"), and the human capital approach. The approaches that are given the most credence at the present time are the human capital and the "willingness-to-pay" approaches.

"Willingness to pay," based on direct measurement of what individuals say they would pay to avoid a given outcome, is still in the developmental stage. The human capital approach is the most commonly used approach in cost of illness studies.[2] Valuation according to human capital (ie, the present value of future earnings) is reliable and consistent, but not without shortcomings. The human capital approach places less value on the lives of the very young (whose earnings are so far into the future that their present value is low), and the lives of the very old (whose expected future earnings may be zero). Under this approach men are often valued more than women, because of their higher labor force participation and higher average earnings. Thus, calculations of the costs of sports injuries will necessarily estimate higher indirect costs for those sports dominated by youth and men as opposed to those sports primarily engaged in by the older population and by women.

Another major problem with the human capital approach is how to value the productivity losses resulting from premature death and/or disability of housewives. Housewives' services have no market value. However, ignoring the value of housewives' services results in an underestimate of the cost of those injuries that affect the female population. In recent years this problem has been resolved by assigning to housewives an imputed value based on the market value of the task they perform. Some studies have gone even further and also added the imputed value of housework to the present value of earnings of individuals in the labor force.[3]

Second, the methodology focuses on the economic contributions of individuals in the calculation of indirect costs of injuries and illnesses. The methodology itself makes no claim that these are the only contributions that matter or the only costs that are important. Certainly pain and suffering, disfigurement, loss of self-esteem, psychological and emotional adjustments necessitated by the occurrence of a sports injury, eg, blindness due to an ice hockey injury, are important and real and should be included in any assessment of the overall costs. Such costs, however, are difficult to quantify and thus are not generally included in calculations of economic costs. Economic cost estimates do, however, serve to highlight an important aspect of illness and injury, namely, the opportunity cost of sustaining such injuries in a society that must decide how to allocate its scarce resources.

PROTECTIVE EQUIPMENT: AN APPLICATION OF COST-BENEFIT ANALYSIS

In the context of the framework of analysis developed in this chapter, the old adage "an ounce of prevention is worth a pound of cure" must be qualified. The economist, recognizing resource constraints, would suggest that "an ounce of prevention is worth a pound of cure" only if the benefit derived from the ounce of prevention is greater than or equal to the benefit derived from the pound of cure.

In fact, in order to convert estimates of the total economic costs of a specific injury, eg, eye injuries in hockey, into a calculation of the expected benefits of the use of protective devices such as hockey masks, two pieces of information are necessary: 1) the costs of the eye injuries incurred in the absence of protective devices, and 2) the effectiveness of the devices in terms of preventing or reducing the seriousness of eye injuries in hockey. With a knowledge of both of these factors, it is possible to estimate the averted costs; that is, the benefits of a particular research and development, information dissemination, or even subsidization program directed towards the prevention of these sports injuries.

In order to estimate benefits, the expected costs of a sports injury must be multiplied by the rate of effectiveness of the protective device or other program. Thus, the calculation of economic costs—both direct and indirect—of specific injuries are a vital input in determining the benefits—both direct and indirect—of a program designed to eliminate or reduce the incidence and/or severity of those injuries. And the benefits of the protective device vary directly with both the cost of the injury (which in turn varies directly with the amount and cost of resources used in treating the injury, the incidence and prevalence of the injury, and the degree of disability associated with the injury) and the effectiveness of the protective device.

In resource allocation decisions involving prevention and protective devices, the decision maker must compare the total expected benefits of the protective device with the total costs of the device. The expected benefits are both direct and indirect and correspond to the direct and indirect costs, appropriately adjusted for the effectiveness of the device, averted. The total cost of the prevention program or protective device would include the value of the resources used in its production (reflected in the price of the protective device) as well as certain intangible costs that might be associated with the use of the device, eg, discomfort or perceived stigma when viewed from the player's perspective. The ratio of benefits to costs will be higher in cases where the cost of the protective device is relatively small and the effectiveness of the device in terms of preventing expensive injuries is relatively large.

In order to illustrate the issues presented in this section, it is useful to consider a specific example relating to ocular injuries in hockey and hockey face protectors. Paul F. Vinger, made a study of fairly typical ocular injuries suffered by 38 hockey players during a three-year period. For this group of injured players, the estimated initial direct costs* involved in their treatment were, on average, $1586 per injured person. Assuming that 4% of all hockey players incur such injuries, the expected direct benefit from the use of hockey masks can be valued at $63.44 (.04 × $1586). When we compare this potential saving ($63.44) with the cost of a hockey mask ($20), we see that it is cost-beneficial to use the protective device. If, in this calculation, we include estimates of indirect, societal and social costs averted through the use of such protective devices, the benefit/cost ratio becomes even greater.

SUMMARY AND DIRECTIONS FOR FUTURE RESEARCH

Research in the area of cost-of-injury appears to be directed towards the following areas: quantification of patient suffering in particular and social costs in general; valuation of different qualities of life; and development of more comprehensive and consistent data bases. The methodology of this type of analysis is fairly well developed to date; the binding constraint in the application of this methodology is the lack of reliable and consistent data.

Thus, if state-of-the-art methodology is to be applied fruitfully to the estimation of the economic costs of sports injuries, those involved in the treatment and/or prevention of sports injuries must develop and maintain a reliable data system upon which to base further research.

REFERENCES

1. Smart, C.N., and Sanders, C.R. *The Costs of Motor Vehicle-Related Spinal Cord Injuries.* Washington, DC: Insurance Institute for Highway Safety, 1976.

2. Cooper, B.S., and Rice, D.P. *The Economic Cost of Illness Revisited.* Washington, DC: US Department of Health, Education and Welfare, 1976.

3. Mushkin, S.J. et al. Cost of disease and illness in the United States in the year 2000. *Publ Health Rep.* 93:495-588, 1978.

*Estimates provided by Dr. Vinger did not include follow-up costs and were computed in 1973 dollars. The authors converted the direct cost estimates to fiscal 1980 dollars.

SUGGESTED READINGS

Berry, R. *The Economic Cost of Alcohol Abuse and Alcoholism, 1971.* Contract HSM 42-73-114(NIA). Washington, DC: National Institute of Alcohol Abuse and Alcoholism, March 1974.

Klarman, H.E., Francis, I., and Rosenthal, C.D. Cost effectiveness analysis applied to the treatment of chronic renal disease. *Med Care.* 6(1):48–54, 1968.

LeSourd, D.A., Fogel, M.E., and Johnston, D.R. *Benefit-Cost Analysis of Kidney Disease Programs.* Research Triangle Park, NC: Research Triangle Institute, 1968.

Lipscomb, J. *The Willingness to Pay Criteria in A Public Program Evaluation.* New York: Pergamon Press, 91–139, 1979.

Little, Arthur, D., Inc. *Estimated Economic Costs of Medical Events Known or Suspected to be Related to the Administration of Certain Vaccines.* Cambridge, Mass: Arthur D. Little, Inc. (In preparation).

Mishan, E. Evaluation of life and limb. *J Political Economics.* 79:687–705, 1971.

Mushkin, S. Health as an investment. *J Political Economics.* 70(5), Suppl, Part 2:129–157, 1962.

Paringer, L.C., and Berk, A. *Costs of Illness and Disease, Fiscal Year 1975.* Washington, DC: Public Services Laboratory, Georgetown University, 1977.

PHS Task Force of Costs of Illness. *Guidelines for Cost of Illness.* Washington, DC: National Center for Health Statistics, March 6, 1979.

Pliskin, J.S., Shepard, D.S., and Weinstein, M.C. Utility functions for life years and health status. *Operations Research.* (In press).

Prest, A.P., and Turvey, R. Cost benefit analysis: a survey. *Economic J.* December: 683–735, 1965.

Rice, D.P. Estimating the cost of illness. Health Economics Series No. 6. US Department of Health, Education and Welfare, Public Health Service. Washington, DC: US Government Printing Office, May 1966.

Rice, D., and Hodgson, T. *Social and Economic Implications of Cancer in the United States.* Presented to the Expert Committee on Cancer Statistics, WHO and International Agency for Research on Cancer, Madrid, Spain, June 20–26, 1978.

Schoenbaum, S.J. et al. Benefit-cost analysis of rubella vaccination policy. *N Engl J Med.* 294:306–310, 1976.

Schoenbaum, S., McNeil, B., and Kavet, J. The swine-influenza decision. *N Engl J Med.* 295:759–765, 1976.

Vinger, P.F. Ocular injuries in hockey. *Arch Ophthalmol.* 94:74–76, 1976.

Weinstein, M.C., and Stason, W.B. *Hypertension: A Policy Perspective.* Cambridge, Mass: Harvard University Press, 1976.

Zeckhauser, R. Procedures for valuing lives. *Public Policy.* 23:419–464, 1975.

Zeckhauser, R., and Shapard, D. Where now for saving lives? *Law and Contemporary Problems* 40:5–45, 1976.

CHAPTER 6
Risks and Gains

Arnold E. Reif, DSc

Participation in sports provides much fun and delight and gives us the satisfaction of mastering skills and keeping our bodies fit. We feel refreshed by the relaxation and sense of release provided by an activity that requires our full concentration and represents a complete change from work. Whatever our motives for participation, we hope that it will leave us better off in mind, body and spirit,[1] certainly not worse off.[2]

Most sports require the taking of risks. In order to make sound decisions about which sports to take up as being relatively safe, and which to avoid because of high risk, we need comparative data on the risks of popular sports. The main objective of this chapter is to illustrate how such data can be provided in a form in which they are easily understood. A table of the benefits provided by different sports is also given in the hope that it will permit the choice of sports giving the best rewards at minimal risk. Finally, it is relevant to look at the psychology of risk-taking, and examine the question of what can be done to discourage excessive risk-taking.

RISKS

To permit a broad overview of approximate risks inherent in different sports, it is essential to keep the classifications simple. However, for people interested in a specific sport, a more detailed secondary classification of risks exclusive to that sport can be constructed.

Types of Injury

Five different classifications have been chosen.

Death directly related to the sport. An example is death from drowning following a boating mishap.

Death from heart attack due to overexertion. Such deaths are common to a great variety of sports.

Long-lasting injury requires at least one year for repair, or is permanent. An example of maximal insult is a spinal injury that leaves the victim paraplegic. An example of minimal injury is a compound fracture that requires more than a year to heal.

Temporary injury causes at least three days' loss of work, but at worst takes less than one year for near-complete repair. A bad sprain is an example.

Minor trauma requires fewer than three days out of work before healing. Examples are bruises caused by a blow from a racquet or from falls.

Degree of Risk

The degrees of risk have been classified, in the first instance, per unit time of participation in the sport (Table 6-1). Ranges of risks each covering a tenfold increase have been assigned numbers from 0 to 10, with range 0 to 1 denoting least and range 9 to 10 denoting most risk.

We lack definitive statistics on how often a given sports activity is performed each year by an average participant, and how many years constitute a "lifetime" of activity. An arbitrary choice is 10 days per year of participation and 25 years for the lifetime. Of course, these figures represent "ballpark" values. Nevertheless, they are adequate for an overview of comparative risks. The last two footnotes in Table 6-1 indicate that risk levels values below 0 and above 10 may occur. The former represent virtually no risk; the latter represent statistical likelihood, or the probability of more than one injury, in the case of injuries.

The description of the risk level in the last column of Table 6-1 may seem excessively conservative for a single day of participation. Viewed, however, on the basis of lifetime participation (fourth column of Table 6-1) it seems appropriate.

Classification of Victims

When sufficient data for a given sport are available, a five-step classification of victims is desirable. The most relevant categories are beginner, intermediate, expert, competitor, and professional.

When data for separate categories are not available, a single risk value that includes all participants must suffice.

Other classifications that can be useful when an individual sport is considered are: age ranges of participants with emphasis on the young and the old, sex, disabilities, contributing personal characteristics such as obesity, and contributing personal habits such as smoking or drug use.

Validity of Risk Estimate

Each risk estimate contains a different degree of error. Errors are made in reporting and diagnosis of injuries, tabulation of data, and are inherent in small or nonrepresentative samplings of the test population. Table 6-2 gives a subjective description of validity. From the user's point of view some data may be inapplicable to the type of person or to the circumstances of participation that one is interested in.

Table 6-1
Classification of Risk Odds Per Unit Time of Participation
Risks increase by powers of 10.

	Risk odds			
Risk score*	*Per day*	*Per year*	*Per lifetime*	Description of risk score
0†	1:10,000,000,000	1:1,000,000,000	1:40,000,000	Risk almost absent
1.0	1:1,000,000,000	1:100,000,000	1:4,000,000	Ultra low risk
2.0	1:100,000,000	1:10,000,000	1:400,000	Extremely low risk
3.0	1:10,000,000	1:1,000,000	1:40,000	Very low risk
4.0	1:1,000,000	1:100,000	1:4000	Low risk
5.0	1:100,000	1:10,000	1:400	Medium risk
6.0	1:10,000	1:1000	1:40	High risk
7.0	1:1,000	1:100	1:4	Very high risk
8.0	1:100	1:10	2.5:1	Extremely high risk
9.0	1:10	1:1	25:1	Ultra high risk
10.0‡	1:1	10:1	250:1	Ultimate risk

*Risk scores have the advantage of substituting a single figure between 0 and 10 for risk odds. Values of *risk score* are calculated from risk odds per day as 10 − $\log_{10}$(risk odds per day), and from risk odds per year as 9 − $\log_{10}$(risk odds per year). For instance, if the risk odds per day are 1:2000, the risk score is 10 − $\log_{10}$(2000), which is 10 − 3.30, or 6.7. To reverse this process and obtain risk odds from risk score, the formula *risk odds per day* = antilog(10 − risk score) is used, or else *risk odds per year* = antilog(9 − risk score). For instance, if the risk score is 7.3, the risk odds per day = antilog(10 − 7.3) or antilog2.7, which is 500, so that the risk odds per day are 1:500; to obtain risk odds per year, reduce the risk odds per day by a factor of 10, from 1:500 to 1:50. Or alternatively, use the formula risk odds per year = antilog 9 − 7.3) or antilog1.7, which is 50, to give risk odds per year of 1:50.

†Risk scores below 0 have negative values when determined according to the above footnote.

‡Risk scores above 1:1 denote higher than even chances of the stated accident, or else the possibility of multiple injuries.

Table 6-2
Estimated Validity of Risk Figures

Estimated reliability	Description of reliability	Estimated deviation of risk figure from true value of risk (by percent)
A	High accuracy	30
B	Good accuracy	60
C	Fair accuracy	120
D	Poor accuracy	250
E	Very poor accuracy	500

Comparison of Risks Between Different Sports

Different types of injury, the degree of risk, and the validity of risk estimates, are defined above. These definitions can be used to compare sports for which risk data are available (Tables 6-3 through 6-6). No attempt at completeness has been made. The purpose is purely to demonstrate the application of the present approach to the problem of risk comparison.

Risk estimations reported on the basis of fractional values of risk levels in logarithmic form are unfamiliar on first view (see footnote to Table 6-1). With increasing familiarity this method of expressing risk may be useful for professionals who work in the area of sports medicine. The major advantage is a brief and precise number to express risk, and the concept that 0 represents zero risk, while 10 represents statistical likelihood of injury.

In Table 6-5, unit risk has been assigned round figures closest to the lowest risk rate among the various sports under consideration, as explained in subheading to the table. By this strategy, a direct comparison of the risks assumed in different sports is possible. For example, death for dedicated mountain climbers (those who often undertake difficult climbs) is 490 times as likely as for students who play high school football.

Another useful way to look at risks is on the basis of lifetime participation (Table 6-6). Unfortunately, sufficient data were not available to permit a subdivision of risks between long-term disability and mere "injury." Death is of course the

Table 6-3
Comparison of Risks of Different Types of Sport and Activity*
The degree of risk is expressed as a number ranging from 0 to 10, as explained in Table 6-1. An estimate of the accuracy of the risk score is given by the letter, with accuracy ranging from A to F, as detailed in Table 6-2. The superscript numbers represent the reference used to derive the risk score.

Sport	Death	Injury or long-term disability	Minor injury that requires medical attention†
Automobile use	5.4B[3]		
Boating¶			
Canoes and kayaks	4.9A[4]		
Motorized boats	4.6A[4]		
Sailboats (all types)	4.4A[4]		
Boxing (professional)	5.7C[5]		
Hang gliding¶	6.2D[5-8]	7.2D[8]	
Football (high school)	4.1B[5,9]		
(college)	4.5B[5]	7.7D[10,11]	8.7C[11]
Motorcycling	6.0B[3]		
Mountain climbing (dedicated experts)	6.8D[10]	7.6D[10]	
(all climbers)	5.8C[5]		
Mountain hiking	4.8D[12]	5.8D[12]	
Parachuting	6.2C[5,8]		
Sailplaning (gliding)	5.8C[5,8]		
School athletics (girls' high school)			8.3C[13]
Scuba diving (nonprofessional)	5.6C[5]		
Skiing, downhill (recreational)	2.8C[3]	7.5B[14]	
(racing)	4.4C[7]		
Snowmobiling	5.1C[6]	7.4C[6]	8.1C[6]
Surfing		5.8C[15]	

*Emphasis was placed on obtaining scores correct on a per year basis. When statistics based on per day participation were used, it was assumed that there were 10 days of sports participation per year, except in the case of Football and School athletics, for which 25 days of participation per year were assumed.
†Medical attention by nurse or physician required.
‡The figures for boating assume the following number of people per boat: for canoes and kayaks, 1.8; for sailboats, 3.0; for motorized boats, 2.4. Motorized boats include all types of boats with motors except sailboats.
¶Deaths for 1977 and 1978 corrected to 24 and 38, respectively, from data provided by Director, National Injury Information Clearing House, Consumer Product Safety Commission, Washington, DC.

Table 6-4
Risk Odds for Types of Sport or Activity Per Year of Participation*

Sport	Death	Injury or long-term disability	Minor injury that requires medical attention
Automobile use	1:4,000		
Boating			
Canoes and kayaks	1:13,200		
Motorized boats	1:24,000		
Sailboats (all types)	1:38,000		
Boxing (professional)	1:2200		
Hang gliding	1:560	1:56	
Football (high school)	1:81,000		
(college)	1:33,000	1:18	1:2.1
Motorcycling	1:1,100		
Mountain climbing (dedicated experts)	1:167	1:23	
(all climbers)	1:1750		
Mountain hiking	1:15,700	1:1570	
Parachuting	1:570		
Sailplaning (gliding)	1:1710		
School athletics (girls' high school)			1:5.3
Scuba diving (nonprofessional)	1:2400		
Skiing, downhill (recreational)	1:1,430,000	1:30	
(racing)	1:40,000		
Snowmobiling	1:7600	1:40	1:8.0
Surfing		1:1750	

*The data presented here are identical in every way with those given in Table 6-3, except that they are expressed here as risk odds, instead of as risk scores. Thus, the sources of the data and their estimated accuracy are as given in Table 6-3. All four of the footnotes of Table 6-3 apply here also.

most severe risk, but long-term, including permanent, disability is also highly undesirable. It would therefore be most useful to have separate data on this classification. Also, data were not at hand to classify separately death from heart attack due to overexertion.

GAINS

Whenever we take a risk, we consciously or unconsciously balance risk against gain.[16-18] Play is a change from work, a chosen activity that gives real pleasure. Often it is practiced in surroundings far more lovely than those of the work place. In addition, the following advantages can be considered.

Exhilaration One can experience a powerful sense of exhilaration in sports such as skiing or surfing. Work may provide similar delights, but far less frequently or predictably.

Challenge A sport such as jogging is a challenge to one's will and endurance. Most sports include a great deal of challenge.

Competition For many people, few events are as exciting as a competitive sports meet. This is especially true for the competitors.

Learning new skills Some of the pleasure of a sport is progressing in learning its skills. It is an avenue of life in which mastery is clearly demonstrable, and often rewarded.

Social rewards At school, being on a major team confers social standing often in excess of its importance. However, there are real friendships and closeness to be shared with team members. Sports also serve a vital usefulness in cementing family bonds when activities are enjoyed by parents and children.[18]

Healthfulness Sportsmen appreciate the feeling of fitness at the end of time spent in sports participation. Time spent this way is amply refunded by increased energy and powers of concentration. It is also necessary to use our bodies to

Table 6-5
Comparative Risks of Different Sports or Activities Per Year of Participation*
Relative risk figures for each category of injury are based on a value of 1 assigned to the lowest risk. Relative risk differs for each category.

Sport	Death	Injury or long-term disability	Minor injury that requires medical attention
Automobile use	360		
Boating			
Canoes and kayaks	110		
Motorized boats	60		
Sailboats (all types)	38		
Boxing (professional)	650		
Hang gliding	2,600	31	
Football (high school)	18		
(college)	43	97	3.8
Motorcycling	1,300		
Mountain climbing (dedicated experts)	8,600	76	
(all climbers)	820		
Mountain hiking	91	1.1	
Parachuting	2,500		
Sailplaning (gliding)	840		
School athletics (girls' high school)			1.7
Scuba diving (nonprofessional)	600		
Skiing, downhill (recreational)	1	58	
(racing)	36		
Snowmobiling	190	44	1
Surfing		1	

*The data presented here are identical with those in Table 6-3, except that they are presented as relative risk rather than as risk odds.

avoid muscle-wasting.[19,20] It is necessary to imitate experts in a sport not only in related skills but in fitness skills.

Weight control It is important to the athlete to achieve proper body weight. For most people that means keeping weight down or reducing. Physical exercise burns up calories. In addition, performance is a powerful incentive to watch both the quantity and the quality of food that is eaten.

Smoking Within sports there is strong peer pressure to quit smoking. The loss of lung capacity associated even with only a little smoking is incompatible with most sports.

Self-image Perhaps most important, sports participation improves self-image. Feelings of adequacy, effectiveness, vitality, resourcefulness, and success engendered by achievement in sports will be manifested in other areas of one's life.

Can Sports Extend Life?

Perhaps the most important factor in determining longevity is genetic background. No one can change that. Changeable factors are the amount of exercise we take, the quantity and quality of food we eat, and whether and how much we smoke and drink.

The group of men with the longest lifespan in our country are postmen. On the average, they walk about 12 miles on each work day. Most physicians believe that a program of long-continued moderate exercise such as this prolongs life.[19,21,22] Long-term indolence as well as extreme exertion may shorten it.[23] Those over 40 years of age who take up exercise should have a physical examination, and, as necessary, stop smoking, control their blood pressure, and start a weight-reduction program—then initiate exercise very gradually.[19,24]

Most cardiologists emphasize five major risk factors in heart attacks: smoking, cholesterol-rich diet, high blood pressure, fatness, and sedentary living.[19,20,24–26] Effective participation in many sports requires participants to stop smoking and to trim down if overweight (see Table 6-7). The life prolongation achieved by this will outweigh life loss through participation in low-risk sports.

Table 6-6
Risk Odds for Different Sports or Activities on a Lifetime Participation Basis*

Sport	Death	Injury or long-term disability	Minor injury that requires medical attention
Automobile use†	1:80		
Boating			
Canoes and Kayaks	1:530		
Motorized boats	1:960		
Sailboats (all types)	1:1,500		
Boxing (professional)‡	1:220		
Hang gliding	1:22	1:2.2	
Football (high school)¶	1:20,000		
(college)¶	1:8300	1:4.5	1.9:1
Motorcycling	1:22		
Mountain climbing (dedicated experts)	1:6.7	1.1:1	
(all climbers)	1:70		
Mountain hiking†	1:320	1:32	
Parachuting	1:23		
Sailplaning (gliding)	1:68		
School athletics (girls' high school)¶			1:1.3
Scuba diving (nonprofessional)	1:96		
Skiing, downhill (recreational)	1:57,000	1:1.2	
(racing)‡	1:4000		
Snowmobiling	1:300	1:1.6	3.2:1
Surfing		1:70	

*These data are identical with those in Table 6-3, except that they are calculated for 25 years of participation.
†Based on 50 years of participation.
‡Based on 10 years of participation.
¶Based on 4 years of participation.

Table 6-7
Comparative Merits of Different Sports

	Exhilaration	Challenge	Opportunity to exhibit expertise	Degree of mixed participation	Fitness training provided	Obesity, smoking discouraged	Self-image
Boxing (professional)	B	A+	A	F	A	A	A
Hang gliding	A+	A+	A	C	D	D	A+
Football (student)	A	A+	A	C	A	A	A
Mountain climbing							
(dedicated)	A+	A+	A	C+	A	A	A+
(all climbers)	A	A	A	B	A	A–	A
Mountain hiking	B	B–	D	A	A	B+	B+
Parachuting	A+	A+	A	B	D	D	A
Sailplaning	A+	A	A	B	D	D	A
School athletics (girls' high school)	A–	A	A	C	A	A	A
Scuba diving (nonprofessional)	A	A	B	A	B	B	A
Skiing, downhill	A+	A	A	A	A–	C	A
Snowmobiling	B	C	C	A	C	D	B
Surfing	A+	A	A	B–	A	B	A

Merits of Different Sports

To compare the attractions of various sports, each of the sports listed in Table 6-7 is classified for merits. The scoring system of A to F is commonly used for grading in schools, with A denoting excellent, B good, C fair, D poor, E very poor, and F failing.

No doubt an anonymous survey of enthusiasts of each of the 12 sports would give a more valid evaluation of their relative merits. Nevertheless, some revealing differences emerge. The three sports with exceptionally high death risk are mountain climbing (technical), hang gliding, and parachuting. They are rivaled in exhilaration, challenge, and opportunity to show off new skills by two sports with low death risk: skiing and surfing. Hang gliding and parachuting compare badly with the other sports in one important attribute: healthfulness, or fitness training. In all three high-risk sports, male participants greatly outnumber females.

Football and school athletics score high on practically all counts except mixed participation. Mountain hiking lacks the spectacular quality of the other sports, but scores high in healthfulness. The largely mechanical sport of snowmobiling not only scores low on health orientation but lacks the showing off of special skills.

Certainly, expansion of Table 6-7 to cover a wider range of sports would be desirable. Still, even in its present form, it should facilitate the choice of a new sport, if used in conjunction with the data on risks in the preceding tables.

RISKS vs GAINS

With regard to participating in sports, some excess risk is justifiable simply on the basis of the healthful effects of exercise. If the sport combines low risks with high benefits, the quality of life will hopefully be improved. Therefore, it seems important that easily understood data on the risks and benefits of various sports be available to the public. This will permit future participants to choose those sports that offer them most benefit and least risk.

What Sports Risks Are Justified by Gains?

For the vast majority of participants, the objective of sports is to experience the benefits described. Normally, most do not stop to think about the risks involved. Are they worth taking?

One must calculate whether the long-term gains exceed the risks. Since the risks with high school and college football are known with some accuracy, definite conclusions are possible (see Tables 6-4 to 6-6).

A spinal injury can leave the victim paraplegic. In student football, roughly twice as many men are permanently disabled as incur death.[7] Still, such serious or fatal accidents are rare. In contrast, approximately one in three participants is likely to suffer a sprain, fracture, or contusion in four years of play. Since no permanent damage results from the great majority of these injuries, they can be accepted as risks worth taking for the other benefits. When all risks are considered, drag racing, drugs, or criminal activities can be far more dangerous than student football.

High-Risk Sports

A rational person will wish to participate in a risky sport only if the result is "high-level wellness" and not "low-level wellness."[2] Thus, the probability of gains must greatly outnumber that of ill effects.

The sport with the highest risk of death is mountain climbing; dedicated participation carries with it a death risk of 1:7. In fact, the death risk in a single assault on a Himalayan peak is 1:20.[27] These risks cannot be justified by most. Why, then, do people love technical mountain climbing? The joys, challenges, and the excitement of climbing are well documented. It is obvious that mountaineers are fully aware of the high death risks, and use them to express their own courage, and to heighten the worth of their achievement.[27-29]

One could ask whether people who engage in high-death-risk sports suffer from peculiarities of character that make them likely to take such risks. Most of us feel that our recreational activities should not be of the type in which a simple mistake can cause our death. When faced with the question of whether or not to participate in a sport with a high risk of death or permanent injury, the rational response is to choose a low-risk sport that offers similar benefits (see Table 6-7).

Change of Risks With Expertise

In general, it can be said that technical climbing is perfectly safe as long as one is properly trained, fit, and uses good equipment and sound judgment. On the first few training trips with competent leaders, beginning climbers will be safe enough. What is not being considered is how risk increases as expertise develops. As this occurs, "uncontrolled" risks, those over which the climber himself has no control, increase drastically. A single serious error by a fellow climber to which he is roped, can result in death. Furthermore, all the uncontrolled risks of large mountains and steep faces—rock falls, slides, avalanches, crevasses, and long-continued storms—take their toll.

Even if expertise reaches such a degree that there is zero chance of injury or death due to self-controlled error, the effect of uncontrolled risks will still be high. As the beginning mountain climber becomes more expert, the pressure on him to attempt more demanding climbs will be great. Thus, he will be assuming the higher risks involved.

A similar gradation of risks, from lower to higher as expertise is acquired, has been described for hang gliding.[8] In contrast, novice parachutists (who have a tendency to fail to pull the rip cord) share maximum risk with the experts. Risks are lowest for intermediately skilled participants.[8]

PSYCHOLOGY OF RISK-TAKING

Several different theories seek to explain risk-taking. For instance, Zuckerman divides people into low and high sensation-seekers.[30] He believes that there are four different types of high sensation seekers: *adventure-seekers* who take up risky but socially acceptable activities such as parachute-jumping; *experience-seekers* who adopt a non-conforming lifestyle; *disinhibitionists* who free themselves from social inhibitions by drinking, partying, gambling, or seeking a variety of sexual partners; and *boredom-fleers* who have a low tolerance for repetitious situations. People who score high marks for one of these four categories are likely to score high on others also. Therefore, Zuckerman thinks that sensation-seeking is a broad trait, which is in part inherited, in part acquired through upbringing and experience. He believes that there is a biological basis for sensation-seeking, since the enzyme MAO (monamine oxidase) which destroys hormones such as noradrenaline that *stimulate* the brain, tends to be present in relatively *low* levels in sensation-seekers. This insures that such hormones will be more effective in sensation-seekers. Further, both male and female sex hormones seem to activate noradrenaline—and sensation-seekers have a higher level of sex hormones than do those who are low on this trait. If Zuckerman is correct, high sensation-seekers get far stronger stimulation from risks than do low sensation-seekers. Finally, his research suggests that sensation-seekers are *not* driven by compulsive neurotic needs.

In contrast, Rosenthal feels that risk-taking constitutes a useful exercise which enhances physical and mental powers, and prescribes it for us all.[31] In his view, it is vital that the risk-taker has the skills to overcome the risk. Otherwise, terror may overwhelm the desired responses to the risk, which are exhilaration, euphoria, and heightened awareness. He thinks that these responses go further than an "adrenalin high", which is a "fight or flight" secretion that speeds up the body's function and gives it more energy. Rosenthal uses risk-taking activities to clear out the problem-solving portion of his mind, giving him a clean slate on which to attack work-related projects with single-minded concentration.

According to Solomon, the same principle that produces junkies and alcoholics also produces social attachment, love, thrill-seeking, power-seeking, overeating, and other forms of addiction.[32] As a necessary adjunct to the "high" that results from the activity, there is pain. For instance, a runner's "high" is an example of pain giving way to pleasure. Withdrawal symptoms, such as when an anticipated thrill-producing activity has to be cancelled, produce the opposite result: pleasure turns to pain and anxiety. This is the cycle which spawns addiction. Solomon believes that endorphins, our own euphoria-producing hormones, are involved in these feelings, and thinks the brain is organized to limit the extent of highs and lows. He argues that one should live moderately, because great pleasures rarely go unpunished.

While the above three views of the psychology of risk-taking seem quite different, all seem to incorporate some correct and useful insights. A certain degree of risk-taking is as normal, healthy, and necessary for human beings as is motherhood. Obviously, there is much variation in the capacity for the enjoyment of risk-taking, as there is in any other of the behavioral attributes of human beings. The challenge lies in engaging in those activities which will produce the maximum benefit for the lowest possible risk. Perhaps the most important benefit is to acquire confidence in our skill and judgment, and in our ability to control fear.[33]

SUMMARY

Many people take up a sport only to discover later, once they have grown to love it, that it is a high-risk sport. Further, the level of risk may rise as one progresses from beginner to dedicated expert, as in the case of mountain climbers. If only the relevant information was readily available, many would shun high-risk sports in favor of low-risk sports which offer comparable benefits.

To remedy this need, simple-to-understand tables of comparative sports risks should be published annually by the U.S. Consumer Product Safety Commission, which already collects and publishes accurate data on sports injuries.[34] Then, safety-conscious sports participants should publish these tables and comment upon them in numerous sports magazines. Further, the benefits offered by various sports should be published alongside the risk data, as in the present report. These benefits could be determined by questionnaires completed by participants all at a particular level of expertise or all just exposed to a single set of conditions commonly encountered in that sport.

The majority of sports participants are neither high- nor low-sensation seekers, but fall somewhere in between and are amenable to reason. It seems high time they had far better data than are available presently, to help them decide in which sports to achieve "high level wellness" with minimal risk. While "nothing risked, nothing gained" is as true in sports as in other endeavors, risking all for sports' sake shows disrespect for the value of life—except for those few for whom their sport *is* their life.

Thanks are owed to Dorothy T. Taylor and Burnham H. Martin of the AMC Research Department for the data on deaths for mountain hiking, and to Edward Lipchus for providing reference 5.

REFERENCES

1. Dunn, H.L. What high-level wellness means. *Health Values* 1:9–16, 1977.

2. Reif, A.E. High-level wellness and low-level wellness: an overview. *Health Values* 2:198–210, 1978.

3. Lee, B.W. Risk assessment. *JAMA*. 246:1196–1197, 1981.

4. U.S. Coast Guard report on recreational boating accidents for 1976 supplied to me in December, 1980 by the Chief, Boating Safety Division, 150 Causeway Street, Boston, MA 02114.

5. Sports hazards. *Statistical Bulletin*. Metropolitan Life Insurance Company. July–Sept, 1979, pp. 3–6.

6. Sampson, P. Physicians find three new sports exhilarating, beautiful, risky. *JAMA*. 239:283–285, 1978.

7. Krissoff, W.B., and Eiseman, B. Injuries associated with hang gliding. *JAMA*. 233:148–160, 1975.

8. Tongue, J.R. Hang gliding injuries in California. *J Trauma*. 17:898–902, 1977.

9. Truex, R., Jr., Quedenfelb, T.C., Burstein, A. et al. The national football head and neck injury registry. Report and conclusions, *JAMA*. 241:1477–1479, 1979.

10. Ferriss, B.G., Jr. Hazards to health. Mountain-climbing accidents in the United States. *N Engl J Med*. 268:430–431, 1963.

11. Hirata, I., Jr. *The Doctor and the Athlete*, 2nd Ed. Philadelphia: J.B. Lippincott Co., 1974, p. 278.

12. Surgenor, S.H. AMC search and rescue: an analysis. *Appalachia* June, 117–125, 1977.

13. Garrick, J.G., and Requa, R.K. Girls' sports injuries in high school athletics. *JAMA*. 239:2245–2248, 1978.

14. Gutman, J., Weisbuch, J., and Wolf, M. Ski injuries in 1972–1973. A repeat analysis of a major health problem. *JAMA*. 230:1423–1425, 1974.

15. Allen, R.H., Eiseman, B., Straehley, C.J. et al. Surfing injuries at Waikiki. *JAMA*. 237:668–670, 1977.

16. Rowe, W.D. *An "Anatomy" of Risk*. Washington, DC: US Environmental Protection Agency, 1975.

17. Lowrance, W.W. *Of Acceptable Risk*. Los Altos, Calif: William Kaufmann, Inc., 1976.

18. Beisser, A.R. *The Madness in Sports*. New York: Appleton-Century-Crofts, 1967, pp. viii, 238.

19. Farquhar, J.W. *The American Way of Life Need Not Be Hazardous to Your Health*. New York: W.W. Norton and Co., 1978, p. 81.

20. Craig, T.T., (Ed.) *Comments in Sports Medicine*. Chicago: American Medical Association, 1973, p. 198.

21. Kannel, W.B., and Gordon, T. Obesity and cardiovascular disease. Edited by W.L. Burland, P.D. Samuel, and J. Yodkin. In *Obesity Symposium*. Edinburgh: Churchill-Livingstone, 1974.

22. Cantwell, J.D. Running. *JAMA*. 242: 1409–1410, 1978.

23. Rennie, D., and Hollenberg, N.K. Cardiomythology and marathons. *N Engl J Med*. 301:103–104, 1979.

24. McIntosh, H.D. Jogging. Thou shalt not

kill (thyself). *JAMA*. 241:2547–2548, 1979.

25. Richmond, J.B. *Smoking and Health. A Report of the Surgeon General.* Washington, DC: US Department of Health, Education, and Welfare, Publ. No. (PHS)79-50066, 1979.

26. Reif, A.E. Public information on smoking: an urgent responsibility for cancer research workers? *J Natl Cancer Inst.* 57:1207–1210, 1976. Addendum: *Natl Cancer Inst Monogr.* 52:123–128, 1979.

27. Whittaker, J.W. The ultimate challenge. *Natl Geographic.* 155:624–639, 1979.

28. Slone, R. Retreat from Devil's mountain. *Mariah/Outside.* 4(1):20–40, 1979.

29. Blum, A. Triumph and tragedy on Annapurna. *Natl Geographic.* 155:294–311, 1979.

30. Zuckerman, M. The search for high sensation. *Psychology Today*. Feb: 38–99, 1978.

31. Furlong, W.B. Doctor danger. *Outside.* 5(6):40–96, 1980–1981.

32. Leo, J. A painful theory on pleasures. *Time*. Nov. 10:112, 1980.

33. Tessman, R. Mind over water. *Whitewater*. 24(3–4):14–34, 1979.

34. U.S. Consumer Product Safety Commission, Hazard Identification and Analysis, National Injury Information Clearinghouse, Washington, D.C. 20207.

CHAPTER 7
Adventure: An Alternative

Ralph R. Kylloe, EdD

... with the chance for adventure, the opportunity for learning ...
Charles Brightbill, 1960

Numerous books and articles have recently appeared that deal with the negative aspects of organized, traditional sports. It is not the intention of the author to further debase activities in which thousands of people earn their living and millions of others find enjoyment. However it is my belief that these activities may not be suited for the majority of our populations. Without doubt many individuals have found satisfaction in highly competitive, sometimes violent, games, and it is not my intention to suggest that we eliminate the opportunity for those who wish to become involved to do so. Nonetheless, as professional people, it is our responsibility to provide opportunities for all segments of the population to become involved in physical activities that can be enjoyed throughout their lives.

The function of this chapter is threefold. The first area of concern is our present physical lifestyle as well as our present physical education curriculum. Second, adventure education is reviewed, not as a substitute for traditional activities, but as a natural growth and expansion of the physical education curriculum. Third, we shall look at research in adventure education. The vast majority of individuals involved in adventure education today, believe strongly in the benefits derived from the adventure experience. Significant research has now been conducted in this area, and a review of this literature may shed light on the effects of the adventure experience. This research falls basically into four areas: research conducted on the Outward Bound experience; research conducted on Outward Bound and corrections; adventure in the educational school system; and adventure for the handicapped person. Also an extended bibliography is provided for those who wish to further explore the area of adventure education.

WHERE WE ARE

Few people today can question the need for physical education and physical experiences in their lives. Physical education literature is replete with studies suggesting a correlation between physical fitness and active mental processes. People who are physically fit live longer and are healthier, enjoy a more positive mental image, are more likely to score higher academically, and appear to be better adjusted and happier.

Joggers and others involved in intense physical activities frequently assert that they experience "highs and euphoria," and research has found that these activities reduce stress and the possibility of many diseases. Researchers at the National Institute for Mental Health have found that depressed patients who undertake a regular program of physical activities often experience mood elevations. Many doctors who are prescribing physical exercise for their patients notice a marked reduction in anxiety and stress. Further, researchers at the Fort Worth Cancer Center are requiring a regular program of physical activities as part of their treatments of numerous forms of malignancies.

Nonetheless, for those skeptics who remain doubtful of the positive outcomes of physical exercise—ask any doctor.

It is indeed unfortunate that the general public cannot be convinced of the great need for and value of physical activity. But do not underestimate the knowledge of your neighbor. The average person is aware of the need for physical activity, but certain people just have a difficult time managing their own physicalness. In much the same way a smoker realizes the debilitating effects of the cigarette, yet continues to indulge in this self-destructive practice.

Despite the present fitness craze, statistics indicate that Americans are in poor shape. In 1954, Dr Hans Kraus and Dr Sonja Weber, both of the Posture Clinic at Presbyterian Hospital in New York, developed a test that looks at overall physical fitness. The test includes touching one's toes with straight legs, doing one sit-up with straight legs and then one with legs bent, raising the legs off the floor for 10 seconds while lying in the prone position, and a few other simple tasks designed to measure physical ability.

The test was then administered around the world. Samples of people were drawn from rural, urban, and suburban regions, and the findings analyzed.

The first results were shocking. In 1955, 24% of American children could not do one sit-up, nearly half of the Americans tested could not touch their toes.[1] It was found that 58% of the Americans tested could not pass the test while about 8% of Europeans failed.

In 1977 the Kraus-Weber test was again administered throughout the world. These results showed that the European failure rate stayed the same, 8%, but the overall failure rate in this country rose to 85%.

The United States Health Department reports that approximately one-third of American children are overweight, and 40% of Americans over age 35 have a weight problem.

As a further indication of our poor physical condition, the American Heart Association reports that this year nearly one million Americans will die from heart attacks while another four million will suffer from heart disease. Although we have the most sophisticated and advanced medical and communications technology of any country in thc world, we are rank twelfth in life expectancy.

Although we are now entering the period called "the post-industrial society and the age of leisure," we apparently know very little about how to use our "free time."

The Federal Communications Commission recently reported that 97% of all American households, or 73,307,000 homes, have at least one television set turned on for at least six hours per day. That represents approximately 439.8 million hours of television viewing per day. Other reports indicate that preschoolers view about 40 hours per week while schoolchildren average about 30 hours per week. The average adult spends about three to four hours per evening watching television.

At the same time the Scholastic Aptitude Test scores and the reading scores of our students continue to drop.

Could there possibly be a correlation between unhealthy leisure time pursuits and the way physical education and activities are introduced to our children? Are we failing to teach activities that place emphasis on fun and group cooperation rather than winning at any cost? Are we providing activities that are likely to be engaged in later in life? Is an individual likely to participate in activities that were unpleasant for him or her as a youngster?

Dr John Cheffers of Boston University, a former Olympic coach, equates much of today's physical education with what he calls the "dodgeball society." Two teams are chosen. Usually the physically unfit person, the one who needs the exercise the most, is chosen last. (What does that do to his self-image?) Then play begins. Within a short time those who are in poor condition are eliminated and literally denied the right to further exercise until those who are already in shape decide who the winner of the contest is. It seems obvious, then, that out of a class of 30 students, three or four will dominate while the rest fall more and more into the role of spectators. These principles control most of our traditional physical education activities.

Terry Orlick, sport psychology researcher from the University of Ottawa, says, "Games themselves have become rigid, judgmental, highly organized, and excessively goal-oriented. There is no freedom from the pressure of evaluation and the psychological distress of disapproval. In the end, the focus on squeezing the most out of every individual leaves no room for plain old fun."[2] Orlick further says, "The games are now beginning to destroy even the winners. Children are encouraged in the delight in others' failures. They hope for it, they help it happen, because it enhances their own chances of victory....As the kids grow older, they have been so conditioned by the importance of winning that they can no longer play for fun."[2] It may be that they no longer play, and instead join the millions of others who spend their hard-earned free time as armchair quarterbacks.

Think of it another way. If a child is asked to shoot five baskets in front of his classmates and he misses all five, there is the likelihood that he may not have the greatest opinion of physical education.

Although a rather dim overview of traditional physical education has been presented, to suggest that most sports educators are unaware of these concerns would be inaccurate. Fortunately, many schools recognize the need to expand their curriculum and allow for greater individuality among their students. Significant government funds are being allocated to explore new curriculum areas such as coed classes in jogging, bicycling, human movement (dance), canoeing, camping, cross-country skiing, and many other activities that do not emphasize winning.

Along with these changes, the vocabulary of the physical educator is changing to include such ideas as self-concept, group cooperation, and trust. With the introduction of adventure activities into the school curriculum, students are indicating their preference for these activities through better attendance, increased communication with both their fellow students and teachers, and a willingness to respond, in a positive way, to new and exciting challenges.

ADVENTURE EDUCATION – AN ALTERNATIVE

The philosophical foundations of adventure education were developed by Kurt Hahn.[3] Born into a Jewish family of the German intelligentsia in 1886, Hahn received his initial education in Berlin where he favored the classics as well as Plato, both of which, he later professed, strongly influenced his life.

In the 1920s Hahn, with the aid of Prince Max of Baden, helped to establish the Salem School in Baden-Baden. With its strong moral foundations, the institution thrived and was dubbed the "school for princes" by the aristocracy of Europe. Under Hahn's guidance the school expanded. Then Hahn was arrested for severely criticizing the newly appointed German government and challenging the Salem students to break with the government's new leader, Hitler.

Influential friends petitioned his release, and Hahn quickly found his way to England where the same friends persuaded him to open a new school on the coast of Wales. However, those were bad times for England, and the competition for students was fierce. Nonetheless, the Gordonstoun School opened with a few children from his followers who recognized his philosophical and educational capabilities.

His new students, however, were not the cultured and aristocratic models the Salem School once tutored. These were students who were failures and misfits from other schools. Consequently, the Gordonstoun School found itself dealing with a high percentage of "frail, difficult and mediocre boys."

Within a short time the school became quite successful under Hahn's philosophy of: 1) building up the physical fitness of each child; 2) restricting the amount of team games in favor of individual skill development; 3) providing a genuine opportunity for self-discovery by encouraging the individual to spend time with a favorite hobby, such as the cello, or with a sport such as rock climbing; 4) allowing the child to meet with both success and failure; and 5) including periods of extended silence.

During World War II the school was moved to a new location to allow the military the use of the buildings. After this, the structure and philosophy of the program intensified greatly. Hahn added seamanship and mountaineering to the curriculum because "he felt it was necessary to introduce youth to danger (in a positive sense) and adventure and to provide a learning environment that would provide the moral equivalent to war."[4] And although Hahn recognized its value, he "never advocated adventure as an end in itself, but rather as a training vehicle through which youth would mature."[5]

Unfortunately, the war years were difficult times for educational institutions. Gordonstoun saw a one-third reduction in its student body and a financial crisis that nearly closed the school altogether. Yet these were times when Hahn developed the ideas that would lead to Outward Bound. After the war Hahn and his students returned to the school site and, with much physical effort, managed to reopen its doors. Once again, under Hahn's direction, the school prospered. Today it is a solid institution with well over four hundred students.

In 1941, Hahn was approached by Lawrence Holt, the head of a large merchant shipping line. He expressed deep concern over the large numbers of young seamen who perished in the water and lifeboats after being torpedoed. Holt said, "These youths lacked the feel for the wind and the weather. They could not rely on their own inner resources."

Hahn proposed that they join forces and develop a new kind of curriculum: primarily a one-month course in small boat training, orienteering; search and rescue expeditions at sea, athletics, and a final expedition on the open sea. The philosophy for the curriculum would follow Hahn's ideas of "Experience Therapy," which basically stated, "An individual in today's technological society [the year was 1941] needs the opportunity to test and challenge his basic human potential in order for the individual to realize and discover themselves."

Holt was favorably impressed and generously provided funding and a staff. Within a short time the first Outward Bound school opened at Aberdovey, Wales in 1941. The school proved to be a positive experience for those who chose to enroll and endure the physical challenges. The program was so successful that within eight years several more Outward Bound schools opened in rapid succession at various locations around the world. In 1963 the first American Outward Bound school opened in Colorado.

Since 1941, 28 Outward Bound schools have opened around the world. In this country over 70,000 people have attended the wide range of programs offered by seven Outward Bound schools.

Although today we are better able to describe the educational objectives of Outward Bound in terms of self-concept, group cooperation, concern for others, and so forth, the basic philosophical premise of Outward Bound is still Hahn's original aim, "to build character through adventure."

Although the philosophical framework of all Outward Bound schools is the same, the curriculum that each school follows is primarily indicative of its environmental setting. For instance, the Colorado school deals mainly with mountaineering, while the Hurricane Island school on the coast of Maine provides adventure activities on the open seas during the summer, and winter camping during the frozen New England months. The Minnesota school offers extensive canoeing activities, while the southwest school in Arizona offers extended desert experiences. Both the North Carolina school and the northwest school in Oregon, offer backpacking and river-running activities. The Dartmouth College, New Hampshire school offers courses in bicycling and canoeing. The schools, however, are not restricted to these particular activities. Rock climbing, ropes course activities, map and compass work, caving, white-water kayaking, canoeing and rafting, cross-country skiing, snowshoeing, shelter building, endurance running, solo experience, and numerous other outdoor activities are also used often.

These activities and others are offered to a wide range of people including educators, adults over 30, business executives, special populations, the helping professions, women's groups, and special interest groups. The majority of the standard courses are open to anyone 16½ years or older. These programs are offered for periods of 4 days to 26 days. One school offers not only a trek through the Himalayas but a full semester of other activities as well.

The growth of adventure education throughout the world, and particularly in North America, has been rapid. Not only has Outward Bound expanded its programs but also numerous other agencies and organizations have emerged that offer adventure activities as their main program as well.

In 1975 Alan Hale of Mankato State College, Mankato, Minnesota, prepared a directory of programs in outdoor adventure activities. At that time the directory listed 203 organizations, including Outward Bound, that offered adventure experiences. That included 47 colleges and universities and 49 elementary and secondary schools that offered academic credit for an experience from an accepted adventure program. Also included were 30 to 40 agencies that offered experiences for particular factions such as drug dependents, youth offenders, religious groups, special populations, and other interest groups. At that time the growth of adventure education was considered by many to be phenomenal. Today, just a few years later, the directory is out of date.

Although exact figures are not available, the Association of Experiential Education (AEE) estimates that there are between 3000 and 4000 organizations and agencies in this country alone that are providing adventure experiences. They also state that there are approximately 200 to 300 educational institutions that offer academic credit for an approved adventure experience.

On a worldwide basis, one travel agency boasts of having contact with over 2000 adventure agencies that can provide anything from camping in northern Iceland to falconry vacations in Pakistan.

Along with the growth of outdoor schools, the public seems to have taken to the adventure experience as well. One survey suggests that in 1978 there were over 58 million individuals camped out for one night or more in this country alone, as compared to about 17 million a decade ago. Additionally, the National Park Service estimates that in 1982 there were over 400 million visits to the National Park System.

In addition to various private agencies offering adventure activities, many educators and administrators, convinced of the positive aspects of the adventure experience, have instituted adventure programs in a variety of educational institutions including elementary schools, junior and senior high schools, prep schools, and colleges and universities.

In New England, Karl Rhonke of Project Adventure has built over 50 ropes courses in eastern Massachusetts alone. Also, he has advised many other schools on the introduction of the adventure concept into the regular school curriculum. There are between 70 and 100 schools in eastern

Massachusetts providing adventure experiences as an extension of their physical education curriculum. The transition to the modified Outward Bound program has been occurring primarily at the sophomore level. The adventure program in many schools lasts for the duration of the academic year. The following year, although many schools prefer to continue the adventure program, the regular physical education classes are reinstated.

The basic adventure curriculum adopted by the school may include initiative problems, map and compass work, ropes course activities (Figures 7-1 and 7-2), cross-country skiing and snowshoeing, extended hiking, canoeing, camping, and mountaineering trips, and a wide range of other cooperative, physical activities. (For the most complete reference source of these and hundreds of other creative ideas, see *Cowstails and Cobras* by Karl Rhonke.[6]) The majority of these experiences can be divided into a series of 45-minute class periods. The "aim of many of these activities is to allow the students to view themselves as increasingly capable and competent. By attempting a gradual series of activities which involve physical or emotional risk, and succeeding (or sometimes failing) in a supportive group atmosphere, a student may begin to develop true self-esteem."

Many schools, because of budget restrictions, have been unable to fully explore outdoor and adventure education on their own school sites. Consequently, because of a strong desire to explore this area of education, numerous institutions have developed creative solutions for their restrictions.

The Peabody, Massachusetts, school system found a solution through its town recreation and parks department. The city had recently purchased a 200-acre apple farm within the town limits and, with considerable communication and cooperation between the two city departments, an environmental and adventure education program was developed utilizing the newly acquired site. The cooperative used municipal tree workers to build a ropes course and other needed equipment while the school board provided the necessary funds for a part-time staff and transportation. Today, the program serves the ten elementary schools with each school in attendance at the site for a one-week period. High school volunteers are trained to conduct short classes in environmental education and graduate students in adventure education provide

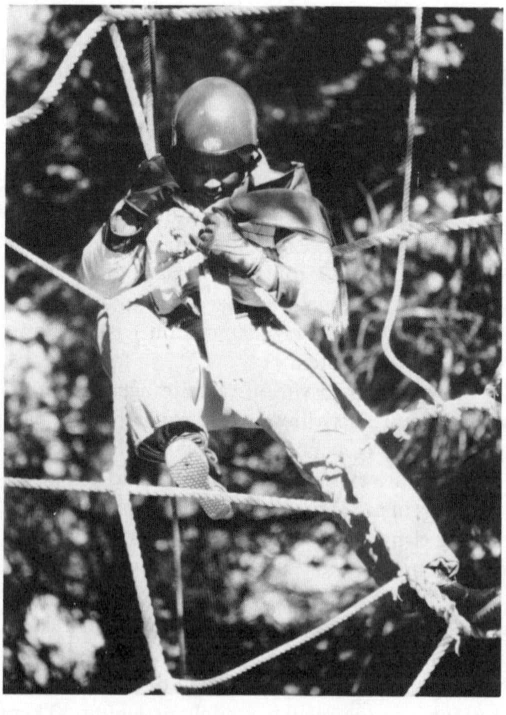

Figure 7-1 Participant on a ropes course.

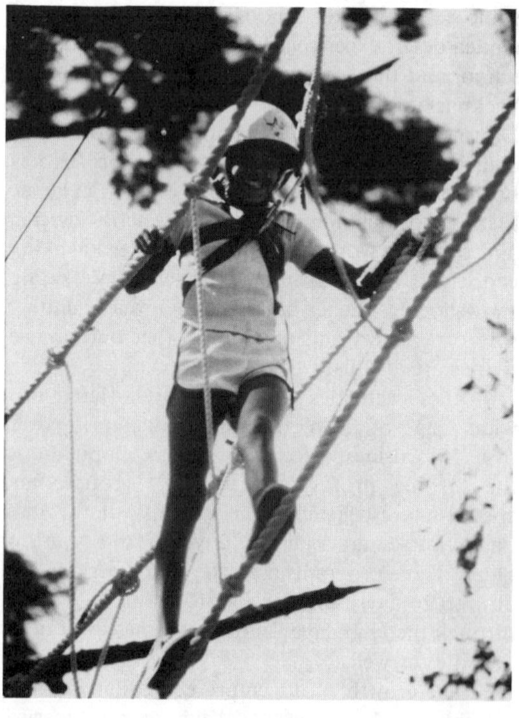

Figure 7-2 Crossing a ropes course bridge.

the adventure experiences. The town has found the arrangement to be working well and has plans for a year-round facility that could be used by various town groups including scouting groups and other youth agencies.

Sargent Camp, located in Peterborough, New Hampshire and owned by Boston University, is another alternative for educational institutions. This progressive organization provides year round residential and nonresidential environmental and adventure experiences for hundreds of organizations and groups in New England. The camp employs interns (often college graduates) as instructors to maintain low budgeting, and provides academic experiences for numerous elementary schools, high schools, prep schools, colleges, and universities. Adventure activities include skiing, snowshoeing and winter camping, rock climbing (Figure 7-3) and rappelling (Figure 7-4), white water rafting, kayaking and canoeing, extensive ropes course activities, and other experiences.

Along with these activities, Sargent Camp has developed two innovative programs. One is the inclusion of people with special needs into many of the adventure activities. The other is the "Executive Challenge" program, which provides long- and short-term adventure experiences for the business executive. Recently, managers from the Polaroid Corporation endured both a summer and winter program and expressed considerable enthusiasm for the entire concept.

Adventure, then, has grown considerably during the last decade. So much so that one cannot help but ask, "why?"

Dr Jerry Fain of Boston University and president of the National Therapeutic Recreation Society, suggests, "The reason adventure is so popular today is that technology has altered our lives in such a way that we need experiences which remind us that we can control our own existence. In a natural setting we can cook and camp wherever and whenever we want. We can also sleep and recreate at our own pace and not at the dictates of our fast-moving and complex society. In essence, we can begin to take real control of our own lives" (personal communication).

Another explanation is offered by John Miles of Western Washington University. In a recent article published in the *Journal of Physical Education and Recreation,*[7] Miles states, "Obviously people

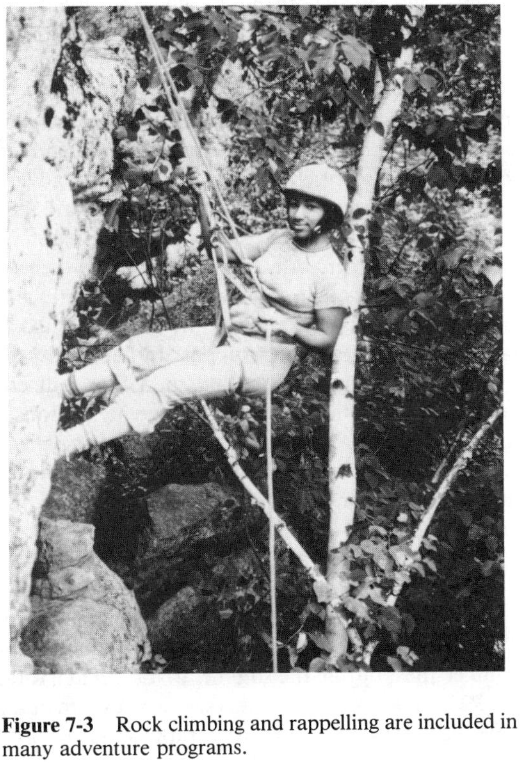

Figure 7-3 Rock climbing and rappelling are included in many adventure programs.

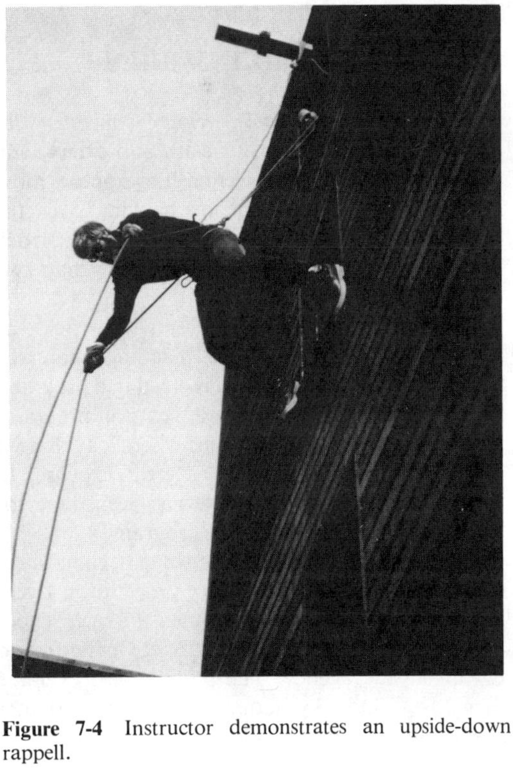

Figure 7-4 Instructor demonstrates an upside-down rappell.

engage in these activities [adventure] and go to these places [wilderness] for their unique natural values, qualities which they do not experience in their daily lives. Having confronted self and met a spiritual and physical challenge, a person may become more secure in their identity, more confident in themselves."

Abraham Maslow describes these same experiences as "peak experiences."[8] He suggests that at these times the individual feels more integrated, more intelligent, more perceptive, wittier, and stronger than at other times. He is no longer wasting time fighting with himself. The person in this state feels at the peak of his powers. Maslow further suggests that these experiences allow the individual to realize that he can grow and go beyond his society-oriented limits.

Dr Marvin Zuckerman, Professor of Psychology at the University of Delaware, suggests that sensation-seeking is a response to our body's need for a maximum state of arousal. In his recent article in *Psychology Today* Zuckerman states, "I believe that it [sensation-seeking] has a biological basis we share with animals." In the same article he describes how certain levels of monoamine oxidase, androgens, and estrogens play an important role in man's quest for adventure and sensations.[9]

ACCIDENTS AND INJURIES

Certainly the most serious concern with adventure programming is health and safety, and rightfully so. To the observer nothing appears more life-threatening than someone hanging over the edge of a high cliff with nothing but solid rock below and support from nothing more than two thin-looking ropes.

Among professionals within the field of adventure nothing is more plaguing than the thought of injury to anyone involved in a program. Having directed two large adventure programs myself, I speak from experience when I say that we go to great lengths as well as great expense, to insure that everything possible has been done for the safety of all involved in a program.

Outward Bound, for instance, is continually reviewing and revising its safety procedures. Every year the procedures and equipment of each school are evaluated by the national office and by an outside agency. The schools also evaluate themselves and, by request, have yet another agency do the same. In addition, each year the entire organization is examined carefully for safety concerns by a nationally recognized association of retired business executives.

Furthermore, if any injury or near-injury occurs, a hearing is held by both internal and external groups to insure complete understanding of the event and to prevent the recurrence of a similar situation. As a result of these elaborate precautions taken by Outward Bound, and many other organizations as well, there have been few injuries and, according to Dr Betty van der Smissen, attorney and Professor of Recreation at Pennsylvania State University, few insurance claims and even fewer lawsuits. According to their main office, with the exception of inflation increases, Outward Bound has never had an increase in insurance rates due to the nature and type of their programming.

Because of the present state of the economy, however, and the general concern over litigation, the acquisition of specific information relative to injuries and accidents has been difficult. The information that has been collected is presented here in hopes of furthering acceptance of adventure programming by those in charge of program development.

As stated earlier, those of us who have contact with adventure programming go to great lengths to not only develop ourselves as competent and safety-conscious (both physically and mentally) professionals, but also to provide continual training to those employed by us in a teaching capacity. As a rule, we do not provide "assembly line" adventure experiences or "cheap thrills" for people who voluntarily come to us seeking rejuvenation and the opportunity to enrich themselves. We view adventure as an attempt to introduce humanistic and self-developmental teaching concepts into the realm of education and growth. Furthermore, we believe that individuals can go beyond their self and society-imposed limits, if activities are conducted in an atmosphere of group support rather than peer pressure. We recognize that people need encouragement rather than discouragement. Consequently professional adventure educators place significant emphasis establishing meaningful interpersonal communication and fostering personal growth.

Following are case studies of the numbers of injuries at nine Adventure programs.

1. Underway Program (now named the "Touch Of Nature" program) at Southern Illinois Universities, during the summer of 1972 had a total of 722 students enrolled in various programs that involved rock climbing and rappelling, caving,

ropes course work, extended camping, and other general adventure activities. During the many thousands of hours of programming two injuries were sustained by students, one sprained ankle and one cut finger that required no stitches. During that time four instructors received cuts to various parts of the body but none required stitches.

2. Glenbrook South High School, Glenview, Illinois has a program that deals primarily with underachievers and serves 90 students per year. Classes meet three times a week for nine weeks followed by a three-day adventure weekend that includes rock climbing, ropes course work, caving, and camping. The program has operated for five years and reports no injuries.

3. Boston University, Sargent Camp, Peterborough, New Hampshire, for the past four years has provided hundreds of year-round environmental and adventure programs to thousands of resident and nonresident campers. Programs have included rock climbing and rappelling, white water canoeing, rafting and kayaking, cross-country skiing and snowshoeing, winter camping, mountaineering, extended camping, and extensive medium and high ropes course work, as well as environmental studies. Injuries include two major accidents. One involved a concussion, back strain, and chipped teeth resulting from misusing equipment. The other involved a fractured ankle suffered during a winter time fall. Also during this time four to six other injuries were reported that involved sprains but no fractures.

4. Hamilton-Wenham Regional High School, Hamilton, Massachusetts, has a model program in New England presently completing its eighth year of programming that includes initiative problems, active games, extensive ropes course activity, winter camping trips, climbing and rappelling, canoeing, and many other extended adventure experiences. The program has served approximately 1500 students and faculty members. There have been five reported fractures, four of ankles and fingers and one of the sternum. Also reported were five minor sprains or strains.

5. Agassiz Village, West Poland, Maine, serves over 1500 low-income youths each summer season and is New England's largest camp. During the 1978–1979 camping season approximately 80% to 90% of the population, including 80 nonambulatory and ambulatory special needs persons, were involved in many different forms of adventure activities including canoeing, ropes course activities, camping. Also approximately 60 older campers experienced extended camping, rock climbing, and rappelling. Five to seven minor injuries were incurred that were related directly to the adventure program. One instructor received a minor cut on the head when struck by a falling stone during a rock climb while supervising observers. She was on the ground and not wearing a helmet. One student received a cut on the leg when she fell on a dead tree. Two sprained ankles and a few cases of poison ivy were also reported.

6. Expedition 735, Melrose, Massachusetts is an agency that provides adventure experiences including white water canoeing, ropes course work, cross-country skiing, rock climbing, and rappelling as well as numerous other adventure activities for schools and youth service agencies in Massachusetts. During 1978, there were 511 participants, and two minor injuries were reported. One person had a nosebleed (which was not related to an activity), and another suffered a minor eye injury after being struck by a projectile.

7. Peabody Outdoor Education Program, Peabody, Massachusetts serves the ten elementary schools within the Peabody school system. Each school uses the site daily for one week. The program includes initiative problems, ropes course work, environmental studies, and other activities. During the 1978–1979 academic year, 600 to 700 children were involved in programs. One injury was reported, a sixth-grader fell while running and received a cut on the hand that required four stitches. Also three to five cases of poison ivy occurred.

8. Medway High School, Medway, Massachusetts has a program that serves the sophomore class with a modified Outward Bound curriculum that includes initiative problems, cross-country skiing, snowshoeing, extended winter camping, ropes course work, extended canoeing and wilderness trips, and indoor wall climbing. The program has been in operation for four years and has involved 350 students and 25 instructors. To date there has been one fracture of the coccyx (no permanent injury), and three minor cases of frostbite.

9. North Carolina Outward Bound School, Morganton, North Carolina, between 1970 and 1976, had over 4000 people attend its courses. Accidents occurred at the rate of one injury for every 80 students who were attending the standard 26-day course. There were no fatalities, and no injuries more serious than a simple fracture.

An analysis of the programming time indicates that these 4000 participants received a total of 104,000 days, or 2.5 million hours, of intense adventure programming.

Report of the American Alpine Club, 1978

The American Alpine Club publishes a yearly report entitled "Accidents in North American Mountaineering."[10] The major climbing areas reported a significant increase in climbing activities, and many areas indicated record numbers of climbs. Solo and winter climbs also showed significant increases. The report states that it is "significant to note that in two major areas (Alaska and Wyoming) the accident rate was one-half that of the previous year." In Grand Teton National Park alone, 8957 climbs were registered, and if one multiplies by the average party size of four, one would see that the number of climber/user days comes close to 40,000. This figure does not include guide service beginner or intermediate days in unregistered nonsummit climbs. "...The total number of climbing accidents (for this area) for 1977 was 11, a ratio which clearly suggests a good level of safe climbing."

An analysis of the reported injuries indicates a surprising number of mishaps due to inadequate equipment (clothing, helmets, etc), failure to properly utilize equipment (non-belay, carabiners, etc), and other accidents that can happen when climbers are not thinking or are improperly trained.

As mentioned earlier, the acquisition of specific information relative to injuries in adventure programs has proven to be difficult. No doubt commercial agencies and schools are concerned with reputation, litigation, and insurance increases. Numerous people have offered information but have asked that sources be kept confidential.

While the figures here are not to be taken as conclusive evidence, they indicate that far fewer injuries are occurring within the adventure setting than might be expected. Many schools have stated that, on the whole, injuries involving an adventure situation are not as frequent as accidents that have occurred within the regular physical education setting. One school stated that while regular physical education serves more students, statistics strongly favor the adventure curriculum on an injury basis.

However, serious injuries and deaths have occurred within the adventure setting. Unfortunately, Outward Bound is presently involved in litigation over the deaths of two students who were caught in a sudden storm while kayaking (May 1980). The determination of safety considerations relevant to adventure programming is cumbersome and inconclusive. What is important to realize, however, is that although accidents and fatalities have occurred in the adventure arena, it is no more dangerous than daily living.

RESEARCH IN EDUCATIONAL SETTINGS

Hamilton-Wenham Regional High School

In 1971, a Title III Elementary and Secondary Education Act (ESEA) grant was awarded to the Hamilton-Wenham Regional High School, Hamilton, Massachusetts, for the development of an innovative, modified Outward Bound program at the school.

As reported in the evaluation findings[11] the objectives of the program included: 1) "to improve self-concept, confidence, and a sense of personal achievement among participants; 2) to increase psychomotor skills especially in the areas of balance and coordination; 3) to overcome pervasive passivity, apathy, and uninvolvement among students."

Also, teachers working with the project developing curriculum and implementing specific programs have had the following goal: "To promote active concern for the student as a social, intellectual, physical, and emotional human being. And to manifest this concern in changes in teaching style, curriculum, and extra-curricular activities."

Curriculum was developed to include innovative workshops in English, history, and science as well as rock climbing and rappelling, bicycling, canoeing, rigorous camping, initiative problems, extensive ropes course activities, and numerous other adventure activities. Extended trips ranged from one day to three weeks.

Four doctoral-level researchers, with considerable research experience in the adventure phenomenon, were enlisted to develop and analyze the research design, which included the following six diagnostic instruments: 1) the Tennessee Self-Concept Scale; 2) the School Climate Survey (a test based on McClelland's Classroom Climate Survey); 3) a Student Description Form (developed by the Independent School Association); 4) a questionnaire designed to measure types and levels of student leisure activities; 5) The American Association of Health, Physical Education, and Recreation Test of Physical Fitness; and 6) the Rotter Scale of Internal vs External Control of Reinforcement, which measures the degree of perceived external control.

The test population included the entire tenth grade class in the school. This study was conducted for two consecutive years using two different sophomore classes. Total population for the two years was 455. Year 1 included 224 students (104 girls and 120 boys). Year 2 included 231 students (108 girls and 123 boys).

Before and after tests were administered during the months of October and June of the two consecutive academic years. English and science teachers also completed the Student Description Form during the before and after testing. Each student also rated himself on the same dimensions of the Student Description Form. Personal and teacher ratings were compared on matched t-tests. The statistical information was analyzed by computer using DATA TEXT. The acceptable level of significance was 0.05.

As stated in these evaluation findings, the major "limitation of this study is the lack of a control group. Changes may thus be a factor of maturation or other unknown variables. On the other hand, the fact that consistent changes among two different groups of students in two consecutive years may indicate a clear-cut effect."

For the sake of clarity and cohesiveness, an abbreviated synopsis will be presented. Full evaluations are available, but are far too extensive to be examined here.

Student goal—"To Improve...Confidence" The success of student goal 1 is shown in Tables 7-1 through 7-5 with excerpts from the various tests.

As reported in the conclusions from Tables 7-1 and 7-2, "These findings indicate that the project did have a marked effect on the self-concepts of students, most strongly on girls ...and that the students perceived themselves to be more in control and less at the mercy of outside forces...." Table 7-3 showed that "Consistently significant increases in positive identity among females may be the result of accomplishments in the physical outdoor realm...." From Table 7-4 it was concluded that

Table 7-1
Statistically Significant Changes, Year 1
Rotter Scale, combined boys and girls, maximum score is 23

Before Test		After Test			
$\bar{X}$	SD	$\bar{X}$	SD	t-test	p
10.80	3.48	10.1	3.75	−2.22	.028

Table 7-2
Tennessee Self-Concept Scale, Year 1
Maximum score, 100

	$\bar{X}$ diff	SD	t-test	p
Total conflict (M)	−5.37	14.9	−3.43	> .001
Self-criticism (F)	−1.86	6.93	−2.34	> .023
Total positivity (F)	1.96	8.06	2.12	> .038
Positive identity (F)	2.48	9.65	2.24	> .029
Positive behavior (F)	2.07	7.98	2.26	> .027
Moral self (F)	2.77	10.13	2.39	> .020
Family self (F)	2.42	8.96	2.36	> .021

Table 7-3
Tennessee Self-Concept Scale, Years 1 and 2
Positive Identity (F)

Year 1			Year 2		
$\bar{X}$ diff	SD	p	$\bar{X}$	SD	p
2.48	9.65	.029	2.05	8.60	.039

there was "Improvement in scores of Achievement Motivation over the two years among females...." And the data in Table 7-5 led the researchers to conclude that "The revised questionnaire indicated ...that males and females saw themselves as more willing to try new things. These attitudes reflect growth in confidence and overcoming fear of change and risk-taking."

Student goal—"To Increase Psychomotor Skills" Some conclusions from the American Association of Health, Physical Education, and Recreation (AAHPER) Test of Physical Fitness are shown in Table 7-6.

As reported in the final evaluation of student goal 2: "Students in classes in two consecutive years improved significantly on all dimensions of physical functioning (except the flexed arm hang for females) as measured on the AAHPER Test of Physical Fitness. It should be noted that the relationship between physical fitness and positive self-concept has been documented elsewhere."

Student goal 3—"To Overcome... Passivity..." Tables 7-7 through 7-10 show the results of student goal 3.

As reported in the final evaluation of the data in Table 7-7 "In self-reports, the females' list of

Table 7-4
School Climate Survey
Achievement Motivation (F)

Year 1			Year 2		
$\overline{X}$ diff	SD	p	$\overline{X}$	SD	p
0.54	2.24	.040	.481	2.079	.042

Table 7-5
Significant Changes in Attitude and Values, Year 2
Student Questionnaire

		$\overline{X}$ diff	SD	t-test	p
Willingness to take a chance	M	−0.04	1.06	−0.30	NS
	F	0.36	1.19	2.69	.009
Willingness to try new things	M	0.30	1.12	2.44	.017
	F	0.31	0.88	3.18	.003

Table 7-6
Significant Changes Among Sophomores on All Dimensions for Years 1 and 2

	Year 1			Year 2		
	$\overline{X}$ diff	SD	p	$\overline{X}$ diff	SD	p
Sit-Ups	4.56	5.06	.001	1.33	5.78	.006
300 Yard	−5.33 sec	10.26	.001	−4.61 sec	3.78	.001
Standing Broad	3.84	6.83	.001	3.15	6.81	.001
50 Yard Run	−1.24 sec	5.97	.017	−0.89 sec	5.10	.041
Pull-Ups (males)	1.44	1.47	.001	1.30	1.79	.001
Flex Arm Hang (females)	0.38 sec	1.55	NS	−0.24 sec	1.90	NS

Table 7-7
Student Questionnaire
Total number of activities listed by students (F)

Year 1 (n = 224)			Year 2 (n = 231)		
$\overline{X}$ diff	SD	p	$\overline{X}$	SD	p
2.88	3.32	.001	1.67	3.59	.001

Table 7-8
Student Self-Description Form
Participation in discussion

Year 1 (Females n = 74)			Year 2 (Males n = 80)		
$\overline{X}$ diff	SD	p	$\overline{X}$ diff	SD	p
0.29	1.19	.037	0.32	1.05	.008

Table 7-9
Parent Questionnaire
Effect of participation on child

	Year 1 (n = 103)	Year 2 (n = 78)
Positive	80%	90%
Negative	3%	1%
Neutral, don't know	17%	9%

Table 7-10
Volunteer Program
Number of students volunteering

Year 1	Year 2	Year 3 (to date)
30	130	104

activities (such as jobs, glee club, athletics, hobbies) were significantly longer after participation in the year-long program. These findings tend to indicate a decrease in overall passivity and an increase in risk taking and ability to work with groups." From Table 7-8 it is concluded that "Self-ratings on participation in discussion showed significant improvement in both years. Females the first year and males the second year rated themselves as significantly more talkative by the end of the year. Thus they saw themselves as more willing to take the risk of speaking up in class and actively participating, rather than passively absorbing." Table 7-9 shows that, particularly in year 2, the parents indicated "that they viewed the project as having a more positive effect on their children. Their comments most frequently mentioned 'growing confidence,' 'a refreshing enthusiasm,' and 'a more positive attitude' as changes they had observed and attributed to the program." And from Table 7-10, which shows a marked increase in the number of volunteers, it is concluded that "The growth in numbers of students involved in the volunteer program indicates a trend toward active involvement, a willingness to try new things, and a willingness to assume a responsible job."

Teacher involvement The final report states that "in both the first and second year over 50% of the faculty at Hamilton-Wenham were actively involved in project-sponsored activities."

Outside observation During the spring of 1973, the USOE Validation Team investigated the project for a three-day period and gave the program a rating of 100. Their study concluded, "...the impressive educative power fundamentally in the depth, subtlety, and sensitivity of its basic objectives and approach. The positive effect of this project on the affective educational climate of Hamilton-Wenham Regional High School cannot be missed by any on site observer. The project is positive; it is necessary; it works...."

Medway High School

By law, all public schools operating in the New England area must undergo an accreditation process by the New England Association of Schools and Colleges at ten-year intervals. This process was completed at the Medway High School, Medway, Massachusetts, during the spring of 1977.

Although the report commended the school on several areas it concluded that there was far too much "departmentalization" and far too little communication within the school setting. The report recommended, "provisions be taken to formulate a standing curriculum committee for the purpose of updating and articulating the entire program." The report also suggested a complete "revitalization" of the entire physical education program concluding that the present program was found to be "boring to both the students and the instructors."

After considerable effort on the part of faculty committees, and with consulting services provided by Project Adventure, an Interdisciplinary Physical Education Curriculum program (IPEC) was developed to meet the problems that were listed in the accreditation report.

Curriculum was developed around the adventure concept, and numerous departments contributed time and effort to the program. A Title IV

ESEA grant was funded during the beginning of the 1977–1978 academic year for development of the IPEC program.

The program included initiative problems, cross-country skiing, snowshoeing, mountaineering, canoeing and winter camping expeditions, ropes course activities, cardiopulmonary resuscitation training, indoor wall climbing, and outdoor cooking, as well as English and science activities.

Although the goals of the program are quite lengthy, a brief synopsis of the objectives includes: 1) to involve instructors from various departments within IPEC; 2) to develop a ropes course; 3) to introduce to students "life skills," such as skiing and camping; 4–9) to develop problem-solving abilities, to be able to meet a crisis effectively, and to deemphasize the importance of winning; 10) to involve girls as well as boys; and 11) to involve students with special needs.

An evaluation team from Boston University was enlisted to develop and analyze the research design. Diagnostic instruments included; 1) the Tennessee Self-Concept Scale; 2) the Cooper-Smith Self Concept Scale; 3) the Platt Adventure Behavior Scale (PABS) (an observer system to measure growth along ten adventure variables); 4) a questionnaire designed to measure attitudes toward physical education, seasonal activities, and winning; and 5) extensive interviews of administrators, instructors, student leaders, and others involved.

The self-concept scales were administered on a pre and post schedule. Interviews were held several times throughout the academic year with relevant individuals. The PABS scale was used four times during scheduled classes. Because the entire sophomore class was involved in the program, no control group was used. However, because the program was to be evaluated for three consecutive years, clear patterns would become visible. Classes met twice every six days.

Conclusions of the program follow.

Top administrators when interviewed asserted: 1) That "the IPEC program was a viable solution to the curriculum problems at the school; 2) That the program has facilitated growth in many areas including group cooperation, self-concept, self-reliance, interpersonal relations, and life-saving abilities for not only the students but the instructors as well; 3) That the program has been a positive experience for the staff; 4) That the program should be continued and expanded."

Instructors when interviewed said: 1) That "the program has added excitement and rejuvenated the staff who chose to become involved; 2) ...has added excitement to the lives of the students; 3) ...has had a significant and positive impact on the students; 4) ...has created positive feelings between staff members; 5) that the program should be expanded and continued; 6) that the students are doing better academically as well as socially."

Students when interviewed said: 1) "The program has generated positive feelings among those students involved in the program; 2) the program provided information that was relevant to their lives; 3) the program has allowed the students to see their teachers as 'real people and not just adults that stand and lecture for hours'; 4) that the students now 'feel better about themselves'; 5) that the program has allowed themselves, as individuals, to mature, and are now capable of better judgments."

For the sake of expediency, only brief parts of the final evaluation (which is over 100 pages) are presented here.

Objective 1 sought to involve numerous departments and instructors within the IPEC program. As stated in the evaluation, "approximately 95% of the faculty participated...during some phase of the program, while 36% of the faculty and administration made a continuing contribution."

Also reported in an interview with the school assistant principal was the fact that there were only one or two cases of unexcused absences during the entire academic year involving approximately 150 students. "Normally," he commented, "there would have been hundreds of cuts during this same period."

Objectives 7 and 8 identify self-esteem, trust, and mutual support as significant goals for the program. The evaluation reported, "There was a 17.2% positive change in students seeing themselves as leaders on the post-test," while "the Adventure Behavior Scale indicates a positive growth in self-concept when students are faced with new situations within the IPEC program. There was also a dramatic change in student attitude toward helping other students ...(pre $\bar{x}$ = 19.23, post $\bar{x}$ = 36.69)."

The curriculum included cardiopulmonary resuscitation (CPR) training for all sophomore students and was taught within the regular framework of the IPEC program. All sophomore students, including one special-needs individual (who participated in canoeing and skiing), received certification in CPR. The training later proved to be invaluable to one sophomore who succeeded in saving her father's life twice during one year because of her CPR training.

The evaluation design for the second year included extensive interviews with not only a random sample of students, but with their parents as well. During the midyear interview[13] "70% volunteered that they preferred the IPEC program to the regular physical education program," while all students interviewed expressed strongly "a sincere fondness for the program and a desire to see the program continued after the sophomore year."

At the midyear evaluation 70% to 80% of parents interviewed, "strongly supported the IPEC and their children's involvement." And parents used such adjectives as "enriching," "more trusting," and "much more cooperative" when describing the program and their children's reaction to the new experiences.

It appears then, that adventure programming can and does have a significant impact on the educational setting. In 1971, Dr Joseph R. Schultz, professor at Mankato State College, Mankato, Minnesota, published an extensive report, *An Analysis of the Impact of Outward Bound on Twelve High Schools.*[14] The schools were from various parts of the country and the students themselves, were from varying socioeconomic backgrounds. In his concluding remarks, Schultz points out that "as an increasing number of students complain about the sterile curriculum and demand more relevant and individual programs, the Outward Bound [adventure] process offers a dynamic and realistic alternative." Furthermore, Schultz suggests that the adventure experience can act as a catalyst in relation to curriculum and human relations, "...because the quality of the relationship between students and teachers is improved [more trust, sensitivity]...the atmosphere or climate in the classroom is altered and different types of activities or topics can be pursued or different techniques can be used."

Schultz continues by stating, "the [adventure] activities stimulate a climate of acceptance, knowledge, and tolerance... Students have found a sense of accomplishment and reward, and teachers have discovered new dimensions in their teaching. [Consequently] these individuals have become excited about education and their role in education." Schultz concludes, "Outward Bound [adventure] represents a process which has the potential to help the schools become more relevant and help them begin the process of change toward humane, sensitive institutions concerned with the education of children and adults."

ADVENTURE AND CORRECTIONS

The question of juvenile crime and delinquency has proven to be a difficult issue for modern society. As recidivism rates at the national level remain high, 50% to 60%, those who are responsible for rehabilitation are questioning the value of incarceration, training, release, and parole as an effective means of coping with this problem. Traditional treatments are now being seen as increasingly expensive and often seem to plunge youthful offenders further into the realm of antisocial life styles.

Available literature describes the juvenile delinquent as having, "low self-esteem, inability to communicate, lack of confidence, inability to cooperate, ...low threshold of frustration, and lack of skills related to adult functioning."[15]

During the summer of 1964, the Massachusetts Department of Youth Services received five scholarships for the Colorado Outward Bound School. After carefully screening a number of youths, the chosen boys were told that they would be returned to the custody of their parents upon completion of the course. "The group returned exhilarated by their experience, and all who met them were impressed enormously with the experience's effect upon them, particularly on their attitudes about themselves and the future."[16]

The following summer, at the expense of the Department, 40 boys were sent to the Colorado Outward Bound School. The effects were similar to that of the five boys who attended the year before. The group was carefully followed for the next six months, and after that time, 4 (10%) of the 40 boys had been recommitted to a correctional facility. Under normal circumstances, (the traditional treatment method), 15 to 16 boys would have been recommitted.

There is no doubt that these findings had to be observed under a controlled setting. In 1966, 60 boys were sent to the Outward Bound School, while 60 more boys were committed to the traditional training facility as a control group. The Outward Bound group attended a 26-day course while the control group was incarcerated for periods of six months to a year or more. Recidivism was operationally defined as recommitment to a juvenile or adult institution for a new offense.

Researchers Francis Kelly, EdD, and D.J. Baer, "found a 20% recidivism rate for the Outward Bound group after one year's release and a 42% recidivism rate for those in the control group after one year's release."[16]

Based on these figures and the fact that the Outward Bound course costs about $600 per individual vs $3000 to $4000 for each individual in attendance at a training facility for one year, the Department of Youth Services sent 120 more boys during the next two consecutive summers. Under similar research design, statistics continued to strongly favor the experimental group after one year's release.

Long-term Effects

Kelly and Baer completed a five-year follow-up on the subjects of the 1966 study and results indicated an increase in recidivism after the first year. As reported after five years, "While the difference in recidivism rates continue to favor the Outward Bound group, it is no longer statistically significant (38% vs 53%). An important finding here is the greatest increase in recidivism after the first year in the Outward Bound group occurred at the end of the second year of parole."[16]

Kelly concluded that basically the negative effects of the youth's environment has the ability to erode the benefits gained at the Outward Bound course. He continued by suggesting that these same "youngsters might have been helped by a community-based Outward Bound adaptive program serving to reinforce and consolidate the gains achieved at the Outward Bound schools."[16]

Homeward Bound

In 1970, the state of Massachusetts, with the assistance of Outward Bound, developed the adventure-based Homeward Bound program. Located in Massachusetts, the structure and curriculum of the new program was similar to that of the Outward Bound programs. However modifications were made from information gained during the several years of affiliation with Outward Bound. Each boy was informed that the program was voluntary, rugged, limited in number of openings, and, once the course was begun, it must be completed. Once the six weeks of program were completed, each boy was released to the custody of his parents.

Research findings indicate a close approximation to the earlier Kelly-Baer reports in that within fourteen months of release 20.8% of the Homeward Bound group had been recommitted while 42.7% of the control group were recommitted.

Along with these two organizations, several other agencies have developed adventured-based alternatives to incarceration. Numerous other research reports indicate similar findings.

The question of effectiveness is often difficult to evaluate, especially when dealing within the affective realm. Youthful offenders (as well as adult violators) are not objects that can be removed from society, and once returned, be expected to conform to its rules without radical change and growth within themselves. All too often we expect far too much from individuals with limited experiences. Our responsibility should be to provide experiences that will add to their self-esteem and their own ability to see themselves as positive people who can effect change within their own lives. Unfortunately, incarceration has been shown to be a method of protecting society from these individuals rather than institutions providing growth and rehabilitative-oriented experiences.

Adventure programming does not pretend to be a panacea. Many boys have had to drop out of adventure programs or, once completing them, have again fallen victim to their own inescapable environment. It is clear, however, that there is no simple answer to this problem.

It has been suggested, however, that the adventure experience meets the youthful offender in his own arena—Action. For an individual with limited communicative skills, talk therapies and group counseling seem to be of little use. The adventure setting can provide "activities that are challenging, exciting, exhilarating, where the results are immediate and irrevocable, are ready to be grasped and understood. They speak deeply into the need to feel competent, to exert their large muscles, to assert their 'machismo' in socially acceptable ways. The experience is often seen as a 'rite de passage,' helping to clarify the confusion of emerging adulthood."[15]

Nold and Wilpers conclude that the Outward Bound group "commits significantly fewer crimes, they are less serious, they spend less time in detention, and there is a considerable savings in cost to the state." Furthermore, "the evidence is conclusive that wilderness training can provide a valuable alternative to incarceration, and it can be an effective method of rehabilitation, provided that it is not overinflated in claims and overloaded with unrealistic expectations."[15]

RESEARCH IN OUTWARD BOUND

In 1977, Arnold Shore compiled a one and three-quarters-inch thick document entitled "Outward Bound: A Reference Volume," which contained an approximately 1400-item bibliography of literature relevant to the adventure experience. Many of the items were research studies, dissertations, evaluations, assessments, and other research efforts as well as numerous articles, personal interpretations, and descriptive exposés. To say the least, then, the adventure experience has been explored and well documented.

While the goals of the adventure program remains "to develop character," researchers, cognizant of this objective, have guided many studies in the direction of the psychology of the individual and how it is affected by the adventure experience.

Although many studies have been completed, the two studies reported were chosen for their completeness and excellence as determined by an outside observer. Statistical analyses and data are available but are not presented for the sake of brevity. Unfortunately, any interpretation or synopsis of lengthy research analysis and findings is bound to discredit the research effort. My apologies to those authors whose studies may suffer under my attempt at conciseness.

S.M. Koepke, 1977 (unpublished data) argues that self-concept is partially related to stress. Since an Outward Bound course can significantly increase stress and anxiety, the experience of adequately meeting the adventure challenge with coping behavior rather than defensive behavior may thus affect the overall self-concept of the participant in a positive manner.

To test this hypothesis, Koepke utilized Gough and Heilburns' *Adjective Check List* to determine self-concept levels, while anxiety was examined through use of the State-Trait Anxiety Inventory of Spielberger, et al. Both instruments were utilized in the traditional pre-post design and analyzed using nonparametric statistical techniques that included the Wilcoxon Matched-Pairs Signed-Ranks test and the Mann-Whitney U test to determine whether or not unmatched pairs belonged to the same population. This study included 11 girls and 33 boys who participated in a standard summer Colorado Outward Bound course (n = 44).

Findings

In summary, "Following the Outward Bound course participants ascribed significantly fewer unfavorable adjectives to their real selves and found themselves less likely either to solicit sympathy from others (succorance) or to express feelings of inferiority through self-criticism (abasement)." Furthermore, "The comparison of real and ideal self-concepts on the post-test indicated higher ideal self scores for self-control, personal adjustment, achievement, dominance, endurance, and order; the ideal self scored lower in number of unfavorable adjectives checked and succorance." "The discrepancies between real and ideal self-concepts were found to be smaller (significantly) on the post-test for defensiveness, number of unfavorable adjectives checked, self-confidence, personal adjustment, dominance, introspection, nurturance, affiliation, aggression, succorance and abasement..." (Koepke, unpublished data).

According to this study, because of the Outward Bound course, students basically felt better about themselves and had a more realistic and positive approach to their life. Numerous other significant findings were reported within the study but are too lengthy to mention here.

Wetmore in 1977 studied, "...the degree to which a change in the self-concept of adolescent boys is 1) influenced by an Outward Bound experience and 2) related to differences in age, socioeconomic status, race, educational level, residential locale, sports background, and specific course attended at Outward Bound."[17] The sample included 272 adolescent boys from varying backgrounds who ranged in age from 15.5 to 19.5 years. All boys attended a standard 26-day Hurricane Island Outward Bound course.

Self-concepts were examined by use of the Tennessee Self-Concept Scale on a pre-post and six-months-post schedule and means were analyzed through T-tests at the 0.05 level of significance. Student critiques were completed six months after the end of their specific course. Also, the semantic differential scale was completed by instructors on the last day of their contact with the subjects.

As reported in the conclusions, "Results indicate a distinct positive statistically significant change (0.05) in the self-concepts of the boys while they were in attendance at the school."[17] The post-post test results indicated a still significantly higher increase but that some decrease had occurred six months after the completion of the course. Students were also asked to complete a questionnaire six months after completion of the course. One hundred twenty-four boys responded from the original 272 subjects and 95% of the returned questionnaires indicated favorable effects of the Outward Bound experience on their lives. Furthermore, many of the respondents claimed that the Outward Bound experience had improved their relations with people and increased their self-awareness and self-confidence. Results did not indicate a relationship between backgrounds and success in relation to the course and study objectives.

ADVENTURE AND THE HANDICAPPED

With the coming of Public Law 94-142, the Education for the Handicapped Act, a new consciousness has entered the area of education and adventure as well.

In the past, the special needs person had considerable difficulty finding his rightful place not only within the work force but in the world of leisure as well. Often the special person found education and themselves being placed in front of televisions for endless hours of media viewing.

As Perske pointed out in 1972 "Many who worked with the handicapped, impaired, disadvantaged, and aged tend to be overzealous in their attempts to 'protect,' 'comfort,' 'keep safe,' 'take care,' and 'watch.' Acting on these impulses at the right time can be beneficial, helpful, and developmental. But, if they are acted upon exclusively or excessively, without allowing for each client's individuality and growth potential, they will overprotect and emotionally smother the intended beneficiary. In fact, such overprotection endangers the client's human dignity and tends to keep him from experiencing the risk-taking of ordinary life which is necessary for human growth and development."[18]

With these thoughts in mind, C.C. Roland developed a pilot study (unpublished data) to answer the following questions: 1) "Can handicapped children, including the severely physically handicapped, be involved in an adventure program with participation on a ropes course? 2) Can handicapped children be mainstreamed in the adventure program with normal children? 3) Can attitudes be changed?...and 4) Can an adventure experience be a growing experience for the handicapped child?"

The research design included two groups of ten children. Each group contained five handicapped and five normal children. All normal children were interviewed before and after for attitudes toward the handicapped. Each group was rated during activities with an observation rating system known as IRG II that measures involvement.

After two weeks of adventure programming that included ropes course activities, new games, and initiative problems, the following conclusions were reached: "handicapped children can definitely be involved in this type of programming; handicapped children can be mainstreamed into the adventure program, providing the instructor is willing and capable; remarkable attitudinal changes (in a positive sense) took place toward the handicapped children from the normal students; and the experience was perceived as very positive by all the campers involved."

Programs

Outward Bound in Minnesota has run programs for the handicapped for the last four years and research on it will be published this year. The program follows the traditional Outward Bound model, and many people with a variety of handicaps including blindness, cerebral palsy, multiple sclerosis, single and double amputations, paraplegia, individuals recovering from polio, and numerous others have attended this progressive workshop. Programs are also run for the hearing impaired. Initial reactions to these programs have been very good because they instill new confidence into participants (Figure 7-5).

Agassiz Village, West Poland, Maine, mainstreams many special needs individual into several adventure activities including rock climbing, ropes course work, canoeing, and many other areas. Many of these individuals climbed 50 feet up a tree and descended some 350 feet down a giant zip line (Figure 7-6). For many it was their first time off the level ground, and all who chose to participate were extremely excited.

Other organizations have developed that provide numerous adventure activities, but research into this area is lacking.

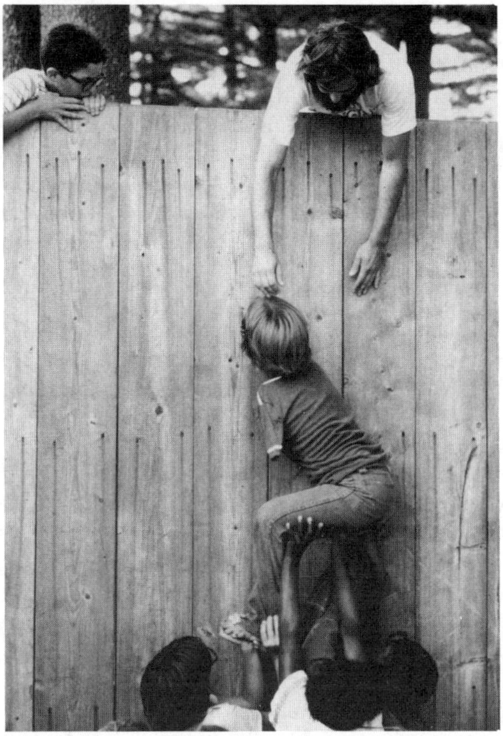

Figure 7-5 Triple amputee being helped over a 12-foot climbing wall.

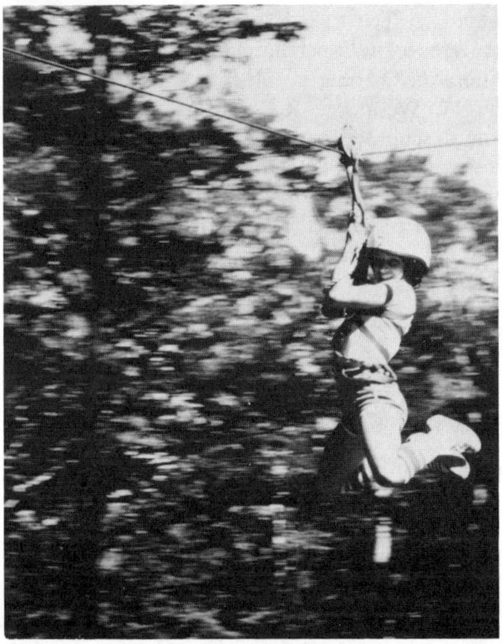

Figure 7-6 Descending a zip line requires much inner strength.

CONCLUSION

As mentioned earlier, considerable research has been conducted on the adventure experience, and a few studies have been presented here to allow the reader a glimpse into the mountains of data now available on this subject. The results examined are indicative of a general body of research findings. However, there have been studies where little or no change was observed.

Numerous scales, tests, questionnaires, and diagnostic instruments have been developed over the years and many of these tools have been used by professionals in an attempt to evaluate particular experiences. And this, as many individuals with research backgrounds are already aware, is no easy task.

The human psychic and affective behaviors are elusive and dramatic phenomena. Furthermore, they are incredibly difficult to define, let alone measure. Along with this they are subject to rapid change due to often minute and incomprehensible variables. Items such as weather, diet, rest or stress, bio-rhythms, physical condition, attitude, obscure past experiences, and endless other variables can play significant unobservable roles in the human personality.

All too often we, as researchers, attempt to define and evaluate individuals at the 0.05 level of significance while using factoral analysis of variance. And all too often we fail to comprehand the real significance of an event on an individual.

I do not mention this to discredit or invalidate research that has already been completed. I do suggest this because the tests that we are precently using often are not capable of exploring and examining real human qualities and growth. Unfortunately, administrators, granting and funding agencies, dissertation chairmen, and others often require these boring and unimaginative figures as justification for the existence of particular programs.

I suggest that the whole area of testing and evaluation needs to be carefully examined and that new techniques and methods, such as participant observation rating scales, be further incorporated into basic research designs.

FINAL COMMENTS

The adventure education field is in its infancy. Many problems will arise and will need to be resolved as this progressive and humanistic-oriented profession emerges.

The most important issue facing the field today is the training and certification of its members. Many certification schemes have been developed but they lack the support of the profession at large. To achieve this end, standards of competency need to be developed with the aid and consensus of experts and practitioners from within the field itself.

It is furthermore urged that the profession, rather than waiting for governmental regulation, define and establish principles and standards that will allow itself to be recognized as a group concerned with the growth and safety of those who come seeking adventure.

REFERENCES

1. Kelley, G. What's wrong with this child? *Boston Magazine* 69(10):84–137, 1977.

2. Orlick, T. *The Cooperative Sports and Games Book*. New York: Pantheon Books, 1978, p. 5.

3. Stewart, W.A.C. *Progressive and Radicals in English Education 1750–1970.* Fairfield, NJ: Augustus M. Kelley Publishers, 1972, p. 323.

4. Templin, G.A., and Baldwin, P.W. The evolution and adaption of Outward Bound. In *Kurt Hahn and the Development of Outward Bound: A Compilation of Essays.* London: Routledge and Kegan Paul Ltd, 1970, p. 6.

5. Rohrs, H. *The Educational Thought of Kurt Hahn.* London: Routledge and Kegan Paul Ltd, 1970, p. 128.

6. Rhonke, K. *Cowstails and Cobras.* Hamilton, Mass: Project Adventure, 1977, p. 7.

7. Miles, J. The value of high adventure activities. *J Phys Ed Recreation.* 49(4):28, 1978.

8. Maslow, A.H. *Toward a Psychology of Being.* New York: D. Van Nostrand Company, 1968, pp. 103–114.

9. Zuckerman, M. The search for high sensation. *Psychology Today* 11(9):38–99, 1978.

10. Williamson, J.E., and Whalley, E. *Accidents in North American Mountaineering 1978.* Vol. 4, No. 1 Issue 31. New York: American Alpine Club and Alpine Club of Canada, 1978, pp. 3–4.

11. Project Adventure. *Summary Statement.* Projects Grant Application for ESEA Title III, Section 306, 1974, for Hamilton-Wenham Regional High School, Hamilton, Mass.

12. Kylloe, R.R., and Lahnston, A. *I.P.E.C. Interdisciplinary Physical Education Curriculum.* 1977–1978 Annual report at Medway High School, Medway, Mass.

13. Kylloe, R.R. *I.P.E.C. A Mid-Year Look.* 1978–1979 Mid-year evaluation of adventure program at Medway High School, Medway, Mass.

14. Schultz, J.R. *An Analysis of the Impact of Outward Bound on Twelve High Schools.* Reston, Va: Outward Bound, Inc., 1971.

15. Nold, J., and Wilpers, M. A nation without prisons. Edited by C.R. Dodge. In *Outward Bound in Corrections.* Lexington, Mass: Lexington Books, 1975.

16. Kelley, R.J. Outward Bound and Delinquency: A Ten-Year Experience. Presented at the Conference on Experiential Education. Estes Park, Colorado, October, 1974.

17. Wetmore, R.C. Influence of Outward Bound school experience on the self-concept of adolescent boys. Doctoral dissertation, Boston University, 1972.

18. Perske, R. The dignity of risk and the mentally retarded. *Mental Retardation* 10(1): 24–26, 1972.

SECTION III
Medical and Allied Health Aspects

CHAPTER 8
Women in Sports

Christine E. Haycock, MD

When a surge of women entered into vigorous sports in the United States in the early 70s, there was much speculation regarding their injury potential. Inquiries came from coaches and physical education directors as to what might be expected. An investigation of the literature in 1973 indicated that very little was known about possible types of injuries to women. There was a question as to whether they would be different from those sustained by men.

Inquiries were especially directed toward the breasts and reproductive organs. Despite any evidence that women would suffer serious or disabling injuries to these organs, old myths which had been perpetuated to discourage women from participating in "unladylike" active sports still persisted. Even knowledgeable physicians made unwarranted assumptions.

Nonetheless, the 1970s saw an outpouring of women, particularly at the collegiate level, into competitive sports. They came from backgrounds in sports in which little was known of conditioning, or pre-sport warm-ups. Many had never had adequate coaching, training, or equipment.

The editors of *The Physician and Sports-medicine* were also interested to see what injuries might be occurring among female athletes. In 1974, Joan Gillette, the first certified woman athletic trainer, surveyed physical education departments; the results were published in the journal.[1]

The American Medical Association's Committee on the Medical Aspects of Sports published a statement endorsing the unlimited participation of women in sports. Following this, Dr Donald Cooper, a committee member, brought Ms Gillette and the author together and they conducted two additional surveys among college women. These surveys[2] indicated that the number of injuries to women in athletics was initially higher than to men. This was believed to be primarily because of poor conditioning and training. The types of injuries seen were essentially the same as men. The majority of problems were in the knees and ankles, with women sustaining a higher incidence of shin splints and chondromalacia.

Despite much investigation, the exact mechanism involved in shin splints remains undetermined. It is felt to be an overuse syndrome in which minute periosteal tears in the muscle attachments to the anterior tibia and perhaps actual small stress fractures in the area occur. It is an annoying and painful condition where only rest plus nonsteroidal anti-inflammatory agents appear to alleviate the problem.

Chondromalacia is more complex involving a roughening of the cartilage of the undersurface of the patella due to improper tracking of this structure in its glide path. Many factors play a role and the wider *Q* angle of the femur in relation to the pelvis in the female may contribute to it, but weakness of the attached musculature is probably more important, therefore, good conditioning of particularly the quadriceps and hamstring muscles is the best preventive measure.

Women joggers are particularly susceptible to achilles tendon problems, especially those who began running after having worn high heels most of their lives. Tendonitis is common, and rupture may occur if improper shoes, a poor running surface (rough, uphill or downhill), or bad running form are used. Playing basketball and volleyball where a lot of jumping is involved may cause achilles rupture due to the violent dorsiflexion of the feet combined with a push-off on that flexed foot.

Strengthening and stretching exercises, especially those of the triceps surae muscles (gastrocnemius and soleus) are important to prevention, in addition to proper shoes, etc.

A condition known as "carpal tunnel syndrome" is seen more often in women in general, and among female athletes it may be the result of repetitious-type motions of the wrist as in softball pitching, golf or tennis. It is an entrapment of the medial nerve at the wrist under the carpal ligament resulting in pain, numbness and tingling in the thumb and first and second fingers, which is worse at night. Simple surgery excising a portion of the carpal ligament usually relieves the problem.

Low back pain in young female gymnasts requires special investigation for spondylolysis, a congenital condition in which there is a disruption of the continuity of the lamina of the spine between the posterior facet joints usually at L_4 and L_5. This allows slippage of the body of the superior vertebra anteriorly on the lower vertebra with instability and pressure on the nerve root and resulting spondylolisthesis. If left untreated, disc disruption and even stress fractures can occur. Activity must be stopped and the girl fitted with a modified scoliosis-type brace. Severe cases may require surgery.

Screening of young women for scoliosis (lateral curvature) at the grade school level is a must and if found, early corrective bracing is important. They may continue in many sporting activities with the brace. The author suggests that more details on these and other injuries should be sought in other chapters in this book.

It was noted, however, that despite the increasing numbers of women participating (the number doubled between 1973 and 1975), the percentage of injuries had already begun to decrease. Rapid improvement in conditioning and training probably accounted for this. It was also noted that women were not suffering many severe fractures or head injuries since they rarely participated in collision sports such as football and ice hockey. This trend has continued, and injury rates have dropped further.

The most common injuries occurred as might be expected in sports such as basketball, softball, gymnastics, track and field, field hockey, etc, where contact between players often occurred, or falls from apparatus used in the sports, or the stress of running and jumping events would precipitate such injuries.[3]

Albom[4] stated that "the difference in injuries that often exists between men and women is.... often not related to a structural or physiological difference. Instead it is due to the different sports activities that men and women pursue." Garrich[5] writing about high school female athletes states that, "generally, the type and frequency of injuries were comparable with those seen in noncontact boys' interscholastic sports."

Dr. James Anderson[6] reporting on the physical fitness programs for women at the U.S. Military Academy at West Point noted that while the first class of cadets had 119 young women, only 65% could do one complete pull-up. Within six months, working on their own, 86% could do at least one. The second class had 50% able to do one on admission, and later 70% of the class of '81 could do one. Following classes have done even better as conditioning and upper limb strength have improved.

Women no longer reject the use of weights in training, nor do they fear "building muscles" the way their predecessors did. The extreme of this is now represented by the women participating in body building contests. As a result of better preparation of their bodies for athletic endeavors, less injuries and improved performance by women athletes can be expected.

THE BREASTS

The original survey by the author appeared to show no injuries to the breast. A separate inquiry, not using the term "injury," asked about discomfort to the breasts. This showed that a large number of women were indeed suffering discomfort, resulting primarily from poorly designed brassieres.

The primary problems associated with the brassieres were contusions and abrasions from hooks, allergies to synthetic materials, the bra slipping up over the breasts, and straps slipping off the shoulders. So-called "runner's nipple" from rubbing against the bra seam also occurred. If no bra was worn, the breasts rubbed against the shirt and caused the same problem.

The author, Gail Shierman of the University of Oklahoma, and Ms Gillette filmed some women athletes running on a treadmill. They were filmed wearing no bras, then their own bras, and then with bras that were individually fitted. This last bra was not of an ideal design, but did limit the motion of the breasts. In that respect it proved comfortable for the larger-breasted woman. It was shown that for optimum comfort and safety a bra should restrict breast motion.[7,8]

In addition the authors pointed out that the bras should be made of firm, nonallergic materials (at least 55% cotton) to prevent stretching of the cloth that would lead to bouncing of the breast and irritation of the nipple, yet allow absorption and evaporation of sweat. The straps should be constructed to come close to the midline in the back to prevent slipping off of the shoulders, and the binding band below the breast should be either wide or of a cling-to-the-skin type material to prevent riding up. Only enough elastic in the lower band of the bra to permit unrestricted breathing should be used.

Based on this study and other published criteria a number of bra manufacturers in the United States have designed sport bras that should eliminate the problem.

Direct blows to the breast may result in hematomas. The immediate application of ice to the area will minimize this, but if a large area is involved it should be drained to prevent infection once the bleeding has stopped (usually in 48 hours). Prevention of infection by careful cleansing of any contusions or abrasions is important to avoid breast abscess formation.

Any lumps or masses detected after a blow to the breast should be brought to the attention of a physician if they persist, or if the mass may have possibly been there prior to the blow, to rule out the possibility of malignancy. (Blows to the breast do not cause cancer.)

GENITALIA AND REPRODUCTIVE ORGANS

There are only isolated reports of injuries to the gynecologic system. Injuries of the vulva occur from falls on the balance beam in gymnastics, and vaginal tears from forceful douches occurring when water skiers fall while traveling at high speed. A study on abdominal trauma included several cases of pelvic fractures and pelvic injuries. Despite severe pelvic fractures none of the women sustained any injuries to the reproductive organs. The exception was one patient who was pregnant and suffered an abortion as a result of the injury. There have been very few reported injuries to the reproductive organs associated with trauma to the pelvis. Where the entire pelvis was crushed the injuries were often fatal.

One can conclude that injuries to the reproductive organs of female athletes are unlikely unless the woman is pregnant beyond the first trimester. The reproductive organs are very well protected by the bony structure and only a direct blow or penetrating injury is likely to cause damage.

Uterine injury is more easily sustained when the organ rises up out of the pelvis after the fourth or fifth month of pregnancy. Therefore it is advisable for a pregnant athlete to refrain from any type of collision sports beyond that time. However, no restrictions for noncontact sports are required if the pregnancy is progressing in an uncomplicated manner. Reports have been made of women who have run up to five miles a day within 24 hours of delivery without apparent ill effects.[9,10]

Gold medals have been won in the Olympics by pregnant athletes. However, it would not be advisable for a woman who is not already active in a strenuous sport before she becomes pregnant to begin such a sport once she is.

A well supervised exercise regimen that will strengthen the abdominal and back muscles is certainly a valuable asset for any woman who faces the stress of delivery. Such programs are widely available.

Menstruation

Gynecologists are aware that a sudden stressful event in the life of a woman with normal menstrual periods can bring about cessation of menses.

It has also been noted that women athletes in intense training develop either amenorrhea or irregular periods. Studies show this to be of no consequence. Once stressful training is discontinued the menstrual cycle returns to normal and the woman is able to become pregnant. The same phenomenon is true for women training as ballet dancers. It is an expected physiologic response and causes no distress.

Perhaps a degree of anxiety arose among the athletes because of the delay in onset of menses among the younger women. Their periods did not begin until age 16 or even 18 because of stressful training, dieting, and associated emotional factors. After a let-up in training menarche occurs. Late menarche does not preclude successful pregnancy.

Statistics indicate that 85% of the women who entered West Point, and who were under both physical and mental stress, developed amenorrhea within a few months of arrival. By the end of two years of training all except 7% had resumed normal menstrual cycles and reported fewer side effects such as backache, headache, and dysmenorrhea. A combination of good physical conditioning and proper diet can probably bring about an improvement in patients with menstrual difficulties.[11]

Shangold[12] has pointed out, however, the necessity of endocrine studies in those women who persist in amenorrhea beyond the normal expected onset date (12.8 years)—certainly by age 18, or in those women who had irregular menses prior to the amenorrhea, or who do not regain their cycles within a few months of the reduction of intensive training. Ullyot mentions that amenorrhea associated with lactation is probably a form of natural birth control, but it is also necessary to rule out pregnancy in the face of continued amenorrhea in previously normally menstruating athletes.

Dombovy[13] believes amenorrhea is not a disease but could be of benefit to the athlete by reducing menstrual flow. She points out that athletes who flow heavily during their menses should be checked for anemia, and iron supplementation should be used if mild anemia attributable to no other cause is found. Dietary intake should also be checked for iron content. Occasionally the hematuria seen in marathon runners may add to this problem.

There appears to be no contraindication to the use of birth control pills in women athletes providing they have been on the pill for several months prior to competition. Initial mild early side effects could be a problem if the pills were started just prior to an important competition.

A great deal has been written recently on the psychology of the female athlete. Women do have psychologic problems associated with sports. However, beneficial release of anxiety and aggression during competition are more important than any adverse factors involved in competitiveness among athletes.

REFERENCES

1. Gillette, J. When and where women are injured in sports. *Physician and Sportsmedicine* 3(5): 61–63, 1975.

2. Haycock, C.E., and Gillette, J. Susceptibility of women athletes to injury. *JAMA*. 236(2): 163–165, 1976.

3. Haycock, C.E. *Sports Medicine for the Athletic Female.* Oradell, N.J. Medical Economics, Book Division, 1980.

4. Albom, M. How injuries occur in girl's sports. *Physician and Sportsmedicine* 4:2, 46–49, 1976.

5. Garrick, J.G. Girl's sports injuries in high school athletics. *JAMA* 239:21, 2245–2248, 1978.

6. Anderson, J.L. Sports and physical fitness program for women at the United States Military Academy. *Proceedings of the 20th AMA Symposia*, June 1978.

7. Haycock, C.E. Breast support and protection in the female athlete. *AAHPER Research Consortium Symposium Papers.* Vol. 1, #2, 1978.

8. Haycock, C.E., Shierman, G., and Gillette, J. The female athlete–does her anatomy pose problems? In *Proceedings of the 19th Conference on the Medical Aspects of Sports.* Chicago: American Medical Association, 1978.

9. Hale, R.W. Women and sports: keeping up with female athlete's needs. *Contemp Ob/Gyn.* 13(4):84–95, 1979.

10. Dressendorfer, R.H. Physical training during pregnancy and lactation. *Physician and Sportsmedicine* 6(2):74–80, 1978.

11. Women at the military academies. Symposia. *Physician and Sportsmedicine* 7(4):41–80, 1979.

12. Shangold, M. Evaluating menstrual irregularity in athletes. *Physician and Sportsmedicine* 10:2, 21, 1982.

13. Dombovy, M.L. Amenorrhea. *JAMA*. 243:20–28, 1980.

CHAPTER 9

Injuries Involving the Head and Neck: Experimental and Biomechanical Aspects

Voigt R. Hodgson, PhD

The head and neck are unquestionably the most important and difficult parts of the body to protect in those sports requiring protection. Other vital parts such as heart, lungs, and spleen, have overlying soft tissue and/or ribs to protect them, and are not as prominently situated. Questions that arise when considering head-neck protection are: 1) what are the criteria to be used for evaluating a protective device; 2) what are the tolerable limits of these criteria; 3) what are the potential impact surfaces; 4) what kinematics are involved; 5) how much protection is required compared with how much can be tolerated in terms of size, weight, vision, and mobility; 6) how will the protection of one part affect another?

HEAD INJURY PROTECTION

Cerebral Concussion Tolerance Criteria

Design and evaluation of helmets is based on experimental and clinical evidence of skull fracture and concussion. Sports requiring headgear are: football; box lacrosse; bobsledding; car, motorcycle, and boat racing; bicycling; skiing; hockey; water skiing; skate boarding; polo; and competitive horseback riding. These sports have varied impact potential but all require protection against skull fracture.

Skull fracture is the most basic injury against which a helmet should be designed. By its very construction it provides protection for the scalp and brain. Gurdjian and Schawan noted that 80% of patients admitted to the hospital with linear skull fractures experienced cerebral concussion (CC).[1] From this observation came the first direct end point on which to base a tolerance level for human head impact.

Lissner et al devised the Wayne State University (WSU) Cerebral Concussion Tolerance Curve,[2] shown in Figure 9-1. All the data points used to construct the curve, including cadaver heads dropped to produce linear skull fracture, were indirectly related to CC in the human. Considerable medical and biomechanical subjective decisions went into its derivation.[3] Despite shortcomings, it was the original benchmark. The most commonly used head injury indices, such as the Head Injury Criterion (HIC) and Severity Index (SI), are based on the WSU Curve.[3]

The original curve is considered to be the CC tolerance limit in terms of linear acceleration and time. Head injury criteria are necessary to use with the curve because it is acceleration- and time-related. Most impacts from injury produce *complex pulses* that cannot be directly compared to the tolerance curve. An acceleration-time integration procedure is used, in which the acceleration is raised to a power of 2.5 in both SI and HIC procedure is: $\text{HIC} = (t_2\text{-}t_1)\ [1/t_1\text{-}t_2 \int_{t_1}^{t_2} A(t)\ dt]^{2.5}$ where t is pulse duration and A(t) is resultant acceleration (measured by gravity, or g) measured at the center of gravity of the head. The HIC procedure is: $\text{HIC} = (t_2\text{-}t_1)\ [1/t_1\text{-}t_2\ {}_{t}\ll^{t_2} A(t)\ dt]^{2.5}$ where t_1 and t_2 are the initial and final times (sec) during the pulse for which HIC attains a maximum value.

Gadd[4] set an upper SI limit of 1000 as representing a dangerous CC level for concentrated impact. Derivation of the curve is asymptotic to roughly 40 g for long duration pulses. Patrick et al suggested 80 g as the limit for distributed impacts.[5] Gadd followed this with a 1500 SI limit

The head and neck injury research on which this paper is based was supported by the National Operating Committee on Standards for Athletic Equipment.

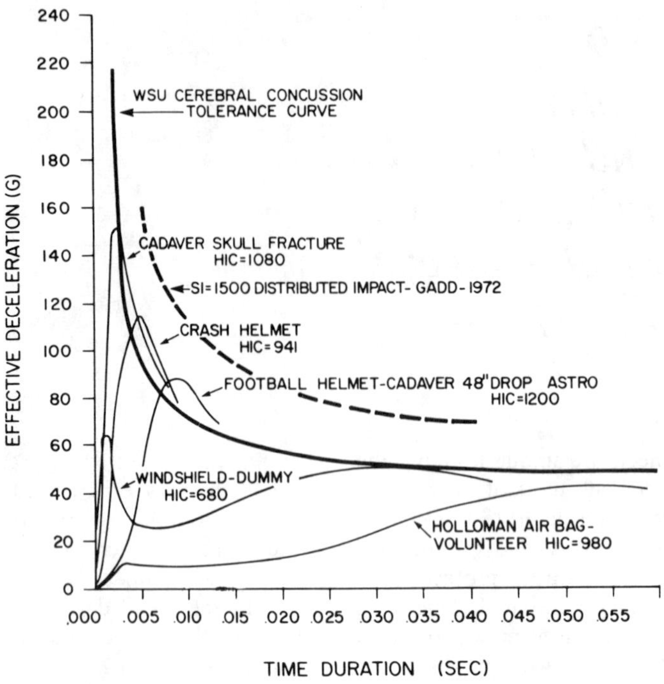

Figure 9-1 Concussion tolerance curves for concentrated and distributed (helmet) impact, with response curves of typical impact situations and associated head injury indices, to demonstrate validity.

for distributed impacts in which the skull fracture hazard is not present. This is based upon other considerations including volunteer airbag impact results.[6] The foregoing are often used on human surrogates (cadavers and dummies) to evaluate a protective device or system. Occasionally, in cases of distributed impact, they are used on human volunteers up to judiciously determined injury levels.[6]

The original acceleration-time data used to construct the short duration part of the WSU curve were based upon average acceleration. The uniform acceleration lasts over the effective duration of a pulse. It produces the same velocity change as would be obtained by integrating the area under the pulse. Thus, both the concentrated and distributed SI curves (Figure 9-1), can be plotted on a kinematics chart relating uniform acceleration, time, velocity changes, and stopping distance (Figure 9-2). Assume the distributed impact curve (SI = 1500) indicates tolerable limits for a sports participant. Designers can gauge the amount of stopping distance needed for a given change in velocity in a given time, to avoid possible concussion. Such a stopping distance is the theoretical minimum, possible only with 100% efficient material, which is not available.

There recently arose out of the Society of Automotive Engineers Human Biomechanical Simulation Subcommittee, a position paper on Head Injury Criterion (HIC) levels, in which percentage of population expected to experience a severe brain injury vs HIC levels, was plotted.[7] The HIC values can be transformed to approximate SI for football helmet drop-test type impacts.[8] This plot will allow HIC or SI values to be selected as design goals or standard compliance limits that reflect the degree of severe brain injury risk willing to be accepted for the specific environment being considered.

Protective Helmet Design Considerations

Material efficiency Efficiency = A_u/A_p, where A_u is the uniform negative acceleration possible for a given distance and impact velocity. A_p is peak acceleration measured on a rigid body which strikes a material of the same thickness (distance) overlaying a rigid plate at the same impact velocity. This ranges between 20% and 45% and varies with thickness, impact velocity, and temperature. Every material has an optimum thickness for energy ab-

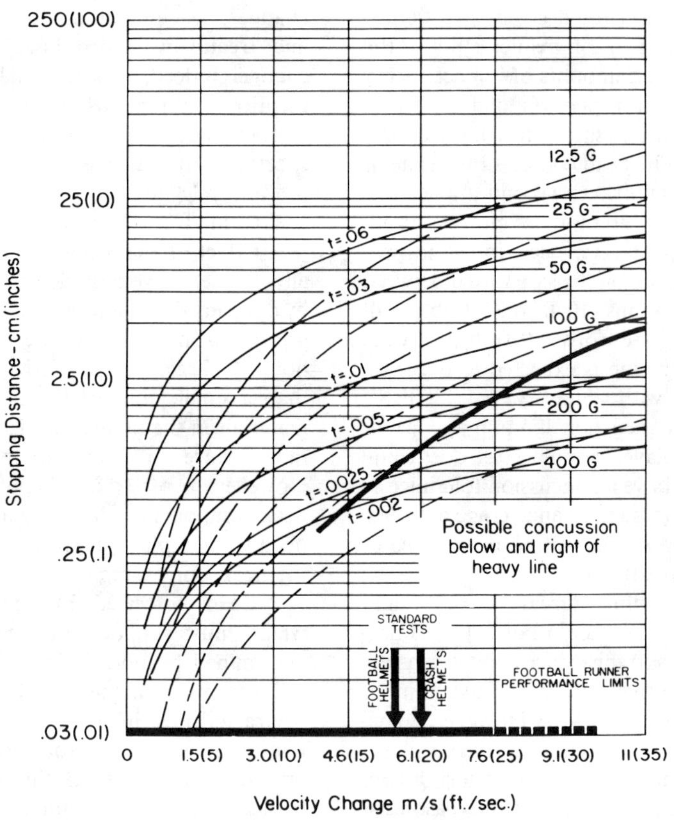

Figure 9-2 Kinematics chart on which is plotted the concussion tolerance curve for nonconcentrated impacts (SI = 1500) (see Figure 10-1) used in the *NOCSAE* football helmet standard. Given a stopping distance and velocity change requirement, the time duration and average acceleration (from which head injury criteria can be computed) are determined. This is the ideal against which to gauge a helmet's performance.

sorption and linear head acceleration tolerance limits. Some of the best materials at low to normal temperatures can be dangerously soft under elevated temperature conditions.

Comfort The most efficient materials are usually also the stiffest. In a limited space therefore, a very efficient material cannot be tolerated next to the scalp because of uncomfortable high pressure points. Part of the space must be taken up by a layer of comfort foam. Some space must be allocated to air, since at 20°C (68°F), roughly 25% of body heat loss is from the head. This is despite the fact that the head comprises only about 7% of total body surface area. Most heat loss is due to evaporation. It is aided by the pumping action of the helmet bouncing on the head, forcing air out around the lower edges.[9,10] Coleman and Mortage[11] showed a significant difference among football helmets with web suspension systems (lower air temperatures around the head), and those with form-fitting inflatable, and hammock suspension systems.

Shell deflection Ideally, the shell would not deflect, leaving the space between head and shell available for energy absorption (EA) and material deformation. However, such a shell would tend to be heavy and rigid, posing a threat of neck injury to the wearer, and a general injury hazard to opponents.

Energy absorption (EA) space Even when "bottomed" (the condition where the material can absorb no energy, ie, deformation becomes negligible as force increases excessively), foam EA thickness is considerable, depending upon the area it covers. Consequently, the effective stopping distance may be on the order of only one-half the unloaded thickness of the EA. In this respect, suspension helmets have an advantage over foam liners in space utilization for a given shell deflection. However, if a suspension helmet is put to the test of absorbing greater amounts of impact energy than the combined shell suspension load-deflection capabilities, a sudden transition in head acceleration can occur when the head contacts the inside of the shell in what amounts to a second impact.

Human tolerance variation Among a group of seven embalmed cadavers, peak forces to produce linear skull fracture on the side varied between 4.67 and 15.0 kilonewtons (1050 to 3360 lb), with an average of 8.5 kilonewtons (1910 lb).[12] In the average person concussion is expected to occur on distributed impact with intensity of 1500 SI. However, tolerable concussion limits may vary as widely among the player populace as does skull fracture. Some may have a concussion tolerance as low as 300 to 400 SI (assuming an average acceleration tolerance spread similar to the peak force to produce fracture spread).

Cerebrovascular injury threat It is thought that concussion is the threshold brain injury. Football experience attests to this, since concussions are vastly more common then cerebrovascular injuries or contusions to the brain surface. However, an occasional atypical accident occurs in which a player suffers a serious brain injury without losing consciousness until much later. Part of the reason for this has nothing to do with equipment or the sport itself. The rate of cerebrovascular disease among 15- to 24-year-old men in the United States, about 70% of which are cerebral hemorrhages, runs between 1 and 2 per 100,000.[13] The average death rate due to head injury among 1,200,000 junior and high school football players for the 1964–1970 seasons was 1.56 per 100,000, almost all of which were caused by subdural hematomas.[14] Probably some football players have low tolerance for cerebrovascular injury.

It appears, however, that even among the football population, which may include low-tolerance individuals, helmet changes that produce better linear acceleration impact attenuation relative to a concussion standard, can also help reduce the incidence of subdural hematomas. It is conjectured by numerous people that subdural hematomas are related to angular acceleration. During the 1971–1983 period during which time the NOCSAE football helmet research program has had an influence on new and used helmets, death due to head injury declined by 64% compared to the 1964–1970 period, for which statistics were available for high school players.[14] It should be emphasized that there are many factors such as rules changes, teaching techniques, rules enforcement, and treatment, which have also contributed to change. Indeed, it is essential that the previously mentioned limitations on equipment and unknown factors about head injury be recognized in all sports. Head gear must be removed from offensive use and relegated to its proper role of protecting against inadvertent impact.

Effect of the helmet on the neck Traditionally, helmets have been designed to protect the head by covering the cranium in such a way as to prevent injuries from penetration and excessive acceleration. A larger helmet provides more protection than a smaller one of the same construction and materials in the same head size, because it provides more space in which to brake head motion. However, increased inertia puts an added strain on neck components when they are forced to stop the head when a player is struck on a blind side below the neck, for example.

Load perceived by the neck components, which must support and decelerate the head, is determined by both weight and center of gravity (CG) location of the head-helmet combination.[15] Characteristics inherent in shell geometry, EA materials, and neck protection, work to increase weight and raise the CG, thus increasing the hazard of neck injury. For example, EA foams generally become more efficient as the density (weight/unit volume) and/or thickness are increased. If shells are made larger they must also be made thicker to maintain rigidity. Consequently there is increased weight and probably a rise in the CG, as well as reduction of the field of vision. Raising the helmet to include more crown EA for increased neck axial compression protection, introduces more inertia and leverage for shear and flexural neck loading. Even though minimum standards are set at 1500 SI, most manufacturers strive toward lower SI test performances to provide what they believe to be a safer product. This usually leads to either stiffer, or larger and heavier helmets.

Other head protection devices or design considerations that directly or indirectly may affect neck injury are face mask, chin strap, helmet edge location, and surface hardness.

Face masks are required in football primarily to protect the teeth.[16] They have become mandatory in some levels of ice hockey and box lacrosse, primarily to protect the eyes.[17,18] There are various types and all can impinge on other surfaces, or be illegally grabbed to act as a lever on the helmet to flex or twist the neck. Their effectiveness in transmitting loads to the neck depend, in turn, upon standoff, rigidity of the mask, rigidity of attachment, helmet fit, and chin strap design, ie, two or four points of attachment, and strength. This threat to the neck may be more apparent than real. Torg et al have published a study of 209 football-related neck injuries, 73 of which resulted in permanent cervical quadriplegia.[19] They divided the causes into eight categories and found that none of these serious injuries was due to the face mask acting as a lever. No relation between the mask and lesser injuries was discussed.

Cutting the shell higher in the rear as advocated by Schneider[20] exposes more vital areas of upper neck as well as allowing more neck extension that a longer skirt would help to limit. The neck is much less able to resist extension than flexion because of differences in muscle mass and leverage.[21]

The hard, smooth shell has been criticized as a source of injury to opponents. Solutions to this problem have appeared in the form of permanent or slip-over soft covers. Concern for serviceability and the effects on the neck of added helmet weight and size have kept them from being adopted.

NECK INJURY PROTECTION

Background

Injury to the neck is caused in essentially four ways: 1) slowly applied loads to the head and/or neck, as in wrestling; 2) direct impact to the neck; 3) inertial loading of the head, eg, a blind-sided blow to the body; 4) impact to or by the head. Although serious injury can occur in the first instance, rules rather than equipment are used for protection. The second and third ways can produce a variety of pulled muscles, strained ligaments, and pinched nerve injuries that are difficult to diagnose, treat, or analyze biomechanically. Paralyzing injuries to the cord are primarily caused by the fourth method. They occur when loads are applied by impact with relatively large masses. A tap on the head by a pipe will be reacted to almost exclusively by the inertia of the head. A dive into the bottom of a swimming hole, or running into an opponent's chest with the crown of the head, will produce sustained loading of the cervical spine. Because of the sometimes catastrophic nature of this (fourth) type of loading and the vague understanding of mechanics and tolerable levels, it is felt that, in a limited space, it is best treated exclusively. This will be done by discussing static loading as a lead-in to understanding dynamic loading of the cervical spine.

Static Loading

Anatomic consideration The cervical cord is sheathed in a system of vertebrae, intervertebral discs, ligaments, and muscles that provide adequate protection and movement for ordinary loads and tasks. Statically, the CG of the head falls slightly forward of the base of support of the head, which is supplied by the atlas (C1) reaction against the occipital condyles. Consequently, a slight amount of posterior muscle tension is required to keep the head from nodding into flexion when one is seated or standing erect. In addition to the static moment resisted by the muscles, the axial component of load (head weight plus axial component of muscle force) is transmitted to the two concave superior articulating surfaces (permits the rocking "yes" gesture) on either side of the atlas. (There would also be a small shear force acting on the neck to counteract the horizontal component of muscle forces.) Load is in turn passed through the smoother articulating surfaces between C1 and C2 that permit the gliding "no" gesture. Vertebra C1 does not have a body but C2 does, and transmits the load to C3 through the uppermost intervertebral disc and articulating facets mounted on either side and slightly to the rear of the vertebral body. Vertebrae C3 to C7 are similar in construction and transmit the axial load in the same manner as between C2 and C3. Axial load below C2 is thus transmitted over a triangular area comprised of the body and facets.

The facets have been found in test specimens to carry anywhere from 0% to 18% of statically applied compressive loads.[22] (In intact cadavers loaded by means of caudocephalad acceleration, they have been found to share up to 33% of the load in the lumbar region.[23]) The intervertebral discs serve to form bonds of connection between vertebrae, distribute the load over the end plates of the bodies, and prevent rapid force buildup (absorb shock). They do this by virtue of pliable annular fibers enclosing the nucleus pulposus, which is highly elastic and contains fluid ranging from 70% to 90%. In the cervical region from the inferior surface of C2 through C7, the discs make up about 25% of the length. They are thicker ventrally in the cervical region, thus contributing to the cervical curve that is normally convex anteriorly from C2 through T2. The cervical spine also has a slight lateral curvature, convex toward the dominant hand.[24,25]

The integrity of the cervical spine from excessive relative movement between adjacent vertebrae is maintained by strong longitudinal ligaments connected to the skull and running anteriorly and posteriorly along the bodies. Also, a group of five ligaments connecting the laminae, spinous, and transverse processes, and a complex of ligaments and membranes connecting occipital bone, atlas, and axis contribute to the maintenance of integrity. Basic movements in the cervical spine are: 1) flexion, or bending ventrally, which is the most extensive, and is limited by chin contact with the chest in normal movement; 2) extension, or bending dorsally, limited by the anterior longitudinal ligament, and spinous process-ligament interference; 3) lateral flexion, in which the sides of the discs are compressed, and in which motion is limited by resistance offered by the surrounding ligaments; and 4) rotation, allowed predominantly between C1 and C2, but also by twisting of the discs and gliding motion, allowed between the inferior facets of C2 through the inferior facets of C7. This movement is limited by capsular ligament resistance.

Shear force vulnerability Shear forces are resisted only by ligaments between the occipital bone and C1, and C1 and C2.[21] Below C2 the facet joints are slanted at approximately 45° as viewed from the side. Bone-to-bone interlocking surfaces are formed, which, along with ligaments, resist shear forces. Shear forces arise from head-loading that produces bending—a transverse-to-cervical axis component—or that applies torsion, and therefore rotation to the neck. Farfan has found that the disc and longitudinal ligaments share equally with the two facets, including their capsular ligaments, about 90% of torsional strength of the cervical spine. The remaining 10% is contributed by the interspinous ligaments.[26]

Roaf[27] investigated the question of why on one occasion a relatively small force produces a serious dislocation or slipped disc, whereas, on another occasion a much larger force produces only a relatively minor vertebral crush. He found the discs, joints, and ligaments to be very resistant to compression, distraction, flexion, and extension, but very vulnerable to rotation and horizontal shearing forces.

He achieved uniform results from loading 18 spinal units (two vertebrae, an intervertebral disc, two posterior articulations, and a number of ligaments), in compression. A force of 6.23 kilonewtons (1400 lb) was reached before the load fell off slightly, coincident with bulging of the end plates, which caused blood to be squeezed out of the cancellous bone of the vertebral body. He considered this latter action to be an important shock-absorbing mechanism in the spine. The intact disc was found to be more resistant to vertical compression than was the vertebral body, which failed at 7.12 kilonewtons (1600 lb). When he held the spinal unit in slight flexion and applied a rotational force, the posterior ligaments, joint capsules, and posterior longitudinal ligaments tore in that order, resulting in a typical dislocation. He was unable to succeed in producing pure hyperflexion (when disruption of posterior ligaments occurs) injuries of a normal intact spinal unit. Before the posterior ligaments ruptured, the vertebral body was always crushed. He calculated that the pressure at the anterior vertebral body edges (fulcrum) was three to four times as great as tension in posterior ligaments, whose breaking point was cited as being about 1.78 kilonewtons (400 lb). Pressure on the disc nucleus was therefore, 5.34 to 7.12 kilonewtons (1200 to 1600 lb), which exceeds the breaking point of the vertebral end plate. Very similar results were obtained with extension and lateral bending. Roaf's work confirmed that spontaneous reduction of rotation dislocations can occur. Radiologic examination alone will fail to reveal the extent of damage and degree of spinal instability. In general, he found that rotation forces produce dislocations, and compression forces produce fracture.

Bauze and Ardran devised an experiment in which entire cervical spines, with basiocciput attached, were subjected to compressive loads with the lower part of the spine flexed and fixed, and the upper spine extended and free to move forward. Bilateral dislocation of the facets was produced without fracture with only 1.42 kilonewtons (319 lb).[28] They found that the maximum load coincided with the rupture of the posterior ligament and capsule, and stripping of the anterior longitudinal ligament, prior to dislocation. Loading was described as a combination of vertical compression, flexion, and horizontal shear forces.

The results obtained by Roaf, and Bauze and Ardran point out that injuries to the spine are dependent not only on magnitude of loading, but also upon its direction, point of application, and orientation of the spine. Such findings as these make it appear almost impossible to determine tolerance levels on which to base the design of neck protection under conditions where head impact is common and mobility essential. It should be kept in mind that these experiments utilized partial spines with special loading conditions designed to discover the mechanics of cervical spine failure.

Dynamic Loading

Limitations of muscle protection There are common loading situations in which rotation is minimal, and also where neck musculature can prevent excessive shear forces from reaching the spine. As noted by Mertz,[21] articulation of the neck and head is accomplished through muscle pairs that are attached to the skull, individual vertebrae, and torso. These pairs, which are symmetric with respect to the midsagittal plane, respond in various group actions to produce desired movement of the head and neck. Similarly, in some situations a performer can anticipate and use the leverage of these muscle groups to help resist rotational and bending movements of the spine caused by headloading, thereby preventing the spine ligaments from being stretched or torn. Obviously, neck muscles strengthened by exercise will provide more protection for the spine against bending and torsional head-loading.

Foust et al[29] have found that neck extensor muscles in the 18- to 24-year-old, 80th to 99th percentile group, seated erect, can exert about 191 newtons (43 lb) when the head is loaded horizontally through its CG, compared to 162 newtons (36.3 lb) by flexor muscles. They deduced that these values may represent about 80% of maximum available physiologic strength capacity. Muscle reflex times were in the 58 to 74 msec range, and muscle activation was in the 57 to 75 msec range.

If loads are applied through the head with a major SI (compressive) component offset from the cervical axis but with negligible rotational effect, the tendency will be to compress and bend the cervical column. With impulsive loading, the neck muscles, which cannot resist spinal compression, and which require considerable time to activate relative to time to peak impact force (25 to 30 msec),[30] may not even be involved in trying to maintain the spinal alignment, depending upon whether the load is anticipated or not. Even if anticipated, the loading may be too great for the muscles to resist, and bending of the cervical spine will occur in the direction dictated by load eccentricity from the cervical axis and curvature of the spinal column at impact. Construction of the neck allows ample overall movement in the normal cervical spine, to the extent of motion limiting contact of the head with chest in flexion, shoulders in lateral bending, and tissue interference in rotation and extension. However, under the action of an eccentric compressive load, excessive stresses can occur in the spine even before reaching head rotational motion limiting contact, such as chin with chest. Once bent, it is easier for the compressive component of load to cause further buckling of the cervical spine.

Effect of head rotation restriction by loading surface Situations arise in sports in which a participant runs into, or is struck on the crown of the head by a relatively large mass moving at moderate speed, such as running into another player or meeting with an obstacle, ie, skating into ice hockey boards, diving onto an underwater surface, falling onto a mat or trampoline. Loading on the head or helmet prevents or restricts head rotation with respect to the neck, most of which normally occurs between the skull and C2. Consequently, the head cannot rotate to a limiting position that would transfer some of the load into the trunk.[21] Since the trunk mass, and therefore inertia, is relatively much greater than that of the neck, and since the thorax is so much more rigid than the neck, the work of absorbing the energy of impact to the crown must be done primarily by the cervical spine.

If the loading is on the crown, somewhat anterior to the cervical axis and symmetric about the midsagittal plane, a situation that commonly arises in football, it is similar to the static loads applied to a complete human cervical spine by Bauze and Ardran.[28] They described the loading as creating a combination of vertical compression, flexion, and horizontal shear forces at the juncture where forward bilateral dislocation of the facets was produced, at only 1.42 kilonewtons (319 lb). In their experiment, if lateral tilt or axial rotation occurred as well, a unilateral dislocation was produced.

Roaf noted that most human injuries are the consequence of rapidly acting forces, but on the few occasions when he applied a rapidly acting force, the general pattern of response was similar to the pattern when slowly acting forces were used. Consequently, it is theorized that head-gripping action by the dynamic loading surface is one of the reasons for the occasional catastrophic injury that occurs at impact intensity levels similar to, or even much lower than, the multitudes of collisions that happen routinely. For example, in the 1977 football season, Mueller and Arnold[31] reported 17 catastrophic head and neck injuries among high school, college, and sandlot players. Of these eight died and nine were reported with varying degrees of paralysis. There were 10 to 12 neck injuries in this group, the number of which is uncertain, but at least 1,500,000 high school and college players are included. Comparing the huge numbers of apparently violent blocks and tackles involving the head and neck that must transpire in the course of a season, to the ease with which Roaf,[27] and Bauze and Ardran[28] produced dislocation in cervical spine specimens, leads one to conjecture why more are not seriously injured. It is even more puzzling considering the head loads that can easily be developed in situations where the crown of the head strikes a surface with the spinal axis aligned perpendicular to the surface, ie, the neck is compressed between impact surface and the body.

Vulnerability of the Neck to High Compressive Loads

It is apparent that excessive crown loads can be achieved at energy levels far below those often generated on the football field. For example, considering one-half the mass of a .89 kilonewtons (200 lb) player running at 9.1 m/sec (30 ft/sec), the kinetic energy is 1900 joules (1400 ft-lb).

Based on the above findings four theories can be devised:

1. The necks of live young players are much stronger than tests on cervical sections of cadavers would indicate;
2. The neck is a very good energy absorber;
3. Large amounts of kinetic energy are rarely absorbed by the neck; or
4. A combination of player control, training, rules of the game, and neck design usually work to protect the neck from head-loading that causes ligaments to fail in shear.

Some reasons for support or rejection of these theories may be found in the results described by Mertz et al,[30] pertinent parts of which are summarized in the following section.

Tolerance to Axial Compressive Neck Loads

An injury reference curve was constructed for high school football players based upon axial compressive neck loads and time duration, measured in a Hybrid III dummy under injury-simulating conditions. The reference proposed is a straight line starting with coordinates of 0 msec and 6.67 kilonewtons (1500 lb), sloping to 35 msec and 1.11 kilonewtons (250 lb), and constant at 1.11 kilonewtons for durations greater than 35 msec (Figure 9-3). The peak value of 6.67 kilonewtons (1500 lb) determined by accident reproduction with a dummy (which had been calibrated for neck response on the basis of cadaver and volunteer horizontal sled tests,[15]) fell between the 6.23 kilonewtons (1400 lb) first load drop-off, and ultimate load of 7.12 kilonewtons (1600 lb), obtained by Roaf from static compression tests of a cervical spine unit (uniform results claimed on 18 specimens).[27]

These correlations indicate that theory 1 is erroneous at least for axial compressive loads. This might be expected since pure axial compressive loading involves the strength of the vertebra. Theory 1 may still be true for other than axial loads, where muscle strength may assist in preventing excessive bending or rotation from stretching or tearing ligaments. For theory 2 to be true would require the neck to deflect much more than it is capable of compressing in the axial direction. Roaf showed a deflection of 3.8 mm (0.15 inch) at ultimate load for one spinal unit (two vertebrae and a disk). There are roughly four units in the cervical spine and consequently total deflection to failure would be on the order of 15.2 mm (0.60 inch). Using the first drop-off load of Roaf 6.23 kilonewtons (1400 lb), this means the neck could absorb about 95 joules (70 ft-lb) of energy in the axial direction. Consequently, theory 2 is out of the question.

More than likely theories 3 and 4 are primary reasons for the extremely low incidence of neck injury in football. In the Hybrid III dummy tests, a dynamic tackling block was used to deliver impacts to the helmeted head. The block was a padded cylinder that could rotate on its vertical axis, and also about a horizontal pipe along which it was propelled. As a consequence it was difficult to deliver a flush impact to the stationary dummy head that was necessary to produce high axial neck forces. Similarly in the field, a tackler (which is the most dangerous role[19,31]) rarely meets a ball carrier head-on in such a way as to absorb all of the energy of the runner at full speed. When it does happen there is usually much more stopping distance available than the allowable neck axial deflection, to absorb energy.

The foregoing determinations concerning neck loading based upon cadaver, dummy, and cervical

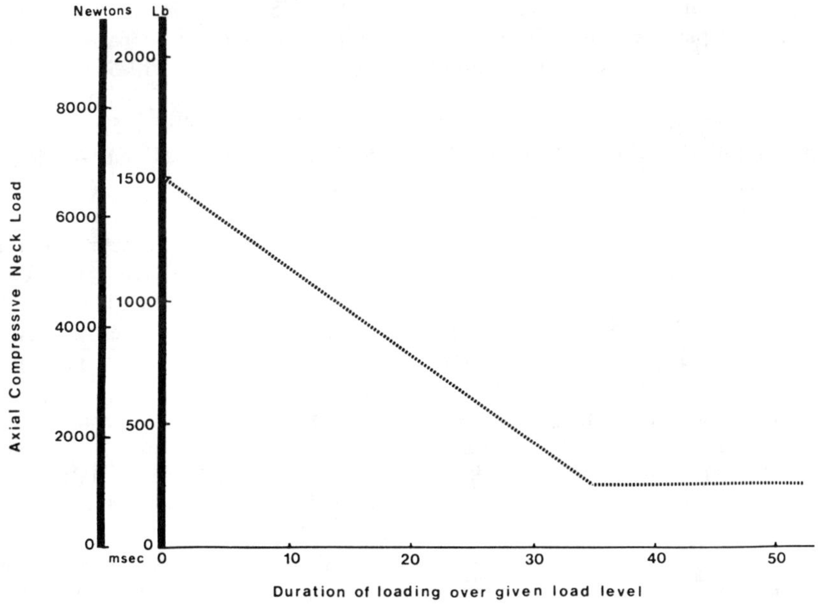

Figure 9-3 Proposed neck injury reference for axial compressive neck forces in high school football players.

section studies, have been approximated by at least one field accident. Torg et al[32] reported the case of a defensive back hitting a ball carrier in the chest with the anterior crown of the helmet. Both players dropped vertically to the ground. The tackled player had the wind knocked out of him, but the tackler suffered unilateral dislocation between the articular processes of C3 and C4. Film coverage of the event was very good both laterally and from behind the tackler. The relative velocity was 9.8 m/sec (32.2 ft/sec) and the victim was stopped in 60 msec from time of contact. Average deceleration of the body and the average axial force on the neck was calculated to be 18 g and between 3.5 and 6.2 kilonewtons (790 and 1390 lb), respectively. Automotive injury researchers consider a 7.5 cm (3 inch) chest deflection measured in a human surrogate to be AIS 3 (Abbreviated Injury Scale), which is a threat to life.[33]

Of all the items listed in theories 3 and 4, changing rules and techniques may be the most important of all neck protection devices, mechanical or schematic. Mueller and Arnold investigated the effect of 1976 football rules changes in the National Collegiate Athletic Association and the National Federation of State High School Associations, which made it an infraction of the rules to use the helmeted head as the initial point of contact when blocking and tackling.[31] Their preliminary results demonstrated that the rules changes have "dramatically reduced the number of fatalities associated with catastrophic head and neck injuries."

Since their report, paralyzing neck injuries have been reduced from an annual average of 21.1 during the 1971–1976 seasons, down to 10.8 from 1977 through 1983, among high school and college football players.

One of the most compelling reasons for keeping the head out of football has been demonstrated in a head spearing simulation with the Hybrid III dummy. It was found that there is a critical location of contact on the front of the helmet, which, if the head is lowered to strike an opponent above this point, the neck is trapped in a bent attitude. Axial compression and the bending moment resisting couple can be combined in the dummy neck to produce what would be human spine failure load levels, according to Figure 9-3, at only 3.3 m/s (11 ft/sec). If the dummy's head makes contact in a head-up position, the head is knocked aside or up and the neck is not trapped into absorbing its own body energy, which is instead taken out through the chest or shoulder. Translated to the field, this critical position is roughly making contact no higher on the helmet than 76mm (3 in) above the front rim, with the body in a stable football running attitude. It is all too often mentioned in the neck injury registries that the injured player lowered his head, either intentionally, or perhaps flinching, while tackling, blocking, or running with the ball. Mueller and Blyth reported the head down attitude in 6/7 cases of paralyzing neck injuries in 1982 and 8/11 cases in 1983, among high school players, the remaining cases being unknown.[34,35] The numbers permanently paralyzed have remained rather uniform during the 1977–1983 period. If further reductions are to be made, the rules must be augmented by coaching and/or equipment aimed at keeping the head up.

Playing heads up football is not only safer than hitting with the head down, but can be done very effectively. Sweeney High School, Sweeney, Texas, has used a chin roll designed to keep the head up, on its entire offensive and defensive units for several years and has been in or near the state class AAA playoff finals in 1982 and 1983 (Personal communication, Bob Pyssen, head coach and athletic director).

CONCLUSION

Head injuries can be and are being reduced in sports, particularly football, by virtue of new and used helmet improvements, new rules, and teaching changes. Helmet improvements have been achieved by adjusting head sizes, materials, construction, and quality control measures to fit test method and performance requirements that are tuned to existing head injury knowledge and field kinematics. Rules and teaching techniques have been instituted that recognize the limitations of equipment in terms of physical characteristics and ability to prevent all forms of brain injury in all situations among participants with a wide range of tolerance.

Paralyzing neck injury has been reduced by almost 50% as a result of the 1976 rules changes prohibiting initial contact by the helmet in blocking and tackling. Further reductions may be possible through coaching and the use of equipment designed to keep the head up.

REFERENCES

1. Gurdjian, E.S., and Schawan, H.K. Management of skull fracture involving the frontal sinus. *Ann Surg*. 95:22–23, 1932.

2. Lissner, H.P., Lebow, M., and Evans, F.G. Experimental studies on the relation between acceleration and intracranial pressure changes in man. *Surg Gynecol Obstet*. 3:329–338, 1960.

3. King, A.I. Survey of the state of the art of human biodynamic response. Edited by K. Saczalski, G.T. Singley, III, W.D. Pilkey et al. In *Aircraft Crashworthiness*. Charlottesville, Va: University Press of Virginia, 1975, pp. 83–120.

4. Gadd, C.W. Criteria for injury potential. In *Impact Acceleration Stress,* Publication 977. Washington, DC: National Academy of Science, 1962, pp. 141–145.

5. Patrick, L.M., Lissner, H.R., and Gurdjian, E.S. Survival by design—head protection. In *Proceedings of the Seventh Stapp Car Crash Conference*. Springfield, Ill: Charles C Thomas, 1965.

6. Gadd, C.W. Tolerable severity index in whole-head, nonmechanical impact. Presented at Proceedings of the Fifteenth Stapp Car Crash Conference. Cironado, California, November 17–19, 1971.

7. Position Paper on HIC Levels. Prepared by U.S.A. Delegation, ISO/TC22/SC12/WG6, AFNOR, France, 1983.

8. Hodgson, V. R. Improving head crash protection. *Proceedings of the Twenty First Annual Symposium, Safe Association*. San Antonio, Texas, Safe Association, Nov. 5–8, 1983.

9. Goldman, R.F. *Physiological Studies on Headwear*. Natick, Mass: US Army Natick Clothing and Personal Life Support Equipment Laboratory.

10. Fonseca, G.F. *Heat Transfer Properties of Military Protective Headgear*. Natick, Mass: US Army Natick Clothing and Personal Life Support Equipment Laboratory, 1974.

11. Coleman, A.E., and Mortage, A.K. Ambient head temperature and football helmet design. *Med Sci Sports*. 5(3):553–558, 1970.

12. Hodgson, V.R., and Murray, T.L. *Breaking Strength of the Human Skull vs Impact Surface Curvature*. Washington, DC: US Department of Transportation, 1973.

13. *Cerebrovascular Survey Report,* Revised. Washington, DC: National Institute of Neurological and Communicative Disorders and Stroke, and National Heart and Lung Institute, 1976.

14. Hodgson, V.R. NOCSAE helmet tests are tougher: here are the steps that make the standard work. *Athletic Purchasing and Facilities*. 2(2):26–28, 1978.

15. Mertz, H.J., Jr., and Patrick L.M. Investigation of the kinematics and kinetics of whiplash. Presented at Proceedings of the Eleventh Stapp Car Crash Conference. Anaheim, California, 1967.

16. *Football Rule Book, The National Alliance Edition*. Elgin, Ill: National Federation of State High School Associations, 1975.

17. *Face Protectors For Ice Hockey and Box Lacrosse Players.* Rexdale, Ontario, Canada: Canadian Standard Association, 1978.

18. *Face Guard Standards.* Philadelphia: American Society for Testing and Materials, 1979.

19. Torg, J.S., Truex, R., Jr., Quedenfeld, T.C. et al. The national football head and neck injury registry. *JAMA.* 241(14):1477–1478, 1979.

20. Schneider, R.C. *Head and Neck Injuries in Football: Mechanisms, Treatment, and Prevention.* Baltimore: Williams and Wilkins, 1973.

21. Mertz, H.J., Jr. Neck injury. In *Biomechanics and Its Application to Automotive Design.* New York: Society of Automotive Engineers, Inc., 1973.

22. Nachemson, A. Lumbar interdiscal pressure. *Acta Orthop Scand.* 43(suppl), 1960.

23. King, A.I., Prasad, P., and Ewing, C.L. Mechanism of spinal injury due to caudocephalad acceleration. *Orthop Clin North Am.* 6:19, 1975.

24. White, A.A., and Pajabi, M.M. *Clinical Biomechanics of the Spine.* Philadelphia: J.B. Lippincott, 1978.

25. Gray, H. *Anatomy of the Human Body,* 9th American Ed. Edited by C.M. Goss. Philadelphia: Lea and Febiger, 1975.

26. Farfan, H.F. *Mechanical Disorders of the Low Back.* Philadelphia: Lea and Febiger, 1973.

27. Roaf, R. A study of the mechanics of spinal injury. *J Bone Joint Surg.* 42B(4):810–823, 1960.

28. Bauze, R.J., and Ardran, M.A. Experimental production of forward dislocation in the human cervical spine. *J Bone Joint Surg.* 60B(2):95–106, 1978.

29. Foust, D.R., Chaffin, D.B., Snyder, R.G. et al. Cervical range of motion and dynamic response and strength of cervical muscles. In *Proceedings of the Seventeenth Stapp Car Crash Conference.* New York: Society of Automotive Engineers, Inc., 1972.

30. Mertz, H.J., Jr., Hodgson, V.R., Thomas, L.M. et al. An assessment of compressive neck loads under injury producing conditions. *Physician and Sportsmedicine* November, 1978.

31. Mueller, F.O., and Arnold, D.C. Catastrophic head and neck football injuries. *Physician and Sportsmedicine* October, 1979.

32. Torg, J.S., Truex, R.C., Jr., Marshall, J. et al. Spinal injury at the level of the third and fourth cervical vertebrae from football. *J Bone Joint Surg.* 59A(8):1017–1019, 1977.

33. American Medical Association. *The Abbreviated Injury Scale (AIS),* Revised. New York: Society of Automotive Engineers, Inc., 1976.

34. Mueller, F. O., and Blyth, C. S. *Annual Survey of Catastrophic Football Injuries, 1977–1982.* Department of Physical Education, Chapel Hill, University of North Carolina.

35. Mueller, F. O., and Blyth, C. S. *Annual Survey of Catastrophic Football Injuries,* 1977–1983. Department of Physical Education, Chapel Hill, University of North Carolina.

CHAPTER 10
Injuries Involving the Head and Neck: Clinical and Anatomic Aspects

Francis X. Rockett, MD

The clinical evaluation of an injured athlete must proceed expeditiously and be based on long recognized principles. Chief among these is the Hippocratic prohibition: "First, do no harm."

Whenever the injury of a player involves loss of consciousness, the examining physician simultaneously moves in three spheres: 1) he conducts a rapid baseline assessment of the player's physical condition, 2) assures an adequate airway, and 3) plans for transportation of the player from the field to an area where more detailed evaluation and treatment can be carried out. From the instant of injury, all observations are used to answer the most important question in neurology: what is the rate and direction of change in relation to time? This question is represented by the mathematical formula, $\triangle_t$. The simple mnemonic is the key to clinical evaluation of any head- or neck-injured patient. It determines the rapidity with which a patient must be evacuated or operated on; it prevents unnecessary hospitalizations; it is the basis for determining when and if a player returns to active competition.

In order to assess change, the initial examination determines the following:

1. Is the patient conscious?
2. Is the patient breathing?
3. Is the patient moving all extremities?
4. What is the least stimulus to which the patient will respond?

From these basics, more detailed observations of neurologic signs can be made while arrangements for transportation from the field are made.

Obviously, common sense plays a large part in determining the manner in which an injured player is removed from the site of his injury. A swimmer, unconscious after striking the end of the pool while turning, is handled quite differently than a golfer struck in the temple by a ball. In the case of the swimmer, the risk of drowning is added to the possibility of a neck injury, which cannot be evaluated until after the patient is transported from the pool. Since the swimmer is unconscious, he cannot tell the examiner if sensation is lost or if there is pain in the neck. Usually at poolside, there is a kickboard that is pressed into service to support the patient's head and neck while he is being taken from the pool. This can be further used as a spine board to secure the head during transportation and while an adequate airway is being established. Transportation of the patient to a point where x-rays can be obtained will then proceed in a more orderly manner. Transporting the golfer does not have nearly the urgency that transporting the injured swimmer has. Nonetheless, in moving the unconscious golfer, care must be taken to ensure a patent airway and also to prevent further injury by his being thrown from a bouncing golfcart.

In handling unconscious helmeted players, it should be remembered that the helmet makes an excellent traction device. If there is any question of neck injury, the helmet can be used to apply gentle traction to the patient's neck; the chin strap serves as the halter, and the earholes or edge of the helmet serve as a point of attachment for weights, or as a means of securing the head in position while the patient is being moved on a spine board. A helmet should never be removed forcibly. There is usually no need of it and its removal may cause additional damage to an unsuspected neck injury.

If a spine board is not available, more than adequate assistance is readily available at most team events and the players on either or both benches can be pressed into service. By locking hands to the elbows of players standing opposite them, they can make a very adequate and secure surface on which to transport an injured player.

Another person, at the head, applies traction to the helmet, or otherwise secures the head and neck from unnecessary movement until x-rays have been taken. It is important to remember that additional injury most often occurs during transportation, and care should be taken not to move too fast or in the wrong direction.

Once the initial assessment is made and basic life support is assured, a detailed survey of the player can be conducted in a more appropriate setting. Whether this is beneath the stands, in the field house, or in the back of an ambulance on the way to a hospital is not important; what is important is to make clear observations and determine how the patient is progressing.

CONCUSSION

In the case of a concussion, the player is usually unconscious or at least badly confused from a blow that causes force to be transmitted to the reticular activating substance in the brain stem. The effect of transfer of energy is to interfere with function of this area of the brain for a varying period of time. Clinically, it is manifested by a brief period of unconsciousness with associated changes in pulse, respiration, and blood pressure that are usually extremely short-lived. As the cells in the brain stem begin to function, consciousness, motor power, and coordination of activity are regained.

There exists a period in which memory formation is interrupted, giving the patient amnesia to a greater or lesser degree. The duration of the amnesia is directly proportional to the extent of injury and duration of unconsciousness. By custom and definition, concussion has come to mean a temporary and totally reversible event. Obviously, there are degrees of concussion. On one extreme is the brief episode of confusion and disorientation that players often refer to as a "ding" or as having their "bell rung"; the other extreme is the concussion associated with a player being unconscious for periods of many minutes.

There is no question that some examining physicians can tell that a patient has had a concussion and that nothing else is going to happen. This degree of injury is a grade I concussion, and sometimes the patient is allowed back into action even on the same day. There are other instances in which the examining physician cannot be certain that something else is not occurring simultaneously. For example, while a player is recovering from a concussion and is clearly improving in terms of his memory, orientation, balance, and coordination, he may also be slowly bleeding inside the head from a surface blood vessel that was torn at the time of injury. This may be completely asymptomatic until it develops enough of a mass to cause headache, produce signs of increased intracranial pressure, or to produce signs of local irritability of the brain. The only way that one can be certain that bleeding is not occurring, is with the passage of time, or by tests such as CAT (computerized axial tomography) scanning. Localized compression may be manifested by a seizure, by loss of function of one or more extremities, or by inability to talk. Frequently, increasing lethargy and confusion are the first signs of increasing pressure. The period in which the player appears to be quite normal is called the lucid interval. During this time there is no way of recognizing what is about to happen.

In many sports, it is virtually impossible to identify the mechanism of injury. In football, it can usually be detected by reviewing the game films. In reviewing the films it is of considerable interest to note how inaccurate the player is in his recollection of the injury. Observations of the people on the sidelines are often equally inaccurate.

Review of game films indicates that concussions can be caused by a variety of injuries. Not only do blows to the head produce the syndrome, the same clinical state can be reproduced by a player's receiving a blow to the midportion of his chest by an oncoming player's head. It can also occur when a player has his neck forcibly rotated by an opponent's grasping his face mask and twisting. It is seen with hyperextension injuries of the neck. All of these injuries interfere with the blood supply to the brain and produce a state indistinguishable from that produced by a blow to the head.

Returning to Play After Concussion

It is possible for a player who has received a concussion to return to play after the attending physician is certain that there is no additional injury and once the player has recovered completely from the effects of the concussion. However, in any injury to the contents of the skull, swelling usually does not occur immediately. Within 12 hours after the injury the patient might begin to develop edema of the brain depending on a number of factors. It is not unusual, therefore, for the player to develop a headache some hours after injury. He should be observed closely during the night following injury, and checked before resuming play. Under no circumstances should he be left alone through the night, in case his condition deteriorates from an expanding intracranial mass.

Until he is headache-free at rest, he should not resume any strenuous activity. Once that point is reached, he then may begin light workouts and running. If the headache recurs while he is running, he should refrain from activity and wait until the headache has subsided. Once he is able to perform calisthenics and run without headache, dizziness, or light-headedness on change of position, and if no additional neurologic signs have developed, he may then resume contact sports.

Occasionally, a player who has received a head injury will develop migraine headaches. These must be distinguished from the headaches of increased intracranial pressure and can be treated separately. The player can resume sports once it is certain that the headaches are indeed migraine, and not due to an expanding mass lesion such as a subdural hematoma.

Repeated Concussion

The question of whether a player should be allowed to resume athletics after repeated concussions is frequently asked and requires careful evaluation of circumstances. If, by repeated concussions, one means once a year, then there is probably no danger to the player; however, if a player is sustaining concussions more frequently, it is imperative to evaluate the situation carefully. If game movies or television tapes are available, a review will often resolve the problem of why injuries are occurring. It can demonstrate to the player and the coach the fact that the player is using his head unwisely, illegally, or both. It may also show that the player is not wearing his equipment properly. Thus, inspection of equipment is in order to be certain that it fits, and to check that the player is wearing it correctly.

In evaluating players with repeated concussions, it is also important to look for the mental "set" of the patient. It is sometimes apparent that players do not want to continue their sport, but because of external pressures, feel trapped into a situation, the only way out of which is by the so-called honorable route of receiving an injury.

It is extremely important to review videotapes or game films in every instance in which a player is hurt. Not only is this helpful to the player, it is educational for both the coach and the physician. Study of these films or tapes form the basis for changes in rules, equipment, and coaching techniques. Unfortunately, they all too frequently document that injury is caused by a breakdown in the concept of sportsmanship.

HEMORRHAGES

Intracranial bleeding is the leading cause of death from head injury in sport. There are essentially three types of potentially fatal intracranial bleeding conditions to which the examining physician must be alert in every instance in which a player receives a head injury.

The most rapidly progressive, yet correctable, one is caused by a tear in one of the arteries in the covering of the brain. This usually takes the form of an extradural hematoma. It is often, but not always, associated with a fractured skull. It is very frequently associated with a lucid interval in which the player regains consciousness and normal function from the concussive effect of injury, but subsequently loses consciousness and function because of the rapid buildup of pressure inside the head. Unless this pressure is relieved surgically, the patient will die in a relatively short time.

The second type of bleeding occurs under the dura. It is either associated with a tear of the vessels bridging from the surface of the brain to the sinuses in the dura, or occasionally is caused by oozing from contused brain surface. The tear in the vessels is usually due to a shearing of these bridging vessels and a contusion to the impact of the surface of the brain against the inner surface of the skull during a deceleration injury. If a patient has to be operated on within 24 hours because of a subdural hematoma, the mortality rate is extremely high because of associated damage to the brain tissue itself and edema in vital parts of the brain stem.

The third type of intracranial bleeding that occurs in association with trauma is within the substance of the brain. Again, this is usually caused by contusion. However, in rare instances it may be associated with rupture of a vascular lesion such as aneurysm or arteriovenous malformation. Death may occur extremely rapidly with intracerebral bleeding, even before a patient can be transported to a hospital. Because of the reaction of the family, teammates and, indeed, of the entire community, to the death of an athlete, it is strongly urged that anyone associated with such an unfortunate event obtain a complete autopsy. Only in this way can the innumerable rumors that spring up be silenced, and the guilt felt by the player's family and associates be assuaged. In many instances findings that would in no other way have been available, show that the cause of death is quite different than anticipated.

SEIZURES

The occurrence of seizure in a head-injured patient is always disconcerting to both player and spectators. In unhelmeted players, a blow to the head of sufficient force may precipitate a seizure, depending on a number of factors. The closer to the motor strip, the rolandic area, of the brain that a contusion occurs, the more likely it is to produce a convulsion. If the skull is broken and a fragment of bone is driven into the cortex, a seizure is very likely to occur. If the player has a tendency toward, or actually has, epilepsy, he may have a seizure resulting from a lesser blow because of his reduced seizure threshold. Occasionally, in an adolescent, the hyperventilation of vigorous sports activity is enough to precipitate a seizure for the first time even without a blow to the head.

Before moving the player, attention should be directed to the airway. Next, care should be taken to prevent the player from hurting himself. Under no circumstances should one put one's finger in the convulsing person's mouth. The force developed by the patient's jaw when they are tonically contracted is enough to amputate the finger of one who unwisely attempts to open the patient's mouth. If the patient has already bitten his tongue, it it best to turn his head so that saliva and blood can run out of his mouth or nose. In a very short time, the seizure will end, the patient will relax, and then he can be transported from the playing field to the aid station or ambulance.

Although a depressed skull fracture is often the cause of seizures, and palpation of the head will often reveal a depression, it is easy to be fooled by the edge of a subgaleal hematoma. This collection of blood in the scalp often begins so gradually that the edges are not appreciated. The soft central portion yields to the palpating finger, giving the impression of a depression in the bone. Obviously, x-ray examination is necessary to make the final diagnosis.

As mentioned, not all seizures that occur on the playing field are caused by contusion of the brain. There are youngsters with epilepsy who for their own reasons want to participate in team, contact, and individual sports. Whether they should be allowed to do so in any particular sport should be determined by such factors as outlined by McLaurin.[1] Among these are degree of control, frequency and type of seizure, and the presence of associated disorders that might affect the patient's ability to play a particular sport. For example, the person with major motor seizures, well controlled with medication, can obviously play and enjoy sports far better than a youngster with multiple attacks of "petit mal," poorly controlled by medication, who experiences short periods of lapse of attention or lapse of postural control.

RETURN TO PLAY AFTER MAJOR HEAD INJURY

In the instance when a player survives a major injury, such as a hemorrhage or a contusion, the question of returning to contact sports often arises. In this, as in all medical decisions regarding a team and its players, the team physician must have the final decision. In consultation with the team physician the following guidelines may be helpful in deciding when a player should return to active play. The neurologic examination should be normal; the deficit that indicated that the patient had a contusion must have cleared. All vasomotor symptoms should be cleared; that is, the patient should no longer get light-headed on sudden change of position. Headache should be gone. If the patient had seizures, or if the injury was severe, return of the electroencephalogram to normal should also be expected. It is not likely that a player who had a seizure will return to contact sport. One must also takc into consideration the player's level of competition. A professional athlete is not treated the same as a junior high school player. At the college and high school levels of competition, one must be guided by the concept that the primary goal of the player is to improve the contents of the skull, not to damage them.

NECK INJURIES

The most devastating injury that can occur to an athlete is tetraplegia. The likelihood of recovery is extremely small and is determined by the degree of injury to the spinal cord. Although tetraplegia can result from an injury to the cord that is of sufficient force to cause only a concussion of the neural elements, the condition of the player at the time of injury is the same as in those whose cord is severed. By improper handling of a broken or dislocated neck, it is possible to convert a recoverable case of tetraplegia into a permanent one. There is no way of differentiating recoverable from permanent tetraplegias at the time of injury. There is also no way of determining whether or not the bony spinal column is stable or unstable until x-rays can be obtained. The mechanism of injury is rarely known at the time of injury in a sport such as rugby or football, while it is usually patently obvious in gymnastics or other individual sports. Needless to say, it is much easier to know exactly how to handle a neck-injured player who is conscious and able to talk, if the exact mechanism of the injury is known, and if x-rays of the vertebral column are available. Such luxuries are rarely afforded at the instant of injury when critical decisions must be made regarding the handling of the player.

The player who is unconscious is much more difficult to handle. The temptation to flip him onto his back, throw his chin upward, and begin mouth-to-mouth resuscitation must be avoided lest, in so doing, an already damaged spinal cord is severed. When running to the side of a fallen player, the first step in proper treatment is—think tetraplegia. One can never diagnose that which is never considered. From that instant, before even touching the player, all thoughts and procedures must be to prevent additional injury to the spinal cord. To establish an airway, look before turning the patient; he may have a very adequate airway and turning may not be necessary. If and when the patient can be turned, it is essential to have enough help. Then working as a unit, with the head and neck held neutrally, neither flexed nor extended, and with gentle traction applied, the patient is slowly turned onto the spine board or other flat surface. If the player is helmeted, the helmet is left on to take advantage of this excellent traction device. If necessary, the face mask is taken off with bolt cutters or screw drivers but the helmet is left in place with the chin strap securely fastened. With the patient secured in the supine position it is possible and desirable not to move him again until the full extent of his injuries have been assessed and the necessary stabilization procedures carried out. After plain x-rays have been obtained and evaluated, cervical myelogram can be performed with the patient still supine. This procedure, if indicated, is performed by puncturing the spinal subarachnoid space between the first and second cervical vertebrae, and approaching the spinal canal from the lateral aspect of the patient, using fluoroscopy to control the position and depth of the needle. Once the subarachnoid space is entered and before the surface of the cord is touched with the fine-gauge needle, a water-soluble contrast agent such as metrizamide is introduced and the cervical subarachnoid space is filled. If fluoroscopy shows no obstruction to the flow of the contrast material, the patient can be turned carefully while other x-ray views or tomograms are obtained. If fluoroscopy shows a complete block, surgery can be performed, the obstruction removed, and stabilization procedures begun—all without having to change the patient's position from supine. This capability has surely contributed to the recovery of patients who, in the past, would have been operated on after being turned prone while anesthetized. It is virtually impossible to prevent motion of the unstable spine under these circumstances. Since most of the data on the effects of early surgery on tetraplegia have been on patients operated on while in the prone position, perhaps better results will become evident from operating on those who have not been turned.

The neck-injured player who is conscious is handled differently. In such a case, it is possible to assess the extent of injury and to enlist the patient's cooperation in transportation.

If the neck injury is sufficient to produce tetraplegia, his neck muscles will develop spasm which will help hold the bony elements in a stable relationship. Any motion that produces pain must be avoided; depend on the patient to tell whether he is being hurt as he is being moved. All movements are made slowly and stopped immediately if the patient reports any pain or increase in symptoms. Again the helmet and spine board are used, traction is applied, and the player is transported slowly to the facility where further studies will be performed and treatment begun. Under no circumstances should the spine be manipulated on the field without x-rays. Definitive treatment will depend on evaluation at the hospital.

Because of the superb physical condition of many athletes and their tendency to minimize painful injuries, it is possible for one to fracture a cervical vertebra and show no more signs than if the injury were a sprain. Because of the potential for serious spinal cord injury, x-ray examination should be readily available and freely used. It is also possible for a player to tear ligaments and to rupture discs in the cervical spine without there being any x-ray evidence of such an injury. Therefore, the careful clinical evaluation must be combined with x-ray evaluation in assessing the extent of injury.

Clinical evaluation consists of inspecting the neck area visually, noting how the player holds his head, palpating the neck muscles, and observing the range of motion of the neck. Subjective feelings of altered sensation are especially important clues to injury of neural elements. Correlation of the player's observations with motor, reflex, and sensory testing is necessary to determine the site of neural injury. Development of numbness or pain radiating into an upper extremity after a neck injury indicates injury to a nerve or nerve root. Careful testing is necessary to determine the level of the injury. The sensation of an electric shock passing through thc trunk when the player flexes his head is a sign (Lhermitte) of compression of the cervical spinal cord. The intense, searing pain often described by players as a "burner" is indication of injury to the nerve root at the point of its emergence from the intervertebral foramen. It is important to differentiate this peripheral injury from nerve root injury because of rupture of the cervical disc between the fifth and sixth cervical vertebrae. Often this can only be done by myelography. The natural history of the "burner" is one of progressive damage beginning during the first years of a player's experience, at which time the sensation is intense but fleeting. As the player, usually one who frequently hits with his head, has more experience, the pain will radiate down the outer aspect of the arm to the base of the thumb. It will last 10 to 20 seconds. The injury is easily detected since the player can be seen running to the sidelines grasping his arm and shaking his hand. By senior year in high school or first year in college, inability to flex the elbow develops, and the pain lasts longer. By the end of the player's career, whether in college or with the professionals, he will develop lasting weakness of the biceps and deltoids with lesser weakness of the teres major. At surgery, the lesion is at the point of emergence of the fifth and/or sixth nerve root where it crosses the posterior lamella of the transverse process of the vertebra and enters the fascial plane between the anterior and medial scalene muscles. Here, external scarring of the root to the surrounding tissue indicates repeated injuries that fix the nerve root and compress the root against the transverse process whenever the neck is stretched away from the point of fixation. This stretch can be either in extension, lateral flexion, or by depression of the shoulder while the head and neck remain fixed. Early recognition of symptoms, correction of the player's hitting practices, the use of a high collar to prevent lateral stretching, or changing the player's position, should prevent development of the full-blown syndrome characterized by weakness of the upper arm and constant pain on use of the arm, on or off the playing field.

Other soft tissue injuries to the neck involve the blood vessels. The carotid arteries are relatively exposed and are subject to trauma from direct blows. The term "close-lining" describes the injury in which the neck of the injured person strikes a relatively fixed and narrow resistance. A horseback rider's neck striking a tree branch, or a football carrier's neck striking a stiffened forearm of an opponent, are examples of this type of injury. If the intima of the carotid artery is damaged by this blow, a clot forms at the site of injury and either causes showers of emboli to migrate to the small vessels in the brain, or the clot enlarges causing thrombosis of the artery and infarction of the cerebral hemisphere. The vertebral arteries are protected by a bony covering. In hyperextension of the neck, it is possible to compress the artery between the base of the occiput and the first or second vertebrae. Schneider[2] has documented the devastating effect of this type of injury to the vertebral artery caused by striking the face mask against the knee or by driving the face mask into an oncoming player thereby severely hyperextending the neck.

Studies on the mechanisms of injury to the head and neck such as those by Schneider[2] and more recently by Torg et al[3] indicate that the incidence of severe head injuries is decreasing in football. The above studies unhappily show that there is an increase in the numbers of serious neck injuries leading to tetraplegia. Other sports, such as rugby, show an alarming increase in the incidence of tetraplegia as recently reported by Silver[4] in the *British Medical Journal,* and confirmed by many subsequent letters to the editor. These clinical studies amply document the risks to the players' necks of certain practices such as "spearing" or vertical compression of the spine by deliberate striking with the crown of the helmet. From the National Athletic Head and Neck Injury Registry comes incontrovertible evidence of the many different ways that tetraplegia can occur.[3] From studies such as those by Reid et al[5] on the field, and by Hodgson et al (see Chapter 9) in the laboratory, comes information that indicates the limits to which the head and neck can be subjected. Hodgson's conclusion that it is not possible to protect the neck from the maximum forces to which it is subjected in contact sports, is in direct opposition to the statement of

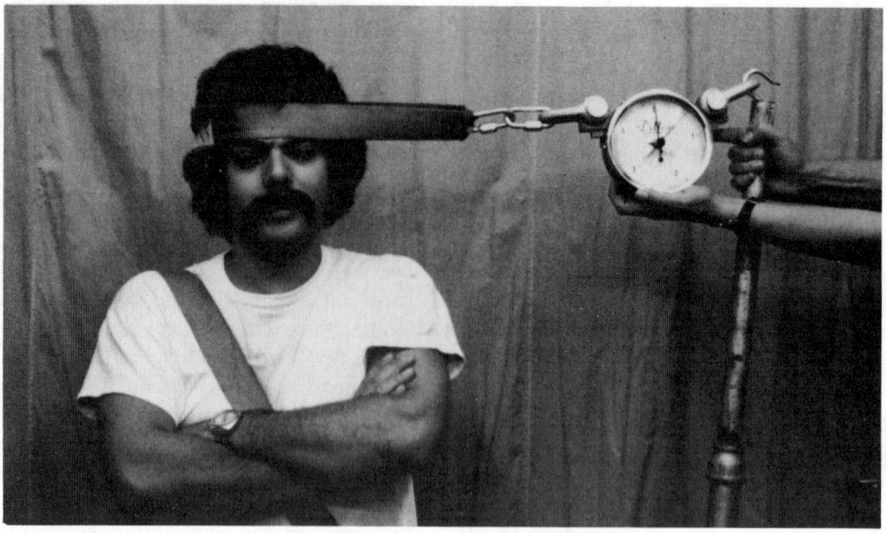

Figure 10-1A Demonstration of the pulley system used at Harvard University.

the NFL Management Council that suggests professional players' necks can be conditioned to withstand these forces.[6]

Return to Play After Neck Injury

It has been documented by Albright et al[7] that a high percentage of high school and college football players have preexisting neck injuries. Since reinjury carries such a high risk of serious damage, it is problematical to know when and if an injured player may resume play.

For those players who have sustained a fracture of the vertebral body, pedicles, or facet joint, and who have healed completely, contact or collision sports should be prohibited. For those players who have sustained a spinal cord injury and have recovered completely, further contact or collision sports are prohibited.

Tetraplegia, even on a transient basis, indi-

PC Age 20 Neck Size 16½ 6'1" 205 lbs. OG

	To Anterior	To Posterior	To Left	To Right
9 /1 /74	35	40	25	25
		Injured 10/14/72		
10/15/72	15	10*	15*	10
10/31/72	15	15	20	12
11/6 /72	35	20	30	27

*Pain

Disability 23 Days
Vertical Study

Figure 10-1B Example of a neck profile chart.

cates a severe dysfunction of the spinal cord. No player who has experienced this symptom should be allowed back to collision sports until and unless a complete evaluation of the spinal cord, its coverings, and its blood supply has been conducted and is negative. It is extremely unlikely that a complete evaluation in a case of transient quadraplegia would be negative and, therefore, it is extremely unlikely that a player who has experienced even a temporary tetraplegia would be allowed back into collision sports or other sports which put the neck at severe risk.

Those players who have sustained soft tissue injury to the neck involving pain-sensitive structures, develop a protective muscle spasm that can often be detected by examination. Once the spasm has gone and the neck is comfortable at rest, the player usually begins to press for return to participation. At Harvard University, we have a system for detection of preexisting injury, and determination of when an injury has healed, and therefore when a player can safely return to contact.[8] Each player is tested by pulling weights on a pulley system attached to a head-band (Figure 10-1A). The player pulls in flexion, extension, and to each side. The maximum weight he pulls is recorded and becomes his neck profile. If a new player cannot pull in one direction to a degree recognized as usual, but pulls normally in other directions, it invariably develops on further inquiry that he has had a previous neck injury. This will be treated and corrected before he is allowed to play a contact sport. If a player sustains an injury during the season, he will not return until he is able to perform up to the level of his previously recorded neck profile (Figure 10-1B). Similar data can also be obtained with a cybex unit. This easy documentation has helped trainer, coach, player, and physician to agree on the safe time for the player's return to action. It is particularly helpful in letting the physician and trainer know that their treatment has been successful.

REFERENCES

1. McLaurin, R.L. Epilepsy and contact sports. *JAMA*. 225:285–287, 1973.

2. Schneider, R.C. *Head and Neck Injuries in Football: Mechanisms, Treatment, and Prevention*. Baltimore: Williams and Wilkins, 1973.

3. Torg, J.S., Truex, R., Quedenfeld, T.C. et al. The National Football Head and Neck Injury Registry Report and Conclusions, 1978. *JAMA*. 241:1477–1479, 1979.

4. Silver, J.R. Rugby injuries to the cervical cord. *Br Med J*. 1:192–193, 1979.

5. Reid, S.E., Tarkington, J.A., Epstein, H.M. et al. Brain tolerance to impact in football. *Surg Gynecol Obstet*. 133:929–936, 1971.

6. Cushing, D. NFL expands roughness rules. *Physician and Sportsmedicine* 7:17, 1979.

7. Albright, J.P., Moses, J.M., Feldick, H.G. et al. Nonfatal cervical spine injuries in interscholastic football. *JAMA*. 236:1243–1245, 1976.

8. Gibbs, R. New methods of evaluating the recovery of neck injuries in football. Presented at the Annual Meeting of the American College of Sports Medicine, New Orleans, May, 1975.

CHAPTER 11
Injuries to the Face, Ear-Nose-Throat, and Airway

Kent S. Wilson, MD

> Athletics are hazardous. In sports requiring vigorous activity, injuries are bound to occur....Educators should exert every effort to assure that the potential for injury is kept to the absolute minimum.[1]

Study of the mechanism and prevention of facial and laryngotracheal injury in athletics is extremely important because of the vital structures involved, and the great potential for prevention of injury. Athletic injuries are preventable because stereotyped athletic activity causes predictable types of trauma and disease. Hence, there exists the possibility of intervention to reduce both sports trauma and sports-related diseases. These considerations are of utmost importance in the facial and laryngotracheal area because four of the five senses (hearing, vision, olfaction [smell], and taste), as well as two vital organ systems (airway and digestive tract) are contained within the area. Maintaining the cosmetic integrity of the face and neck is also important for the individual's pyschologic and social well-being.

STRUCTURE AND FUNCTION

The facial skeleton maintains the soft tissue structure of the face and superior neck. It is a combination of dense, structural bone formed into several buttresses, interconnected by extremely delicate, thin sheets of bone. The upper one-third of the facial skeleton is the frontal bone and forms the base of support for the middle one-third of the face. Buttresses protrude from the lateral aspect to unite with the dense zygoma (cheek bones), and extend medially to unite with the nasal bones. The middle one-third of the face (maxillary bone) supports the nose and maintains patency of the nasal chambers as well as supporting the upper jaw. The maxillary and ethmoid sinuses are hollow spaces that communicate with the nose and lie within the maxillary and ethmoid bones of the middle one-third of the face. The lower portion of the facial skeleton is formed by the mandible, or lower jaw, which supports the teeth. The function of the mandible is not only to support the teeth for masticatory purposes, but also to support the larynx and trachea and maintain patency of the upper airway and digestive tract (Figure 11-1).

The facial musculature provides mobility to the facial structures for respiration, mastication, and expression. The skin covers the musculoskeletal components of the face and contributes significantly to the functional and cosmetic integrity of the face as a whole. The ear includes the external ear, or pinna, the cartilaginous portion of the ear that projects from the side of the head. It also includes the external auditory canal or skin-lined duct between the external environment and the tympanic membrane. The tympanic membrane (ear drum), is mobile, with a consistency similar to parchment, and lies on the inner aspect of the external auditory canal. The tympanic membrane is connected by three small bones or ossicles (malleus, incus, and stapes) to the inner ear. These ossicles lie in the middle ear cleft, which is an air-filled cavity, connected by the auditory tube to the nasopharynx or upper part of the throat. These structures provide a mechanical means of transforming sound waves in the air into mechanical motion as the tympanic membrane vibrates, and this motion in turn is transmitted through the lever system of the ossicular chain to the inner ear where fluid waves are formed (Figure 11-2).

The fluid waves inside the inner ear cause motion of a highly specialized sense organ (organ of Corti). Stimulation of this results in the neural discharge of encoded impulses by the eighth nerve to higher brain centers where the impulses are interpreted as sound. It is critically important that the

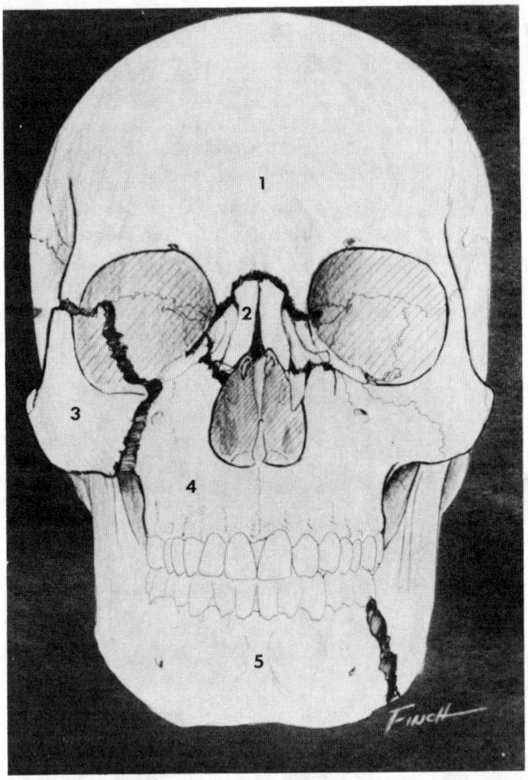

Figure 11-1 Facial skeleton. 1. Frontal bone. 2. Nasal bone. 3. Zygoma. 4. Maxilla. 5. Mandible. The facial bones are injured in direct relation to their degree of projection from the facial plane. The nasal bones are most frequently injured, followed in order by the mandible and the zygoma. The maxilla and frontal bones are the least frequently fractured of the facial bones. (Courtesy Dr Eugene Rontal.)

middle ear be air-filled in order that transmission of mechanical motion from the tympanic membrane to the inner ear can be conducted efficiently. Abnormalities that impair the mobility of this mechanism, such as obstruction of the external auditory canal, perforation of the ear drum, fracture of one of the ossicles, or filling of the middle ear cleft by fluid, all decrease the efficiency of sound conduction, and hence result in hearing loss.

The inner ear also contains the end organ of the balance, or vestibular system. This includes the semicircular canal system as well as the saccule and utricle. Disruption of the internal ear may result in vertigo (dizziness) if this mechanism is injured.

The nose is the primary organ of olfaction and respiration. The olfactory epithelium occupies the upper portion of the nasal chambers. Processes that prevent air circulation to this portion of the nose will result in loss or diminution of the sense of smell. Injuries that result in distortion of the internal nasal structure obviously may cause respiratory obstruction. The respiratory system begins in the nose and includes the oropharynx, or throat, larynx, trachea, and bronchopulmonary tree of the lungs. The digestive tract, which begins in the oral cavity, traverses the pharynx, or throat, and includes the esophagus and, ultimately, stomach. The pharynx, or throat, is an area in which, in the human, the airway and digestive tract cross. Because of this junction, anatomic integrity and neuromuscular coordination of the pharynx is extremely important. Injury to the pharynx that results in incoordination or anatomic disruption, may permit oral or pharyngeal contents to enter the respiratory tract. This could cause asphyxiation.

INJURY CLASSIFICATION

Tissues of the head and neck are subject to several types of trauma. A contusion (commonly called a bruise) is a soft-tissue injury sustained by a blow that does not disrupt the epithelial, or skin, surface. An abrasion, or scrape, is an injury to the skin surface in which the superficial layers may be removed, but complete transection of the skin surface does not occur. Lacerations, or cuts, are those injuries that result in division of the skin and, in some cases, the subcutaneous tissues. Fracture refers to a break in the continuity of a bone.

There are many causes (etiologies) of sports injury. The most common is a physical trauma (such as a direct blow) that may result in soft tissue contusion, abrasion, laceration, or bony fracture. These frequently occur in hockey, football, and other contact sports. Fluid pressure changes may also cause injury, such as when failure to equilibrate pressure, either air or water, results in rupture of the tympanic membrane or the delicate membranes of the inner ear, as occurs in scuba diving. Infections with bacteria, viruses, and fungi are common causes of sports-related disease, such as epidemic herpes simplex skin infection in wrestlers. Both thermal and chemical types of trauma may be sustained by the athlete, although these will not be discussed. It is apparent, then, that there is a variety of physical agents with which an athlete must contend if safety in any sport is to be achieved. The athlete's attitudes, behavior, and training; coaches' and officials' attitudes rules of the activity and physical facilities, all may affect risk of injury.

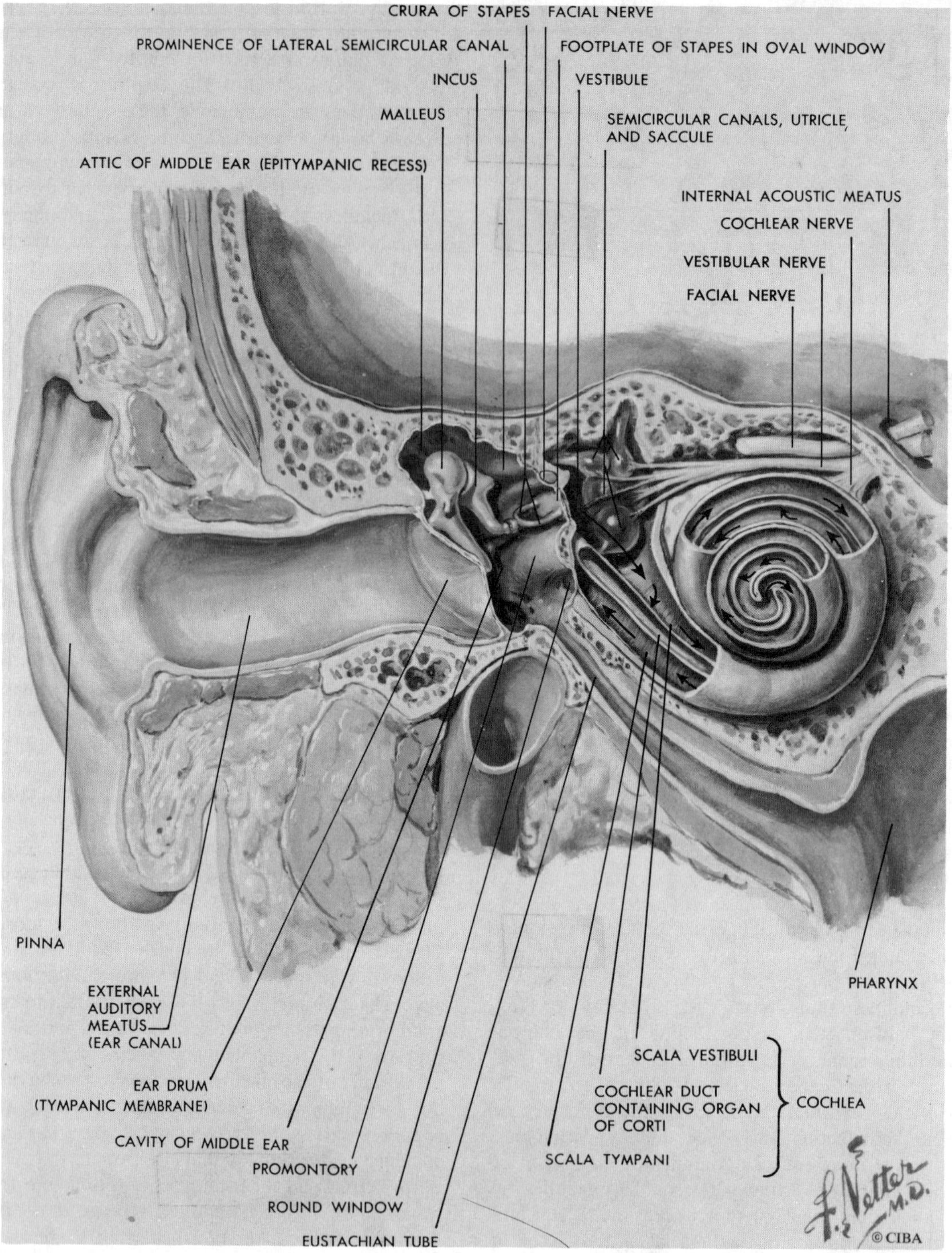

Figure 11-2 Anatomy of the ear. © Copyright 1962 Ciba Pharmaceutical Company, Division of CIBA-GEIGY Corporation. Reproduced, with permission, from *Clinical Symposia,* illustrated by Frank H. Netter, MD. All rights reserved.

INJURY DISCUSSION BY ANATOMIC AREA

The facial skeleton is the supporting structure for several sense organs, the aerodigestive tract, and the facial skin and musculature. When injuries result in fracture of the facial skeleton, severe sequellae, both short- and long-term, can result if the injury is not diagnosed properly, and either first aid or definitive therapy are not appropriate.[2-5]

Frontal Bone

The frontal bone is a dense structure occupying the superior one-third of the anterior head. It contains a hollow air space, the frontal sinus. Because this hollow structure may have rather thin walls, fractures into the sinus can occur. The frontal bone is usually fractured by a force applied from directly anterior, resulting in displacement of the anterior wall of the sinus. Sometimes, with great forces applied, the posterior wall of the sinus can also be injured, with exposure or disruption of either dura (brain covering) or brain. When a fracture of the outer table of the frontal sinus has occurred, there will usually be a depression of the forehead, although soft tissue swelling can mask this. There will frequently be epistaxis (nasal bleeding). If a laceration has been sustained, the fractured bony fragments may be either palpated or visualized in the depths of the laceration. Radiographic examination, either with standard x-rays or with planigrams, may demonstrate fracture of the anterior table or the posterior table. If the injury has been severe these tests will show pneumocephalus, or air within the intracranial space.

Initial management of this injury involves preservation of the airway, and control of hemorrhage if epistaxis is profuse. Rapid transfer to a diagnostic center is required after stabilization, since sophisticated diagnostic techniques may be required. Definitive management usually requires surgery.

Maxilla

The maxilla occupies the central middle one-third of the face. It forms the floor of the eyes' orbits and foundation of both upper jaw and external nose. It also forms and maintains the internal structure of the nose. It is hollow laterally; the spaces are called maxillary sinuses.

Fractures of the maxilla were first categorized by Le Fort, as a result of cadaver studies done near the turn of the century. He found that the maxilla, depending upon the mass, velocity, and vector of the injuring force, usually fractured in a stereotyped way. Should the blow strike the inferior maxilla, a shearing force tends to separate the palate from the superior portion of the maxilla, creating a Le Fort I fracture. This might occur if a hockey stick or puck struck the lower portion of the upper jaw. The patient may report that the teeth do not fit properly (malocclusion) and epistaxis may occur because the fracture line usually traverses the floor of the internal nose. Physical examination usually demonstrates either displacement or mobility of the palate, and there may be lacerations in the inferior portion of the nose at the fracture site.

Should the blow fall somewhat higher in the mid-facial region, the central middle one-third of the face may fracture in a Le Fort II fashion, in which case the nasal bones and middle and lower portions of the maxilla are separated from the zygoma and frontal complex. Primary symptoms include epistaxis, hypesthesia (numbness) of the cheek because of contusion of the inferior orbital nerves, and mobility of both nose and palate. If a severe blow should strike the face anteriorly and be widely distributed, a Le Fort III fracture may result. The zygoma and maxillary-ethmoid complex are completely separated from the frontal bone and cranial vault in this injury. Essentially, the middle one-third of the face is completely separated from the upper one-third of the facial skeleton. Examination usually demonstrates massive edema, and the entire middle one-third of the face will either be displaced or mobile on palpation (Figure 11-3). Careful attention should be directed to eye examination because of the possibility of soft tissue injury to the globe or orbital content, especially in Le Fort II and III fractures.

Several initial management principles are applicable, and must be kept in mind with any maxillary fracture. First, efforts must be directed at airway preservation, since these fractures traverse the nose and paranasal sinuses, and bleeding may be profuse. This may involve removal of bone fragments or other debris from the mouth and throat, suction removal of clots, and/or placement of an oral airway. Second, an attempt must be made to achieve hemostasis. Usually these injuries result in initial epistaxis that resolves spontaneously, although on some occasions intermittent

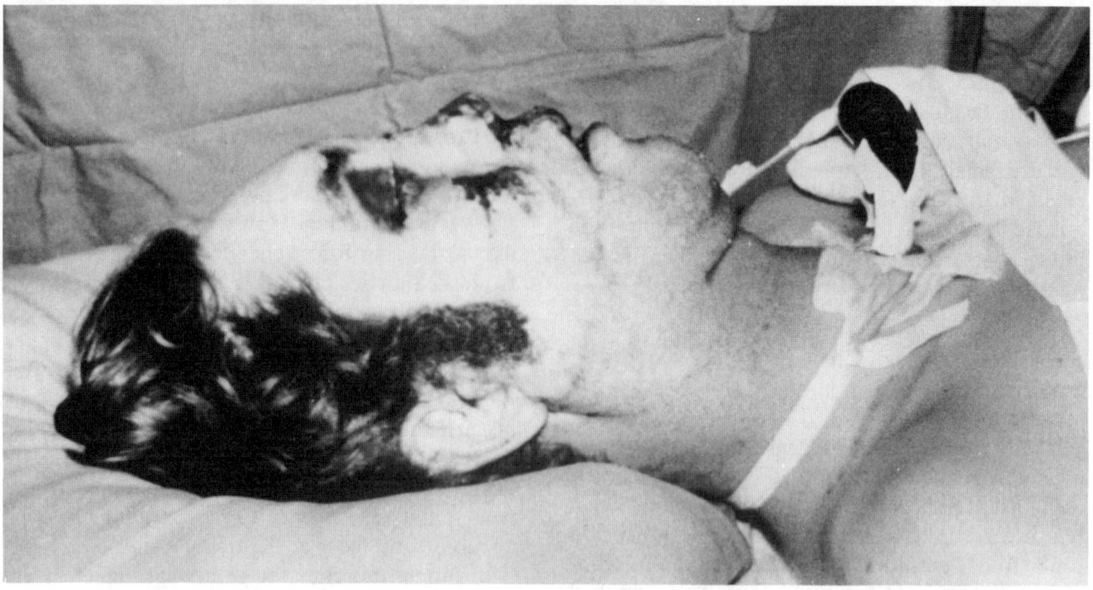

Figure 11-3 Maxilla fracture. When a severe blow has been sustained, the entire middle one-third of the face (Le Fort II or III fracture) may result. This figure demonstrates Le Fort III fracture with displacement of the middle one-third of the face posteriorly and flattening of the facial profile. Soft tissue injury with contusions and nasal bleeding are apparent.

bleeding occurs. Should epistaxis be profuse and uncontrollable by conservative means such as pressure, gently blowing the nose to remove clots, application of vasoconstrictive medication, and the suction removal of clots, anterior and/or posterior nasal packing may be required. Third, it is necessary to determine the extent of any intracranial injury, providing no higher priority abdominal or thoracic injury has occurred. Treatment of these injuries usually requires hospitalization and most frequently involves surgery.

Nose

The nose is the most commonly fractured facial structure because it is the most prominent and has a relatively weak structure. Proper care of the fractured nose is extremely important because of its function as a respiratory and olfactory organ, and because of its cosmetic importance. One need not go through life with a deformed, obstructed nose as "the price for playing the game." The nose is composed of the anterior cartilaginous portions of the septum and tip (lobule), and the more posteriorly placed nasal bones and bony portions of the nasal septum.

A blow to the nose may fracture or dislocate only the cartilaginous portion of the nose, just the bony portion of the nose, or both. Epistaxis following a blow to the nose is the most frequent symptom, and nearly universally indicates that fracture with some displacement has occurred. Bleeding can usually be controlled by compression of the external nose. If nasal deformity is apparent, fracture almost certainly has occurred. Most frequently, one nasal bone will be displaced toward the midline and the entire pyramid of the nose opposite the injury will be displaced away from the midline. This can usually be detected by its appearance and by palpation. Detection of the frequently nondiagnosed nasal septal fracture requires one to grasp the nasal septum between the thumb and forefinger and displace it bilaterally in order to demonstrate mobility at the inferior suture. Internal examination of the nose should be carried out to detect lacerations or septal hematoma (a clot inside the septum). Initial management of a nasal fracture involves preservation of the airway and control of hemorrhage. This may require anterior and/or posterior nasal packing, but usually pressure or the application of a vasoconstrictive medication, following suction removal of clots, suffices.

Mandible

The mandible is the second most frequently injured of the facial bones (Figure 11-4). Because

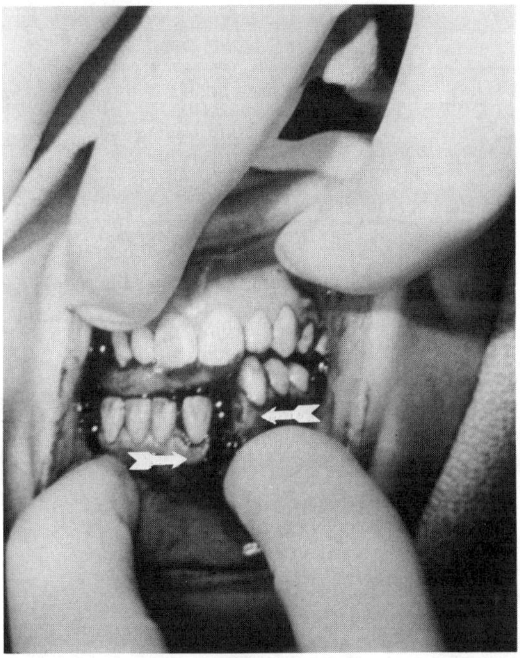

Figure 11-4 Mandible fracture. Bleeding and discontinuity of both mandibular bones and overlying soft tissues exist (arrow).

the mandible has a semicircular structure, usually two fractures result from a blow impinging upon the mandible. A patient who has a mandible fracture may complain of anesthesia about the chin if the mandibular nerve has been damaged, malocclusion, or intraoral bleeding.

Initial management requires maintenance of the airway by removing chipped or broken teeth, blood clots, and other foreign material that may be in the oral cavity. Usually bleeding is not a problem.

If a severe fracture of the mandible has occurred that has made the structure unstable, the tongue and mandibular fragments tend to fall posteriorly obstructing the oropharyngeal airway, and anterior traction on the mandibular fragments must be maintained.

If ready access to a treatment center is available, usually no special support for the fractured fragments is required. However, if the patient must be transported a considerable distance, consideration must be given to a "Barton bandage," a roll bandage that acts to support the fractured fragments and reduce pain. It may be made by taking an elastic two-inch wrap and rolling it in a vertical fashion beneath the chin and over the top of the head. A second bandage is then rolled horizontally from the back of the head to the forehead, and the two bandages pinned together at the temples.

If the patient's state of consciousness is altered and he is unable to protect his airway, or if bleeding is significant, transfer should be accomplished with the patient in either the knee-chest or some other dependent position to keep the airway clear. The Barton bandage should not be used.

Zygoma

Fracture of the zygoma, or cheek bone, is the third most common facial fracture. It is the third most prominent facial structure and its buttressing structures are relatively weak. Should a blow fall on the body of the zygoma, displacement will usually occur, with contusion of the infraorbital nerve resulting in hypesthesia of the cheek. Flattening of the cheek profile will be apparent if displacement is significant. Eye injury must be ruled out early in evaluation of these patients, since it occurs regularly with these fractures. Failure to detect it may have severe visual consequences.[6] Should a blow fall over the zygomatic arch, depression of the temple region will occur. Initial management involves only the application of ice to control edema in the soft tissues, and transfer to a hospital for definitive therapy.

Table 11-1 summarizes the symptoms and findings when significant facial bone injuries have occurred.

FACIAL FRACTURES

Initial Management

First aid of the facially injured athlete requires orderly assessment of the injury and provision of care. The first priority in the case of facial fracture is preservation of the airway. Many fractures will cause nasal bleeding and may result in fragments of bone or teeth being present in the airway. Every effort must be made promptly to cleanse the airway of clots and fragments and guarantee its patency. In severe middle one-third facial fractures, or in severe nasal fractures, the normal nasal airway may be completely obstructed, making maintenance of an oral airway critical. In situations where intracranial injury has resulted in altered consciousness, efforts must be made to prevent the tongue from falling posteriorly and blocking the

Table 11-1
Symptoms and Findings of Facial Bone Injuries

	Symptoms	Examination findings
Maxillary fracture	Pain with chewing Lip and cheek anesthesia Diplopia (double vision) Flattening face Malocclusion	Palpable fracture fragments Middle one-third mobility Subcutaneous emphysema (air beneath skin) Malocclusion Extraocular muscle dysfunction
Nasal bone fracture	Epistaxis Nasal obstruction Pain and swelling Decreased smell sensation	New deformity of external nose or septum Intranasal bleeding Septal hematoma
Mandible fracture	Skin damage over fracture site Mandibular deformity Pain with mastication Lower lip anesthesia	Mobile fracture fragments Palpable irregularity at fracture site Intraoral lacerations Malocclusion
Zygoma fracture	Diplopia Cheek anesthesia Cheek flattening Epistaxis	Palpable fracture Cheek anesthesia Extraocular muscle dysfunction

airway. This may require insertion of a curved device.

The second priority is control of hemorrhage in the injured region. Frequently, fractures of the zygoma and maxilla or frontal bone, traverse either the maxillary, ethmoid, or frontal sinuses, and cause hemorrhage into the nose. Obviously, fracture of the nose may also result in hemorrhage. Usually the nose can be kept clear of clots by having the patient blow his nose frequently or by removing the debris with a suction device. Compression of the external nose will control hemorrhage in most cases when a bleeding point is on the anterior septum or external nose. More severe bleeding may require packing, and consideration of hospitalization.

Intracranial injury such as concussion, intracranial bleeding with loss of consciousness, or gross leakage of clear spinal fluid through the nose, requires maintenance of airway, control of hemorrhage, immediate neurosurgical evaluation, and transfer as promptly as feasible for hospitalization. Whenever transportation is considered, patency of the airway must be kept in mind. This may require placement of the patient in a lateral or knee-chest position with the oral cavity and nose dependent.

Mandible and maxilla fractures will occasionally result in cervical spine injury or fracture. This possibility should be kept in mind when transportation is considered, so that the cervical spine may be immobilized.

Definitive Management

Definitive care of facial fractures requires that the fractured fragments be replaced in as nearly normal a position as possible, and maintained in that position until healing has occurred. When a fracture of the frontal bone has occurred, most frequently a surgical procedure to expose it is required. The fractured fragments are usually elevated to a normal position and fixed in place with wire sutures or appropriate absorbable dressings.

The basic principle that is applied in treatment of mandible or maxilla fractures is that the teeth are used to splint the fractured fragments in the appropriate position for healing. Arch bars may be affixed to the teeth that will unite the upper and lower jaw. This fixation may be sufficient to hold the fractured fragments in relatively normal position while healing occurs (Figure 11-5). In severe fractures of the mandible, with many fragments, it may be necessary to make a surgical incision over the fractured fragments and wire them together, in addition to uniting the upper and lower teeth. In fractures that involve the maxilla, not only are the teeth united, but special wiring devices that unite the fractured fragments may be applied (Figure 11-6).

Fracture of the zygoma sometimes may be treated by closed reduction; that is, a procedure in which no incisions are required to replace the

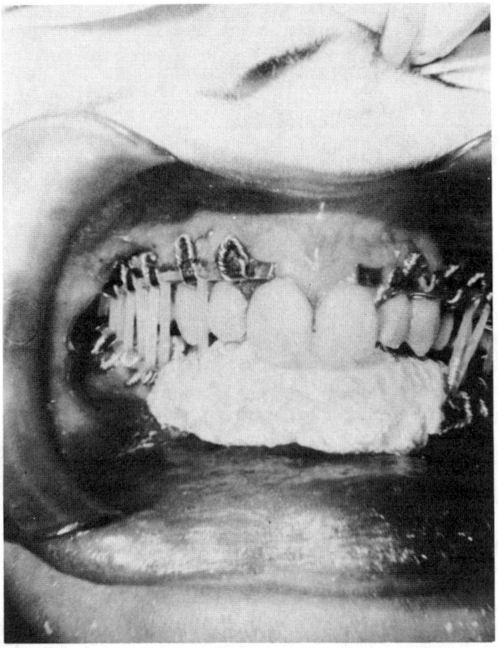

Figure 11-5 Mandible fracture, repaired. This figure shows the arch bars that have been applied to the teeth, and demonstrates the principle of the maxillary dental arch splinting the mandibular dental arch during the healing phase. The white dental dressing over the central mandibular teeth is providing fixation for a reimplanted incisor tooth.

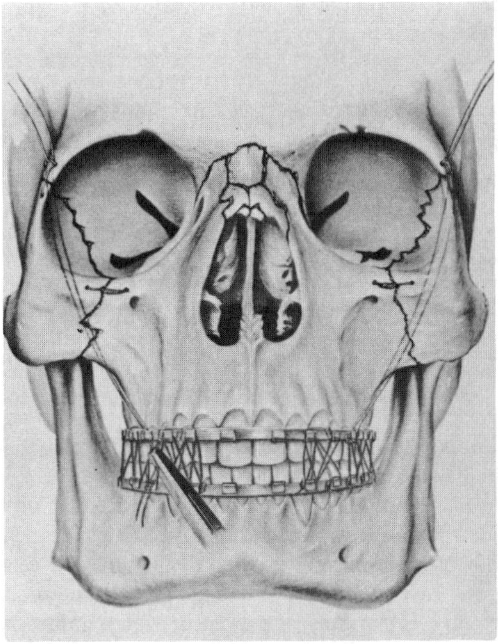

Figure 11-6 Extensive repair may be required in severe maxillary fractures. Individual bone fractures have been wired, the teeth have been approximated with arch bars, and the stable frontal bone has been united to the upper dental arch with suspension wires. From: R. Dingman and P. Natvig. *Surgery of Facial Fractures.* Philadelphia: W.B. Saunders, 1974. Reproduced with permission.

zygoma in satisfactory position for healing. More severe fractures may require that incisions be made over the fracture sites and wire sutures applied to maintain the bones in appropriate position. When fracture of either the nasal bone or nasal septum has occurred, closed reduction may be possible. This procedure involves displacing, either manually or with instruments, the fractured bone and cartilaginous fragments to their normal position, and splinting them until healing has occurred. If displacement of the fractured fragments is significant, incisions may be required to replace them in nearly normal position under direct vision. Intranasal dressings are applied.

Antibiotic treatment is appropriate in most facial fractures because of contamination by oral or nasal bacteria. Care following the repair of the facial fracture is usually minimal, but certainly requires adequate protection of the injured part from reinjury. If the athlete is to return to competition before complete healing, efforts must be directed to providing appropriate protective equipment for the duration of the healing process. Special attention also must be given to particular problems such as methods of opening the jaws when they have been wired together. This is important, since if the athlete were to vomit, he would be unable to rid the oral cavity of the vomitus, might aspirate the stomach content, and be asphyxiated.

METHODS OF FACIAL PROTECTION

What means exist for preventing facial injuries such as fractures, lacerations, and contusions? It has been apparent from antiquity that if the face could be separated mechanically from the injuring agent, no injury would result. This method of injury prevention relies upon the fact that forces directed at the delicate facial structure may be distributed, and therefore dissipated, over a wide area of the structurally stronger frontotemporal region.[7] The end result of this method of prevention is a helmet with facial protective device. Evidence exists from 1500 to 1200 BC that such

Table 11-2
Protective Equipment and Reduction of Facial Injury

Year	Protection	No. of players	Facial and dental injury	Incidence (%) per 100 players
1954	No face masks or dental guards	15,714	356	2.26
1955	Face masks introduced	15,714	288	1.83
1959	Face masks mandatory; few dental guards	22,969	275	1.20
1963	Face masks and dental guards mandatory	30,357	143	0.47
1966	Face masks and dental guards mandatory	34,398	115	0.33

devices were employed in battle. By 500 BC the Corinthians had developed a very sophisticated helmet for protection of both the head and face that provided satisfactory vision and protection.[8] Helmets with facial protectors evolved throughout the centuries, first as a means of defense in war, and more recently as a means of preventing facial injury in sports.

Those methods of facial injury prevention that do not rely upon facial protective equipment, usually rely upon altering the playing conditions at the level of the players', coaches', or officials' behavior, or the physical conditions under which the competition occurs. Rules changes designed to decrease the risk of injury in a sport may be directed at players' or coaches' behavior as can rules interpretation and enforcement by officials. A recent rules change in professional hockey penalizes the third man into a fight. A Canadian Amateur Hockey Association rules change penalizes high sticking, and calls to outlaw the slapshot. These are directed at modifying behavior to reduce injury rates. Hayes[9] has reported a 25% reduction in facial injuries in hockey leagues that legislated against fighting. Rules changes that mandate safer physical facilities or playing equipment may also be employed to reduce facial injury. Suggestions to modify the hockey stick to make it safer would fall in this category.[10]

Application of facial protective equipment can significantly reduce the injury rate. The data in Table 11-2 graphically demonstrate that face masks and intraoral dental guards can markedly reduce the frequency of facial injury in football.[11]

Similar figures demonstrating the protective effect of helmet-face mask combinations in North American hockey have been presented by Pashby.[12] The widespread use of full facial protective equipment (helmet, face mask, and intraoral dental guard) resulted from recognition that significant injury risks, especially of eye injury, resulted from participation. It was also recognized that specific agents, namely the stick and the puck, caused most hockey injuries.[13-15]

The requisites for a satisfactory facial protector are that it provide maximum protection with minimum weight, and that impairment of physiologic function be minimized consistent with the competitive risk at hand. Facial equipment must be relatively heavy for football; fencing, hockey, and lacrosse, where mass and velocity are smaller, require lighter weight facial protective equipment. Numerous materials are available for the fabrication of facial protective equipment, including plastics and combinations of coated or uncoated wire or mesh. Fortunately, standards exist for major sports facial equipment that assure the purchaser of adequate protection with each mask.

Football facial protectors are primarily fabricated of covered, heavy-gauge steel rod. Hockey facial protectors are most frequently made of either clear plastic or wire mesh covered with plastic material. Selection of facial protective equipment should be determined by risk of injury and potentially injuring types of trauma. Football linemen usually select maximally protective, full cage, face masks, since weight and slight visual impairment are of minimal consideration when compared with the necessity for maximum protection (Figure 11-7). Football backs and receivers usually sacrifice some protection for decreased weight and increased visibility when selecting double bar, or "half cage," face masks. These players may be injured either by forearm blows delivered to the mandibular region from below (Figure 11-8) or from objects impinging on the face over the upper bar of the mask.[16]

Ice hockey players, when required to do so,

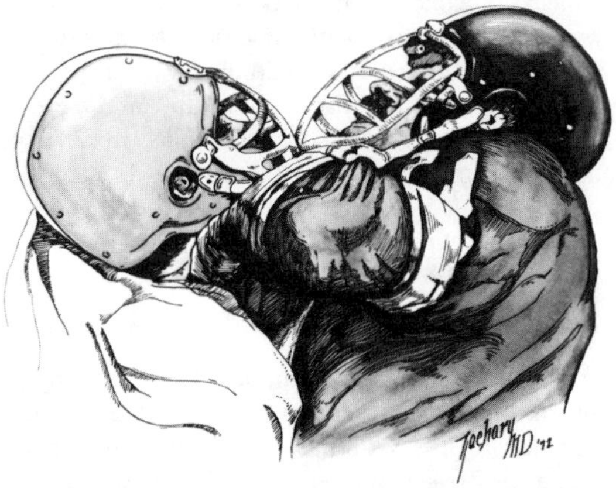

Figure 11-7 Even with full facial protection, techniques of blocking that involve forearm contact to the neck and submandibular region may occur as demonstrated here, and result in laryngotracheal or mandibular injury.

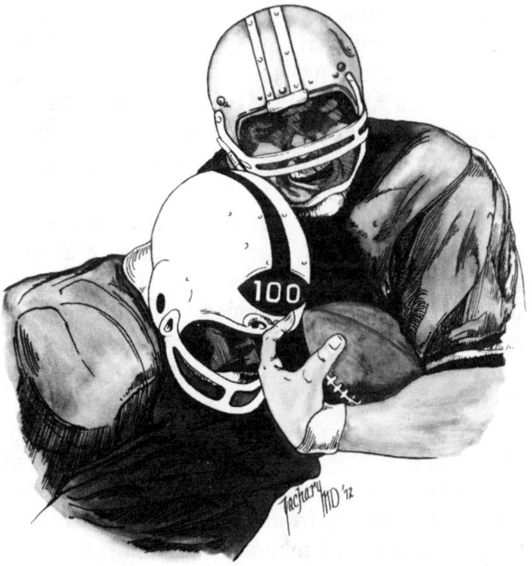

Figure 11-8 Contact of the helmet with the jaw may result in soft tissue injury, or dental or mandibular fracture. The ball carrier would be better protected by a face mask extending below the level of the mandible. Blocking and tackling techniques that rely on initial contact by the helmet, as demonstrated here, have been discouraged by rules changes and recognition by coaches that they are potentially harmful.

usually select maximally protective face masks that do not require the facial skeleton for support. Hockey goalies have historically selected masks that do require the facial skeleton for support, in spite of the fact that fractures and soft tissue injuries have occurred with these masks. These injuries could have been prevented in many cases by a helmet-mask combination that transmitted the impact to the frontotemporal region by the helmet. Fortunately, a trend toward cage masks that do not require facial skeletal support, is emerging among goalies.

Charges have been made that facial protection has resulted in new blocking and tackling techniques. These may encourage more violence in football, and as a result increase the risk of injury, especially to the cervical spine.[17,18] The argument that facial protection equipment predisposes to more violent play, such as spearing or butt-blocking, or that it exposes the player to the risk of cervical spine injury because of excessive torsion being applied to the helmet, must be carefully scrutinized. In the first instance, it is apparent that evolution of face tackling, butt-blocking, and spearing techniques, in which the head is used as the primary point of contact, became feasible only after introduction of the plastic helmet in the early 1950s, and subsequent application of full facial protective masks. It is clear that application of this safety equipment effected a reduction in both intracranial injury and facial injury. If secondary behavioral changes have placed the cervical spine at risk, then these behaviors should be (and, indeed, have been) addressed by rules-making bodies. Rules in football have been passed (and are being enforced) that prohibit manipulation of the face mask, butt-blocking, and face tackling. More importantly, the National Football Coaches Association has resolved that these techniques are potentially injurious and will not be taught in the future.[19] Clear advantages of increased facial safety afforded by the modern helmet-face mask combination should not be sacrificed without careful consideration of the risks involved to all anatomic areas.[20]

EAR

Injuries to the external ear are common in some sports, especially wrestling and boxing. The most frequent external injury is the hematoma or "cauliflower ear." Recent rules changes have mandated the use of wrestling head-gear that protects the external ear from trauma. Unfortunately, in spite of this, injury continues to occur on an occasional basis. The characteristic injury results when a blow is received and bleeding occurs between the cartilage of the external ear and its overlying covering membrane, the perichondrium. If untreated, the blood clot that forms will mature to fibrose, or may become infected. Should fibrosis occur, deformity of the external ear by the mass of tissue will result. Deformity would also result from infection and cartilage necrosis.

First aid for this injury involves immediate compression of the area to minimize extravasation of blood. Definitive therapy involves aspiration of the hematoma initially, and application of a compression dressing. This is satisfactory in most cases; however, occasionally surgical exposure of the area, with removal of fibrous tissue and clotted blood, may be required. Use of wrestling headgear is protective.[21]

Afflictions of the external auditory canal are of two major types, and both usually result from swimming. The external auditory canal is the skin-lined tube that leads from the external environment to the tympanic membrane. Formation of osteomas in the external auditory canal is a significant problem and appears to be related to swimming in cold water. These smooth bony growths, which develop from the lining membrane of the bone of the external canal, form on the walls of the external canal. They may reach sufficient size to obstruct partially the external auditory canal, and may increase the likelihood of external otitis. Should they become bothersome, they may be removed surgically without a great deal of difficulty.[22]

The most common ear canal disorder is external otitis. When the external canal is frequently moistened, as in swimming or frequent showering, bacterial infection may occur. Infection may be triggered by minor trauma, such as scratching the canal with a bobby pin or cotton-tipped stick, or the use of ear plugs. External otitis causes pain and a sensation of fullness in the ear; if it is severe, temporary hearing loss as a result of obstruction may occur. When it occurs, the first requirement is to cleanse the external auditory canal of all debris, usually infected desquamated skin or ear wax. This is best accomplished by suctioning with the aid of the operating microscope. An antibiotic steroid otic drop is extremely helpful. If swelling of the canal skin is severe, application of a wick that will medially displace the drop may be required. In most modest cases of external otitis, removal of the debris and instillation of an antibiotic steroid-containing ear drop will usually result in healing. Severe infections may require systemic antibiotics or even surgery.

Prevention of external otitis requires that the external canal be kept dry. If situations exist in which the ear canal must be moistened, then appropriate otic drops with bacteriostatic and drying properties are used. Acid-alcohol drops are especially effective for prevention, and several drops should be instilled in each ear after efforts have been made at drying the canal.[23,24]

The Tympanic Membrane-Middle Ear

The tympanic membrane-middle ear mechanism can be injured by objects doing physical violence to the external canal, tympanic membrane, or ossicles that enter by the external canal, or by pressure changes in which hydraulic gradients are developed between the external and internal environment resulting in rupture of the tympanic membrane. Perforation of the tympanic membrane may be suspected when a blow has been sustained and sensations of pain, muffled or depressed hearing level, and tinnitus (ringing in the ear) are present. Bleeding from the external auditory canal usually occurs.

Initial management requires medical consultation to establish diagnosis. All foreign material should be kept out of the ear. When perforation of the tympanic membrane has been identified, if the perforation is small, management may consist of observation only, to make sure that spontaneous healing occurs. If the perforation is moderately large and the likelihood of spontaneous healing small, during the acute phase (first 12 hours following injury) margins of the perforation should be repositioned and splinted in proper position using otologic surgical techniques.

Disruption of the ossicular chain with fracture or dislocation of one of the ossicles must also be considered. This syndrome may occur following direct trauma to the external ear, and the tympanic membrane may be either perforated or intact. If, following the trauma, conductive hearing loss is present without other signs, otologic consultation and sophisticated diagnostic evaluation will be required. These injuries are most frequently seen following water skiing accidents in which the side of the head strikes the surface of the water, or in which a blow to the side of the head closes the ear canal, and tympanic membrane rupture occurs because of increased pressure. These injuries can be prevented by using ear plugs that obstruct the external auditory canal.

Occasionally, changes in depth without clearing the eustachian tube while skin or sky diving, can result in tympanic membrane rupture or middle ear barotrauma.[25] These injuries result from processes that cause swelling in the nasal or paranasal sinus lining membranes, or the nasopharynx and auditory tube. Such processes as allergic rhinitis, adenoid enlargement, or viral or bacterial upper respiratory infections, may result in auditory tube dysfunction. The auditory tube is unable to be opened to allow air pressure between the external environment and middle ear. If one is unable to ventilate the middle ears, then activities that involve significant pressure change should be avoided so that the effect of middle ear barotrauma (hemorrhage, fluid formation, or tympanic membrane rupture) will not occur. Prevention of these problems requires avoidance of the activity when the auditory tube is impaired. Treatment of the primary condition may include antibiotic therapy, or topical or systemic nasal decongestants, as indicated.

The inner ear is a delicate, membranous structure suspended in a fluid environment. There are two basic types of injuries to which this structure is subject. One involves significant pressure changes that may rupture various membranes and cause leakage of the inner ear fluids, which will result in temporary hearing loss. Mixing these fluids may cause permanent hearing loss. The other type of injury does little if any physical damage to the membranous structure of the inner ear, but does significant damage to the neural structures that are the sound wave receptors. This injury can cause hearing loss as well.

Injuries to the inner ear are usually detectable because they cause hearing loss, tinnitus, and occasionally vertigo either following great pressure change or significant acoustical insult. Initial management involves protection from further insult and removal from the damaging stimulus.

Prevention of diving injuries is a matter of diver education including appropriate methods of ascent and descent. Prevention of noise-induced hearing loss as a result of shooting or other intense noise exposure, requires an awareness of the damaging potential of high intensity noise and the necessity for either ear muffs or ear plugs for protection.[26]

LARYNGOTRACHEAL INJURY

The larynx and trachea constitute that portion of the airway responsible for voice formation, protection of the lower airway, and passage of air from the upper to the lower respiratory tract. The larynx and trachea occupy the middle and lower central neck. Their exposed position there puts them at significant risk of injury, as testified to by John Garrett, former goalie for the Minnesota Fighting Saints professional hockey team. When asked about risk associated with playing his position, he indicated that the throat was the only part of the body that standard goalie equipment did not protect. "You wonder if you should be struck in the throat, if the trainer can keep you breathing." He said, "I have been struck on the Adam's apple and could not talk for a couple of weeks, but I have never had anything traumatic happen."[27]

No doubt a significant injury occurred in his case. The trachea acts as a passive conduit for air, but the larynx is a rather kinetic muscular structure, in which the epiglottis passively covers the glottic (vocal cord) orifice during the act of swallowing. The muscular constituents of the larynx close the vocal cords during swallowing to obstruct the airway. The vocal folds, when approximated and moved by an air blast, resonate to cause phonation.

Injury to the larynx and trachea is life-threatening. Any blow to the neck that results in shortness of breath, hoarseness, loss of voice, or hemorrhage, requires immediate investigation.

Initial management is dictated by the severity of the injury and is directed at preservation of the airway. If injury is severe and total airway obstruction has occurred or appears to be occurring, emergency endotracheal intubation or emergency tracheostomy will be required. In less urgent situations, in which only hoarseness and mild air hunger may be present, transfer to a hospital setting for evaluation by a laryngologist is necessary. If significant injury to the larynx has been sustained, tracheostomy to bypass that portion of the airway, and open reduction with the approximation of all tissues in as nearly anatomic position as possible, is required.[28,29] This principle of immediate exploration for documented laryngotracheal injury is widely accepted. Injuries may be prevented by the use of laryngotracheal protectors such as those currently employed by some hockey goalies and baseball catchers.

SKIN

Preservation of the head and neck skin integrity is crucial because of its functional importance in relation to the eye, ear, nose, and oral cavity. Function of these organs is vitally dependent on the integrity of the epithelium (skin). The facial skin is fundamental to cosmetic appearance and, therefore, injury demands careful attention so that repair will result in minimal scarring and deformity.

The skin surfaces of the head and neck may be injured in several ways. The most common injuries are mechanical, caused by blows or lacerations with sharp objects. Both thermal and chemical burns may occur, but are not considered in detail here because of their relative infrequency in athletics.

Several factors must be borne in mind when a soft tissue injury in the faciocervical region has occurred. Initial consideration must be control of hemorrhage, which is usually accomplished by compression and prevention of further injury. The next consideration relates to assessment of severity of the injury. This includes estimation of the extent of injury and the necessity for care. If a contusion or superficial abrasion has occurred, healing without further treatment may be expected. In severe abrasions with full-thickness skin removal, consideration must be given to tetanus prophylaxis, careful wound cleansing, employing bland soaps and copious irrigation, and assessment of whether spontaneous healing will result in closure or whether primary repair by suturing or skin grafting may be required.

Lacerations may be simple, small, and superficial, or more severe, both in length, depth, and involvement of underlying vital structures. Simple, linear, superficial lacerations that traverse only the epithelium and superficial soft tissues should be treated by careful cleansing and, depending upon the severity of injury, closure with adhesive strips or suturing. Hemostasis may usually be obtained by pressure alone. More severe lacerations with copious hemorrhage or involvement of underlying structures such as the seventh nerve, parotid duct, or lacerations in vital areas such as the eyelid or nasal tip, require accurate surgical approximation under the best possible conditions, with careful follow-up to insure that healing is appropriate.

Facial soft tissue injuries may be prevented by interposing barriers between injuring objects and the cervicofacial skin, as is demonstrated with helmet and facial protective equipment in the section on facial fracture. In addition, in those sports in which either the activity of the sport or structural parts of the playing surface cause risk, the problem should be addressed by rules or structural changes that might lessen this danger.

An athletically related disease process involving the skin that requires special attention, is epidemic herpes simplex infection in wrestlers. Herpes simplex is a viral disease that may cause cold sores and widespread vesicular dermatitis. Epidemic infection as a result of superficial skin injury, and transmission from wrestler to wrestler as a result of skin contact, has made it apparent that any wrestler with superficial herpes simplex (cold sores) should not compete until the infection has completely resolved.[30]

CONCLUSION

The facial and laryngotracheal structures are at risk in many sporting activities. Only through epidemiologic study of individual sports and athletic situations, will the risks to the athlete be accurately assessed so that appropriate preventive measures may be instituted.

The author wishes to thank Mr John Wirth for valuable research and editorial assistance.

REFERENCES

1. Blyth, C.S., and Mueller, F. O. An epidemiologic study of high school football injury in North Carolina, 1968–1972, final report. US Consumer Product Safety Commission. Washington, DC: US Government Printing Office, 1973.

2. Shumrick, D.A. (Ed.) Maxillofacial and related injuries. *Otolaryngology Clinics of North America.* Philadelphia: W.B. Saunders, 1969.

3. Mathog, R.H. (Ed.) Maxillofacial trauma. *Otolaryngology Clinics of North America.* Philadelphia: W.B. Saunders, 1976.

4. Zaydon, T.J., and Brown, J.B. *Early Treatment of Facial Injuries.* Philadelphia: Lea and Febiger, 1964.

5. Dingman, R.O., and Natvig, P. *Surgery of Facial Fractures.* Philadelphia: W.B. Saunders, 1964.

6. Meyerhoff, W.L., Wilson, K.S., and Christiansen, T. Treatment of the traumatized orbital floor. In *Proceedings of the Second International Symposium on Plastic and Reconstructive Surgery of the Head and Neck.* New York: Grune and Stratton, 1975, pp. 136–141.

7. Helmets, face guards, and better football. Editorial. *Physician and Sportsmedicine* 1:32, 1973.

8. Gurdjian, E.S. *Head Injury from Antiq-*

uity to the Present, with Special Reference to Penetrating Head Wounds. Springfield, Ill: Charles C Thomas, 1973, pp. 58–67.

9. Hayes, D. Winter sports hazard—covert considerations. *Physician and Sportsmedicine* 3:71–76, 1975.

10. Nagobads, V.G. Hockey injuries—the pro is hit the hardest. *Physician and Sportsmedicine* 1:55–57, 1973.

11. *Football Mask and Dental Guard Study.* Wisconsin Interscholastic Athletic Association Bulletin. November 11:36, 1967.

12. Pashby, T.J. Eye injuries in Canadian hockey. Phase II. *Can Med Assoc J.* 117:671–678, 1977.

13. Wilson, K.S. et al. Facial injuries in hockey players. *Minn Med.* 60:13–19, 1977.

14. Horns, R.C. Blinding hockey injuries. *Minn Med.* 59(4):255–258, 1976.

15. Vinger, P.F. Too great a risk spurred hockey mask development. *Physician and Sportsmedicine* 5:70–73, 1977.

16. Rontal, E., and Rontal, M. Maxillofacial injuries in football players, an evaluation of current facial protection. *J Sports Med Phys Fitness.* 11:241–245, 1971.

17. Schneider, R.C. et al. Serious and fatal football injuries involving the head and spinal cord. *JAMA.* 177(6):362–367, 1961.

18. Albright, J.P., Moses, J.M., Feldick, H.G. et al. Nonfatal cervical spine injuries in interscholastic football. *JAMA.* 236(11): 1243–1245, 1976.

19. Cooper, D.L. Commentary: high school football injuries. *South Med J.* 69:1257, 1976.

20. Alley, R.H. Head and neck injuries in high school football. *JAMA.* 188(5):418–422, 1964.

21. Cooper, D.L., and Fair, J. Treating cauliflower ear. *Physician and Sportsmedicine* 4:103, 1976.

22. DiBartolomeo, J.R. Exostotic ear tumors, sea water sport peril. *Physician and Sportsmedicine* 4:60–63, 1976.

23. Eichel, B.S. Otologic hazards of water sports. *Physician and Sportsmedicine* 2:43–45, 1974.

24. Lee, S. Athletic hazards related to otolaryngology. In *The Medical Aspects of Sports.* Proceedings of the 15th National Conference. Chicago: American Medical Association, 1974.

25. Strauss, M.D., and Cantrell, R.W. Ear and sinus barotrauma in diving. *Physician and Sportsmedicine* 2:39–43, 1974.

26. Odess, J.S. The hearing hazard of fire arms. *Physician and Sportsmedicine* 2:65–68, 1974.

27. Hockey's most visible and vulnerable player. Editorial. *Physician and Sportsmedicine* 3:85–90, 1975.

28. Shumrick, D.A. Trauma of the larynx and lower airway. Edited by M.M. Paparella, and D.A. Shumrick. In *Otolaryngology. Vol. 3, Head and Neck.* Philadelphia: W.B. Saunders, 1973.

29. Montgomery, W.W. *Tracheal Stenosis. Surgery of the Upper Respiratory System.* Vol. 2. Philadelphia: Lea and Febiger, 1973, pp. 373–444.

30. Millikan, L.E. Those viral skin infections can run wild. *Physician and Sportsmedicine* 3:38–44, 1975.

CHAPTER 12
Eye Injuries

Paul F. Vinger, MD

The eye, exposed and fragile, was not designed to withstand the forces of most sports. The National Society to Prevent Blindness (NSPB) estimates that about 167,000 eye injuries, of varying degrees of severity, occur to school-age children each year. Two-thirds of these injuries are sports-or play-related and 90% are preventable.[1]

The National Electronic Injury Surveillance System (NEISS) of the Consumer Product Safety Commission estimates that 1.7% (42,112) of the 3,610,286 sports- and recreational equipment-related injuries treated in United States emergency rooms in 1982 were eye injuries (Table 12-1). The NEISS figure is lower than that of the NSPB because NEISS data does not include those patients seen in private offices or clinics, however both NEISS and NSPB agree that the majority of sports eye injuries involve youths.

The tendency for children to hurt their eyes while playing is not unique to the United States. Playing accidents are the most common cause of perforating ocular injuries in Israeli children[2]; Nigerian youth suffer most of their severe eye injuries at play.[3]

Many eye injuries lead to blindness (Table 12-2), yet there frequently is a significant delay between the time of injury and evaluation by a physician.[4,5]

The role of accident prevention has been stressed as a necessary element in the continuing education of pediatricians, but this emphasis is lacking to the general public.[6] Everyone must be convinced of the need to protect themselves, and especially their children, from eye injuries in sports and play. An injury that results in chronic disability costs more, both in dollars and suffering, when it involves a child with many years of life expectancy. Ninety percent of these eye injuries could be prevented with protective equipment or modification of the rules of certain sports. The need for more participation in prevention of eye injuries is apparent.

The chief goal in the preservation of sight in sports is the protection of the eye from accidental trauma.[7]

MECHANISMS OF EYE INJURIES

Direct Blow to the Eye

A blow by a sharp object, such as a shard of glass (Figure 12-1), will result in surface or imbedded foreign bodies or clean, usually well-defined, abrasions or lacerations.

Prognosis is relatively good in a laceration of this type provided the contents of the globe are not expressed through the laceration by forceful lid closure.

A blow by a blunt object smaller than the orbital opening, such as a golf ball or hockey stick (Figure 12-2), will result in transmission of great forces to the delicate internal ocular structures. Ragged rupture of the globe secondary to injury by a blunt object has the worst prognosis for recovery of useful vision.[8] To produce eye injury, less energy is required with high speed and small mass missiles (BB shot) than with low speed and large mass missiles (basketball).[9]

With a blow by a blunt object larger than the orbital opening, such as a tennis ball, elbow, or fist (Figure 12-3), the forces transmitted to the floor of the orbit often fracture that thin bone. This "pressure release valve" usually prevents rupture of the globe, but there is a high incidence of hidden internal ocular injury in these cases.[10] Objects larger than 4 inches in diameter have less potential for eye injury, as the orbital rim absorbs much of the energy, but do deform enough to cause serious eye injury (see Soccer) (Figure 12-3).

Blows to the Skull with Indirect Injury to Eye Structures

Trauma almost anywhere on the head can result in visual problems. The exact nature of the visual field defect helps the physician to localize the lesion (Figure 12-4).

Table 12-1
Estimated Number of Product-related Eye Injuries Treated in Hospital Emergency Rooms for Selected Sports: United States, 1973–1978, 1982

Sport	Total 1973–1978	1973	1974	1975	1976	1977	1978	1982
Total	126,268	16,743	17,417	18,047	22,385	25,268	26,408	30,823
Baseball	36,419	5288	5416	4755	5371	6918	8671	9189
Basketball	19,869	2127	3370	2563	4037	3466	4306	7541
Tennis, badminton, squash	18,049	1679	1719	2751	3519	4699	3682	3976*
Football	11,961	1620	2018	1439	2275	2291	2318	2350
Bicycling	7856	1069	1244	1783	923	1138	1699	3160
Sportsball, not specified	11,382	1293	730	1318	3297	3137	1607	—
Gas, air, spring-operated guns	8081	1267	1552	1489	1288	1150	1335	1866†
Hockey, all kinds	6717	1832	1037	1251	651	629	1317	892
Volleyball	3028	332	34	315	438	1095	814	458
Soccer	2906	236	297	383	586	745	659	1665
Swimming								1262
Boxing								330

Note: From this table the following can be seen:

1. Hockey injuries decreased from 1973 to 1982 as a result of protective face masks. No face or eye injuries occurred to players wearing certified face protectors.
2. Although hockey injuries have decreased dramatically to players wearing face protection, a significant problem remains for unprotected players.
3. An upward trend of injuries in baseball, basketball, football and soccer.
4. A steady stream of injuries from airguns and cycling
5. A steady increase in sports-related eye injuries

*Squash, racquetball and paddle ball = 2229; tennis and badminton = 1747.
†1980 data not added in 1982 total.

Unpublished data from the Consumer Product Safety Commission provided to the Operational Research Department, National Society to Prevent Blindness, New York.

Although many of these injuries are not direct injuries to the eye, they can result in temporary or permanent visual loss, and are frequently seen by the ophthalmologist. The huge forces required to produce these injuries can be encountered in the collision sports, skiing, bicycling, and motor sports.

THE ANATOMY OF PROTECTION

The eye is exposed to injury frontally and laterally (see Figure 12-1). From the front, the bony orbit will permit easy entry of an object smaller than 35 mm (1.4 inches).[11] When viewed from the side, about half of the eye lies anterior to the lateral orbital rim, thus even a large flat object (the blade of a hockey stick) approaching from the side will strike the globe. The eyelids offer little protection against huge forces in most sports.

The strongest bone of the orbit is the supraorbital rim, a part of the frontal bone. Since forces transmitted to the frontal bone have a tendency to be dissipated down the lateral orbital arches into the mass of the face, the frontal bones are desirable areas for the transmission of energy loads from protective devices. The lateral and inferior orbital rims are sturdy, but less desirable areas for the acceptance of large energy loads. The weakest bones of the orbit lie between the two eyes. Somewhat stronger, but still weak, are the floor and roof of the orbit (Figure 12-5).[12]

Protective devices should protect the eyes from lateral as well as frontal blows. Forces from resultant blows should be transmitted, through the protective device, primarily to the strong frontal bones. The protective device should have enough

Table 12-2
Canadian Ophthalmological Society Survey of Eye Injuries in Canadian Sports: Reported Number of Injuries and Blinded Eyes, by Sport

	1972–73	1974–75	1976–77	1977–78	1978–79	1979–80	1980–81	1981–82	1982–83	1983–84	Total
Hockey	287(20)	257(43)	90(12)	52(8)	43(13)	85(21)	68(20)	119(18)	115(13)	123(12)	1239(180)
Racket sports			48(3)	12(1)	28(1)	58(1)	102(3)	100(3)	88(5)	111(3)	547(20)
Baseball			19(2)	2	2	10	15	41(5)	68(3)	56(3)	213(13)
Ball hockey			24(3)	8	9(2)	27(2)	22(4)	10(2)	19(3)	25(2)	144(18)
Football (soccer)			13(1)	2	3	1	8	4	27(1)	22(1)	80(3)
Golf			5(1)	0	1	1	0	5(4)	7(2)	3(2)	22(9)
Volleyball			3(3)	0	0	6	3	2	3	4(1)	21(4)
Broomball			2(2)	0	0	2	2	3	3	2	14(2)
Basketball			0	1	0	0	2	4	3	5	15
Skiing			1(1)	1	3(2)	0	0	3(2)	0	2(1)	10(6)
Lacrosse			3	1	1	0	0	0	3	4	12
Hunting			0	0	0	4(1)	0	0	1	5(2)	10(3)
Water polo			1	0	0	0	3	1	0	0	5
Snowmobiling			2(1)	0	1	0	0	1(1)	0	1	5(2)
Other sports			5	0	0	7	0	5(1)	6(1)	9(2)	32(4)
Total	287(20)	253(43)	216(29)	79(9)	91(18)	201(25)	226(27)	298(36)	342(28)	372(29)	2369(264)

( ) = Blind eyes.
Study is continuous poll of members of Canadian Ophthalmological Society by Thomas Pashby, MD.
Note: No hockey injuries occurred in players wearing CSA certified face protectors. High percentage (41%) of injured eyes blinded as result of golf; 2223 (94%) of eye injuries were from hockey, racket sports, baseball and soccer.

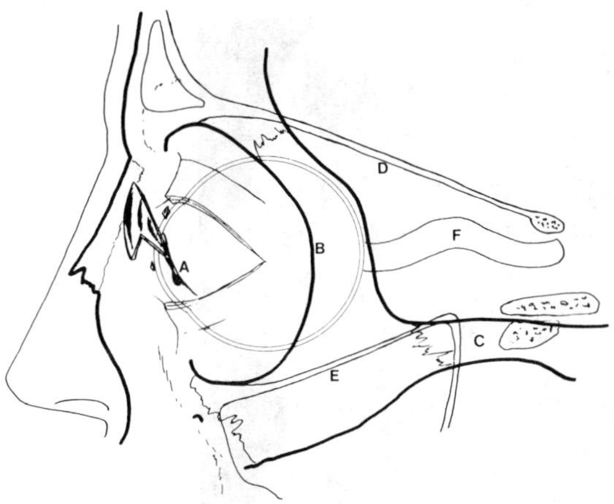

Figure 12-1 Direct blow to the eye (left eye, side view) by a sharp object (glass), with corneo-scleral laceration and iris prolapse (A). The drawing illustrates exposure of eye to injury from the side. The globe is relatively undeformed by the impact. (B) Lateral orbital rim, (C) zygomatic arch, (D) roof of orbit, (E) floor of orbit, (F) optic nerve.

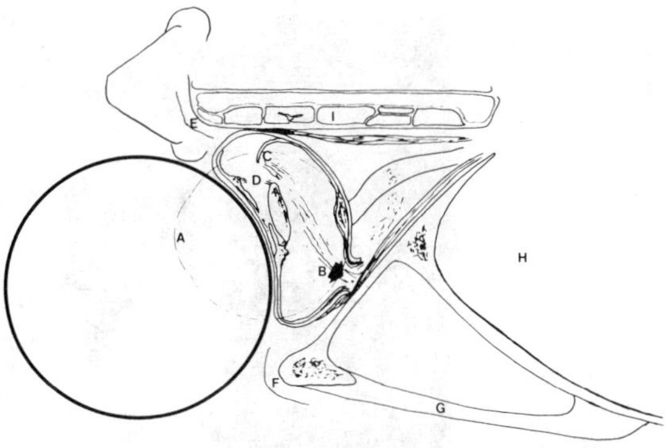

Figure 12-2 Direct blow to the eye (left eye viewed from the top) by a blunt object smaller than the orbital opening (golf ball). (A) Deformation of the globe by impact (normal position shown by dotted line). (B) Increase in diameter of the globe with release of greatly increased intraocular pressure by perforation. (C) Retinal tear caused by traction on vitreous base. (D) Rupture of lens suspensory ligaments. (E) Line drawn from medial orbital rim to lateral orbital rim (F) leaves about 35% to 50% of eye (A) unprotected by bone in blows from lateral side. (G) Zygomatic arch. (H) Temporal fossa (location of tip of temporal lobe of brain). (I) Ethmoid sinuses.

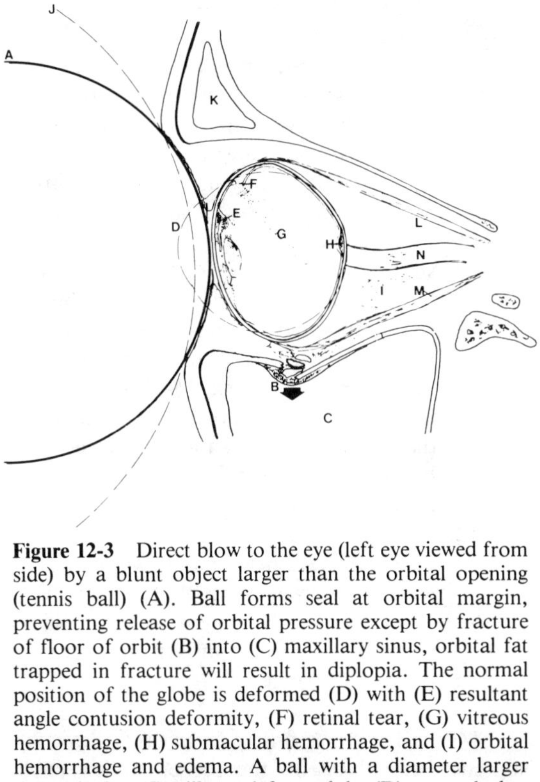

Figure 12-3 Direct blow to the eye (left eye viewed from side) by a blunt object larger than the orbital opening (tennis ball) (A). Ball forms seal at orbital margin, preventing release of orbital pressure except by fracture of floor of orbit (B) into (C) maxillary sinus, orbital fat trapped in fracture will result in diplopia. The normal position of the globe is deformed (D) with (E) resultant angle contusion deformity, (F) retinal tear, (G) vitreous hemorrhage, (H) submacular hemorrhage, and (I) orbital hemorrhage and edema. A ball with a diameter larger than 4 inches (J) will not deform globe (D) as much, but injury is still likely with objects larger than 4 inches in diameter. (K) Frontal sinus, (L) superior rectus muscle, (M) inferior rectus muscle, (N) optic nerve.

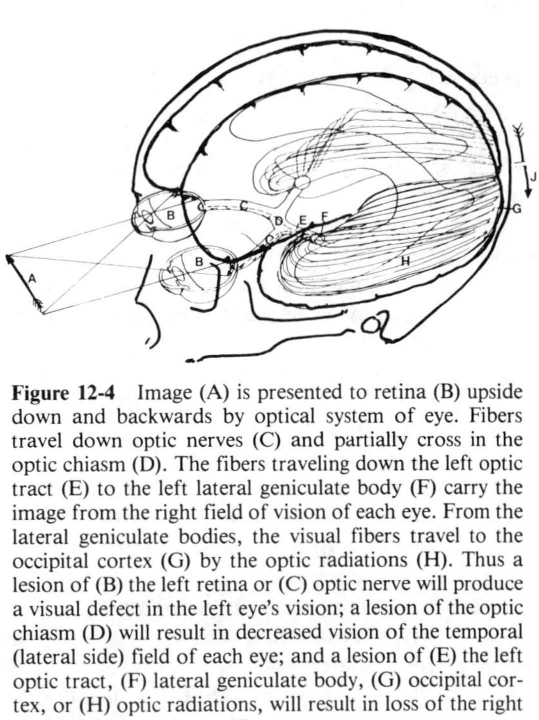

Figure 12-4 Image (A) is presented to retina (B) upside down and backwards by optical system of eye. Fibers travel down optic nerves (C) and partially cross in the optic chiasm (D). The fibers traveling down the left optic tract (E) to the left lateral geniculate body (F) carry the image from the right field of vision of each eye. From the lateral geniculate bodies, the visual fibers travel to the occipital cortex (G) by the optic radiations (H). Thus a lesion of (B) the left retina or (C) optic nerve will produce a visual defect in the left eye's vision; a lesion of the optic chiasm (D) will result in decreased vision of the temporal (lateral side) field of each eye; and a lesion of (E) the left optic tract, (F) lateral geniculate body, (G) occipital cortex, or (H) optic radiations, will result in loss of the right visual field in each eye (J).

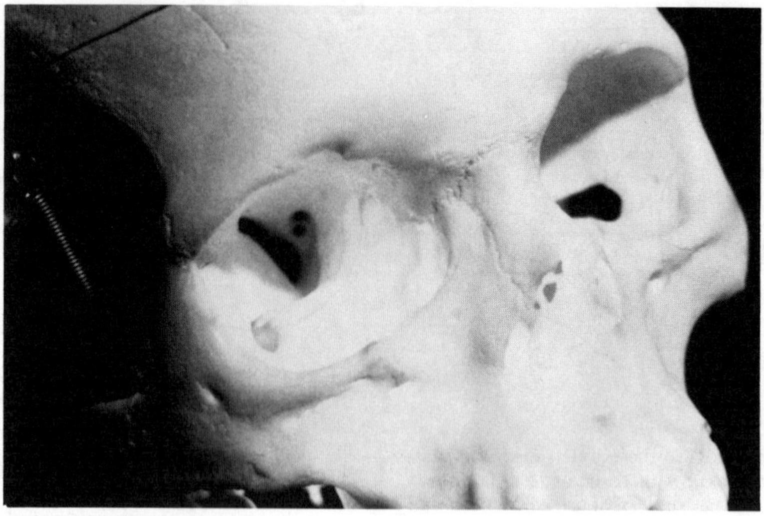

Figure 12-5 Orbital bones: light areas demonstrate the thinness of the medial wall and floor of the orbit. The maxillary sinus also is illuminated. Note the thickness of the bones that form the superior, lateral, and inferior orbital rims.

deflection to increase the duration over which force is dissipated, but be rigid enough to prevent the force from impinging on the eye itself.

TREATMENT OF EYE INJURIES

Necessary Equipment for First Aid

First aid equipment required on the site for eye injuries fits in a small container within the physician's or trainer's bag. Included should be:

1. phone numbers of hospital and covering physicians, especially for away games
2. vision card (mainly as a reminder always to check the vision of an injured eye)
3. penlight
4. hard metal or plastic protective eye shield (to be taped in place for the least suspicion of perforation of the eye)
5. eye patches, sterile
6. tape, transparent or micropore
7. irrigating solution, sterile
8. sterile cotton swabs
9. fluorescein strips, sterile (to diagnose corneal abrasions)
10. antibiotic eye ointment, such as erythromycin 0.5% (the ointment should not contain a corticosteroid)
    CAUTION: never instill an ointment into an eye that may be perforated. Do not instill an ointment into an eye if the player is to be seen within several hours by an ophthalmologist, as ointment interferes with the eye examination.
11. anesthetic eye drops, sterile unit dose, such as proparacaine 0.5%
    CAUTION: the overuse of these topical anesthetics can mask severe underlying pathology and result in permanent scarring of the cornea. Maximum dose is one drop to relieve severe pain for diagnostic or therapeutic use. Never to be used to relieve pain so that a player may return to competition.
12. sterile skin-closure strips
    CAUTION: to be used only with minor lacerations away from the lid margin. With any lid laceration, assume the globe is lacerated until it has been proven otherwise.

Means for transporting an injured player by stretcher should be on the scene. An available telephone should be located, especially at unfamiliar fields. Presbyopic examiners would find a magnifying glass helpful.

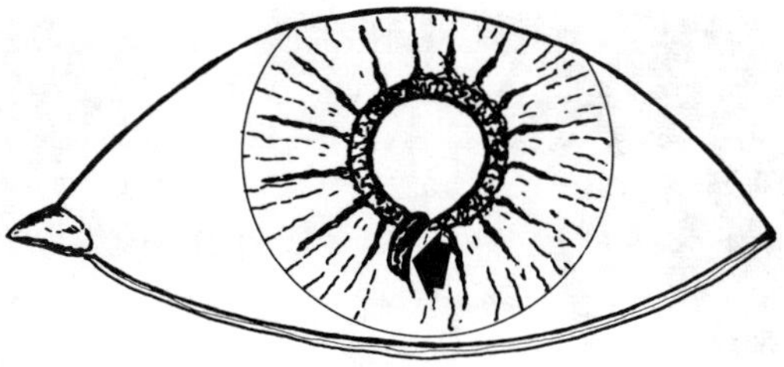

Figure 12-6 Laceration of the cornea with prolapse of the iris. Note distortion of the pupil.

First Aid Evaluation

Initial evaluation of the patient should be carefully performed, as serious eye injuries may not be apparent at first glance.

Check the vision in each eye with the other eye covered. If the player cannot see the 20/20 line on the near vision card, the eye is assumed injured until proven otherwise by an ophthalmologist. Failure to check vision is the most common error of omission on initial examination of an injured athlete.

Look at the pupils with the penlight. Any irregularity of the pupillary border may indicate a laceration of the cornea with prolapse of the iris (Figure 12-6). Unequal or poorly reactive pupils are signs of iritis (inflammation within the eye) and glaucoma (too high pressure in the eye), both potentially blinding conditions.

Look carefully at the cornea, the clear window over the iris (colored part) of the eye. If the iris details are hazy, there may be blood or inflammatory cells between the cornea and the iris (this space filled with fluid, is called the anterior chamber of the eye), or the cornea may be swollen. Any hazy appearance of the iris requires immediate evaluation by an ophthalmologist. Never remove an embedded foreign body from the cornea.

Examine the conjunctiva. An obvious foreign body on the conjunctiva (white of the eye) or under the lid may be removed with a sterile cotton swab without anesthesia. Beware of black foreign bodies. The interior coats of the eye are black. An apparent foreign body may be protrusion of the contents of the eye through a perforation in the sclera (wall of the eye).

Check that both eyes move together in all directions of gaze—right, left, up, down.

Be sure the globe of the eye is intact before proceeding with evaluation of lid lacerations. Never attempt forcibly to open lids swollen closed by edema or hematoma.

For any suspicion of ruptured or lacerated globe patch the injured eye and put a hard shield in place with tape. Patch the uninjured eye, if the player can tolerate this without thrashing. Encourage the player not to squeeze the eyes shut forcefully, as this could express the contents of the eye through the laceration. Keep the player calm and transport him to the hospital or clinic for medical attention.

The primary purpose of the first aid examination is to be sure that the eye is uninjured. When in doubt, remove the athlete from competition and seek medical, preferably ophthalmologic, evaluation.

First Aid Treatment

There are several ocular injuries that may be treated at the scene (medications for physician use only).

Foreign bodies beneath the lids or on the conjunctiva may be removed with irrigation or a sterile swab. After removal, antibiotic eye ointment may be applied to the globe. Play may be resumed.

Superficial corneal foreign bodies may be removed (after topical anesthesia) with a forceful stream of irrigating solution or a gentle stroke of the moistened sterile cotton swab. Corneal foreign bodies that remain in place after these maneuvers should be removed by an ophthalmologist. Removal of an embedded corneal foreign body with a needle or spud should not be attempted on the athletic field. After removal, antibiotic eye ointment and a firm, double eye patch should be applied to the closed eye. The patient should be seen by an ophthalmologist the next day to check for possible secondary infection or incomplete healing. Play should not be resumed.

Corneal abrasions may be diagnosed by a fluorescein strip; the abraded area will stain bright green. Be sure the pupil is normal, the anterior chamber is clear, and the globe is intact. One drop of topical anesthetic and antibiotic eye ointment should be instilled to the injured eye. The eye should be patched and ophthalmologic follow-up arranged as described for corneal foreign bodies. Play should not be resumed.

Small lid or brow lacerations that do not impair lid function and that spare the lid margin may be closed with a sterile closure strip after appropriate cleansing of the area. Be sure the laceration does not penetrate the entire thickness of the lid, and that the globe is intact. Play may be resumed at the discretion of the physician.

Immediate referral to the ophthalmologist is required for:

1. embedded corneal foreign bodies
2. haze or blood in the anterior chamber
3. decreased vision, constriction, or loss of a portion of visual field
4. irregular, asymmetric, or poorly reacting pupil
5. diplopia (double vision)
6. lacerations involving the lid margins or impaired lid function
7. suspected perforation of the globe
8. broken contact lens or shattered eyeglasses.

In addition, the ophthalmologist should examine at a later date all blunt trauma to the eye and orbit. Only a complete eye examination can rule out internal ocular injury.

Attempts at treatment by well-meaning, but incompletely trained medical or nonmedical personnel can convert treatable injuries into blind eyes.

Definitive Medical Evaluation and Treatment

Every eye that has suffered a direct or indirect blow should be evaluated by an ophthalmologist to rule out hidden internal injuries that may threaten loss of vision at a later date. Many injuries, easily treated in their early stages, result in loss of vision if left to their own course.

Perforating ocular injuries One-half or more of all ocular enucleations are performed for trauma, with most of the lost eyes a result of perforation of the globe.[13] Perforating injuries that involve a clean laceration of the cornea have the best prognoses, as simple suturing often results in salvage of vision. Ragged perforating injuries from blunt objects can occur at the area of impact or at a distant site (indirect rupture).[14]

The signs of perforation of the globe are often subtle (Figure 12-7). Even apparently minor brow and lid lacerations, remote from the globe, can be associated with its perforation.[15]

Newer surgical techniques are improving the end results, but the prognosis for a perforating injury of the eye is still serious.[13] It is best when

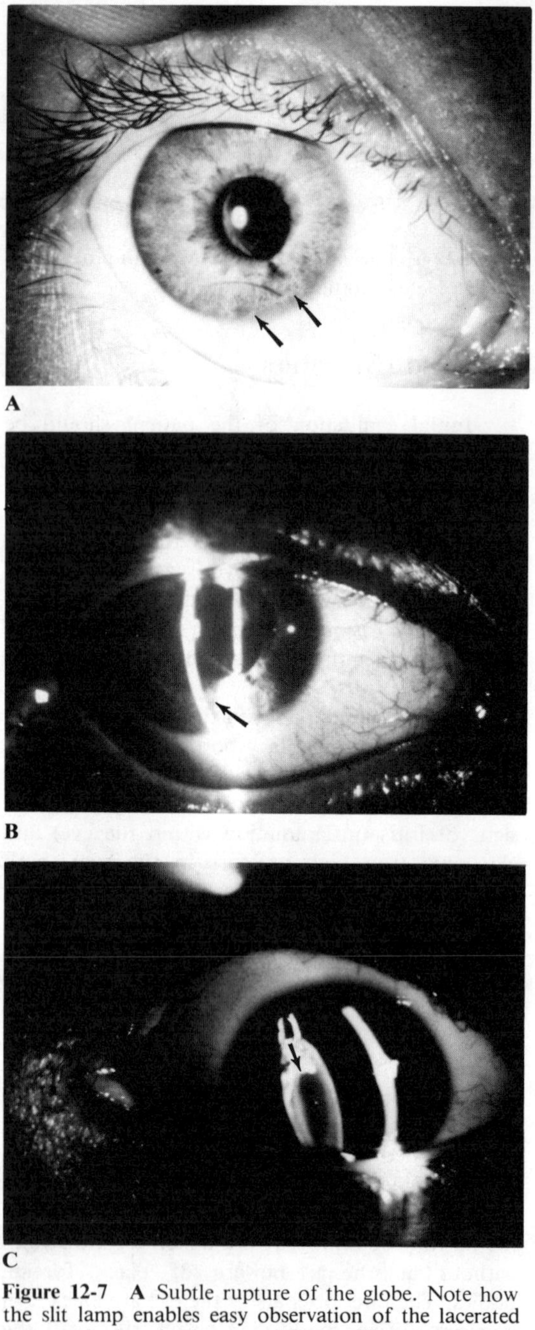

A

B

C

Figure 12-7 **A** Subtle rupture of the globe. Note how the slit lamp enables easy observation of the lacerated cornea, the lens is absent and **B** the cilium (eye lash) is within the anterior chamber. All of these features would easily be overlooked on casual examination. **C** Slit lamp photograph of dislocated lens.

surgery is performed early, and if the ocular contents are contained within the globe. These goals are aided by keeping the patient calm, encouraging him not to squeeze the eyes shut, using a protective shield over the injured eye, and rapid ophthalmologic attention.

Hyphema is bleeding into the anterior chamber of the eye (Figure 12-8). It results from tearing of the major arterial circle of the iris or a disruption of Schlemm canal.[16] Hyphema is often associated with traumatic iridocyclitis (inflammation of the iris and ciliary body). The main direct complication during or after hyphema is glaucoma (elevated intraocular pressure) which results from many causes.[17] Some notable ones are:

1. Blockage of egress of aqueous humor from the eye by entrapment of blood or inflammatory cells in the trabecular meshwork,
2. Blockage of passage of aqueous humor from the posterior to the anterior chambers by adhesions between the iris and the lens (posterior synechiae),
3. Compromise of the iridocorneal angle and trabecular meshwork by adhesions of the iris to the cornea (peripheral anterior synechiae), or scarring secondary to angle contusion deformity. Angle contusion deformity, present in up to 94% of patients with hyphema, results in late-onset glaucoma in 9%, especially when over one-half the circumference of the iridocorneal angle is injured.[18]

Thus every case of hyphema requires careful monitoring of intraocular pressure, observation with the slit lamp for adhesions and inflammatory response, and gonioscopy. Glaucoma may develop years after injury and result in loss of vision in a potentially salvageable eye. Inflammation usually is controlled with topical corticosteroids and cycloplegics. Pupillary block is relieved by dilating the pupil or surgery. Glaucoma is treated with a variety of medications or surgery.

Initial treatment of hyphema usually consists of complete bedrest in the hospital with one or both eyes patched. The injured eye is carefully monitored by the ophthalmologist for complications.

Prognosis is guarded in all cases of hyphema, especially those presenting with more than one-half of the anterior chamber filled with blood, because of the high frequency of associated serious injuries within the eye, especially to the lens, choroid, and retina.[19-21]

Retina and choroid Late blindness following trauma usually results either from the late glaucoma of angle contusion deformity (already discussed), or holes torn in the retina at the time of impact that begin to leak and cause detachment of the retina. The holes may leak immediately or at some future date, long after the initial injury.

Holes in the retina can be treated before they leak and result in retinal detachments; they have the best prognosis when treated early. Trauma is the most common single cause of retinal detachment between birth and age 16; often there is a long delay between the trauma and the diagnosis of retinal detachment.[5]

The importance of careful examination of the peripheral retina (Figure 12-9) in all patients after blunt injury to the eye cannot be overemphasized. The obvious retinal detachment in Figure 12-9 would have been missed by most physicians. The patient was asymptomatic. Only proper examination can detect peripheral retinal lesions. There is a possibility of a long latency period between trauma and detachment associated with the poor ability of some children to communicate in giving a history of decreased visual acuity.[22-24]

Retinal detachment due to ocular penetration has a relatively poor prognosis because continued shrinkage of vitreous membranes often causes redetachment of a previously surgically reattached retina.[25]

A direct blow to the eye can result in severe chorioretinal contusion and scarring with loss of vision[26] secondary to loss of photoreceptor cells.[27] Macular edema may be one of the ocular complications of a flexion-extension (whiplash) type of head and neck injury.[28,29]

Mountaineers at altitudes higher than 12,000 feet (3658 meters),[30] are subject to retinal hemorrhages, probably secondary to hypoxic vasodilation combined with sudden rises in intravascular pressures. The hemorrhages resolve spontaneously with return of normal visual acuity on return of the climber to lower altitude, but the climber may be left with permanent reduction in critical flicker frequency, visual fields, and dark adaptation.[30-32]

Rents in the choroid and Bruch membrane are common complications of contusion injuries of the eye. They usually are concentric with and temporal to the optic disc. If the macula is involved, central vision is immediately and permanently lost. How-

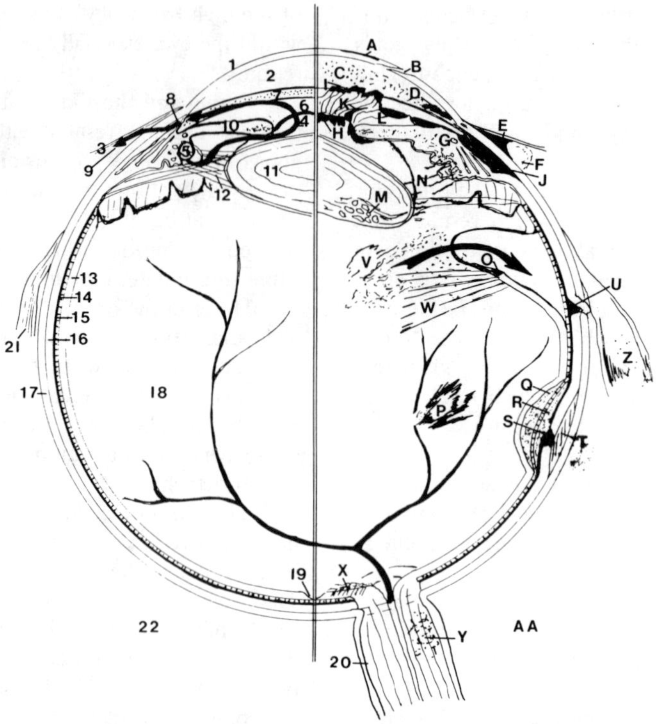

Figure 12-8 Left (numbers) is a normal eye, right (letters) is eye with typical injuries from sports accidents.

1. Cornea: (A) corneal abrasion, (B) corneal laceration.

2. Anterior chamber (filled with aqueous humor–plasma-like liquid): (C) cells and flare in anterior chamber (traumatic iritis), (D) blood in anterior chamber (hyphema).

3. Conjunctiva: (E) subconjunctival hemorrhage, (F) edema beneath conjunctiva (chemosis).

4. Normal aqueous circulation to nourish eye and maintain normal intraocular pressure. Ciliary body (5), through pupil (6) through trabecular meshwork (7) into canal of Schlemm (8) and out through conjunctival and episcleral veins (9): impediments to aqueous production and outflow: (G) ciliary edema, (H) posterior synechiae (adhesions of iris to lens), (I) peripheral anterior synechiae (adhesions of iris to cornea), (J) angle contusion deformity and scarring of trabecular meshwork plus blockage of meshwork with blood and inflammatory debris.

10. Iris: (K) rupture of iris sphincter, (L) iridodialisis.

11. Lens, and (12) lens suspensory ligaments: (M) cataract (opacity of lens), (N) rupture of suspensory ligaments with dislocation of lens.

13. Retina: (O) retinal tear with detachment, (P) retinal hemorrhages, (Q) subretinal hemorrhages or edema.

14. Retinal pigment epithelium: (R) subpigment epithelial bleeding or edema.

15. Bruch membrane: (S) break in Bruch membrane (choroid often also torn).

16. Choroid: (T) subchoroidal hemorrhages or edema.

17. Sclera: (U) scleral rupture with prolapse of choroid.

18. Vitreous: (V) vitreous hemorrhage and inflammation, (W) vitreous traction and fibrosis.

19. Macula: (X) Macula edema with loss of receptor cells.

20. Optic nerve: (Y) hemorrhage, contusion, or edema of optic nerve.

21. Extraocular muscle: (Z) hemorrhage, edema, or contusion of muscle.

22. Orbit: (AA) hemorrhage, edema, or inflammation of orbit.

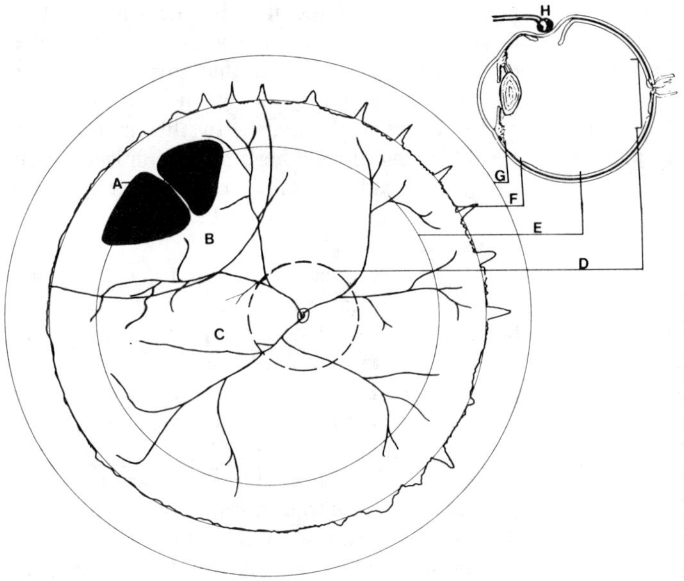

Figure 12-9 Drawing of retina of a player hit with a hockey stick. (A) Retinal hole, (B) detached retina, (C) attached retina, (D) area of retina usually seen by nonophthalmologist using direct (hand-held) ophthalmoscope, (E) equator of eye—absolute limit of view with direct ophthalmoscope easily seen with indirect ophthalmoscope and condensing lens, (F) ora serrata, and (G) pars plana can only be seen by special techniques such as indirect ophthalmoscopy, and (H) scleral depression.

ever, the late development of a subretinal neovascular membrane may result in late macular complications even from choroidal tears away from the macula. All patients with choroidal tears should be followed for this complication. It may be successfully treated with light coagulation of the new blood vessels if they are detected in their early stages of growth.[33,34]

The posterior pole of the eye is involved in other complications of blunt trauma to the eye: preretinal, intraretinal, and subretinal hemorrhages; edema of the retina that could progress to hole formation in the macula area; and hematomas of the retinal pigment, epithelium, and choroid.

Lens and vitreous Trauma is the most common cause of dislocation of the lens that frequently is associated with retinal detachment and glaucoma. Surgical removal of a dislocated lens usually is done to improve vision or to control glaucoma. Surgery is not taken lightly when the lens is dislocated, since it is a relatively high-risk procedure.[35,36]

Traumatic cataracts, with the lens still in normal position, do not pose a large surgical risk; thus restoration of vision is common after removal of a traumatic cataract, provided the cornea, vitreous, retina, optic nerve, and visual pathways are normal.

The vitreous can become opaque with blood, inflammatory cells, or scar tissue. Fortunately, newer types of vitreous surgery are salvaging vision in these formerly hopeless cases.[37]

Blow-out fractures Fractures of the face and orbital rim have been discussed in Chapter 11. Discussion here will be limited to a unique fracture caused either by a sudden increase in the intraorbital pressure or a buckling action of the floor of the orbit that results in breaking of the thin bones of the floor and medial orbital wall behind the intact orbital rim. Blow-out fractures are mostly caused by objects larger than the bony opening (see Figure 12-3).[12]

Most blow-out fractures are treated by observation,[38] but surgery may be required if there is persistent diplopia (double vision), or enophthalmos (sinking of the eye into the orbit).[39]

Surgical repair of the blow-out fracture is within the territory of a number of subspecialists: ophthalmologists, otolaryngologists, plastic surgeons, and oral surgeons. However an ophthalmologist must evaluate the eye before surgical repair. The incidence of intraocular injury with blow-out fracture is up to 74%.[40] Surgery should not be performed until it has been ascertained that there would be no serious risk (such as increased bleeding from an already bleeding retinal tear) from intraocular injury secondary to the original trauma, by the added manipulations of the globe during surgery.[41,42]

Blindness Blindness after eye or head trauma may be transient or permanent. Transient blindness in children is often overlooked[43]; the etiology is uncertain. Some postulate temporary cerebral dysfunction,[44] while others believe a vasospasm farther anterior in the visual system (retina, optic nerves, chiasm, or tracts) is more likely.[45,46]

Concussion to the optic nerve may result in permanent blindness.[47]

Transient blindness of children after head trauma is a real phenomenon. No child should be labeled as hysterically blind, even after apparently minor head trauma, until one is *positive* the child is not truly blind.

The injuries discussed above encompass the vast majority of eye trauma because of sports. Rarer conditions, such as luxation of the globe, complex orbital injuries, and neuroophthalmologic diagnostic problems will not be discussed.

PROTECTIVE DEVICES

A protective device should prevent damaging forces from reaching the eyes. This theory is simple enough, but the practical application can be difficult. As soon as design is begun on an eye protective device for a sport with an ocular hazard, many problems arise. What forces are involved in this sport? Are they high velocity, low mass (hockey puck); low velocity, high mass (player sliding into a goal post); or a combination of the two (bicycle racer collision)? Does a protector have to be designed differently for each type of force? How? Where on the head will these forces be transmitted, and how will it be done? Will the player be killed if the force is transmitted to his brain through the protective device, rather than being dissipated into broken facial or orbital bones as was the case before the protector? Will the protector change the form or appeal of the game? What about design, player acceptance, expense, vision, weight, product liability, full disclosure to the consumer?

These questions cannot be answered by one individual, as expertise at many levels and different areas of interest is required. The best way to design and build a protective device is by a predetermined performance standard to which the protector will be made. Such standards require input from players, coaches, engineers, manufacturers, physicians, and possibly lawyers and economists.

Distribution of Forces

If possible, the best area for distribution of forces when one tries to protect the eyes, is the frontal bones. These bones are the sturdiest about the orbit and have the tendency to transmit energy into the mass of the face by the lateral orbital margins.[11,12] In collision sports such as hockey or football, it is obvious that this result is best achieved by mounting the eye-face protector to a properly designed helmet. In this manner, the desirable goal of total head protection is achieved.

Total head protection, not isolated eye, face, teeth, etc, protection should be the goal for collision sports.

Whenever a large force is transmitted anywhere on the head, the prime consideration must be the ultimate dissipation of this force as it relates to the brain. It is senseless to protect an eye, if in so doing the damaging forces are transmitted directly to the brain. All protective devices for the head and face thus require two areas of consideration: 1) is the primary area of concern (eye, face, teeth, etc) protected; 2) is the transmission of forces such that there is no added risk to the brain?

Forces are best dissipated if they are transmitted over a wide area, and the duration of time over which the force is allowed to act is lengthened.[48] Helmet design must be monitored by comparing predicted forces[49,50] with actual measurements of injury on real players in action.[51]

Sports with less energy potential require less protection. A tennis ball has little potential for injuring the brain, therefore, attention need only be directed toward protecting the eye. In this case, one might consider it acceptable to transmit the forces to the frontal bone (best), or even other less desirable areas (the bridge of the nose, the infraorbital or lateral orbital rims), and still achieve good eye protection. One could accept a cut on the cheek, a broken nose, or even a fracture of the zygoma as far preferable to the potential loss of the eye. For sports such as tennis, trade-offs, style considerations, weight, and visual fields could all interact and result in somewhat less-than-ideal protective devices that would do more good for the majority of players because the players would wear them.

A protective device is effective only when worn by the player. The best designed protective device, if it does not appeal to the tastes of the player, will remain on the dealer's shelf.

AMA SPORTS CLASSIFICATION

Most physicians, in evaluating athletes with loss of a paired organ (eg, eye, ear, kidney, testis) for sports participation, use tables based on the

AMA breakdown of sports into *collision* (eg, football, rugby, hockey, lacrosse), *contact* (eg, baseball, soccer, basketball, wrestling), *noncontact* (eg, cross country, track, tennis, crew, swimming), and *other* (eg, bowling, golf, archery, field events).

These tables suggest disqualification of a one-eyed athlete for collision and contact sports, but not for noncontact and other sports.[52] These tables and recommendations reflect the potential risk of bone, muscle and internal organs to injury in certain sports, but are, for the most part, inaccurate concerning eye injury risk. Thus, the present guidelines are potentially dangerous for some athletes (eg, the one-eyed squash player who would be allowed unprotected participation), while being overly restrictive on others (eg, the one-eyed hockey player who could play with reasonable safety with proper protective equipment).

This chapter hopefully will more accurately present the eye injury potential for most sports and the available eye protective devices so that better guidelines may be developed.

EYE INJURY RISK AND PROTECTIVE DEVICE EFFECTIVENESS FOR SPECIFIC SPORTS

Racket Sports

Over 40 million Americans play racket sports. *All should be wearing eye protectors.* Racket sports are responsible for: 30% to 40% of all sports eye injuries seen in a private ophthalmology practice (Table 12-3)[53]; 23% of all admissions for hyphema to the Massachusetts Eye and Ear Infirmary (Table 12-4); and 29% of all injuries on the racquetball court.[55] Many studies have shown the ocular risk of participating in squash, racquetball, tennis and badminton.[56] The risk of an unprotected squash player suffering a significant eye injury after 25 years of playing three days a week is approximately 25%.[57]

Because of the high risk, several manufacturers have produced eyeguards. Initially, most of these were wire or injection moulded polycarbonate lensless protectors that seemed to offer protection by making the orbital entrance smaller (Figure 12-10). Impact testing with rackets showed that these eyeguards were virtually indestructible, yet injuries were occurring to an alarming number of players wearing lensless protectors.[58]

In 1979 and 1980, the eye safety committees of the Canadian Standards Association and the American Society of Testing and Materials began independent but cooperative studies on the mechanism of existing protective device failure which resulted in the publication, in 1983, of performance standards for racket sport eye protectors.[59,60] The committees determined the speeds of racket and ball (Table 12-5, Figure 12-11), and tested various types of eye protectors by mounting them on a headform, impacting the mounted protector with a ball at various speeds, and using high speed photographs to record the results for analysis (Figure 12-11).

Racquetballs and squashballs penetrated all lensless protectors at speeds above 50 mph (Figure 12-12).[61,62] No lensless protectors thus far manufactured will pass the standards when used for squash and racquetball. However, these protectors have not, as yet, been tested for tennis, paddle ball, badminton and handball. A number of lensed eyeguards are available that will pass the standards and give "state of the art" protection (Figure 12-13).

Protectors will vary for different racket sports as more products are tested to the performance standards. For example, streetwear glasses have been proven dangerous for squash and racquetball, but may, with sturdy frames and streetwear polycarbonate lenses, be adequate for tennis.[63]

Since the standards are new, modification may be necessary if injuries are reported to athletes wearing certified protectors.

Hockey

Ice hockey Eye-face protectors for hockey forwards and defensemen follow the example set by the succesful industrial safety eyewear program and the principles of sports eye injury prevention: 1) An injury problem was recognized; 2) forces were analyzed; 3) performance (hockey) or performance plus design (industry) standards were set by voluntary committees; 4) products were manufactured to these standards and experienced widespread use in the field (Figure 12-14); and 5) injuries were reduced.[64,65]

The full-face hockey protector is one of the most efficient sports protective devices to date. It was designed as part of a total head protection concept—forces are transmitted to a helmet designed to protect the brain.

At first, slightly different approaches were taken by the American Society of Testing and

Table 12-3
Lexington Eye Associates Summary of 263 Sports Eye Injuries 1981–1983, Classified by Type of Sport and Sex and Age of Injured Participant

	Sex		Age Group							Potential
Sport	M	F	0–9	10–19	20–29	30–39	40–49	50–59	>60	Late Complications
Racket sports										
Tennis (52)	24	28		9	7	7	16	8	5	10
Racquetball (22)	21	1	1	3	10	4	3	1		7
Squash (3)	2	1		1	1		1			2
Badminton (2)	2		1	1						1
Paddle tennis (3)	2	1				1	2			
Total 82 (31.2%)										
Hockey (all types)										
Ice (9)	9		1	4	4					4
Street (9)	9			9						1
Floor (6)	5	1	1	4	1					1
Field (1)		1		1						
Total 25 (9.5%)										
Large ball										
Soccer (23)	18	5	2	20		1				9
Basketball (24)	21	3	1	15	4	3		1		1
Volleyball (5)	3	2		4	1					
Speedball (3)	3			3						
Team handball (1)	1			1						1
Bombardment (2)	2			2						1
Total 58 (22.1%)										
Baseball/softball										
Baseball (22)	22		8	13	1					4
Softball (11)	5	6		5	3	3				
Total 33 (12.5%)										
Lacrosse (7)	4	3		7						
Skiing										
Downhill (5)	4	1	2	3						
Cross-country (1)		1					1			
All other sports										
Total 52 (9.8%)										

Older patients tended to be injured in the racket sports.
No tennis injuries were seen in players who were wearing either eyeglasses or a protective device while playing.
Two racquetball players were injured while wearing lensless eyeguards, one wore contact lenses under the open eyeguard. Both felt ball penetrated the guard. One racquetball player who wore plastic lensed spectacles had only periorbital bruising. Though the frames broke, they probably helped prevent more serious injury.
No injuries were seen in racket sports players wearing lensed eye protectors.
No hockey injuries occurred with CSA or HECC approved face protectors.
Two hockey goalies were injured despite moulded face masks.
No injured skiers were wearing ski goggles when injured.
Presently available protective devices would have prevented most injuries.

Materials (ASTM) and the Canadian Standards Association (CSA) hockey face mask standard committees. The CSA[66] insisted from the start on maximal protection—no penetration of the protector was permitted by a 2″ × ¼″ hockey stick blade (Figure 12-15). However, the ASTM[67] allowed a 1% probability of penetration, thus allowing larger openings in the wire mask that (hopefully) would be more acceptable to the athletes (Figure 12-16).

The original ASTM standard did, in fact, perform to the predicted 99% protection level, but the residual penetration injuries (several eyes lost with protectors in place) were unacceptable. The ASTM standard was revised[68] to prevent any chance of penetration by the 2″ × ¼″ hockey stick blade.

The success and widespread use of face masks

Table 12-4
Massachusetts Eye and Ear Infirmary Eye Trauma Admissions March 1979 to February 1980* and Hyphema Admissions February 1980* to September 1980†

Eye Trauma	
Accident (non-sports and non-auto)	35 (32%)
Sports	25 (23%)
Intraocular FBs	21 (20%)
Assault	16 (15%)
Accident (auto/cycle)	10 (9%)
Hyphema	
Total cases	94
Sports	45 (48%)
Sports hospital costs	$39,029

Study of the sports eye injury admissions showed that existing protective equipment would have prevented almost all the injuries. The economic cost of these injuries is apparent.
*Data collected by Vinger.
†Data collected by Slansky, Depperman, Berson, and Kraut.[53,54]

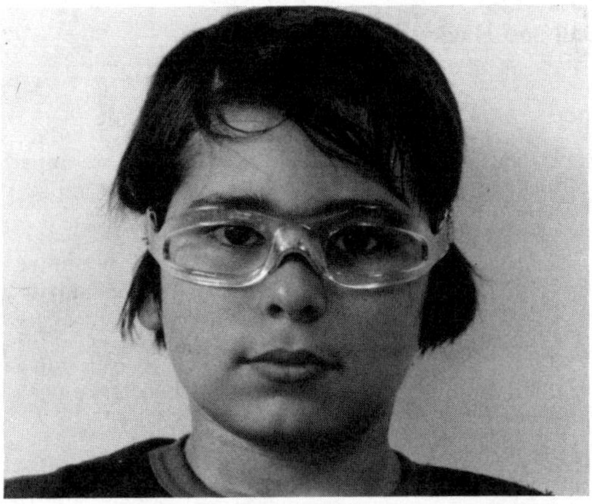

Figure 12-10 Lensless racket sport eye protector.

has encouraged manufacturers to make large investments in polycarbonate full face masks that should gain wide acceptance by the players (Figure 12-17).

Lighter weight helmet/face mask combinations for junior players necessitated development (by the CSA) of a special headform for testing (Figure 12-18).

The form-fitting goalie face mask (Figure 12-19) is a good example of the proven failure of a commonly perceived "safety mask" by careful data collection and laboratory testing. Jacques Plante revolutionized professional goal tending when he had the courage to demand the right to protect himself. The pioneering work and finely moulded masks of Ernie Higgins have prevented many cuts, bruises and fractures—yet the mask is no longer acceptable because: 1) there is little or no protection to the temples and occipital areas of the goalie's skull; 2) players (and the parents of school-age players) often enlarge the eye openings for a larger visual field, thus decreasing eye protection; 3) the form-fitting masks neither spread forces over a wide area, nor substantially lengthen the duration over which a force is allowed to act because they "bottom out" in critical regions[69] and transmit the forces to the brain, face and eye; 4) breathing, heat dissipation, and conversation are markedly compromised; 5) a great range of products exists, from those that are well made with better padding, to cheaply mass-produced, or incompletely fabricated ones with little or no padding. The average player usually owns an inferior mask. Nearly all eye injuries currently seen in protected hockey players involve goalies who are wearing form-fitting masks. This is despite the fact that goalies are far outnumbered by forwards and defensemen.[70]

It is apparent that better protection for goalies lies in a sturdy wire mask-helmet combination (Figure 12-20).[71] With this combination, the head is better protected against blows from the rear and side; the brain is better protected against concussion as energy is dissipated through the helmet and thicker padding; the wire mesh allows for better vision, improved communication, and better protection at less cost. Form-fitting goalie face-masks are no longer permitted by the NCAA and most secondary schools.

Hockey face protectors are now worn by over 1.2 million North American hockey players. These players suffer 70,000 fewer eye and face injuries than they would have were they not protected, with a savings to society of over 10 million dollars in medical bills each year.[1] Economic studies have shown that if every hockey player were given a hockey face protector for free, society would still make a profit in medical expenses avoided by use of the protective device.[72]

Eye and face injuries accounted for two-thirds of all injuries in ice hockey prior to the introduction of mandatory eye and face protection in play

Table 12-5
Ball and Racket Velocities

Sport	Projectile	Velocity (MPH)	Velocity (FT/SEC)
Racketball	Racket – before impact	40–50	65–75
Forehand	– after impact	85–95	125–135
	Ball velocity	85–110	125–160
	Racket – before impact	50–55	75–80
	– after impact	80–90	120–135
	Ball velocity	95–105	140–150
Squash	Racket – before impact	50–60	70–85
Forehand	– after impact	95–110	140–160
	Ball velocity	130–140	190–200
	Racket – before impact	55–60	80–90
	– after impact	85–90	130–135
	Ball velocity	115–120	170–185
Backhand	Racket – before impact	55–65	80–95
	– after impact	80–115	120–170
	Racket – before impact	film poor	film poor
	– after impact	90	130–135
	Racket follow through (after racket higher than shoulder)	15–25	25–35
Tennis	Ball velocity	90–100	135–145
	Ball velocity	85–95	125–135
	Ball velocity	90–110	110–160
Handball	Ball velocity	55–65	85–95
	Ball velocity	60–70	90–105
Badminton	Shuttlecock Velocity	105–117	155–170
Overhead	Shuttlecock Velocity	120–125	175–180
Forehand	Shuttlecock Velocity	130–135	170–200

Studies performed at The Pennsylvania State University by Professor C.A. Morehouse for ASTM Racket Sport Standard 27.

Summary of Procedures: Slides were taken from a 16 mm film which was produced at a frame rate of approximately 400 frames/sec using a Lo Cam camera manufactured by Red Lake Corporation

Films were taken in an indoor archery range so that the main plane of movement was perpendicular to the principal axis of the camera lens. Slides indicated as shots were obtained by tossing the ball to the subject and having him hit it into the indoor archery netting. Slides labeled as swings were taken so that preparatory and follow-through motions would be nearly perpendicular to the lens axis. This was necessary to obtain truer estimates of velocity.

Velocities were obtained by digitizing specific points on the ball and racquet head from the film using a Bendix film analyzer. The coordinates of every second frame were obtained and distances calculated by converting these coordinates from film image distance to real life distances.

A crystal quartz generator was utilized to operate timing lights within the camera at precisely 100 pulses/sec. The lights left marks on the side of the film and by counting the number of frames between successive light marks, an accurate measure of the camera speed was obtained.

Velocities were calculated using the time and distances from the film analyses using a computer program written for a PDP-11 laboratory computer.

sponsored by schools, colleges, and amateur hockey associations. The widespread use of these protective devices has virtually eliminated eye and face injuries to protected players while keeping fun and appeal in the game. It seems that this obvious problem, with its relatively easy solution, should have been soluble in less than 10 years.[73] It is hoped that the hockey model can be applied to eye injuries in other sports, with speedier success in increasing safety for players.

Street/floor hockey Street and floor hockey are played on the street or in the school gym using either regulation or lighter weight hockey sticks and a plastic puck or tennis ball. Protection is rarely worn, even by the goalie. Severe injuries are commonplace (Table 12-6). Testing as to the actual

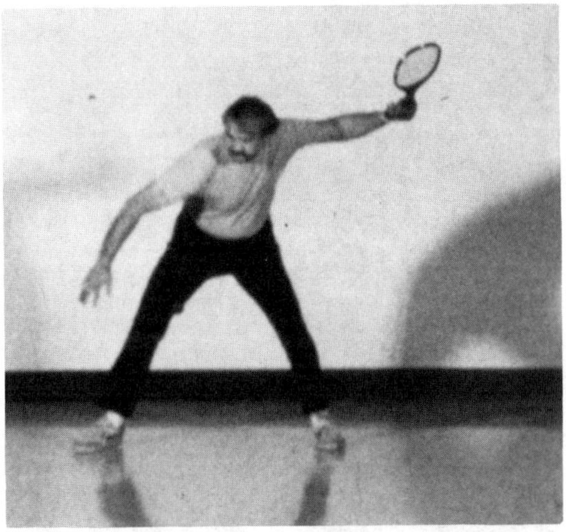

A

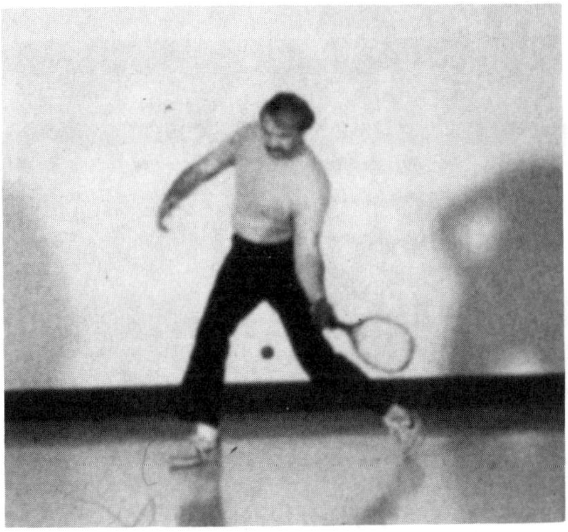

B

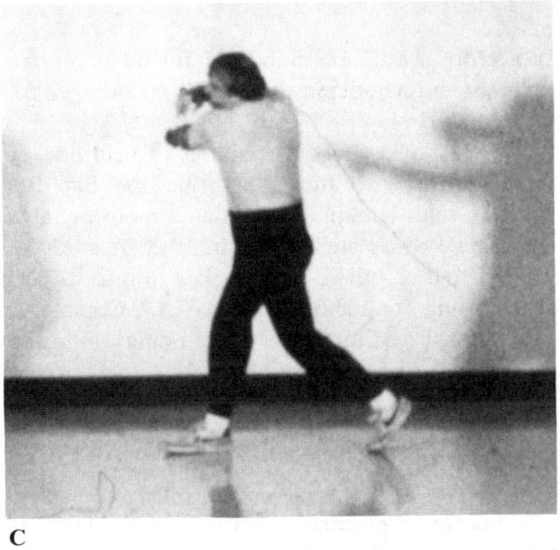

C

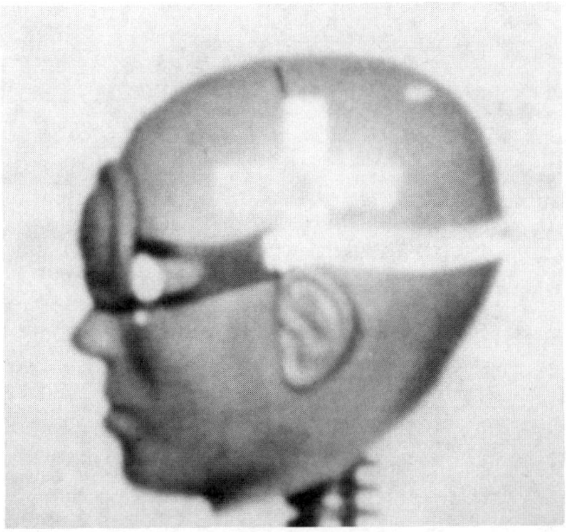

A

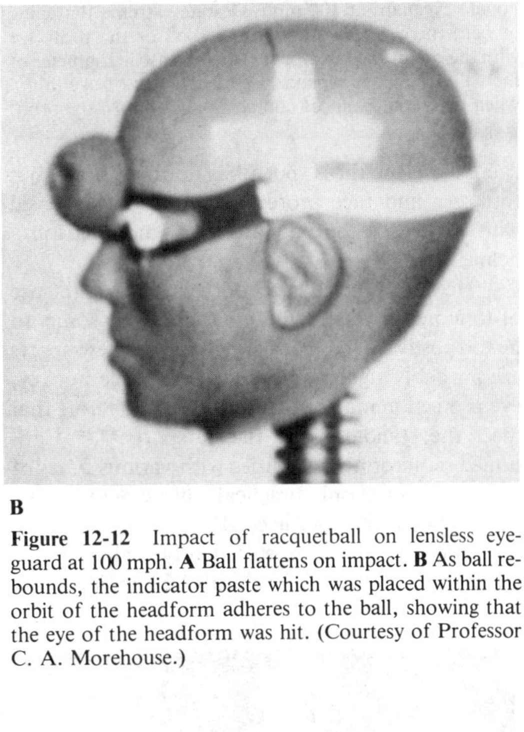

B

Figure 12-12 Impact of racquetball on lensless eyeguard at 100 mph. **A** Ball flattens on impact. **B** As ball rebounds, the indicator paste which was placed within the orbit of the headform adheres to the ball, showing that the eye of the headform was hit. (Courtesy of Professor C. A. Morehouse.)

Figure 12-11 Representative frames from high speed film (see Table 12-10). **A** Racquetball–preparatory to hitting forehand shot. **B** Racquetball–hitting forehand shot. **C** Racquetball–follow through following forehand shot. (Courtesy of Professor C. A. Morehouse).

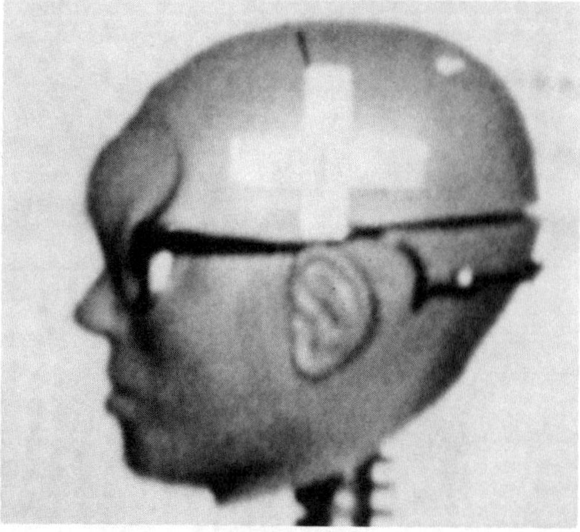

Figure 12-13 Impact of racquetball on lensed polycarbonate eyeguard at 100 mph. Despite extreme flattening of ball, there is no contact of the ball or the protector with the eye of the headform. The increase in diameter of the ball on impact explains the mechanism of eye injury when the initial point of contact is adjacent to the orbit.

energy levels in these sports has not been done, but total eye and face protection would be achieved with an ice hockey full face mask mounted on a helmet.

However, for most school gym classes, the use of total head protection is considered, by some, to be too costly. Since the energy levels in these sports are probably significantly less than in ice hockey, eye protection may be possible with protectors that meet the standards for racket sports.[59,60] Continued monitoring of injuries with various types of protectors is the only practical way of determining the level of protection needed.

The injury rate is sufficiently higher that a minimum requirement for the above mentioned eye

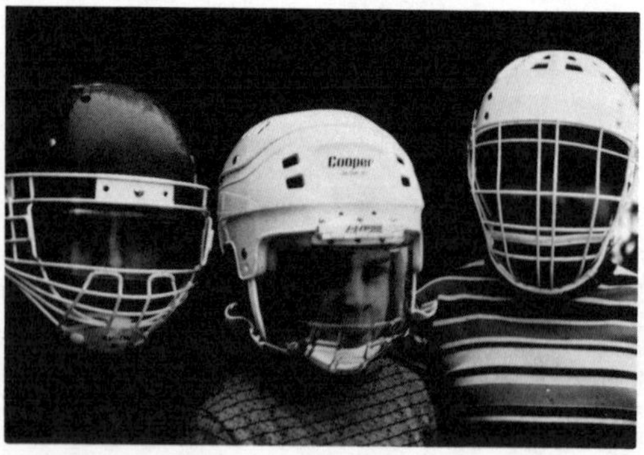

Figure 12-14 "First generation" wire, polycarbonate, and combined wire/polycarbonate hockey face masks.

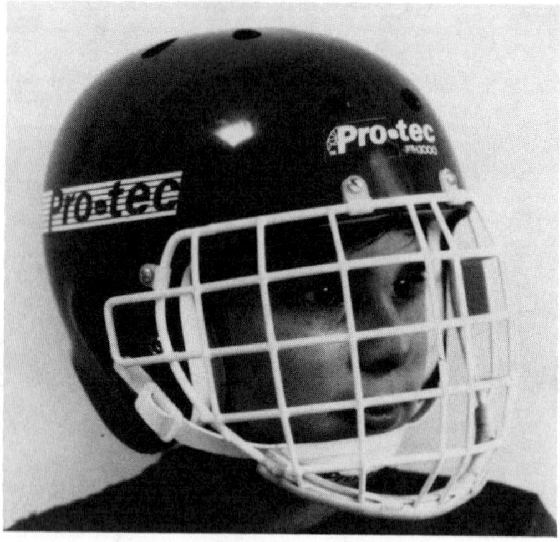

A

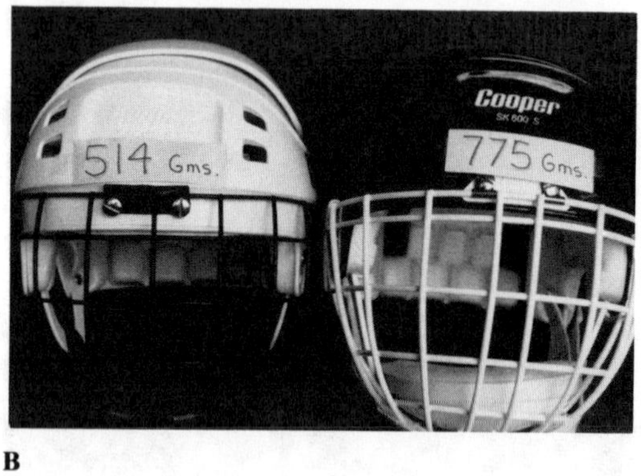

B

Figure 12-15 A,B Wire hockey face masks that will not allow penetration by a 2″ × ¼″ stick. In **B** the face mask on the left is a junior size; the right face mask is an adult size.

protectors should be mandated for all organized amateur and school play and highly encouraged for unorganized play.

Field hockey Tooth injuries in field hockey have increased to the extent that the Big Ten Athletic rules committee mandated mouth guards for female collegiate athletes in 1982. A study of eye, as well as other, field hockey injuries is currently being conducted by the NCAA Committee on Competitive Safeguards and findings on injury rates should soon be available.

Large Ball

Soccer Contrary to prevalent ophthalmology teaching that eye injuries are rarely caused by balls

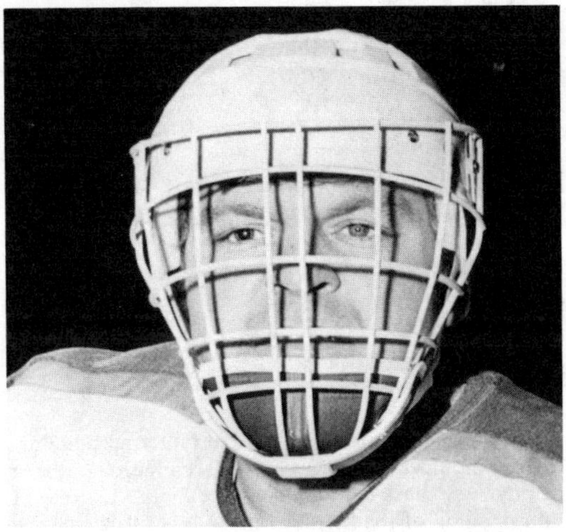

A

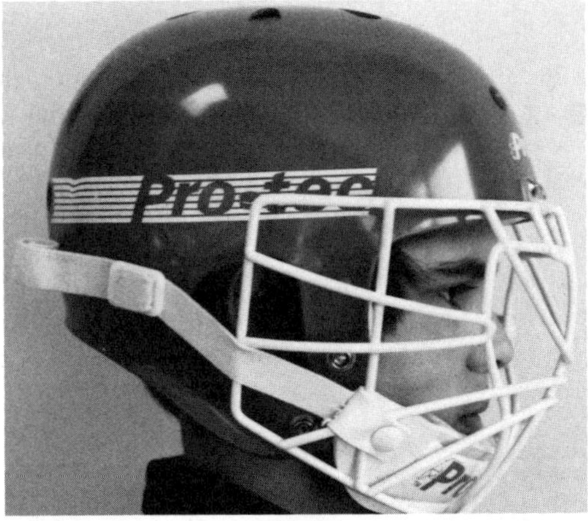

B

Figure 12-16 A,B Wire hockey face masks that have a 1% probability of penetration by a 2″ × ¼″ stick. Although players tended to prefer the more open mesh design, the few serious eye injuries that occurred with the more open mesh masks resulted in modification of the ASTM standard.

larger than 4 inches in diameter,[74] the 8.6 inch diameter soccer ball is responsible for most soccer eye injuries (Table 12-7).[75] How is sufficient energy transmitted from the large ball to the eye to result in retinal detachment and permanent vision loss in many injured players?[76]

It is known that the kicked 14 to 16 ounce (396 to 453 g) soccer ball has a velocity of 60 to 120 kph (37 to 74 mph). The impact energy is sufficiently high that many are concerned about possible brain injury from repeated soccer ball headings.[77]

Are the eye injuries caused by ball deforma-

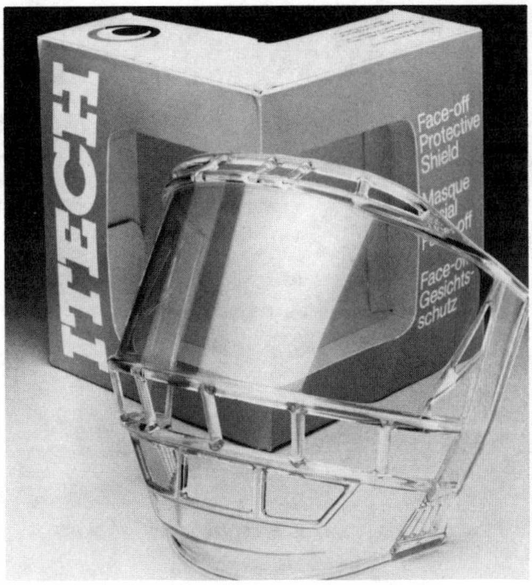

Figure 12-17 State-of-the-art injection moulded polycarbonate hockey face protector (Courtesy of Itech.)

tion? Does underinflation result in more eye injuries than properly inflated balls? Are sports eye protectors currently in use for racket sports sufficient to prevent injury? Should heading the ball be prohibited for certain age groups? What is the incidence of eye injuries in soccer—are they missed in some studies?[78]

Impact testing of balls at varying speed and

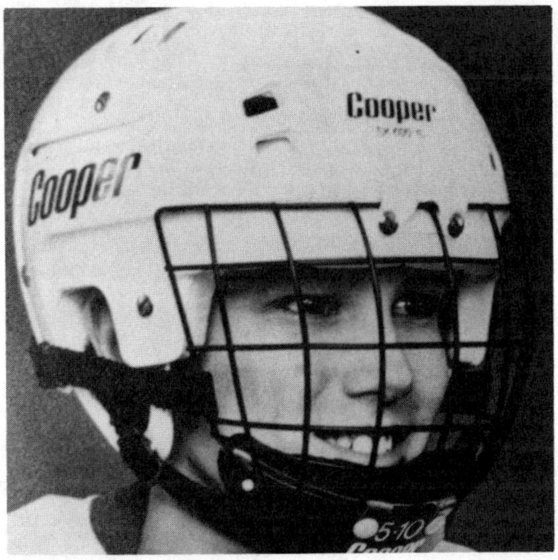

Figure 12-18 Lighter helmet/face mask combinations are more suitable for junior players. (Courtesy of T. Pashby.)

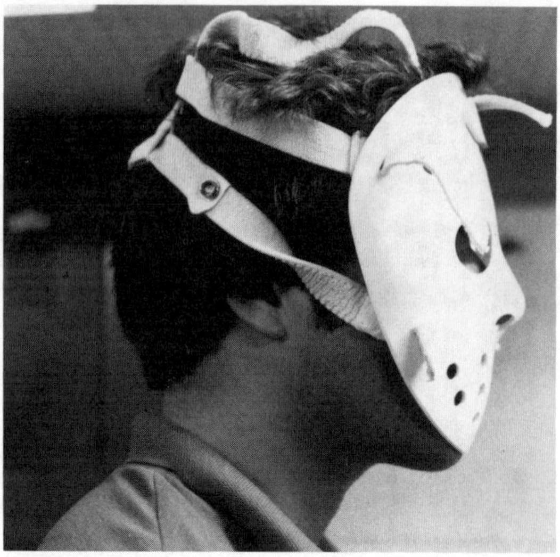

A

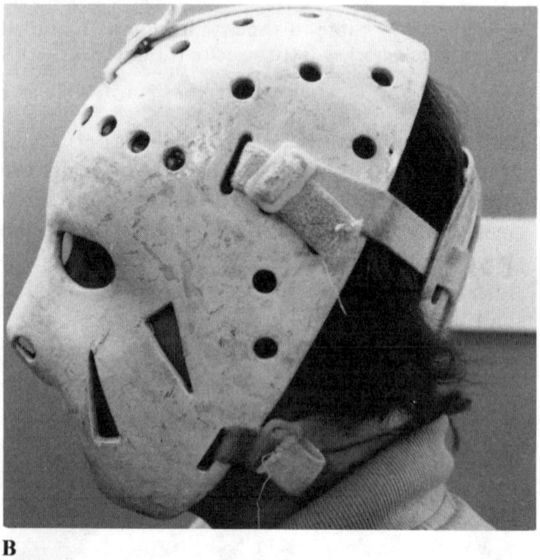

B

Figure 12-19 **A** Mass produced goalie face mask offers essentially no protection. **B** Custom made goalie face protector gives better, but inadequate face, eye, and head protection.

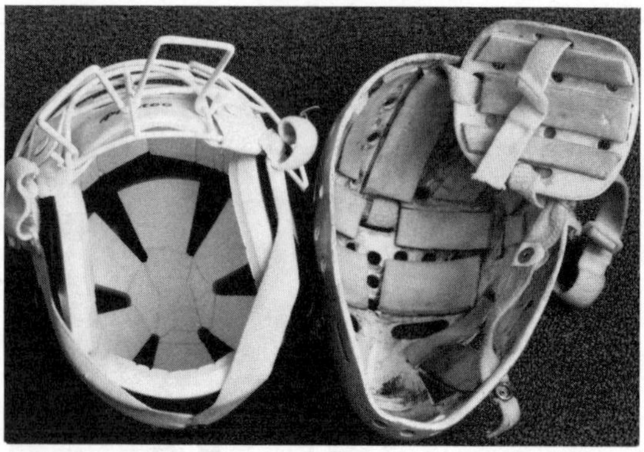

Figure 12-20 Comparison between internal padding of custom moulded goalie face mask (see Figure 12-19B) and helmet/wire mask combination (See Figure 12-16A). The thin padding of the moulded mask is insufficient.

pressures with and without various eye protectors in place, using high speed photography should, in combination with prospective injury studies, answer these questions over the next several years. In the meantime, heading the ball should be discouraged for younger players and sports eye protectors should be encouraged.

Basketball Most basketball eye injuries are caused by opponent's fingers or elbows striking the player's eye, frequently during aggressive play under the boards. Protective devices that meet the racket sport standard requirements are essential for one-eyed, and strongly recommended for other basketball players.

Volleyball, team handball, speedball and bombardment These games also are responsible for some eye injuries, but the incidence is not known at this time.

Table 12-6
Eye Injuries in the Concord Public Schools and the Concord/Carlisle Regional School District 1978–1979 (1½ school years)

Sport	Participants	Eye Injuries	Injury Rate
Floor hockey	4000	10	1/400
Tennis	2000	4	1/500
Soccer	7000	7	1/ 1000
Jump rope	2000	2	1/1000
Football	4000	2	1/2000

Total eye injuries: 55
Sports-related eye injuries: 25 (45%)

The most severe eye injuries (those requiring medical follow-up, hospitalization or permanent loss of function) occurred in floor hockey.
Based upon this data, all students participating in floor hockey were required to wear eye goggles or safety glasses while playing.
Data collected and analyzed by T. Cotton.

Table 12-7
Soccer Eye Injuries seen by Lexington Eye Associates

	Jan. 1977 to Dec. 1980		Jan. 1981 to Dec. 1983	
	Serious	Not Serious	Serious	Not Serious
Mechanism				
Hit with ball	5	3	9	11
Hit with hand, arm, etc	1	1	4	
Hit with head				1
Ran into tree				1
Fell—glasses shattered				1
Total	6	4	13	14
Serious				
Hyphema	1		7	
Angle contusion deformity			7	
Vitreous hemorrhage	2		1	
Retinal tear/detachment			2	
Severe retinal contusion/heme	3		3	
Severe lid laceration/avulsion			2	
Fractured orbit	1		1	
Total	7		23	
Not serious				
Pain but no objective injury		1		3
Corneal abrasion		2		5
Traumatic iritis		5		9
Retinal edema/hemes—cleared		2		7
Subconjunctival hemorrhage		1		2
Periocular contusion/hematoma				3
Multiple ocular glass foreign bodies				1
Total		11		30

Baseball/Softball

Baseball Baseball is the leading cause of sports eye injuries seen in emergency rooms (Table 12-3). Some pitchers throw the ball at speeds up to 100 mph. The batted ball travels even faster. The kinetic energy level of the ball off the bat of Gil McDougall at 120 mph was very high when it struck Herb Score in the eye.[79] The Consumer Products Safety Commission (CPSC) estimates that baseball causes 900,000 injuries per year, of which 170,000 are to the face, eyes, and mouth. They suggest that some sort of facial protection could reduce this group of injuries by 54,000.

In a study of actual injuries to 5 million Little League players, the head suffered 38% of all injuries and injuries to the batter accounted for 22% of the total.

Creighton J. Hale, PhD, the president of Little League Baseball, feels that the CPSC projection of 900,000 injuries each year indicates that additional protective equipment and wider use of the equipment is needed. He has said that substantial injury reduction could be achieved by: 1) eliminating steel spikes; 2) eliminating sliding, or using the breakaway base; 3) eliminating or moving the on-deck circle; 4) screening the dugouts; 5) using face protectors; 6) prohibiting intentional body contact between a baserunner and infielder making a play at a base; and 7) motivating players to use proper equipment.[79]

So that administrators of the sport could take a firmer stand in seeing that appropriate protective equipment is available and used, an ASTM committee (F 8.53—chairperson Lorine Caveness) was formed in 1980 to write a standard specification for youth baseball faceguards. With funding from the American Fund for Dental Health, the Pennsylvania Sports Research Institute (Penn State University, Prof. Chauncey A. Morehouse Prin-

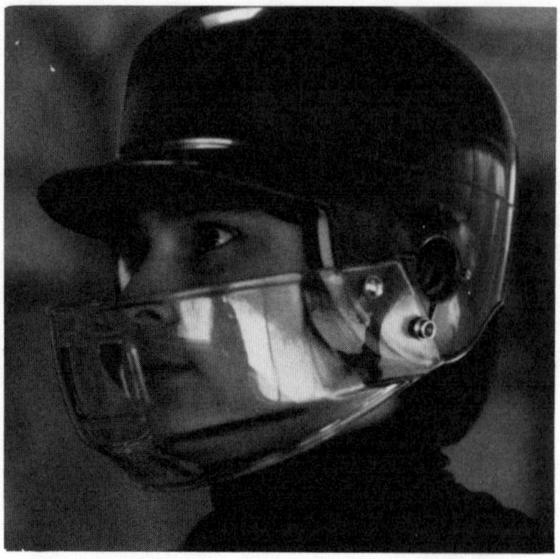

A

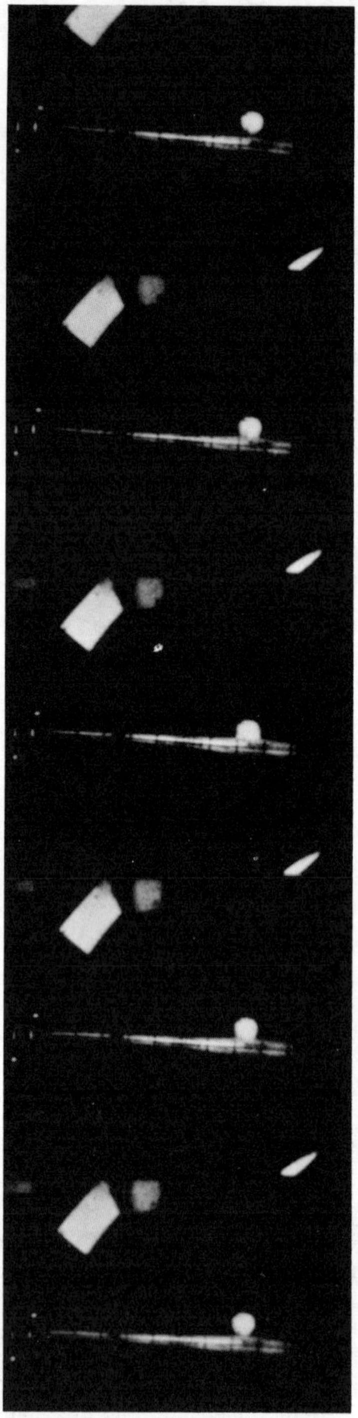

B

Figure 12-21 **A** Baseball face protector. **B** Compression and flattening of baseball when impacted by aluminum baseball bat. The ability of a seemingly incompressible baseball to flatten on impact must be considered when protective devices are designed. (Testing and film by C. A. Morehouse.)

cipal Investigator) was commissioned by the ASTM committee to develop test protocols and procedures. The ASTM standard, which considers any contact between a ball traveling at a minimum speed of 30 ± 2.2 meters/sec (67.1 ± 4.9 mph) with the test headform a product failure, is in the final round of approval and should be ready for final publication later in 1985.[80]

One baseball face protector (Figure 12-21) received the 1983 first place product development award in the National Safety Council awards for achievement in product safety, sponsored by the National Association of Professional Insurance Agents. This product is a good example of cooperation between professional organizations who provide funds in the interest of public health (American Fund For Dental Health), standard development organizations (ASTM), research institutes (Penn State), sports organizations (Little League), manufacturers (Face Guards, Inc.) and those interested in the sport (coaches, athletes, parents, physicians, etc) who came together to help solve an injury problem.

Now that products are available which will prevent injury from baseballs traveling at 90 mph, the field testing on a large scale is ready to begin. The probable first step will be to use facial protec-

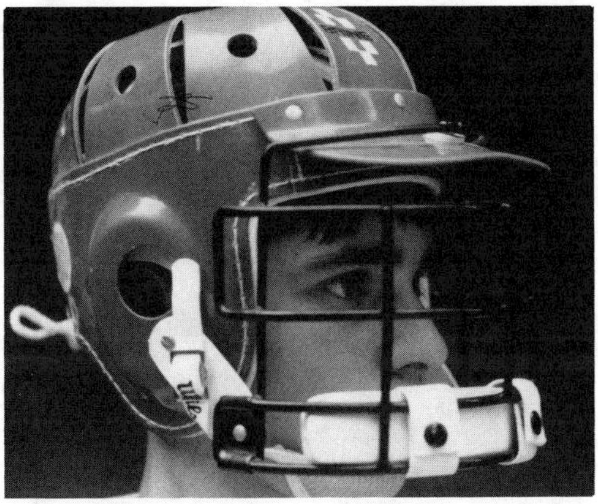

Figure 12-22 Lacrosse helmet with face protector.

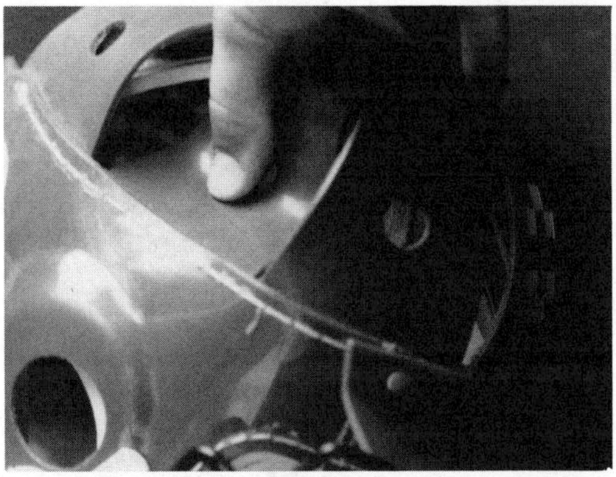

Figure 12-23 Soft helmet may be inadequate for men's (contact) lacrosse, but would be adequate as support for face protector for women's (noncontact) lacrosse.

tors in 5- to 14-year-old batters and evaluate the performance and acceptance rates. The option of using the facemask for baserunners probably will be left open as more data is gathered as to injury mechanisms with and without face protectors. The most effective approach to introducing face protectors to baseball would be along the lines that were successful with the hockey facemask—a somewhat gradual approach to younger players, continued gathering of data, then wider use of the protectors as data proved their worth.

Softball Shattered sunglasses have lacerated globes. Maskless catchers and behind the plate umpires, batters and fielders have all been injured. The incidence is unknown.

Lacrosse Lacrosse, first played by North American Indians with a ball of wood or hair-stuffed deerskin and three to four foot looped sticks, has changed significantly from the original game, which involved hundreds of players and a field several miles long without sidelines, lasted for two or three days, and was used to train warriors in close combat.

Men's Field Lacrosse Men's lacrosse is played on a 60 × 110 yard, marked field. Injuries often occur when defensemen check attackmen with their sticks or bodies. Although the rules forbid blind-siding a player, hitting below the knees and taking uncontrolled swings with the stick, infractions occur. All players are required to wear helmets with face masks and attached chin straps. Prior to 1978, some masks would admit the lacrosse ball (hard rubber, somewhat smaller than a baseball) at speeds approaching 90 mph with resultant face and eye injury. Rules now require a vertical bar that prevents ball penetration.[81] Lacrosse helmets (Figure 12-22) need further study and standardization, since concussions, teeth injuries, facial and jaw fractures and lacerations still account for 9.8% of all men's field lacrosse injuries.[82] Mouth guards, only worn by 10% of players, would help protect the teeth and jaw. The face mask offers good eye and nose protection, since eye injuries and nasal fractures are rare in protected players.[83] If lacrosse helmets were improved to the hockey helmet standard, many serious head injuries, such as epidural hematoma, would be avoided (Figure 12-23).[84]

Women's Field Lacrosse The rules in women's lacrosse do not permit deliberate physical contact, but the stick can be checked. The wooden stick must have a head less than nine inches wide. Only the goalie is permitted the use of protective equipment (helmet, face protector, chest protector, padded gloves and leg guards).

The use of helmets and face protectors for women's field lacrosse is currently a subject of controversy. On the one hand, it is felt that protective equipment is inconsistent with the non-contact nature of women's lacrosse and the concept of a "bubble area" (a zone around the head about 7 inches in all dimensions) where stick penetration is prohibited. On the other hand, as women play with more aggressiveness, it is apparent that the number of face, eye and teeth injuries is growing. Data collected by the United States Women's Lacrosse Association (USWLA) (Table 12-8) show a 6.2% to 9.9% annual incidence of face, eye and tooth in-

Table 12-8
United States Women's Lacrosse Association
Head and Facial Injury Survey

	1980	1981	1982	1983
Colleges reporting	22	95	60	51
College participants	NS	NS	1732	1474
College injuries	82	NS	238(13.7%)	119(8%)
High schools reporting	26	5	31	48
High school participants	NS	NS	1030	1695
High school injuries	46	NS	35(3.4%)	78(4.6%)
USA squad injuries	17	NS	NS	NS
Total participants	1590	NS	2762	3169
Head, face and eye injuries	144(9.1%)	91(?%)	273(9.9%)	197(6.2%)

NS = not stated in report.
Data collected by USWLA Sports Medicine Committee, Roberta Butler, chairperson.

Although many injuries were relatively minor and would not have been reported in less complete studies, many major injuries (skull fracture, concussion, cheek fracture, nasal fracture, chipped teeth, eyeball contusion, eyeball laceration) were reported. No follow-up reports of eye injuries with possible permanent sequellae were reported.

Women's lacrosse, under the present rules, presents too high a risk of head, face and eye injuries to participants. Rule changes and/or full face protection are needed. Since most injuries are accidental, rule changes alone probably will not reduce the injury rate to an acceptable level without changing the basic form or appeal of the game.

Since women's lacrosse is a noncontact sport, there will be minimal risk of a player wearing a helmet/face mask injuring a nonhelmeted player *if the existing rules are enforced by the referees and good coaching practices are used.*

Players, coaches and parents who wish protection should not be banned from use of lacrosse helmets and face masks while officials find other means (rules changes, better coaching/refereeing/training, new helmet-face mask standards, etc) of reducing injuries. If head, eye and face injuries continue at their present rate, despite rules changes, etc, helmets and face masks should be mandated.

jury. So far, USWLA does not agree that these figures represent a high incidence of injury or an unacceptable level of severity.

A significant problem has arisen in Massachusetts, where the Massachusetts Interscholastic Athletic Association (MIAA) saw the potential for injury in women's lacrosse and made helmets with face masks optional for the 1984 season and mandatory in 1985. The Concord-Carlisle High School (CCHS) opted to use helmets and face protectors, in accordance with the MIAA rule, but in violation of the USWLA rule. This has resulted in a threat by USWLA to forbid officials to participate in games where players wear protection and a demand to have the girls play under the boys (contact) lacrosse rules. Many coaches and athletic directors refused to play teams that use protective devices and have forfeited the games, thus effectively prohibiting protected players from participating in the sport. Toward the end of the 1984 season, CCHS officials bowed to the pressure and removed protective headwear to allow CCHS girls competition with the boycotting schools and not risk loss of lacrosse college scholarships (a threat used by some officials to remove protective headgear) for several of their players. The MIAA has held the position that the eye/face/teeth injury rate is too high and the rule for mandatory headgear for the 1985 season is still in effect. A committee has been appointed to choose appropriate protective equipment.

The rationale used by the USWLA and many coaches is that the game will be even more aggressive if protectors are worn and injuries to other parts of the body will increase; some fear helmeted players will injure the unhelmeted in a collision. Complaints about the expense of the helmet/face mask are also voiced. The USWLA insists that better coaches and officials will solve the injury problem.

Proponents of protectors argue that the injury rate is already unacceptable and that most injuries are accidental (Table 12-9), thus will not be eliminated by better coaches and officials. It has been shown in hockey that protective devices are very cost-effective and a good investment. A standard could be written specifically for women's lacrosse helmets and face masks that would correct the problems in existing products; but, while such a standard is being developed, presently available products would certainly reduce eye, face, head and teeth injuries, given the basic non-contact

Table 12-9
Women's Lacrosse
Head and Facial Injury vs Activity

	Passing Catching Cradling	Stick Check *Illegal*	Stick Check Legal	Shot on Goal	Body Check Legal	Body Check *Illegal*	Other
1983 High school	18	33	7	23	3	0	0
1983 College	23	48	21	25	4	4	3
1982 High school	6	10	7	11	1	0	0
1982 College	47	66	57	49	13	6	0
1980 HS + college	47	63	17	27	9	3	0
Total accidental	141		109	135	30		3
Total *Illegal*		220				13	

Data collected by USWLA Sports Medicine Committee, Roberta Butler, chairperson.

Comments:

1. 64% of head, eye, and facial injuries in women's lacrosse are accidental and will not be prevented unless the intrinsic nature of the game is altered by rules changes.
2. Most head, eye, and facial injuries are caused by the stick (1983 survey: stick = 63%; ball = 20%; not applicable = 17%)
3. A helmet with a full face mask would effectively eliminate head and facial injuries in women's lacrosse as it is now played.
4. Since no injuries were reported as caused by the head of a player striking the head or face of the injured player, head to face contact must be rare. It is unlikely that a helmeted player would cause injury to a player who is not wearing a helmet if voluntary protection is allowed for some, but not mandated for all women lacrosse players.

nature of the game (most injuries result from stick and ball impact rather than bodily collision).

This dilemma may, unfortunately, have to be resolved in the courts, when a girl or woman suffers a serious injury that most likely would have been avoided were helmets and face masks permitted.

Box Lacrosse Box lacrosse is played in an enclosed area, such as a hockey rink, with shorter sticks and a lighter, spongier ball than field hockey. Although the rules prohibit wild swinging, hitting from behind, and checking at the head, face and neck, the games can be quite physical. Head and face protection that meets ice hockey standards[33] prevents most eye and facial injury.

Football

Football face guards have been quite effective as they have resulted in an 80% to 90% reduction in facial injuries.[85]

Unfortunately protection of the head and face has encouraged more use of the head as a weapon, resulting in injuries to the offensive player as well as the target.[86] Some think that the leverage transmitted through the protruding mask to the neck by the helmet may be responsible for an increase in cervical injuries.

Presently available football face protectors offer incomplete protection to the eyes and face and decrease visual field.[87] Better eye protection would be achieved if polycarbonate eye protectors that meet the standards for racket sport eye protectors are worn in addition to the face mask (essential for one-eyed football players).

Football needs a performance standard for face protectors that provide for better visibility, better access to the player's face (in case of loss of consciousness), less rotation of the head, less risk to the opponent, and better protection to the player. However, protective equipment alone will be of no value unless coaches, officials, and players make a commitment to safety in their sport by rule changes and the strict enforcement it will take to effect a decrease in injuries.

A modification of a hockey wire or polycarbonate full face hockey protector, hinged at the top of the helmet would be a good starting point. Such a device, sitting closer to the face, might be a partial answer to head, neck, and facial injuries to football players.

Rugby

The incidence of eye injuries in rugby is unknown at this time. As teams use physicians rather than the traditional "magic sponge"[88] to treat injuries, better diagnosis and treatment should allow compilation of more complete data.

Boxing

Boxing is the only sport in which the *intent* is to cause eye or other injury as an aid to winning. Unfortunately, the main eye complications of boxing, angle contusion deformity and retinal tears, are often asymptomatic until vision is lost from glaucoma or long-standing retinal detachment.

Palmer et al[89] examined 55 retired boxers. Of the 110 eyes, there were 9 (8.2%) with angle contusion deformity, 7 had retinal detachments, 2 had choroidal ruptures and 1 optic nerve was atrophic. At the 1968 Olympic games, Dr D. Sime examined 13 boxers with indirect ophthalmoscopy and scleral depression (personal communication). Three eyes had retinal tears and one eye was densely amblyopic.

A number of boxers have been blinded in both eyes by their sport. One tragic example is the 1972 middleweight Olympic medalist, Sugar Ray Seales, who fought over 400 amateur and professional bouts. Despite seven operations for retinal detachment he remains blind, with the lingering impression he was only one or two bouts away from the world middleweight championship.

Because of the high incidence of eye injury in boxing, the Vision Safety and Performance Committee of the United States Olympic Committee recommends an annual ophthalmological examination of every boxer that includes gonioscopy and indirect ophthalmoscopy with scleral depression in addition to the usual complete eye exam. The same examination should be done sooner if the boxer has suffered a severe beating or is symptomatic.

A boxer with prior history of retinal detachment or significant lattice degeneration probably should be banned from future bouts. Despite statements by some ophthalmologists that the retina that has been treated with laser, diathermy or cryosurgery is "stronger than ever," there is no evidence to show this is true. If the retina tears at the posterior edge of the surgical scar, then the athlete has a large, posterior retinal break with a worse prognosis.

Of equal or more concern is the effect of minor and moderate head injury[90–94] that results in brain damage, as evidenced by dementia, memory loss, slurred speech, tremor and abnormal gait in perhaps 15% of professional boxers.[95] More detailed neurologic studies have shown the rate of cerebral atrophy may approach 50% in boxers who have been knocked out.[96] These statistics, plus a number of ring deaths, have stimulated many experts to call for a ban on boxing.[97–98]

Boxing opponents say that boxing is so dangerous that improvements in safety and medical supervision will never eradicate brain damage and death in the ring. Boxing proponents point out that boxing has a far lower death rate (0.13/1000 participants) than some other sports[57] (horse racing—12.8/1000; sports parachuting—12.3/1000; hang gliding—5.6/1000; mountaineering—5.1/1000; scuba diving—1.1/1000; motorcycle racing—0.7/1000; college football—0.3/1000) and is the only sport that requires self-defense in a one-on-one situation. Armed forces view boxing as an essential component of physical education. Many amateur athletes box for love of the sport.

Almost everyone who studies boxing agrees that the social cost of the injuries is too high. If this is the case, there are only two alternatives—ban the sport or make it safer.

Can boxing safety be improved? As far as the eye is concerned, there is no question that eye injuries can virtually be eliminated by changes in glove and headgear design. Boxing gloves and headgear have remained essentially unchanged from the horsehair stuffed leather appliances of 40 years ago. Since the thumb of conventional boxing gloves is smaller than the bony orbital opening, much more force is transmitted to the globe when the eye is hit with the thumb than with the face of the glove. Thumbless gloves and gloves designed with a thumb that cannot be extended beyond a smooth convex anterior face into the "hitch-hikers position" will decrease eye injuries, but certainly not eliminate them since the eye can be deformed sufficiently by the face of the glove to result in retinal detachment, hyphema and angle contusion deformity.

Present helmet/glove combinations permit hooking of the thumb, especially in poorly made gloves where the thumb protrudes beyond the glove face, and can enter the helmet's eye opening with resultant severe injury potential.[99] Newer designs and materials have not been adequately explored nor have standards been written on the basic equipment. However, a combination of a thumbless or fixed-thumb glove design plus more effective headgear is possible and would prevent glove-eye contact and effectively eliminate eye injuries to helmeted boxers.

Protecting the brain, however, is more difficult. Since rotational forces on the head induced by blows cause brain damage and are not eliminated by headgear,[96] blows to the head may have to be banned. Of course, this would eliminate the knockout and a great deal of the crowd appeal in one of the world's biggest money making sports.

Certainly more studies are needed. The forces

transmitted to the eye and brain with various types of gloves and headgear must be determined. Some even argue that the sport would be safer if gloves were eliminated and bare knuckles were again used.[100] This approach would be disaster for the eye.

The United States Olympic Committee task force on head injuries in amateur boxing came to four conclusions at its August 20, 1983 meeting:

1. There is reason for concern that participation in amateur boxing may result in permanent head (brain and eye) injuries.
2. The specific type of injury that is the cause for greatest concern is cumulative permanent brain damage caused by repeated non-knock out (ie, sub-concussive) blows to the head.
3. Present day research techniques (including neurological exams, EEG, CAT scan, PET scan, NMR, evoked responses, neuro-psychological testing, etc) have *not* been shown to recognize early signs of sub-concussive irreversible brain damage. Therefore it is not now possible to determine whether or not amateur boxers, fighting today under the improved medical and safety standards required by the United States Amateur Boxing Federation (USABF), are in danger of receiving clinically significant permanent brain damage during their amateur careers.
4. At this time it is *not* possible to write a research protocol to carry out a long-term prospective study of a sufficient number of boxers (and controls) to provide statistically significant data regarding permanent brain injuries. A pilot study needs to be carried out in order to test the techniques most likely to prove useful. The task force felt these are neuro-psychological testing and, possibly, evoked responses. Physical examination, EEG, and CAT scans were felt to be too crude, while PET and NMR are unstudied in this area and are too expensive to be practical for a large-scale study.

Boxing needs continued ophthalmological and psychoneurological monitoring of all participants on at least an annual basis, with more frequent examinations scheduled in cases of severe trauma or symptoms. Strict protocols for medical ban of an individual from the sport must be written. In-depth studies of the true mechanism of eye and brain injuries in a prospective manner on a large boxing population should be combined with continued work on development and standardization of protective equipment. Officials must be receptive to rule changes. Ringside physicians need the power to immediately stop a contest on their own authority.

Rule changes and protective devices changed fencing from a sport with a mortality approaching 50% to a still exciting, but relatively safe sport. The same can be done for boxing—perhaps to the detriment of the promoters, but certainly in the best interest of the athletes.

Wrestling

The incidence of eye injuries in college wrestling is low. The average college team with 25 players and 2600 athlete-exposures should expect one or two eye injuries each season with a significant injury every nine or 10 seasons. Although the incidence of eye injuries in wrestling is low, the lack of reliable eye protective devices makes protection of the one-eyed wrestler impossible. Wrestling is not recommended for one-eyed athletes.[101]

A teenage 12 diopter myope who lost an eye to a giant retinal tear suffered while wrestling continued to wrestle only to lose the remaining eye the following year to a giant retinal tear secondary to a wrestling injury (patient of Dr Matti Paavola, Tampere, Finland).

Water Sports

Swimming Immersing the cornea in water produces approximately 42 diopters of hyperopia and an unaided visual accuity near 20/4000.[107] For man to see clearly underwater, the only alternative to placing a strong spherical lens (64.5 diopter in air) in front of the eye is to place an air space in front of the eyes. Into this air space, the fine tuning of any preexisting ametropia may be obtained with contact lenses, various types of spectacles or lenses ground or bonded to the front surface of the goggle.[102] Significantly ametropic competitive swimmers have better judgment of critical racing turns, can see competitors, and have visual communication with coaches if their ametropia is corrected. Several goggle and goggle-cap combinations that incorporate prescription lenses are available.

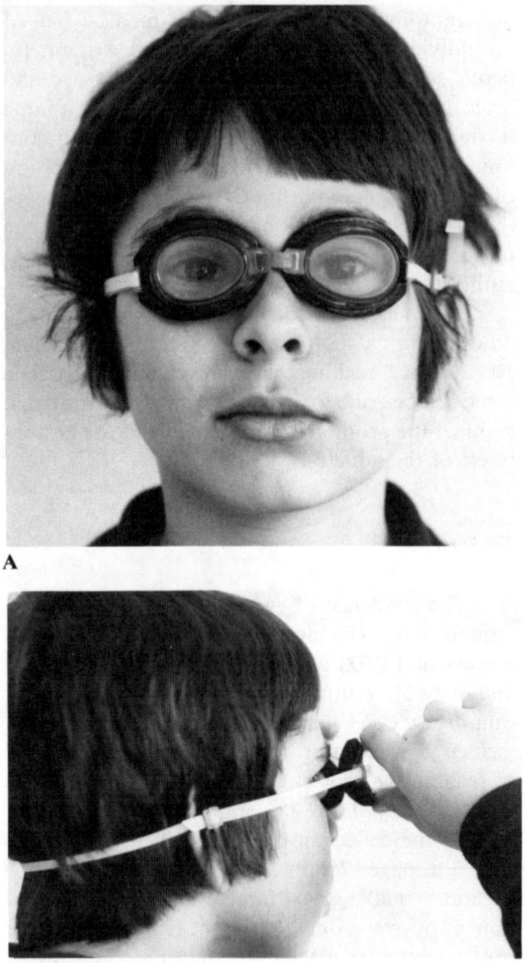

A

B

Figure 12-24 **A** Swim goggles. **B** Note potential for eye injury and need for improvement in strap design.

Since surface swimmers breathe through both nose and mouth, most prefer goggles with elastic straps over face masks, which interfere with breathing through the nose. The main disadvantage with some goggles is the combination of the elastic strap with a sharp edge of the moulded plastic that becomes exposed if the rubber foam cup becomes loose. Several cases of ruptured eyes have been reported in which the goggle was stretched from the face to be "cleared." The goggle then slipped from the wet hands of the swimmer and rebounded toward the eye(s); propelled by the elastic band, the exposed sharp plastic goggle edge then cut open the eye(s) (Figure 12-24). This problem could be solved by fastening the goggle with a less elastic band, having an easily adjustable tightening mechanism, such as Velcro strips, to fasten the goggle plus replacement of any goggle in which the foam had any tendency to come loose from the plastic lens.[103]

Goggles with tight straps have precipitated migraine headaches;[104] goggles with eye cups smaller than the orbital opening may raise the intraocular pressure.[105]

Swimmers may safely wear soft contact lenses in swimming pools and can avoid lens loss by splashing pool water into the eye(s) with the lenses for approximately one minute so the lenses become hypotonic and adhere to the cornea. The osmotic bond lasts at least 30 minutes after exiting the pool, thus the corneal epithelium may be denuded if the lens is removed prior to that time, unless the osmolarity is equilibrated with normal saline drops for 15 to 20 minutes. Ocean water, on the other hand, has a very high osmolarity, causes soft lenses to move excessively, and results in a high loss factor. Although almost all swimming pools are contaminated to some degree with coliform bacteria, and Pseudomonas occasionally is found in ocean water, infection does not seem to present a great hazard to conscientious soft lens wearers.[106]

Water polo Swim goggles for water polo should be made of polycarbonate for impact resistance.

High diving Significantly ametropic divers who have difficulty seeing the water or pool edge could wear hard, soft or gas permeable lenses. The loss rate is much lower than might be expected because divers instinctively close their eyes as they enter the water.[107]

Deep diving Deep diving consists of hard hat diving (essentially limited to commercial use), skin diving (mask plus snorkel) and Scuba diving (mask plus self-contained underwater breathing apparatus).

The hard hat diver may use spectacles as on land, but the spectacles should have straps or cable temples to prevent dislodgment. Polymethylmethacrylate (hard) contact lenses cause corneal epithelial edema during the decompression phase of the dive by the trapping of nitrogen outgassing from the cornea and precorneal tear film. The resultant ocular discomfort, halos, specular highlights, and decreased visual acuity during and after the decompression phase may be hazardous to the diver. Soft lenses do not result in gas trapping or corneal edema and are probably safe.[108] Gas permeable lenses have not yet been studied.

The best, most practical method to correct ametropia for skin and scuba divers is to bond their corrective lenses with optically clear epoxy to a standard oval face mask made of tempered glass

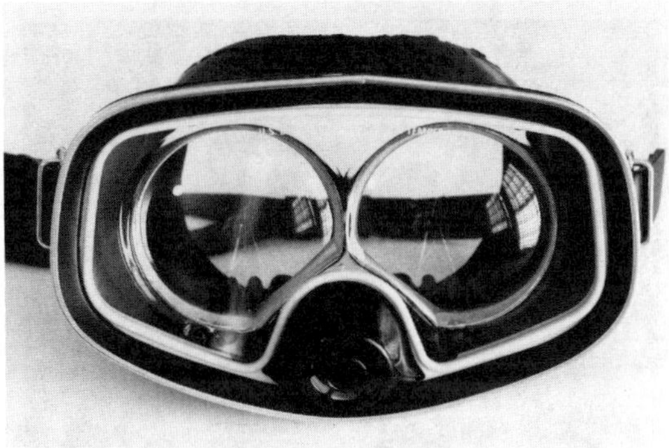

Figure 12-25 Diving mask with bonded prescription spectacle lens.

(Figure 12-25).[109] Contact lenses may be worn under a mask, but they may be dislodged if the mask is flushed with water or in an emergency situation. Because displacement of the contact lens may further impair the diver faced with an emergency, contact lenses are not recommended for snorkel or (especially) scuba divers.

For any dive deeper than 6 to 10 feet below the surface, a face mask is superior to goggles, which at greater depths, often result in ocular and periorbital negative pressure, capillary rupture and hemorrhage.[111]

Saling/yachting The United States Olympic Yachting Committee found that 23 of 44 Olympic yachting hopefuls had pterygium. Many sailors complain of constant eye irritation, the result of wind and salt spray combined with ultraviolet keratitis. Polycarbonate wrap-around, ultraviolet absorbing sunglasses (which may be clear or tinted for comfort) relieve most symptoms and provide eye protection from impact with lines, spars, etc. Competitive sailors are advised to wear a small spray bottle on a short cord around their necks. Water from the bottle is used to clear the sunglass lenses and rinse salt buildup away from the eyes.[112]

Fishing Fishing injuries, some resulting in enucleation,[116] from hooks are fairly common, but whipped pole tips and fishing spears[113] can also result in eye damage. Spectacles, with plastic (preferably polycarbonate lenses), whether in the form of sunglasses or corrective lenses, offer excellent protection and should be worn at all times by anglers.[114]

Golf

Golf is not a common cause of eye injuries, but those that do occur from the ball or club are usually very serious.[115] Golf accounted for 11 (14%) of 80 sports-related injuries that resulted in eye enucleation at the Massachusetts Eye and Ear Infirmary from 1960 to 1980. Golf balls were responsible for 8 of the 11 lost eyes and golf clubs for the other 3. The only sports resulting in more enucleations were BBs (45%) and arrows/darts (15%).[116] The reason for the high enucleation rate is that both a golf ball and the head of the golf club are hard, travel at high speed and can fit within the bony orbit (Figure 12-26), transmitting all of the energy directly to the globe with resultant rupture or disorganization of the eye.

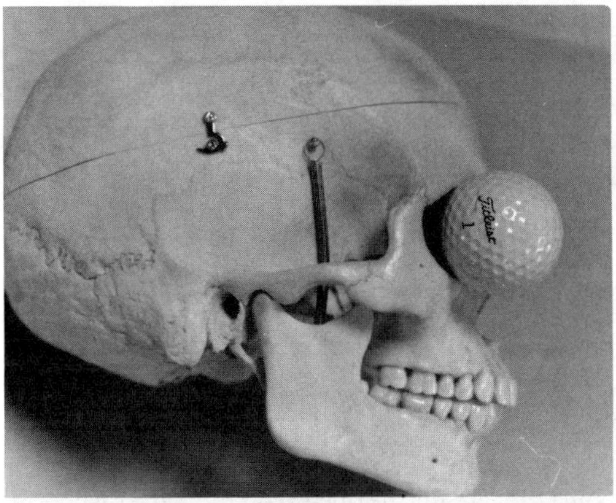

A

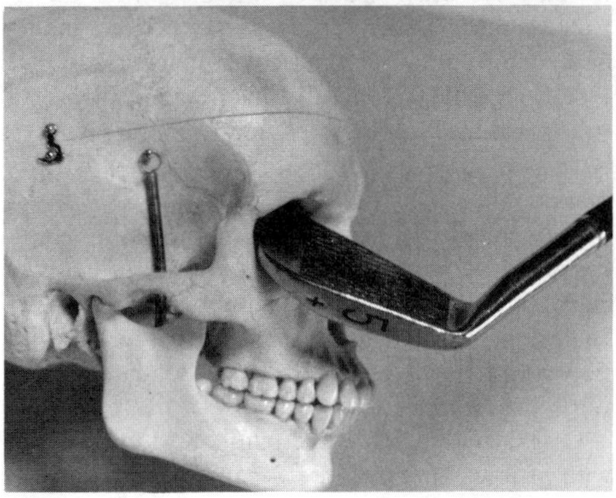

B

Figure 12-26 **A** Penetration of golf ball into orbit. Front of cornea would lie between base and apex of "1" on ball. **B** Golf club injuries to children often result from parent's backswing.

Most people do not realize that liquid center golf balls are very hazardous. If they are cut open the heavy liquid, usually a barium compound, is released under tremendous force. The force is sufficient to penetrate the eye and orbital structures.[117-118] Never cut open a liquid center golf ball.

Most golf injuries could be avoided if golfers check to be sure the way is clear before hitting the ball or swinging the club, with special care to be certain that no curious children are directly behind at the start of the backswing.

Ametropic golfers should have impact resistant polycarbonate lensed spectacles.

Horse-back Riding/Polo

Standards for adequate polo face masks will come too late for the one-eyed polo player who lost his only eye when struck by a mallet, which penetrated a face mask that obviously offered inadequate protection (personal communication, Voigt Hodgson, PhD). Hopefully this tragic incident will spark organized polo clubs and manufacturers to write adequate performance standards for face masks.

Although eye injuries are not a major risk in horseback riding, other than polo, cross country riders frequently suffer corneal abrasions from tree branches overhanging the trail. Spectacles with polycarbonate lenses would offer adequate protection from this risk.

The wide variety and quality of riding helmets, with little or no guidelines for horseback riders to choose adequate protection, has prompted the United States Pony Clubs, Inc. to start the process of organizing an ASTM committee to formalize the writing of a consensus standard for equestrian protective headgear.

In Germany, the Techniche Ueberwachungs-Verein (TUV), a semigovernmental, nonprofit organization that concerns itself with the safety of all types of equipment, established testing procedures for riding helmets and caps. In July, 1982, TUV extended the privilege of their sign of approval, "Gepruefte Sicherheit" (proven safety) to the L.A.S. (Lavorazione Articoli Sportivi in Nembro, Italy) and Three-Day helmets. These helmets, now on the United States market, hopefully will force the rest of the industry to higher levels of product performance.

Cycling

Cyclists would avoid most head, face and eye injuries if they wore adequate head protection whenever they rode. In addition to injuries

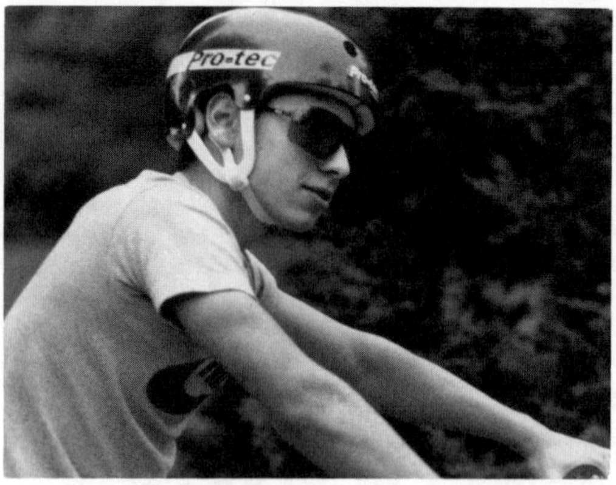

Figure 12-27 Cosmetically acceptable eyewear for cycling and other sports. (Courtesy of Gargoyles, Pro-Tec.)

resulting from falls, many cyclists have constant gritty eye irritation from wind and sun exposure, especially when traveling at high altitude in arid regions. Although a lubricating ointment will give temporary relief from dry eye symptoms, the best protection is a good pair of polycarbonate lenses that shield the eyes from dust, dirt, wind and ultraviolet light. Sore eyes in cyclists is enough of a problem that a bicycling magazine ran tests on available cycling eyewear and found some excellent injection moulded polycarbonate eye protectors (Figure 12-27).[119]

Motorcycling

Full-face helmets provide better facial protection than do "jet" helmets. With the tremendous forces involved in this sport, injury is possible even with the best available protective devices.

Skiing

Cross country skiers are subject to corneal abrasions from tree twigs. Both cross country and downhill skiers can suffer ski pole injuries[120] and snowblindness. Good ultraviolet absorbing goggles (polycarbonate lenses preferable)[121] offer adequate protection.

Snowmobiling

Most eye and facial injuries to snowmobilers can be avoided by a combination of safe driving, avoidance of alcohol and drugs while driving, and full face protection.[122-123] Even careful snowmobilers have been severely injured in the eyes and/or even decapitated when they hit wires that had been placed in formerly familiar terrain since their last trip to the area. Since a fine fence wire is almost impossible to see when travelling at moderate speed during snowfall, the basic design of the snowmobile windscreen should incorporate a sturdy bar to deflect thin wires over the rider(s) heads.

Protection against snowblindness (see mountaineering) and ocular windburn is available with face masks or goggles.

One should exercise the same caution working on a snowmobile battery that should be exercised when working on an auto battery; both can explode.[124]

Mountaineering

Mountaineers at altitudes higher than 12,000 feet (3658 meters) are subject to retinal hemorrhages, probably secondary to hypoxic vasodilation combined with sudden rises in intravascular pressures. The hemorrhages resolve spontaneously with return of normal visual acuity on return of the climber to lower altitude, but the climber may be left with permanent reduction in critical flicker fusion frequency, visual fields, and dark adaptation.[30-32]

The prevention of snowblindness is essential. Snowblindness (photophthalmia) is secondary to overexposure to ultraviolet radiation (UV) which is more intense at higher altitudes because the thinner atmosphere does not filter out as much of the sun's UV as does the thicker atmosphere at sea level. Since ice and snow reflect approximately 85% of UV light, the climber is twice exposed—by both direct and reflected UV. A severe case of snowblindness may be asymptomatic for 8 to 12 hours after exposure, then be totally disabling for several days while the climber is unable to keep the eyes open because of extreme pain, photophobia and lid edema. Mountaineering sunglasses or goggles should filter out at least 90% of wavelengths below 320 nm and be designed to block most reflected light coming from the sides and below. In an emergency, goggles may be made of cardboard with a thin slit. Sherpa and Balti porters have been known to protect their eyes by pulling their hair down over their faces. Mountaineers should understand that UV protection is as important under overcast conditions as it is in full sunlight.[125]

Erythropsia (vision that is temporarily tinged red) is due to retinal overexposure to UV light and eliminated by the use of UV absorbing glasses.[126]

Exercise/Running/Jogging

Most eye injuries incurred while exercising are caused by faulty exercise equipment, expecially elastic cords (used for repetitive resistance exercises) that snap or release from a handle or hook. Manufacturers should write voluntary consensus standards to upgrade the safety of this type of product.

Eye injuries to runners and joggers usually result from striking branches, twigs, pipes, etc., while running in low light conditions in unfamiliar terrain. Running and jogging do not cause a greater incidence of retinal detachment.[127]

Shooting/Archery

It is so rare for elite shooters to be crossed dominant that a right-handed shooter with a dominant left eye should be coached from the start of his/her career to shoot left-handed (or vice versa), since the dominant eye is more important than the dominant hand for shooting accuracy. It is usually stated that pistol shooters need 20/20 *near* visual acuity, probably for sight alignment, while elite rifle shooters usually have the need for 20/20 *distance* acuity.[128-129]

In addition to correcting refractive errors, spectacles are necessary for protection.[130] Polycarbonate lenses have sufficient impact resistance to prevent most accidental injuries to shooters (Figure 12-28). Glass or CR-39 (ordinary plastic) lenses do not have sufficient impact resistance (Figure 12-29, Table 12-10).

Fencing

Although fencing is a relatively safe sport, two recent fatal injuries—penetration of a face mask by a broken foil with intracranial entry through the orbit and penetration of neck over protective bib—and a serious hand laceration with the side of the blade have prompted the formation of an ASTM committee on fencing safety.

This committee is working with experts in penetration resistant fabrics (Kevlar) and designers to write performance standards that give substantially

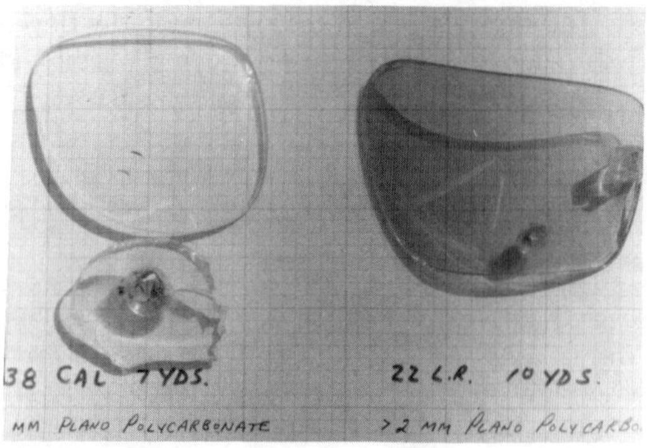

Figure 12-28 Ballistic test of available sports eye protective wear. (Inspector Guy Busa, Lexington Police Dept. 1981). **Left** 3 mm polycarbonate lens, mounted in sports frame (Action Eyes, Bausch and Lomb) shattered when impacted by .38 caliber bullet, but bullet did not pass plane of lens mounted in Action Eyes frame. **Right** injection moulded polycarbonate eye protector (Gargoyles, Pro-Tec) resisted penetration by .22 caliber long rifle bullet.

better protection to the underarm, breast, chest and neck.

As far as eye protection is concerned, the committee felt that the current FIE test is not reliable in that the mask which permitted fatal penetration tested as "good." Standards development will require determining the energy at the tip of a broken foil when thrust by strong fencers, then writing performance standards that will prevent penetration without impeding vision or air flow.

The breakage characteristics of foils will also be studied. Better foils break with a squared rather than a pointed end, but still, the rate of breakage is high. (A competitive fencer usually breaks six or seven blades a season and takes four to five weapons to a match). Some experts believe that metal blades will someday be replaced with fiberglass or carbon-fiber blades, which will be lighter, have fewer breaks and have less lethally shaped break surfaces; others feel that metal blades can be improved with newer metallurgical techniques.

The fact that these few injuries have prompted a complete restudy of the sport speaks highly of the concern of fencing officials for the athlete's safety.

BB Guns/Air Rifles

BB guns and air rifles are not given the respect they deserve as weapons with blinding and killing power.

Surveys by the Consumer Products Safety Commission (NEISS) show that 28,030 injuries from gas, air, spring operated guns, BBs and pellets were seen during 1980 in emergency rooms nationwide, of which 1866 involved the eye. Of the total injuries, 66% were to children aged 14 or younger. Thirty percent of the eye injuries required hospitalization.[132]

Patients that require hospitalization and surgical intervention from BB eye injuries have a high risk of enucleation. Of 32 patients treated with sur-

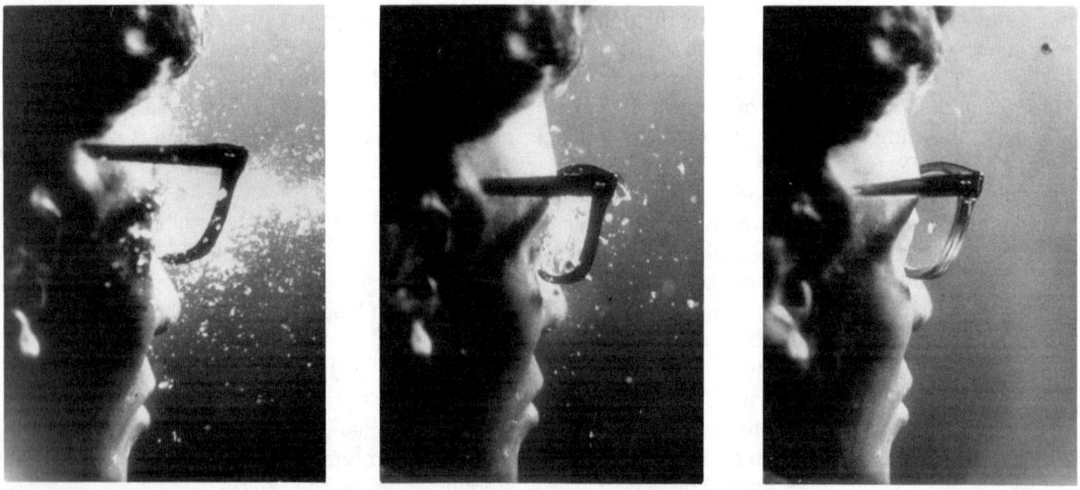

A B C

Figure 12-29 Results of impact of a .177 caliber, .342 gm steel BB delivered at 500–600 ft/sec on 3 mm thick plano samples mounted on head form. (High speed video tape. Gentex Corp. 1982). **A** Tempered glass, **B** CR-39, **C** Polycarbonate.

Table 12-10
Comparative Impact Energies of Missiles and Fracture Energies of Lens Materials

Potential Impact Energy of Selected Missiles	ft-lb
Pitched baseball	21.0
Softball	17.0
Volleyball	3.0–6.0
Average apple, tossed 6 feet	0.75
Human fist	2.0–4.0
Fall (head striking object from 1 to 3 feet)	5.0–15.0
Automobile crash at 20 mph; head striking dash	67.2
3 lb hammer dropped 10 ft.	30.0
BB	0.5–1.5
22 caliber slug	10.0
Flying gravel, (1/8 inch) 30 mph	0.3
Flying gravel, (1/8 inch) 50 mph	0.8
Stone 1 3/4″ × 3/4″ × 1/2″ thrown 30 ft	7.9
Stone 2″ × 1 1/2″ × 1″ thrown 30 ft	8.9
Lawnmower blade throwing small stone 30 ft	6.0–23.0
Grinding wheel throwing chips 2 ft	0.7–28.0
FDA test 5/8 inch steel ball dropped 50 inches	0.15
ANSI Z87-OSHA 1 inch steel ball dropped 50 inches	0.60

	Missile size		
Fracture Energies of Different Lens Types	1/8 inch (ft-lb)	1/4 inch (ft-lb)	1 inch (ft-lb)
Heat treated glass (2 mm)	0.03	0.22	0.36
Chem treated glass (2 mm)	0.07		0.66
Heat treated glass (3 mm)	0.07		2.1
CR-39 (2 mm)	0.22	1.4	0.66
CR-39 (3 mm)	0.37		1.28
Polycarbonate (2 mm)	4.7	13.0	No breaks*

*No failures with forces exceeding 120 ft-lb. Unpublished test: 40 lb steel plate dropped 3 feet with lens bridging two separated 2 × 4 timbers. For 1/8 inch missiles, polycarbonate is 21 times stronger than allyl resin (CR-39); and for larger missiles, polycarbonate is over 100 times stronger than CR-39 allyl resin.

Data supplied by J. Davis, Gentex Corp.

Conclusions:

1. Commonly encountered impact energies will shatter hardened glass and CR-39 spectacle lenses.
2. The ANSI Z87.1-1979 impact energy requirement (for industrial safety lenses) of 0.6 ft-lb is inadequate and not reflective of state-of-the-art polycarbonate technology.
3. Routine testing of polycarbonate lenses at 13.5 ft/lb (4 lb weight dropped 40 inches) has never caused a break or a fracture.
4. Streetwear thickness polycarbonate eyewear far exceeds the impact resistance of industrial thickness hardened glass or CR-39 lenses.
5. Seat/shoulder belts are essential for prevention of eye injuries in automobile crashes.
6. Polycarbonate is the lens material of choice for all athletes and one-eyed patients.

gical intervention at the Wilmer Eye Institute between 1970 and 1981, 22 had penetrating injuries from the pellets—19 of the penetrated eyes were enucleated and the vision in the remaining 3 was worse than 5/200.[133]

Of the 80 eyes removed due to sports injuries at the Massachusetts Eye and Ear Infirmary between 1960 and 1980, 36 were due to BB guns.[116] Some patients suffered loss of the remaining eye from sympathetic ophthalmia.

A standard BB (0.345 gr) will penetrate the globe at speeds higher than 236 ft/sec (72.0 mps) and result in injury at the vitreous base at an average speed of 205 ft/sec (62.3 mps).[134]

Higher powered general purpose air rifles, advertised in children's magazines, may have muzzle velocities as high as 620 ft/sec (189 mps) which is well above the 408 ft/sec (124 mps) velocity required ". . . for penetration of skin, bone, and moderate tissue, or if no bone is encountered, of skin and deep tissue."[135]

For a BB projectile to be beneath the kinetic energy of 0.03 Joule that will result in contusion eye injury, the muzzle velocity would have to be reduced to 43 ft/sec (13 mps). When fired in the horizontal direction from a height of five feet, the BB would travel a mere 24 feet, thus would be useless as a gun.[135]

Since BB guns cannot be made safe and still have any utility, the only means of controlling injuries is to keep them out of the hands of unsupervised children and subject them to the same safety precautions and laws as apply to weapons using gunpowder (firearms). Many states, such as Massachusetts,[136] which classifies BB guns as firearms, have laws regulating the sale and use of BB and air weapons. However, most states still treat these weapons as toys and allow their sale to children.[137]

With supervision, BB and air-powered weapons are excellent training weapons for children who will later move up to the responsible use of their gunpowder-propelled cousins. BB injuries, deaths and blindness will continue as long as children have the feeling they are playing with toys and the true danger of these weapons is not stressed and their use supervised.

Fireworks

Fireworks are a large part of the festivities at many sporting events. Fireworks cause blindness. Extreme caution should be used when in the vicinity of them.

War

While military injuries are not truly sports injuries, the same principles of prevention apply. War injuries were the impetus for my involvement with the prevention of eye injuries. Anyone that sees the result of bilateral blindness on teenaged youth and realizes that the majority of war-related blindness is preventable with slight modifications of existing sports eye protectors could not help but wonder why the military is putting so little effort into this area (some small-scale studies are, however, in progress).

The incidence of eye injuries as a result of maiming weaponry, has increased with each war. Between 6% and 9% of all Vietnam war injuries involved the eye resulting in permanent visual impairment and blindness in thousands of American soldiers.[138]

Even if responsible officials have become hardened to the physical and emotional costs these men have paid, perhaps the economic costs and the cost effectiveness of prevention will result in the widespread use of eye armor.

The main rule in avoiding eye injury is common sense. If you are competing in such a way that you could be hit by a ball, a stick, or the opponent, wear an eye protector. Eye injuries are often hard to fix, and are easy to prevent.

THE ONE-EYED ATHLETE

How can we define "one-eyed"? For the purpose of recommending extra safety precautions, my definition is: *a person is effectively one-eyed when loss of the better eye would result in a significant change in lifestyle due to the poor vision in the remaining eye.*[139]

There is no question that one would have difficulty functioning with 20/200 or poorer best corrected vision in the remaining eye. Since the result of loss of the good eye in this case would be legal or total blindness, with its resultant burden both to the athlete and society, athletes (and the parents of effectively one-eyed children participating in sports) must be well informed of the potential long-term consequences if the good eye were lost. They should also be informed of the risks of injury (without and with various eye protectors) and the possibility of repair of injuries typically seen with the sport in question.

Thus, an athlete certainly should be considered one-eyed if his/her best corrected vision in the involved eye is 20/200 or less, with the other eye found normal by an ophthalmologist. On the other hand, most of us would function fairly well with 20/40 or better vision in the remaining eye. More difficult is advising patients with between 20/40 and 20/200 best corrected vision in the affected eye. The loss of the ability to drive legally in most states would be a significant handicap to most people. The inability to drive would significantly interfere with the jobs available to a youngster when he or she is older. Studies would also be more difficult throughout the school years. Therefore, we could safely conclude that a child is effectively one-eyed when the best correctable vision in the poorer eye is less than 20/40, and an adult effectively one-eyed if they feel the level of vision in their poorer eye would interfere with their life or livelihood if the better eye were lost.

It is only by full discussion of the potential serious long-term consequences of injury to the better eye that the ophthalmologist, the athlete, and the parents can agree on the level of protection necessary for the better eye. The most effective protection is only possible when the athlete understands the risks and is anxious to cooperate in the effort to protect the eyes while still allowing participation and enjoyment of the preferred sport. Having the athlete wear an occluder over the better eye for several days will allow him/her to better evaluate the ability to function with the poorer eye. Usually, if the athlete is sincere and honest with him/herself, it is fairly easy to reach agreement among the athlete, parents, ophthalmologist and sports officials as to whether or not the athlete is effectively one-eyed.

As protective devices improve and more effective sports eye protectors are developed, more and more sports become quite safe even for the one-eyed athlete. The division of sports into collision, contact and non-contact[15] tells little of the risk of eye injury. It is far more dangerous to play a racket sport (noncontact) without an eye protector than to play hockey (collision) with a full face mask. The athlete deserves a true discussion of the risk of eye injury involved in a chosen sport. Unless the patient is especially gifted in a particular sport, or has psychological reasons to participate in a chosen sport, a safer sport (track and field, gymnastics, etc) will usually be chosen.

At this time, the only sport *absolutely contraindicated* for the effectively one-eyed is *boxing* since the risk of serious injury is very high and there is no known effective eye protector.

Sports with higher eye injury risk (Table 12-11) should be discouraged more strongly if the poorer eye has less than 20/200 best corrected vision and the recommendation to the player, parents, and sports/school officials should be to find an outlet for their athletic desires in sports that are more "eye safe." If the player, parents, and possibly their lawyers are persistent and insistent after an informative discussion, they should be required to sign appropriate waivers as dictated by the school committee.

The waiver has a dual purpose: it helps assure that the athlete will wear appropriate protective devices for practices and games; it often affords the only possible legal protection for school committees and members of sports-medical committees faced with the dilemma of the one-eyed athlete who insists (or whose parents insist) he or she play a sport with high eye injury risk. The best medical advice says that this athlete should not, but it seems that there may be confusion in the law.[140] The Massachusetts law reads, "the health and safety of each student must be paramount in every phase of the instructional physical education program," and also "each school shall provide equal opportunity for physical education for all students."[141] Federal law states, "students who can participate in regular physical education programs for all or some aspects of physical education must be placed in such programs."[142] The physician becomes hard put to prove that she/he is not discriminating against the handicapped by excluding the one-eyed student from some sports.

The medical-school committee should specify that the one-eyed athlete wear sports eye protectors that meet the ASTM or CSA racket sport standard for all sports with risk of eye injury for all games and practices. These eye protectors must be worn under the face mask of those sports that usually require a face mask (hockey, football, lacrosse). Baseball face protectors should be used for batting. Face protectors should be required for women's lacrosse (already required for men's lacrosse) and field hockey. A waiver should not be granted for one-eyed boxers. The safety of the athlete is worth a court battle.

For daily wear, off the athletic field, one-eyed people should wear 2 mm center thick polycarbonate lenses mounted in a sturdy street-wear frame (a good compromise between safety and cosmetic acceptance; better options will be available in the future) most of the time to protect the good eye (Figure 12-23). This is especially true of young active people who are subject to injury on or off the athletic field. *The important role of spectacles as a protective device should be emphasized.*

VISUAL NEEDS OF THE ATHLETE

Failure to perform certain athletic feats (catching a fly ball in the outfield) could clearly be related to poor vision. A simple Snellen chart to

Table 12-11
Eye Injury Risk Potential, Availability of Protector, and Adequacy of Protection for One-Eyed Players: Selected Sports

Eye Injury Risk	Sport	Available Protector	Play by One-Eyed with Protector
Extremely High	Boxing	Helmet—needs improvement	Absolutely contraindicated
	Ice hockey	Helmet/face mask[33-35]	OK with CSA or HECC approved face mask*
	Box lacrosse	Yes[33]	OK*
	Men's lacrosse	Helmet/face mask	OK with helmet/face mask (with center bar)*
		Helmet—needs improvement##	
Very High	Squash	Yes[26,27]	Probably OK**
	Racquetball	Yes[26,27]	Probably OK**
	Floor/street/ ball hockey	Possibly#	OK with ice hockey helmet mask*
High	Tennis	Yes[26,27]	OK*
	Paddleball	Yes[26,27]	OK*
	Basketball	Possibly#	Probably OK***
	Baseball/softball	Yes[47]	Would discourage pending further protector tests in the field
	Women's lacrosse	Probably##	OK with men's lacrosse or ice hockey helmet/face shield*
Medium	Badminton	Yes[26,27]	OK*
	Water polo	Probably###	Probably OK with sturdy polycarbonate swim goggles
	Soccer	Possibly#	Probably OK***
	Volleyball	Possibly#	Probably OK***
	Team handball	Possibly#	Probably OK***
	Speedball	Possibly#	Probably OK***
	Bombardment	Possibly#	Probably OK***
	Rugby	Possibly#	Probably OK***
	Polo	Yes—needs improvement	Probably OK with ice hockey face mask[33-35] mounted on good riding helmet
	Football	Yes	OK with full face mask on helmet*

Low	Wrestling	None	Contraindicated
	Skiing	Goggles	OK with polycarbonate ski goggles
	Snowmobiling	Ski goggles[87]	OK with polycarbonate lensed ski goggles
	Men's lacrosse	See above	
	Golf	Probably#	OK*
	Cycling	Helmet – needs standard	OK*
	Fishing	Yes – Eyeglasses (polycarbonate lenses)	OK*
Very Low	Swimming	Probably###	OK with sturdy polycarbonate swim goggles
	Diving	None	Probably OK* (no protector available for high diving – risky)
	Sailing	UV absorbing, polycarbonate	OK*
	Crew	UV absorbing, polycarbonate	OK*
	Track and field	Not needed	OK*
	Hockey (with protector)	See above	
	Box lacrosse (with protector)	See above	OK*
	Women's lacrosse (with protector)	See above	OK*
	Fencing (with protector)	Mask – needs standard	OK with high quality face mask*
	Mountaineering	UV absorbing, polycarbonate	OK*
	Shooting/archery	Polycarbonate eye protectors	OK*
	Running/jogging	Polycarbonate eye protectors	OK*

Risk potential estimates based on combined incidence/severity data plus clinical experience.

*One-eyed athletes should wear polycarbonate prescription glasses or polycarbonate plano eye protectors for *all* sports. This eyewear should meet the ASTM or CSA standards for racket sport eye protectors. When a face guard is worn (as in hockey), the eye protectors must be worn *in addition to the face guard* for added protection.

**Further in the field testing of CSA and ASTM standards for racket sports to be sure they give adequate testing for the one-eyed in squash and racquetball. Blows with the racket are of special concern.

***Racket sport eye protectors[26,27] probably offer adequate protection, but further testing is needed.

#This sport has not been studied in complete detail, nor are there ASTM or CSA performance standards specific to the sport. However, eye protectors that meet the requirements of racket sport CSA[26] or ASTM[27] standards will most likely offer sufficient impact and penetration protection to prevent most eye injuries.

##This sport needs standards for better head and face protection equipment. However, available protective devices should be used while awaiting standards development.

###Some polycarbonate swim goggles appear to offer good impact and penetration resistance; however, no studies have been done.

Table 12-12
Lens Material Properties

Type of Lens Material—2mm	Abrasion Resistance*	Refractive Index	Specific Gravity	VT†	UV‡
Polycarbonate (coated)	0.8	1.586	1.20	92%	380 nm
Cast resin CR-39	7.5	1.498	1.31	92%	350 nm
Glass chemically hardened	0.4	1.523	2.53	92%	290 nm
Glass heat/air hardened	0.4	1.523	2.53	92%	290 nm

*Taber abrasion test. Lower number = more abrasion-resistant.
†Visual transmittance.
‡UV wavelength below which the lens allows 0% transmittance (higher wavelength = more effective ultraviolet protection).

The combination of high index of refraction and low specific gravity makes polycarbonate the lightest and thinnest lens available. For example:

	+3.00 diopter lens, 60 mm round, 2 mm edge		
	Glass	Allyl Resin	Polycarbonate
Center thickness (mm)	4.60	4.73	4.30
Weight (g)	23.6	12.5	10.7

Polycarbonate (as does any high index lens material) has the disadvantage of higher dispersion (NU values: polycarbonate = 30; glass = 58; allyl resin = 58) with an increase in lateral chromatic aberration, sometimes noticeable in lenses over ± 5.00 diopters. Some patients with high refractive errors may require less impact-resistant lenses for desk work. The trade-offs between weight, safety and edge of field color should be discussed with patients with high refractive errors.

Polycarbonate lenses have surface quality at least as good as that of allyl resin lenses and come close to the surface quality of the finest glass lenses. Polycarbonate has excellent resistance to high temperatures, with dimensional stability from −60°F to 25°F.

Polycarbonate lenses have occasional coating specks which are not noticeable to the wearer. Coated polycarbonate lenses are inert to most solvents. The uncoated edge may be attacked. Care should be exercised against carbon tetrachloride.

Polycarbonate lenses are not yet available for: those with prescriptions out of the range (constantly expanding—at this time approximately the range +6.00 diopters to −6.00 diopters with cylinders up to 3.00 diopters); those who need special occupational bifocals (add above, etc); those who require photochromic or progressive addition lenses.

Data supplied by J Davis, Gentex Corp.

test each eye independently (by the coach or the trainer) is a valuable screening test and should be performed on all athletes in a sport that requires good vision for competitive performance. Despite its obvious importance, this simple test is often ignored. Improvement in vision is frequently associated with increased athletic performance.

Contact Lenses

Contact lenses offer advantages for many sports, especially for high ametropes—better visual field, no fogging, stay in place with rapid motion, better cosmetically, etc.

However, contact lenses offer no protection from impact. It must be stressed to patients that protective devices, where indicated, should be worn *in addition to the contacts*. Patients who wish contact lenses for sports use deserve a few minutes discussion of injury prevention.[143]

Sports Sunglasses

The vast majority of sunglasses sold for sports use are deficient in impact resistance and reflected ultraviolet light absorption. The essential qualities that must be present in sports sunglasses are:

1. *Impact resistance* The combination of lens and frame must prevent ocular contact by either the missle or the sunglass lens. Manufacturers should state the sports for which the sunglass is intended. Racket sports sunglasses should meet the impact requirements of ASTM F803-83 or CSA P400-M1982; a softball should not shatter a sunglass designed for all-purpose recreational use, nor should the lens pass through the frame under expected sports impact. Impact performance standards for sports sunglasses which test the lens-frame combination under realistic conditions on anatomical headforms are needed.

2. *Protection from ultraviolet exposure*

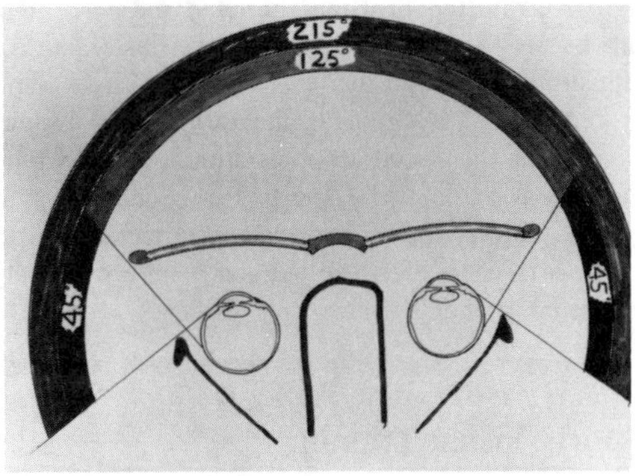

A

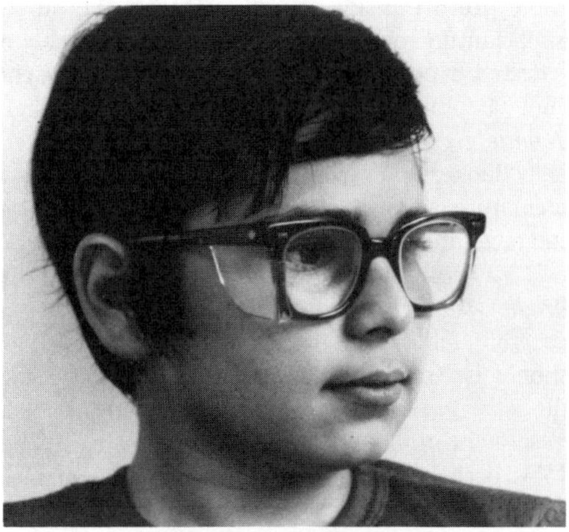

B

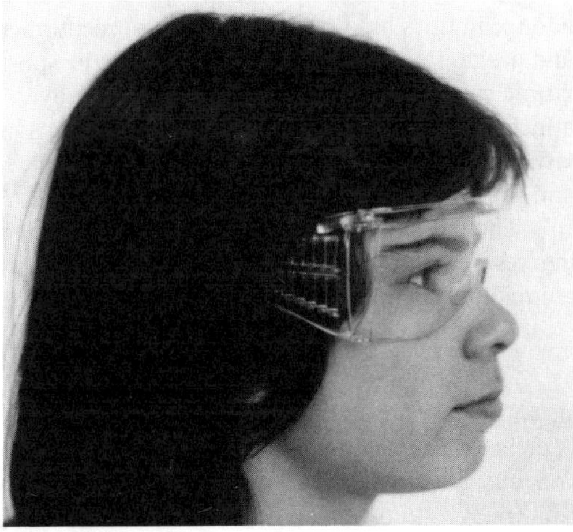

C

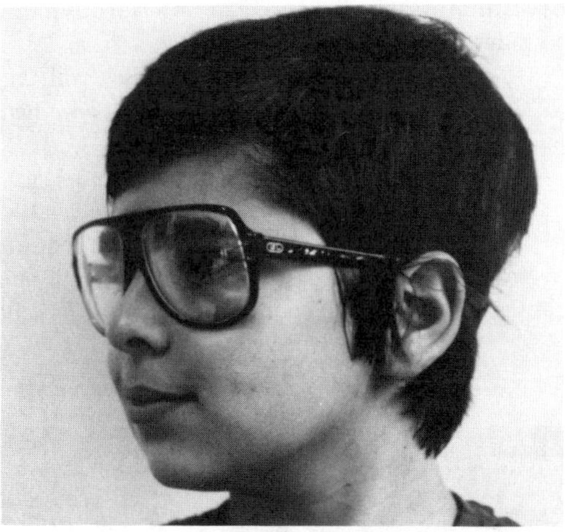

D

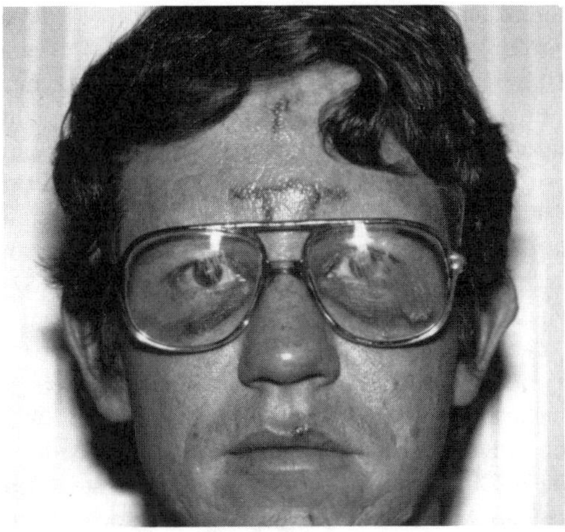

E

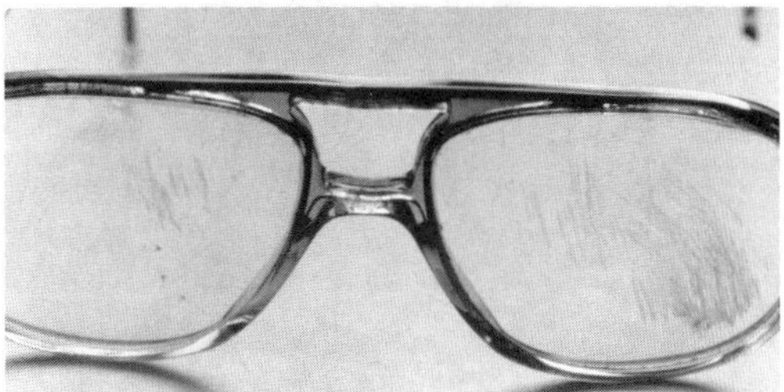

F

Figure 12-30 **A** Industrial safety glasses without side shields leave 90° zone of vulnerability to lateral impacts. **B** Industrial safety glasses with side shields. **C** Polycarbonate industrial eye protector with good lateral protection. **D** Polycarbonate lens (plano or Rx should be mounted in sturdy frame for adequate lens retention. **E** Gentleman wearing polycarbonate Rx lenses in sturdy frame who fell from bicycle. **F** Lenses scratched but did not break.

Protection from side as well as frontal exposure is important in sports where there is a high degree or reflected exposure (mountaineering, skiing, yachting). Prolonged exposure to ultraviolet light *definitely* causes (often incapacitating and potentially dangerous) keratitis, basal cell carcinoma and premature aging of the skin and *possibly* causes cataracts and macular damage.

3. *Prevention of discomfort from glare and bright visible light* For adequate comfort, it is generally felt that no more than 30% of visible light should be transmitted, though this can vary with the activity. In sports where glare is intense, such as in snow or on the water, a factor as low as 10% or 15%, perhaps with polarization, may be preferred.

4. *Aerodynamic efficiency* The drying effects of wind in speed/wind sports (cycling, yachting, mountaineering, skiing, etc) can be prevented by sunglasses designed with aerodynamic considerations.

5. *Light weight* Heavy sunglasses will tend to fly off the face with rapid changes in head position.

6. *Cosmetic acceptability* (Figure 12-31).

It is essential that manufacturers be required to provide the following information on all sunglasses sold for use in sports: the percent of visible light transmitted through the lens; the percent of ultraviolet light (wavelengths specifically stated) transmitted through the lens; additional treatments or coatings (example—polarization) to reduce glare; and the specific sports standards to which they conform and the sports for which the sunglasses have adequate impact resistance as well as the sports for which the sunglasses are definitely not recommended.

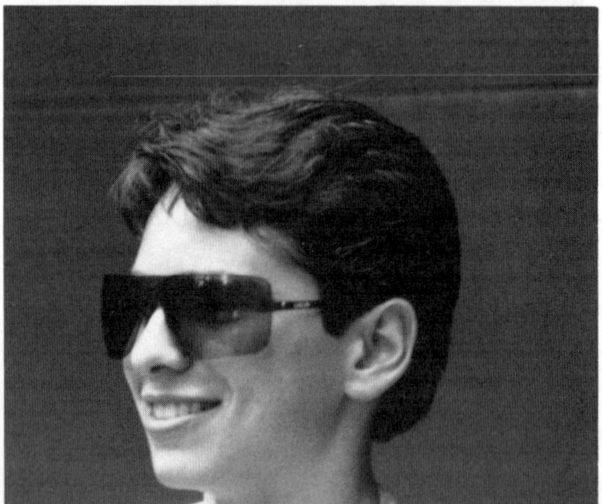

Figure 12-31 Cosmetically acceptable impact-resistant, UV absorbing sunglasses. (Courtesy of Gargoyles, Pro-Tec.)

Sports Visual Training

The use of visual training to improve athletic performance is increasing in popularity as more practitioners (mostly optometrists) enter the field. Most ophthalmologists are unaware of the terms and techniques used by visual training practitioners and are doubtful of claimed results. Can the sports vision specialist really improve a player's overall athletic success by improving certain aspects of visual performance, or are the claims exaggerated and unproven?

The visual parameters included in visual training testing that differ from the usual office examination include:

1. *Vision* Practitioners believe that merely viewing a fast object in motion (baseball, etc) is insufficient. The athlete must look ahead of the action and anticipate with the mind's eye where the ball (puck, shuttlecock, etc) will be in the 0.02 seconds available to pick up the ball (puck, shuttlecock, etc) and determine the plane of the bat (stick, racket, etc) swing.

It is argued that, while *static visual acuity* is important enough to be tested in great detail (several practitioners use the Humphrey Visual Analyzer rather than a phoropter to determine refractive status so as not to obstruct viewing conditions), Snellen testing has little relationship to vision in situations where the athlete, the object of visual regard, or both are moving. The only standardized test for *dynamic visual acuity* is the vision card developed by Arnold Sherman (Figure 12-32), which is viewed as it rotates at 33, 45 and 78 rpm at a distance of ten feet. The smaller letters correspond to Snellen 20/30 and the large letters to Snellen 20/60. Normally, most athletes (with refractive correction in place, if ordinarily used) see the 20/30 letters at 45 rpm. There are no standardized tests to determine dynamic visual acuity with the athlete in motion or with test objects moving in

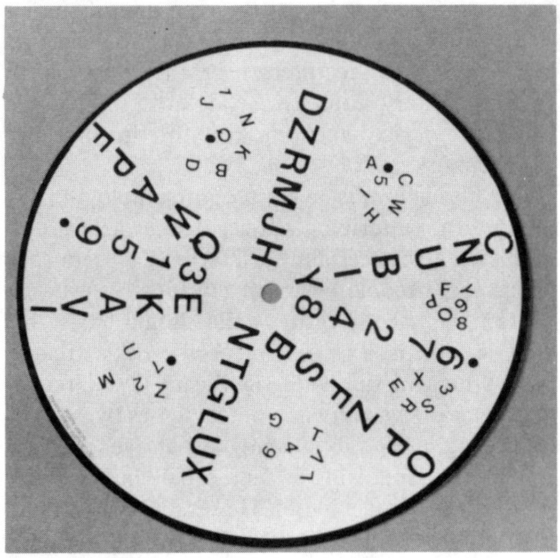

Figure 12-32 Sherman card for measuring dynamic visual acuity.

a linear or variable space, rather than a rotatory flat plane. Training is done, however, with both the athlete and the object to be seen moving in various planes.

2. *Eye tracking ability* While many believe it is impossible for the athlete to track a squash ball at 140 mph or actually see a 90 mph fastball collide with the bat, others say this is not only possible but desirable for better performance. Training methods involve development of fuller range of accurate saccadic eye movements with emphasis on moving the eyes rather than the head. Accommodation, balance, and glare recovery are considered important to eye tracking ability.

3. *Eye teaming and depth perception* refer to the use of both eyes together with accurate steropsis and localization of rapidly moving objects. Test methods for *fusion* are standardized in the Keystone Visual Skills (Davenport, Iowa) and for *stereopsis* in the WIRT and random dot stereograms. A standardized test method for *accommodative facility* (the rate at which accommodation can be stimulated and inhibited repeatedly during a specified period of time) has been proposed.[154] Training methods involve the correct alignment of objects at various distances and angles at progressively increasing degrees of difficulty.

4. *Eye hand coordinator* is divided into the *visual preaction time* (VPT) (the time it takes to fixate and touch an object that moved from the present area of fixation to a random other area) and the *visual reaction time* (VRT) (the number of touches possible as the object is moved to random areas at a fixed rate). Testing is done with the Saccadic Fixator (Wayne Engineering Orthoptic Division, 4120 Greenwood, Skokie, IL 60076). The VPT requires the athlete to press a button next to a red light; the red light then moves randomly to another position on the board and remains lit until the athlete hits that button, and so on. The number of "hits" in 30 seconds is recorded as the VPT. The VRT is then determined by setting the lights to randomly light at the rate of one per second. If the athlete does not press the button within the second, the light moves randomly to another section of the board without a "hit" being recorded. The number of "hits" in 30 seconds is the VRT. A method of combining eye-hand coordination, the visual reaction time and visual preaction time has been called the *Sports Vision Average* (SVA) wherein the SVA = VRT/VPT × 100%. The SVA is proposed as a standardized test to evaluate visual performance compared to athletic performance. Values vary from .506 (modern rhythmic gymnastics) to .759 (ice hockey).[145] Many eye-hand enhancement exercises (shifting of space with prisms, ball bunting, Marsdan ball, Cheiroscopic tracings, stereoscopic pointing) have been reported as useful.

5. *Central-peripheral field awareness* is the ability to be aware of or even concentrate on objects or players eccentric to fixation. On the opposite end of the spectrum is the also necessary aspect of *visual concentration* wherein the athlete must concentrate on the visual task at hand (a basketball free throw, etc) and exclude distractions (crowd noise, other players, etc). *Speed and span of recognition* (the ability to see, often separate, objects quickly and accurately) is important to these skills. There are no standardized measurements for these abilities (other than timed computerized perimetry and standardized visual field testing), but both awareness and concentration can be subjectively improved with various training techniques (such as overcoming the peripheral distraction of a strobe light while performing visual tasks in another area of the visual field and work with a tachistoscope).

6. *Visualization*, the ability to see an image in the minds eye, helps develop muscle memory for the activity by imagining the sequence of steps for proper execution. This has been a popular technique, used by many sports psychologists, to improve performance in highly technical motor activities (ski jumping, figure skating, etc) that has gained general acceptance as improving performance in some athletes.

There is no question that the above visual functions are important for sports performance and activities of daily living such as driving. In any field that is young, there is a rash of case reports that claim extraordinary results, the use of unstandardized test methods and reporting results in a way that does not permit statistical validation. The excesses of some practitioners should not cloud the work that is in progress by many optometrists and psychologists to help answer many questions concerning the role of visual function that is not routinely tested by most ophthalmologists and optometrists. We should keep an open mind on this active area.

Practitioners and researchers in the area of visual training should continue to develop standardized tests and gather data on the normal range of values. Controlled studies, such as those proposed by the Vision Performance and Safety Committee of the United States Olympic Committee should be funded and performed. Visual training may not only prove a valuable technique for improving athletic performance, but the techniques learned may also help in other areas such as macula disease and field loss.[144-154]

LEGAL IMPLICATIONS OF SPORTS EYE INJURIES

It is apparent that malpractice and product liability suits will remain a significant factor in sports eye injuries. Having been involved in a fairly large number of these cases as an expert witness, I believe there are both good and bad aspects to the present legal situation.

The negative aspects—extravagant awards, capricious juries and judges, inconsistency in awards for apparently similar injuries in apparently similar circumstances, long delay in trials so that physicians and manufacturers are often (de facto) held to a state of the art that has advanced since the time of the injury, escalating insurance premiums, a long "tail" on protective equipment that has become obsolete yet is still used by the athlete, lawyers' greed and tendency to instigate suit for high awards—are well known to all physicians and manufacturers and must be corrected by the legal profession.

However, the present legal climate, as much as it desperately needs improvement, does have a significant positive attribute—it is the most efficient check on the small fraction of manufacturers, retailers and health professionals who are inept, incompetent, without conscience or motivated solely by greed. The fact is that the potential of the injured athlete to obtain large awards from the courts has forced manufacturers to gather together to write voluntary consensus standards to upgrade protective devices and help keep inferior products off the market.

Although suits against ophthalmologists for improperly prescribing optical devices are rare[155] at this time, they certainly will increase in frequency as lawyers become aware of advances in eyewear protection that the professional should advise for athletic patients exposed to specific risks. (Example: A high myope with significant lattice retinal degeneration was fit with contact lenses by an ophthalmologist. He subsequently lost an eye to a giant retinal tear following a tennis ball injury while wearing the contact lenses. He is suing the ophthalmologist for failure to prescribe appropriate protective eyewear for use over the contact lenses when exposed to impact.)

The optician, dispensing optometrist and ophthalmologist *must* take a sports, industrial and hobby history and advise appropriate protective eyewear. (Example: A one-eyed myopic lawyer who played racquetball was fit with plastic "safety" streetwear glasses by a reputable optician. He was hit with a racquetball racquet which shattered the plastic lens, resulting in full-thickness corneal laceration in his only eye and a best corrected postoperative vision of 20/40, and is suing the optician for failure to prescribe appropriate protective eyewear for racquetball.)

Manufacturers *must* participate in the voluntary standard-setting process and test their products *before* release to the general public. Devices, advertised as protective, that fail to give adequate protection will result in litigation. (Some litigation examples: lensless racquetball and squash eyeguards that permitted ball penetration at relatively low speed; polo face shield that permitted mallet penetration—player's only eye lost; improperly designed boxing gloves where thumb protruded beyond glove face and caused retinal detachment to helmeted boxer; swim goggles with sharp edges that snapped back and caused corneal laceration; "sport" sunglasses with little impact resistance that shattered when hit with softball, lacerating globe.)

The responsibilities of teachers and coaches of motor skill activities as well as the agencies which sponsor them were further defined in a \$6.3 million award to an injured Seattle high school football player.[156] Although this case involved football, the legal principals would probably apply to all supervised sports. The student *must*: be instructed in appropriate skills, be warned of potential dangers, and have available the latest safety precautions and techniques. (Example: A high school student allowed on the ice in the capacity of hockey team manager during shooting practice was hit in the eye with the puck, resulting in enucleation, and is suing the town and school officials.)

The participants in sports are also not immune from litigation if they act with more aggression than permitted by the rules of the sport or use the sport as an excuse for acts of violence. (Example: A volleyball player blinded an opponent's eye with a finger in what was asserted to have been overly aggressive net-play and is being sued.)

Athletic administrators, coaches, doctors, and equipment manufacturers realize that injuries cannot be entirely eliminated from sports. They are working to at least minimize the risk of serious injury.[157] The best defense in a legal suit seems to be the ability to demonstrate that all concerned were acting responsibly, utilizing state-of-the-art protective devices, playing surfaces, conditioning and training techniques to protect the athlete to an acceptable level of risk considering the nature of the sport.

OPHTHALMOLOGY'S ROLE IN PREVENTING SPORTS EYE INJURIES

National Organizations

Organized ophthalmology and national organizations should recognize that prevention of eye injuries in sports, industry, war and activities of daily living is a valid discipline and is as worthy of consideration and funding as the treatment and study of eye disease from other etiologies.

Despite the proven value of eye protector standards in the prevention of eye disease, national organizations with the word "prevention" in their title have discouraged grant applications for the work of standards writing committees, while freely funding more "basic" research. The concepts that "basic" is more valid than practical research and that the work of full time academicians is more worthy than that of clinicians should be reconsidered.

Individual Ophthalmologists

The ophthalmologist, as any physician interested in public health, has an obligation to the athlete/patient. If she/he sees many injuries from a particular sporting activity, the clinical impression that a potential eye injury problem exists should be conveyed to responsible organizations or officials. The ophthalmologist may be called upon to help gather data and to work with officials to determine the best methods to reduce injuries. The physician frequently underestimates the importance of her/his input in the solution of a problem which, on the surface, seems non-medical.

A brief sport/work/hobby activity description should be obtained from each patient and appropriate eye protectors prescribed. The one-eyed patient deserves a few minutes of discussion on protecting the remaining eye.

Opticians must clearly understand that the referring ophthalmologist expects them to know which frames and lenses offer better protection and that they should suggest safety devices the ophthalmologist may have failed to discuss.

The ophthalmologist should instruct nurses and paramedicals in the emergency treatment and prevention of eye injuries.

Ophthalmology residents should be taught how to prescribe adequate safety eyewear for their patients.

REFERENCES

1. National Society to Prevent Blindness. *Fact Sheet*. New York: National Society to Prevent Blindness, 1978.

2. Scharf, J., and Zonis, S. Perforating injuries of the eye in childhood. *J Pediatr Ophthalmol*. 13:326–328, 1976.

3. Olurin, O. Eye injuries in Nigeria: a review of 433 cases. *Am J Ophthalmol*. 72:159–166, 1971.

4. Bowers, K.D. Young athletes enduring alarming treatment delays. *Physician and Sportsmedicine* 4:57–59, 1976.

5. Antaki, S., Labelle, P., and Dumas, J. Retinal detachment following hockey injury. *Can Med Assoc J*. 117:245–246, 1977.

6. Wheatley, G.M. Childhood accidents prevention and treatment: introduction. *Pediatr Ann*. 6(11):688–695, 1977.

7. Berkow, J.W. Preservation of sight in sports. *Md State Med J*. 20:57–59, 1971.

8. Hahn, H.J.A. Perforating wounds of the eye. *J R Nav Med Serv*. 62:73–81, 1976.

9. Delori, F., Pomerantzeff, O., and Cox, M.S. Deformation of the globe under high-speed impact: its relation to contusion injuries. *Invest Ophthalmol*. 8:290–301, 1969.

10. Leibsohn, J., Burton, T.C., and Scott,

W.E. Orbital floor fractures: a retrospective study. *Ann Ophthalmol.* 8:1057–1062, 1976.

11. Duke-Elder, S., and Wybar, K.C. *System of Ophthalmology.* Vol. 2. *The Anatomy of the Visual System.* St Louis: C.V. Mosby, 1961.

12. Hötte, H.H. *Orbital Fractures.* Springfield, Ill: Charles C Thomas, 1970.

13. Coles, W.H., and Haik, G.M. Vitrectomy in intraocular trauma: its rationale and its indications and limitations. *Arch Ophthalmol.* 87:621–628, 1972.

14. Cherry, P.M.H. Indirect traumatic rupture of the globe. *Arch Ophthalmol.* 96:252–256, 1978.

15. Goldberg, M.F., and Tessler, H.H. Occult intraocular perforations from brow and lid lacerations. *Arch Ophthalmol.* 86:145–149, 1971.

16. Kelman, J.P., Dobbie, G., and Constantaras, A.A. Recurrent traumatic hyphema: a sequel of injury to the Schlemm canal. *Arch Ophthalmol.* 95:484–485, 1977.

17. Layden, W.E. Traumatic glaucoma. *Trans Am Acad Ophthalmol Otolaryngol.* 78:346–350, 1974.

18. Kaufman, J.H., and Tolpin, D.W. Glaucoma after traumatic angle recession: a ten-year prospective study. *Am J Ophthalmol.* 78:648–653, 1974.

19. Rakusin, W. Traumatic hyphema. *Am J Ophthalmol.* 74:284–292, 1972.

20. Read, J., and Goldberg, M.F. Comparison of medical treatment for traumatic hyphema. *Trans Am Acad Ophthalmol Otolaryngol.* 78:799–815, 1974.

21. Beale, H.L., and Wood, T.O. Observations on traumatic hyphema. *Ann Ophthalmol.* 5:1101–1104, 1973.

22. Tassman, W. Retinal detachment in children. *Trans Am Acad Ophthalmol Otolaryngol.* 71:455–460, 1967.

23. Arentsen, J.J., and Welch, R.B. Retinal detachment in the young individual: a survey of 100 cases seen at the Wilmer Institute. *J Pediatr Ophthalmol.* 11:198–202, 1974.

24. Cox, M.S., Schepens, C.L., and Freeman, H.M. Retinal detachment due to ocular contusion. *Arch Ophthalmol.* 76:678–685, 1966.

25. Cox, M.S., and Freeman, H.M. Retinal detachment due to ocular penetration: clinical characteristics and surgical results. *Arch Ophthalmol.* 96:1354–1361, 1978.

26. Richards, R.D., West, C.E., and Meisels, A.A. Chorioretinitis sclopetaria. *Am J Ophthalmol.* 66:852–860, 1968.

27. Sipperley, J.O., Quigley, H.A., and Glass, D.M. Traumatic retinopathy in primates. *Arch Ophthalmol.* 96:2267–2273, 1978.

28. Roca, P.D. Ocular manifestations of whiplash injuries. *Ann Ophthalmol.* 4:63–73, 1972.

29. Kelley, J.S., Hoover, R.E., and George, T. Whiplash maculopathy. *Arch Ophthalmol.* 96:834–835, 1978.

30. Schults, W.T., and Swan, K.C. High altitude retinopathy in mountain climbers. *Arch Ophthalmol.* 93:404–408, 1975.

31. Wiedman, M. High altitude retinal hemorrhage. *Arch Ophthalmol.* 93:401–403, 1975.

32. Rennie, D., and Morrissey, J. Retinal changes in Himalayan climbers. *Arch Ophthalmol.* 93:395–400, 1975.

33. Fuller, B., and Gitter, K.A. Traumatic choroidal rupture with late serous detachment of macula. *Arch Ophthalmol.* 89:354–355, 1973.

34. Hilton, G.F. Late serosanguineous detachment of the macula after traumatic choroidal rupture. *Am J Ophthalmol.* 79:997–1000, 1975.

35. Chandler, P.A. Choice of treatment in dislocation of the lens. *Arch Ophthalmol.* 71:765–786, 1964.

36. Jarrett, W.H. Dislocation of the lens: a study of 166 hospitalized cases. *Arch Ophthalmol.* 78:289–296, 1967.

37. Machemer, R. et al. Symposium: pars plana vitrectomy. *Trans Am Acad Ophthalmol Otolaryngol.* 81:350–450, 1976.

38. Putterman, A.M., Stevens, T., and Urist, M.J. Nonsurgical management of blow-out fractures of the orbital floor. *Am J Ophthalmol.* 77:232–239, 1974.

39. Putterman, A.M. Late management of blow-out fractures of the orbital floor. *Trans Am Acad Ophthalmol Otolaryngol.* 83:650–662, 1977.

40. Aiello, L.M., and Myers, E.N. Blow-out fracture of the orbital floor. *Arch Otolaryngol.* 82:638–648, 1965.

41. Cullen, G.C.R., Luce, C.M., and Shannon, G.M. Blindness following blow-out orbital fractures. *Ophthalmic Surg.* 8:60–62, 1977.

42. Nicholson, D.H., and Guzak, S.V. Visual loss complicating repair of orbital floor fractures. *Arch Ophthalmol.* 86:369–375, 1971.

43. Carmola, J.R., and Harris, B.S. Transient cortical blindness: still an overlooked syndrome? *N Engl J Med.* 282:1325, 1970.

44. Griffith, J.F., and Dodge, P.R. Transient blindness following head injury in children. *N Engl J Med.* 278:648–651, 1968.

45. Bodian, M. Transient blindness after head injury. *N Engl J Med.* 278:966, 1968.

46. Frueh, B.R. Transient blindness following

blunt trauma to the eye. *Am J Ophthalmol.* 71:1034–1036, 1971.

47. Barsky, D. Blindness following concussion of the optic nerve. *J Pediatr Ophthalmol.* 8:195–197, 1971.

48. Bishop, P.J. Head protection in sports with particular application to ice hockey. *Ergonomics* 19:451–464, 1976.

49. Saczalski, K.J., and Richardson, E.Q. Nonlinear numerical prediction of human head/helmet crash impact response. *Aviat Space Environ Med.* 49(1):114–119, 1978.

50. Bishop, P.J. Ice hockey helmets: using a mathematical model of head protection for evaluating standards. *J Safety Research.* 8:163–170, 1976.

51. Hughes, J.R., Wilms, J.H., Adams, C.L. et al. Football helmet evaluation based on players' EEGs. *Physician and Sportsmedicine* 5:73–77, 1977.

52. Meyer, C. Preparaticipation health evaluation. Edited by Smith, N. In *Sports Medicine: Health Care For Young Athletes*, p. 75. Evanston, Ill: American Academy of Pediatrics, 1983.

53. Vinger, P.F. The incidence of eye injuries in sports. *Int Ophthalmol Clin.* 21(4):1981.

54. Slansky, H.H., Depperman, S., Berson, F. et al. Massachusetts Eye and Ear Infirmary, Boston, staff data, 1980.

55. Rose, C.P., and Morse, J.O. Racquetball injuries. *Phys Sportsmed.* 7:73, 1979.

56. Easterbrook, M. Eye injuries in racket sports. *Int Ophthalmol Clin.* 21(4):1981.

57. Reif, A.E., Vinger, P.F., and Easterbrook, M. New developments in protection against eye injuries. *Squash News.* 4:10, 1981.

58. Easterbrook, M. Eye injuries in squash and racquetball players: An update. *Phys Sportsmed.* 10:47–56, 1982.

59. Canadian Standards Association: Racket sports eye protection, preliminary standard P400-M1982. Toronto, 1982.

60. American Society of Testing and Materials: Eye protectors for use by players of racket sports, standard specification F803-83. Philadelphia, 1983.

61. Bishop, P.J., Kozey, J., and Caldwell, G. Performance of eye protectors for squash and racquetball. *Phys Sportsmed.* 10:63–69, 1982.

62. Feigelman, M.J., Sugar, J., Jednock, N. et al. Assessment of ocular protection for racquetball. *JAMA* 250:3305–3309, 1983.

63. Vinger, P.F., and Tolpin, D.W. Racket sports: an ocular hazard. *JAMA* 239:2575, 1978.

64. Vinger, P.F. Eye injuries. Edited by P.F. Vinger and E.F. Hoerner. *Sports Injuries: The Unthwarted Epidemic.* Littleton, MA: PSG Publishing Co., 1981.

65. Pashby, T.J. Eye injuries in hockey. *Int Ophthalmol Clin.* 21(4):1981.

66. Canadian Standards Association: National standard of Canada (CAN 3-Z262.2-M78): Face protectors for ice hockey and box lacrosse players. Rexdale, Ontario, 1978.

67. American Society of Testing and Materials: Consumer safety specification for eye and face protective equipment for hockey players (F513-77) Philadelphia, 1977.

68. American Society of Testing and Materials: Consumer safety specification for eye and face protective equipment for hockey players (F513-80) Philadelphia, 1980.

69. Sze, Y., Thomson, J.C., Norman, R.W. et al. Procedures for the evaluation of hockey goaltenders' face masks. Edited by J.L. Bleustein. In *Mechanics and Sports.* New York: American Society of Mechanical Engineers, 1973.

70. Pashby, T.J. Eye injuries in Canadian hockey: Phase III—Older players now at risk. *Can Med Assoc J.* 113:663, 1975.

71. Norman, R.W., Thomson, J.C., Sze, Y. et al. Relative impact attenuating properties of face masks of ice hockey goaltenders. Edited by R.C. Nelson and C.A. Morehouse. In *Biomechanics IV.* Baltimore: University Park Press, 1974.

72. Tolpin, H.G., and Bentkover, J.D. The economic costs of sports injuries. Edited by P.F. Vinger and E.F. Hoerner. In *Sports Injuries: The Unthwarted Epidemic.* Littleton, MA: PSG Publishing Co., 1982.

73. Vinger, P.F. Eye and face protection for United States hockey players: A chronology. *Int Ophthalmol Clin.* 21(4):1981.

74. Keeney AH: Prevention of eye injuries. Edited by H.M. Freeman. *Ocular Trauma.* New York: Appleton-Century-Crofts, 1979, pp. 337–383.

75. Burke, M.J., Sanitato, J.J., Vinger, P.F. et al. Soccerball induced eye injuries. *JAMA.* 219: 2682–2685, 1983.

76. Verdaguer, T.J. Juvenile retinal detachment. *Am J Ophthalmol.* 93(pt 2):145–156, 1982.

77. Smodlaka, V.N. Medical aspects of heading the ball in soccer. *Phys Sportsmed.* 12:127–131, 1984.

78. McCarroll, J.R., Meaney, C., and Sieber, J.M. Profile of youth soccer injuries. *Phys Sportsmed.* 12:113–115, 1984.

79. Hale, C.J. Protective equipment for baseball. *Phys Sportsmed.* 7:59–63, 1979.

80. American Society of Testing and Mate-

rials: Standard specification for face guards for youth baseball (tentative). Philadelphia, 1985.

81. Kulund, D.N., Schildwacher, T.L., McCue, F.C. et al. Lacrosse injuries. *Phys Sportsmed.* 7:83–90, 1979.

82. Mueller, F.O., and Blyth, C.S. A survey of 1981 college lacrosse injuries. *Phys Sportsmed.* 10:87–93, 1982.

83. Nelson, W.E., DePalma, B., Gieck, J.H. et al. Intercollegiate lacrosse injuries. *Phys Sportsmed.* 10:86–92, 1981.

84. Rimel, R.W., Nelson, W.E., Persing, J.A. et al. Epidural hematoma in lacrosse. *Phys Sportsmed.* 11:140–144, 1983.

85. Wilson, K., and Rontal, M. Facial injuries in football. *Trans Am Acad Ophthalmol Otolaryngol.* 77:434–437, 1973.

86. Torg, J.S., Moyer, R.A., and Nichols, C.E. Unusual fractures caused by football helmet impact. *Phys Sportsmed.* 4:73–75, 1976.

87. Schneider, R.C., and Antine, B.E. Visual field impairment related to football headgear and faceguards. *JAMA.* 192:120–122, 1965.

88. Baake, T. Rugby Medicine: no more magic sponge. *Phys Sportsmed.* 7:139–145, 1979.

89. Palmer, E., Lieberman, T.W., and Burns, S. Contusion angle deformity in prizefighters. *Arch Ophthalmol.* 94:225–228, 1976.

90. McCunney, R.J., and Russo, P.K. Brain injuries in boxers. *Phys Sportsmed.* 12:53, 1984.

91. Rimel, R.W., Giordani, B., Barth, J.T. et al. Disability caused by minor head injury. *Neurosurgery.* 9:221–228, 1981.

92. Rimel, R.W., Giordani, B., Barth, J.T. et al. Moderate head injury: Completing the clinical spectrum of brain trauma. *Neurosurgery* 11:344–351, 1982.

93. Unterharnscheidt, F.J. About boxing: Review of historical and medical aspects. *Texas Rep Biol Med.* 28:421–495, 1970.

94. Unterharnscheidt, F.J. Injuries due to boxing and other sports. *Handbook Clin Neurology* 23:527–593, 1975.

95. AMA Council on Scientific Affairs: Brain injury in boxing. *JAMA.* 249:254–257, 1983.

96. Casson, I.R., Sham, R., Campbell, E.A. et al. Neurological and CT evaluation of knocked-out boxers. *J Neurol Neurosurg Psychiatry.* 45: 170–174, 1982.

97. Hage, P. Boxing: To ban or not to ban? *Phys Sportsmed.* 11:143–146, 1983.

98. Lundberg, G.D. Boxing should be banned in civilized countries. *JAMA.* 249:250, 1983.

99. *Wilbur Cone v. Safe-Play Manufacturing Co., Inc.* United States District Court, Boston, MA, Feb 14, 1983.

100. Ryan, A.J. Eliminate boxing gloves. *Phys Sportsmed.* 11:49, 1983.

101. Powell, J.W. National athletic injury/illness reporting system: eye injuries in college wrestling. *Int Ophthalmol Clin.* 21(4):1981.

102. Williamson, D.E. Correction of ametropia in skin and scuba divers. *Eye, Ear, Nose Throat Monthly.* 49:19–23, 1970.

103. Jonasson, F. Swimming goggles causing severe eye injuries. *Br Med J.* 1(6065):881, 1977.

104. Pestronk, A., and Pestronk, S. Goggle migraine. *N Engl J Med.* 308:226–237, 1983.

105. Joselo, M.M. Goggles increase eye pressure. *Phys Sportsmed.* 11:16, 1983.

106. Stein, H. Swimming with soft contact lenses. *Contact Lens J.* 10:10–12, 1976.

107. Gillilan, R.W. Vision and water sports. *J Am Optometric Assoc.* 51:683–685, 1980.

108. Simon, D.R., and Bradley, M.E. Corneal edema in divers wearing hard contact lenses. *Am J Ophthalmol.* 85:462–464, 1978.

109. Swanson, K.W. Underwater vision. *Contact Lens J.* April:20–22, 1971.

110. Cotter, J. Soft contact lens testing on fresh water scuba divers. *Contact Lens J.* Oct/Dec:323–326, 1981.

111. Craig, A.B. Physics and physiology of swimming goggles. *Phys Sportsmed.* In press.

112. Legwold, G. Pterygium found in Olympic sailors. *Phys Sportsmed.* 11:23, 1983.

113. Tanton, J.H., and Elliott, D.C. Fishing-spear injury of the orbit. *Am J Ophthalmol.* 64:973–974, 1967.

114. Raynor, L.A. Eye protection for anglers. *N Engl J Med.* 307:954, 1982.

115. Millar, G.T. Golfing eye injuries. *Am J Ophthalmol.* 64:741–743, 1967.

116. Portis, J.M., Vassallo, S.A., and Albert, D.M. Ocular sports injuries: A review of cases on file in the Massachusetts Eye and Ear Infirmary pathology laboratory. *Int Ophthalmol Clin.* 21(4): 1981, pp. 1–19.

117. O'Grady, R., and Shoch, D. Golfball granuloma of the eyelids and conjunctiva. *Am J Ophthalmol.* 76:148–151, 1973.

118. Slusher, M.M., Jaegers, K.R., and Annesley, W.H. Liquid center golf balls and ocular injury. *Am J Ophthalmol.* 64:736–740, 1967.

119. De Crosta, T. A sight for sore eyes: cycling eyewear prevents injuries. *Bicycling* Sep/Oct: 40–46, 1983.

120. Eichler, J. Eye accidents due to ski pole

injuries. *Deutsch Gesundheitsw.* 27:375.377, 1972.

121. American Society of Testing and Materials: Standard specification for eye protective devices (Alpine Skiing) F659-80. Philadelphia, 1980.

122. Daniel, R.K., and Midgley, R.D. Facial fractures in snowmobile injuries. *Plast Reconstr Surg.* 49:38–40, 1972.

123. Rigg, B.M. Facial fractures and snowmobile accidents. *Can J Surg.* 20:275–277, 1977.

124. Holekamp, T.L.R., and Becker, B. Ocular injuries from automobile batteries. *Trans Am Acad Ophthalmol Otolaryngol.* 83:805–810, 1977.

125. Wilkerson, J.A. Editor. In *Medicine for Mountaineering.* Seattle: The Mountaineers, 1967, pp. 130–131.

126. DeBenedette, V. Sunglasses for mountaineers: personal experience shared. *Ophthalmology Times* Sept 1:31, 1983.

127. Worthen, D.M. Retinal detachment and jogging. *Ophthalmic Surgery* 11:253, 1980.

128. Landers, D.M. Moving competitive shooting into the scientist's lab. *American Rifleman* April:36–37, 1980.

129. Daniels, F.S. Do the eyes have it? *American Rifleman* March:38, 1981.

130. Gregg, J.R. How to prescribe for hunters and marksmen. *J Am Optometric Assoc.* 51:675–681, 1980.

131. Simmons, S.T., Krohel, G.B., and Hay, P.B. Prevention of ocular gunshot injuries using polycarbonate lenses. *Ophthalmology.* In press.

132. U.S. Consumer Product Safety Commission, National Electronic Injury Surveillance System, 1980.

133. Sternberg, P., de Juan, E., Green, W.R. et al. Ocular BB injuries. *Ophthalmology.* In press.

134. Delori, F., Pomerantzeff, O., and Cox, M.S. Deformation of the globe under high speed impact: its relation to contusion injuries. *Invest Ophthalmol.* 8:290–301, 1969.

135. Preston, J.D. Review of standard consumer safety specification for non-powder guns (ANSI/ASTM F589-78) and non-powder gun projectiles and propellants (ANSI/ASTM F590-78). Mechanical and Textile Division, Engineering Sciences, CPSC, Washington, Feb 8, 1980.

136. Chapter 140, Section 121, Massachusetts General Law.

137. Kerby, C.E. Are we ready to let children shoot? *Sight Saving Review* 23:18–20, 1953.

138. Hornblass, A. Eye injuries in the military. *Int Ophthalmol Clin.* 2(4):121–138, 1981.

139. Vinger, P.F. Preventing ocular injuries. *Am Orthopt J.* 32:56–60, 1982.

140. Ryan, A.J. A dangerous interpretation. *Phys Sportsmed.* 7:43, 1979.

141. Laws and Regulations Pertaining to Physical Education. Publication #11019, Boston, Massachusetts Dept of Education, 1978, Sect. 5.01,7.02.

142. Public Law 94-142, Washington, D.C., 1977.

143. Weis, D.R. Contact lenses for athletes. *Int Ophthalmol Clin.* 21(4):139–148, 1981.

144. Teig, D.S. Sports vision care: the eyes have it! *J Am Optometric Assoc.* 51:671, 1980.

145. Sherman, A. A method of evaluating eye-hand coordination and visual reaction time in athletes. *J Am Optometric Assoc.* 54:801, 1983.

146. Runninger, J. "Eyes on the ball" and oversimplification. *J Am Optometric Assoc.* 51: 667, 1980.

147. Eger, M.J. The "why" of sports vision care results (editorial). *J Am Optometric Assoc.* 51:651, 1980.

148. Garner, A.I. An overlooked problem: athletes' visual needs. *Phys Sportsmed.* 5:75–82, 1977.

149. Sherman, A. Overview of research information regarding vision and sports. *J Am Optometric Assoc.* 7:661–666, 1980.

150. Sherman, A. Prescribing for patients who play. *Optometric Management.* Nov:67–68, 1981.

151. Leibowitk, H.W., and Post, R.B. The two modes of processing concept and some implications. Edited by J. Beck. In *Organization and Representation in Perception.* Hillsdale, NJ: Lawrence Erlbaum Associates, 1982.

152. Revien, L., and Gabor, M. *Sports Vision.* New York: Workman Publishing, 1981.

153. Seiderman, A., and Schneider, S. *The Athletic Eye.* New York: Hearst Books, 1983.

154. Zellers, J.A., Alpert, T.L., and Rouse, M.W. A review of the literature and a normative study of accommodative facility. *J Am Optometric Assoc.* 55:31–37, 1984.

155. Bettman, J.W. *Ophthalmology—The Art, The Law, and A Bit of Science.* Birmingham, AL: Aesculapius Publishing Co, 1984.

156. Adams, S.H., Bayless, M.A. How the Seattle decision affects liability and you. *Athletic Purchasing and Facilities.* July:12–16, 1982.

157. Youth sports injuries: Is the risk acceptable? (staff article). *Athletic Purchasing Facilities* Jan:14–20, 1984.

CHAPTER 13
Injuries to the Teeth

Cosmo R. Castaldi, DDS

Compared to some types of injuries, injuries to the teeth are generally not considered serious; yet teeth have the lowest potential for returning to a normal, healthy state following injury than any other part of the body. A tooth may sustain a mild blow that does not result in any visible fracture. However, within weeks, the pulp—the portion of the tooth that provides the blood and nerve supply—may become completely and irreversibly damaged. For such a tooth to be maintained in a healthy (although nonvital) state requires root canal treatment consisting of removal of all diseased pulp tissue and filling the hollow canal with sterile softened unvulcanized rubber (gutta percha). The technique is exacting and time consuming, and therefore costly. For obvious reasons, prevention must be the prime emphasis of sportsmedicine in relation to dental injuries.

VARIETY OF INJURIES TO THE TEETH

Injuries to the teeth may involve one, several, or in some cases, all of the following structures: crown, pulp, root, periodontal membrane, and supporting bone (Figure 13-1A).

The crown, the visible portion of the tooth, consists of 1) a thin (0.1 to 2.0 mm) hard outer shell called the enamel, which when fractured cannot repair itself, 2) a dense inner structure called the dentine that has a very low potential for repair following injury, and 3) the pulp, a very soft central portion (about the size of a pencil lead) that contains an artery, vein, nerve supply, and lymphatic system all of which also have a low potential for repair following injury.

The root is composed almost entirely of dentine, and contains a hollow canal that extends throughout its length. Covering the root is a thin layer of connective tissue, the cementum, to which is attached the periodontal membrane, an elastic connective tissue that attaches the tooth to the bone and cradles the tooth in the bone socket. Although the cementum and periodontal membrane have good repair potential, a fractured root rarely repairs itself. Even when a repair does occur (Figure 13-1B), it is not true healing, as in the case of a long bone fracture.

The roots of anterior teeth that sustain most dental injuries are incompletely formed under the age of 12 years. For this reason injuries during the early years are additionally complicated. If a tooth loses its vitality following injury, it usually loses its ability to form a normal root. Fortunately, sports-related dental injuries rarely occur under the age of 10 years. However, with the worldwide growing interest in competitive youth soccer, dental injuries in young participants may soon escalate.

Epidemiology

Although the incidence of injuries to the teeth associated with ice hockey and football are well documented,[1-3] the frequency of dental injuries associated with other contact sports such as soccer, basketball, field hockey, street hockey, lacrosse, wrestling, and water polo are not generally known. Table 13-1 reviews some of the major studies of dental injuries in contact sports from 1941 to 1978. Eleven relate to football, six to ice hockey, one to basketball, and one to lacrosse. When players are not wearing any face or mouth protective equipment the highest frequency of dental injuries occurs in ice hockey and lacrosse. There the rate may be three to six times greater than in football. The rate of dental injuries in basketball is much lower than in hockey or football, but is about equal to the rate in football when players are wearing mouth guards. Table 13-1 also shows that the dental injury rate drops to less than 1% when mouth guards are worn.

A careful review of the reports in Table 13-1 raises some questions about the frequency of dental injuries in relation to the use of protective equipment. In six of the studies, it was not certain whether some of the players were using mouth guards; a few may have been, but most were not. In the report of Rovere et al[4] involving professional

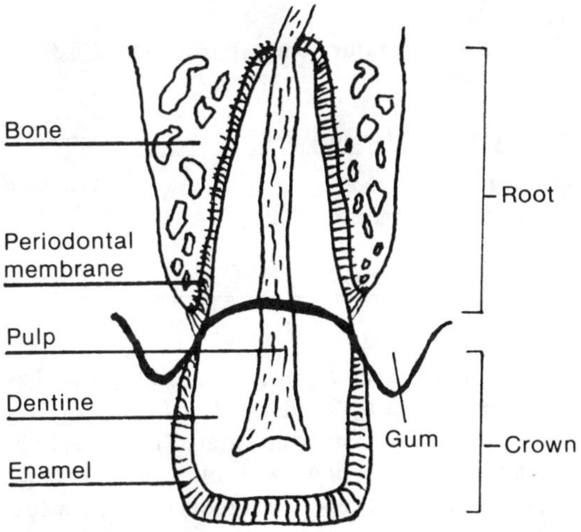

A

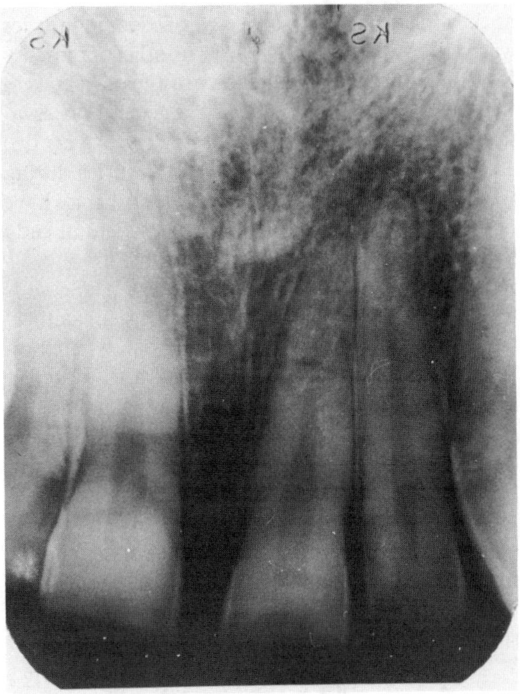

B

Figure 13-1 Anatomy of a normal healthy incisor tooth. **A** An injury may affect one, several, or all of the parts. The pulp may die from a moderate blow even though no fracture occurs. **B** Healed root fracture in 21-year-old professional hockey player who sustained the injury in a game eight years previously. The injured tooth received no treatment.

Table 13-1
Frequency of Dental Injuries in Contact Sports

Study	Year	Sport	Mouth guards worn	Injury frequency (%)
Kramer[13]	1941	Football	Few	1.2
Kramer[13]	1941	Basketball	Few	0.3
Roberts (quoted in Stevens[14])	1954	Football	None	2.3*
Cohen and Borish[15]	1957	Football	Few	3.5
Cohen and Borish[15]	1957	Football	All	0
Roberts[14]	1959–1960	Football	None	1.9†
Roberts[14]	1959–1960	Football	All	0.6†
Anderson (quoted in Stevens[14])	1961	Football	None	1.5
Anderson[14]	1961	Football	All	0.6
Fagan[16]	1963	Football	All	0.5
Marchant et al[5]	1963–1972	Ice hockey	Few	19.6
Stevens[14]	1965	Football	All	0.5
Blyth and Mueller[1]	1968–1972	Football	Most	0.3
Reeves and Mendryk[6]	1969–1970	Ice hockey	Few	8.7
Castaldi[12]	1971	Ice hockey	None	8.3
Castaldi[12]	1973	Ice hockey	All	0
Marchant et al[5]	1973	Lacrosse	Few	10.9
Rovere et al[4]	1973–1976	Ice hockey	?	0.8
Park and Castaldi[8]	1977–1978	Ice hockey	Few	4.8

*No face masks.
†Wore face masks.

hockey players, the frequency of dental injuries was very low (0.8%) compared to other reports.[5,6] Rovere did not indicate that any of the players were wearing mouth guards, but it is a general observation that very few professional hockey players do. The reason the frequency of dental injuries during the period of study (three years) was low may have been because 60% to 70% of the players already had lost one or several upper front teeth.[7]

As indicated in Chapter 1, sports medicine is in great need of adequate mechanisms for gathering injury statistics, not only to pinpoint where preventive measures are necessary, but also to detect design flaws in protective equipment. An example of the latter can be found in two of the studies cited[4,8] in which a design flaw in hockey pants was found related to contusion injuries of the thigh. Until reliable injury reporting mechanisms for all contact sports are established, it will not be possible to determine the need for, and the design of, protective equipment for the mouth in relation to a specific contact sport.

Cause, Mechanism, and Cost of Injuries to the Teeth

Although a number of studies have been concerned with the type of activity engaged in by the player when injuries occur, most reports do not relate the activity to the specific injury. Even in the case of ice hockey and lacrosse, where the injury rate to the mouth and teeth is very high,[5,6] the cause of injury has not been analyzed in detail. Reeves and Mendryk indicated that 59% of all dental injuries were caused by the hockey stick but did not report the cause of injury for the remaining 41%.

Marchant et al commented that internal mouth guards might prevent both concussion and injuries to the teeth, but would not protect against lacerations about the mouth as effectively as an externally worn mouth guard.

Of far more serious consequences than a dental injury is concussion that can result from a blow to the jaw. The force is transmitted along the lower jaw to the base of the skull, and if severe enough, the injured player will be knocked unconscious. This is precisely what happens to a boxer who receives a blow to the lower jaw. Although the need for an internal mouth guard to protect the jaws and teeth from injury has been known to boxers for many years, the relationship between concussion, and failure to wear an internal mouth guard has now been clearly established.[9] Prior to this laboratory study that demonstrated an increase in cranial pressure following a blow to the chin, another study had reported a reduction in concussion and neck injuries in Notre Dame football players when custom-made internal mouth guards were worn.[10]

Table 13-2
Type of Dental Injury and Approximate Cost of Treatment

Type of injury and treatment	Cost range
Corner fracture of tooth	$30 to $100
Complete endodontic (root canal) treatment	$150 to $300
Full crown (capped tooth)	$200 to $400

Cost of Treatment

Although it was reported that the cost of injury to the teeth is drastically reduced when mouth guards are worn, interpretation of the data is cautioned "until a more exacting analysis is made of the cause of such [dental] injuries."[5] In terms of present day dental fees, the cost of care for the treatment of injured teeth is approximately as shown in Table 13-2.

TREATMENT OF INJURIES

Dental

Treatment of dental injuries can be divided into four phases: first aid, short-term, interim, and long-term.

First aid for dental injuries As pointed out previously, dental injuries rarely occur if the player is wearing a face guard as in lacrosse, football, or ice hockey, and even less frequently when the player is wearing both a face guard and a mouth guard.

If a tooth is partially fractured (angle or corner of tooth, Figure 13-2), the best advice for the injured player is to keep his mouth closed. Most players do this anyway because the exposed dentine of a fractured tooth is usually very sensitive to air temperatures, and particularly to the cold temperature at hockey rinks. If the tooth is not dislodged from its normal position and if there is no bleeding

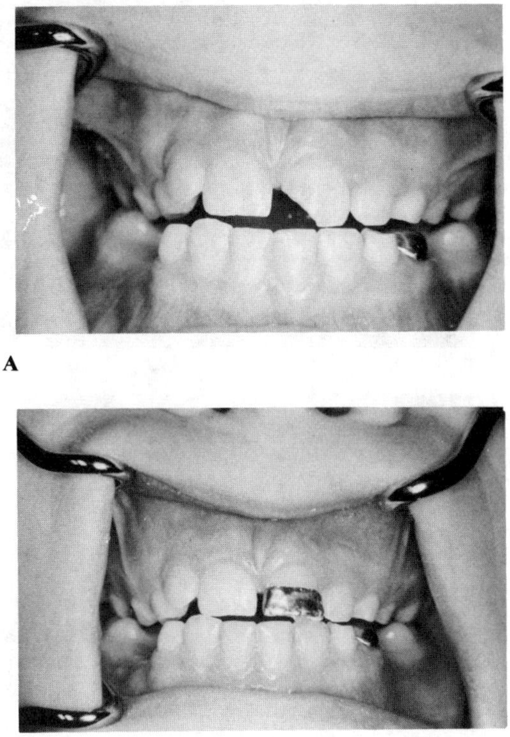

A

B

Figure 13-2 Corner fracture of incisor tooth. **A** Enamel and dentine were fractured but the pulp was not exposed. **B** An orthodontic band was placed on the tooth to protect the pulp for a period of six weeks.

from intraoral or extraoral lacerations, the player may continue playing. Short-term dental treatment can take place at a dental office within 48 hours.

Partially dislodged teeth, Figure 13-3, must be moved back into good alignment as quickly as possible. Teeth that are completely dislodged and appear to have no root fracture should be washed with tap water to remove all dirt and then forced back into their sockets as quickly as possible. One need not be concerned about cleaning off a dislodged tooth in the case of ice hockey injuries because there is very little dirt or debris on artificial ice. If a tooth is dislodged, the player should stop playing, have the tooth repositioned, and be taken to a dentist to have it more securely held in position (splinted) with a wire ligature, orthodontic appliance, or one of the new bond-on plastic materials (Figure 13-4).

It is very important not to carry a dislodged tooth to the dentist. Those who feel squeamish about repositioning a dislodged tooth should know that if it is left out of the mouth dry for longer than

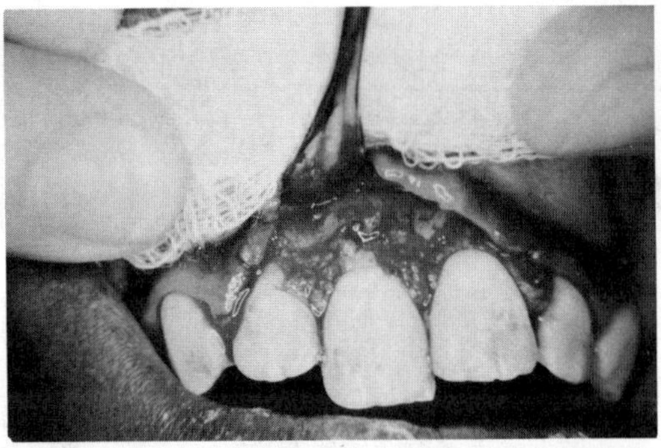

Figure 13-3 Partially dislodged tooth and laceration of gum. First aid is to move the tooth back into its socket and take the player to a dentist to have it stabilized into its normal position, usually by wiring it to adjacent teeth. Player should not continue playing.

30 minutes, its chances of being retained once it is repositioned are very slim.[11] If the person administering first aid finds it difficult to reposition the dislodged tooth correctly, the injured player should hold it in his mouth under the tongue, thus keeping it moist until it is splinted by the dentist.

Equipment for emergency treatment of dental injuries In the vast majority of cases, adequate (but by no means ideal) emergency dental treatment is available at emergency rooms of municipal hospitals where local dentists are on call. In large communities which have dental interns on call after hours and on weekends, emergency care generally will be more efficiently provided, an important factor when time is critical; for example, when one or several teeth have been dislodged.

Some athletic programs, particularly at the advanced college and amateur level, may enjoy the luxury of having a dentist who travels with the team. In the case of amateur hockey teams that play two games in different towns on a weekend, a team dentist can be a valuable asset if adequate emergency equipment and supplies are carried. The University of Michigan School of Dentistry recommends the following for complete emergency care for dento-facial injuries (see Table 13-3).

Short-term treatment of dental injuries Once first aid has been attended to and the injured player is taken to a dentist, the most important part of the immediate short-term care is an x-ray of the injured tooth and adjacent teeth because they may also be injured (see Figure 13-1B). The x-ray will rule out fractured roots and provide an initial record, to which follow-up pictures taken at one-, three-, and six-month intervals, can be compared to determine the status of the dental pulp. Injured pulp may

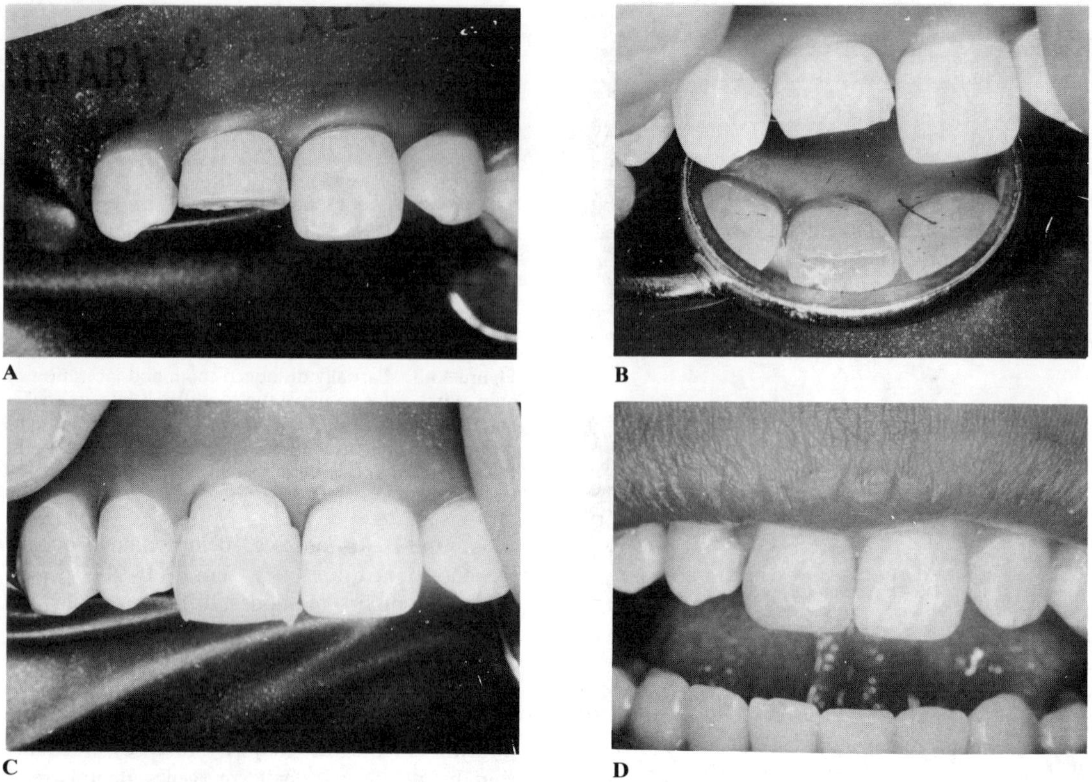

Figure 13-4 Interim repair of fractured tooth. **A** Appearance of tooth before repair. **B** The tooth is tapered to create a narrower neck to which the plastic will adhere. **C** A transparent tooth form holds the soft plastic in place while it sets. **D** The hardened plastic is shaped to reproduce the shape of the tooth before the fracture.

recover completely or it may die and subsequently abscess. Even worse, it may become chronically inflamed and slowly begin to resorb the root. It is impossible to predict the eventual outcome of the status of pulp for at least five years after injury. Thus, good follow-up x-ray records to determine the need for additional treatment, and also to settle insurance claims, are necessary.

After the x-ray is taken, the pulp can be treated with a mild dressing (calcium hydroxide and water paste) in the case of a simple fracture. Or it may be completely removed and necessitate root canal treatment if it is grossly exposed from the injury. To protect the dressing, an orthodontic band is usually cemented in place (see Figure 13-2B). The use of the orthodontic band may be dispensed with in the case of minor fractures, and interim esthetic treatment started. Most authorities agree that injuries that are more severe but do not require immediate root canal treatment should have the interim esthetic treatment postponed for almost a month. The additional trauma to pulp from grinding the tooth to fit the esthetic repair may result in pulp death before it has a chance to recover.

Interim treatment of dental injuries is to improve the injured player's appearance until the outcome of injury to the pulp can be established. Treatment of the fractured tooth involves trimming and shaping the enamel, briefly etching the enamel with a strong acid, and using a bonding agent to attach the white plastic to the tooth (see Figure 13-4). Such repairs bond remarkably well and can remain attached for periods up to five years. They will stain if the person is a heavy smoker or drinks a lot of tea or coffee. Subsequent repairs when necessary, are fairly easily done.

Long-term treatment of dental injuries may not be necessary, but if interim care proves unsatisfactory, the fractured tooth may have to be capped. If root canal treatment was also necessary, the hollowed-out tooth must first be fitted with a metal post cemented into the root canal, which of

Table 13-3
Dento-facial Injury Emergency Kit

Pen Light
2% Lidocaine hydrochloride with epinephrine, 1:100,000 cartridges
Aspirating carpule syringe
Disposable needles, 30 gauge and 27 gauge
Surgical gloves
#4 Mouth mirror
Cotton pliers
Surgical scissors
#4 Hemostat
4-0 Silk sutures with surgical needle
Lidocaine ointment (5%)
Disposable scalpel, #15 or #11
Hydrogen peroxide (shatterproof bottle)
99% Ethyl alcohol (shatterproof bottle)
Tongue depressors (6 inch and 4 inch)
Cotton tipped applicators
Cotton pellets
2 x 2 Sponges
4 x 4 Sponges

#3 Cowhorn explorer
Spoon excavator, #18 or #19
Root canal files
Calcium hydroxide preparation (Life or Dycal)
Formocresol, diluted to 1/5 concentration
Cavit temporary seal and filling

Caulk ZOE
Caulk Fynal
Disposable mixing pads
#24 Cement spatula
Tarno #2 plastic instrument
Tarno #1 plastic instrument
Wesco #25 tapered plugger
Dura Lay kit
Dappen dish
Aluminum crown forms (posterior)
Anterior temporary crown forms

#150 diagonal wire cutters
#110 plier
#347 band removing plier

Hanau torch
Stock mouthguards
Boilable mouthguards
Wet and dry sand paper
Crown and collar scissors, curved
White wax ropes
Irrigating solution
½ tsp salt
¼ tsp baking soda
10 oz. H_2O

While the list may seem extensive, most items are quite small and are easily contained in a small sized attache case.

course complicates the treatment and obviously compounds the cost.

First aid for cuts about the mouth Not all cuts have to be referred to hospital emergency rooms for stitching. Although facial cuts tend to bleed profusely and can be somewhat frightening, first aid can be of great value. Most first aid kits contain individually wrapped 4 × 4 or 3 × 3 gauze sponges. Placing several sponges over the wound with gentle pressure easily controls most bleeding. After bleeding is controlled by pressure (30 to 60 seconds), the gauze is removed to observe the extent and nature of the injury. If, when the facial tissues are at rest the sides of the wound tend to come into close proximity naturally, there is little need for stitching. Experience shows that most such injuries tend to heal with less scarring without stitching since the stitches themselves usually leave small scars. Cuts that remain open when the tissues are at rest, require stitching as soon as possible.

Treatment of the Fractured Jaw

In the case of a fractured jaw, it is usually quite obvious to the person administering first aid that the injury is serious. Rarely is there a fractured jaw without concussion, and in most cases the blow renders the player unconscious. As such, the basic rules of first aid would apply as they relate to the unconscious state. From the standpoint of the fractured jaw the most obvious aspect will be that the teeth are out of alignment and that the injured player is well aware that a part of his mouth is not in its correct position. If there are any teeth that have been dislodged into the mouth, they should be removed and wrapped in a wet 4 × 4 gauze sponge and taken with the player to a hospital emergency room where the jaw can be set. This usually involves wiring the teeth in the closed-mouth position. The only first aid for a fractured jaw is to make sure that the player is comfortable and that a good airway is maintained until arrival at the hospital.

PROTECTIVE EQUIPMENT

There is no question that dental and other oral injuries can be almost completely eliminated using presently available protective equipment (see Table 13-1). However, injuries continue to occur because of:

1. Lack of mandatory protective rules.
2. Failure of officials to enforce mandatory rules.
3. Failure of players to wear protective equipment in practice.

Protective Rules

Although the sport of boxing has long used the internal mouth guard and the face and head protector to reduce the severity of injuries, football was the first team sport to adopt protective equipment for the face in the early 1950s. By 1965, internal mouth guards began to be used more frequently, but it was not until 1974 that the National Collegiate Athletic Association (NCAA) adopted a rule mandating internal mouth guards for football.

Although several reports[5,6,12] indicate a high frequency of dental and face injuries in hockey, it was not until 1977–1978 that mandatory mouth guard and face guard rules were introduced into amateur hockey in the United States and Canada. Regretfully, the rules are not uniformly applied and often are not enforced.

In Canada, all players under 17 years of age who play in the minor hockey division of the Canada Amateur Hockey Association, must wear face guards but do not have to wear internal mouth guards. The Amateur Hockey Association of the United States (AHAUS) requires all players 13 to 19 years of age to wear face guards and internal mouth guards, except in the case of the junior classification (17 to 19 years) when there is a paid gate. The NCAA requires all hockey players to wear internal mouth guards but the rule is not always enforced by the referees.

Table 13-4 illustrates the remarkable effect of a mandatory face guard rule in reducing the prevalence of above the shoulder and dental injuries in ice hockey. Face guards appeared on the market during the 1975–76 season when the percent of above the shoulder injuries reported by the claims department of the AHAUS insurance carrier was 45%. After the mandatory face guard rule in 1978, the above the shoulder injury rate dropped to 25% by 1981 and rose slightly to 28% by 1983. Dental injuries were reduced by 50% but still comprised 7% of all injuries even though a mandatory mouthguard rule was adopted in 1976.

Types of Equipment

The internal mouth guard A great deal of study has been done on the design, fit, and player acceptance of the internal mouth guard. Internal mouth guards may consist of a loose-fitting horseshoe-shaped piece of plastic (stock type), they may be custom-made on a plaster model of the player's mouth, or mouth-formed by using a heat-labile material. Table 13-5 summarizes the findings from a study of 238 Chicago, Illinois high school football players who evaluated all three types.

It is obvious that players much prefer the custom-made mouth guard (Figure 13-5), over the mouth-formed and the stock type. But the cost of the stock type* and the mouth formed† protector varies between \$2 and \$3, while the custom made type will vary between \$20 and \$40. When team budgets are tight, the choice may be between \$60 to outfit a whole football team with stock type mouthguards compared to \$1200 for the same team using custom made mouthguards. For this reason and also because of the inconvenience of obtaining dental models for up to 30 players, custom made mouthguards have fallen out of favor since 1970. However, in 1983, a new organization, the Academy of Sports Dentistry, was formed and one of its major goals is to encourage more widespread use of the custom made mouthguard with its obvious advantages. The intermittent play action of football may not absolutely require a custom-made mouth guard except for the signal-calling quarterback. The same does not hold for ice hockey or basketball where sustained high speed action requires a constant high volume exchange of air by the player. Hayes[17] has shown that there is a significant *reduction* in air exchange in players using a stock type mouth protector compared to the

---

*Right Gard LWS 301.

†Right Gard BSG, Right Gard Corp., Montgomeryville, PA.

Table 13-4
Percent Reduction in Above the Shoulder and Dental Injury Rates* in Ice Hockey Resulting from the Introduction of a Mandatory Face Guard Rule

	1975–76	1976–77	1977–78	1978–79	1979–80	1980–81	1981–82	1982–83
Below the shoulder:								
Pelvis	—	.5	—	.5	—	—	—	—
Thigh	.5	—	2.0	1.0	.5	.5	2.0	—
Leg	8.0	5.0	5.0	4.0	3.0	3.0	3.0	4.0
Knee	7.0	16.0	10.0	14.0	16.0	12.0	10.0	10.0
Shoulder and collarbone	7.0	11.0	12.0	16.0	12.0	12.0	11.0	15.0
Forearm and upper arm	6.0	3.0	5.0	3.0	3.0	4.0	5.0	3.5
Hand and wrist	3.0	7.0	9.0	5.0	9.0	11.0	9.0	5.0
Ankle and foot	5.0	5.0	8.0	8.0	9.0	6.0	5.0	7.0
Chest	1.0	1.0	1.0	—	1.0	—	2.0	1.0
Torn ligament	—	.5	—	1.0	—	3.0	1.0	—
Back	3.0	4.0	3.0	4.0	4.0	3.0	5.0	5.0
Finger and thumb	3.0	2.0	5.0	4.0	5.0	6.0	6.0	5.0
Rib	1.0	3.0	2.0	3.0	2.0	4.0	1.0	3.0
Elbow	3.0	3.0	4.0	.5	3.0	3.0	3.0	5.0
Hip	2.0	1.0	2.0	.5	.5	.5	2.0	2.0
Bruises	1.0	—	—	—	.5	3.0	2.0	1.0
Sprains and strains	4.0	—	—	1.0	1.0	3.0	3.0	5.0
Spleen	.5	2.0	1.0	.5	1.0	1.0	—	—
	55.0%	64.0%	69.0%	66.0%	70.5%	75.0%	70.0%	71.5%
Above the shoulder:								
Head and concussions	—	.5	2.0	5.0	7.5	2.0	2.0	3.0
Skull	2.0	4.0	2.0	1.0	3.0	.5	4.0	2.0
Nose	5.0	1.0	2.0	4.0	.5	1.0	1.0	.5
Lacerations	20.0	14.0	9.0	8.0	7.0	9.0	9.0	12.0
Eye	3.0	2.0	—	3.0	1.0	1.0	2.0	—
Jaw	1.0	1.0	1.0	1.0	—	1.0	2.0	1.0
Neck	1.0	.5	3.0	1.0	2.0	3.0	3.0	3.0
Dental	13.0	13.0	12.0	11.0	8.0	7.5	7.0	7.0
	45.0%	36.0%	31.0%	34.0%	29.5%	25.0%	30.0%	28.5%
Number of claims:	354	367	257	280	265	280	322	308
Number of teams:	3963	4405	4521	4323	3627	4262	4416	4390

*For Claims Department, Sturhahn, Dickenson and Bernard, Inc., Princeton, NJ.
Changes in ice hockey injury rates from the introduction of a mandatory face guard rule by the Amateur Hockey Association of the United States in 1978. Between 1975–76 and 1982–83, dental injuries were reduced by 54% but still continued at a rate of 7% despite a mandatory mouthguard rule in 1975–76 for all divisions up to and including Junior B.

Table 13-5
Player Evaluation of Mouth Protectors

	Custom-made	Mouth-formed	Stock type
Comfortable	85%	46%	30%
Stayed in place	90%	40%	19%
Irritation of gums	25%	50%	78%
Interfered with speech	28%	68%	77%
Interfered with breathing	21%	44%	51%
Choice of protector	87%	11%	2%

From: Bureau of Dental Health Education and Bureau of Economic Research and Statistics. Evaluation of mouth protectors used by high school football players. *J Am Dent Assoc.* 68:430, 1964.

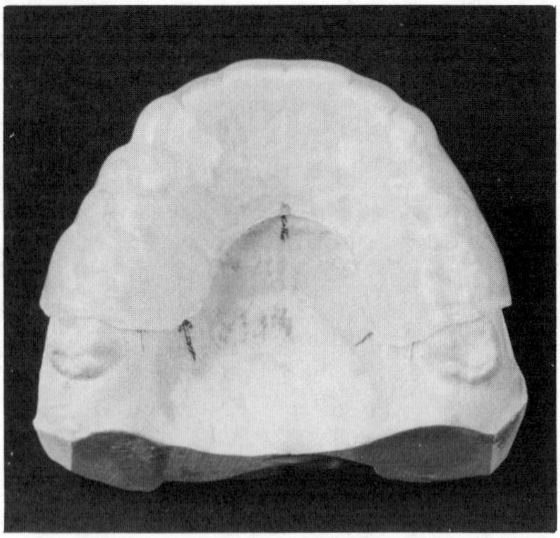

Figure 13-5 The custom-made mouth protector. A piece of clear vinyl plastic is heated and vacuum-formed to a plaster model made from a dental impression of the upper jaw.

custom made one. The reason is probably because the stock type often will not stay in place unless the mouth is closed. Figure 13-6 illustrates three inexpensive mouth-formed protectors, two of which were discarded by the players because of loose fit, and one that has been worn steadily at least once a week during hockey season for over five years. The difference lies in the care and accuracy of fitting. The successful one comes in a kit that contains a hard plastic holding tray used to compress the heated clear plastic material against the teeth and gums while it sets (Figure 13-7). The technique can be handled by a player or a trainer, and if carefully followed will result in a mouth guard that stays in place even with the mouth wide open; the assistance of a dentist is preferred, however.

The face guard While most face guards used in football and lacrosse provide excellent protection against facial injuries, those used in ice hockey are still in the early stages of development. A popular early type was the clear polycarbonate half-face protector that provided excellent protection for the eyes but not for the rest of the face or mouth, where an extraoral mouth guard had to be worn. The reason for the half-face design was to assure good visibility downward toward the ice but also because a full-face design had a tendency to fog. While eye injuries were virtually eliminated except in those rare cases when a stick penetrated beneath the mask (Figure 13-8A), injuries to the mouth and the lower part of the face continued to occur. (Figure 13-8B,C,D).

The wire face guard has been found to give better protection to the entire face than the half-face (clear plastic one), and fogging is not a problem. However, some designs have spaces between

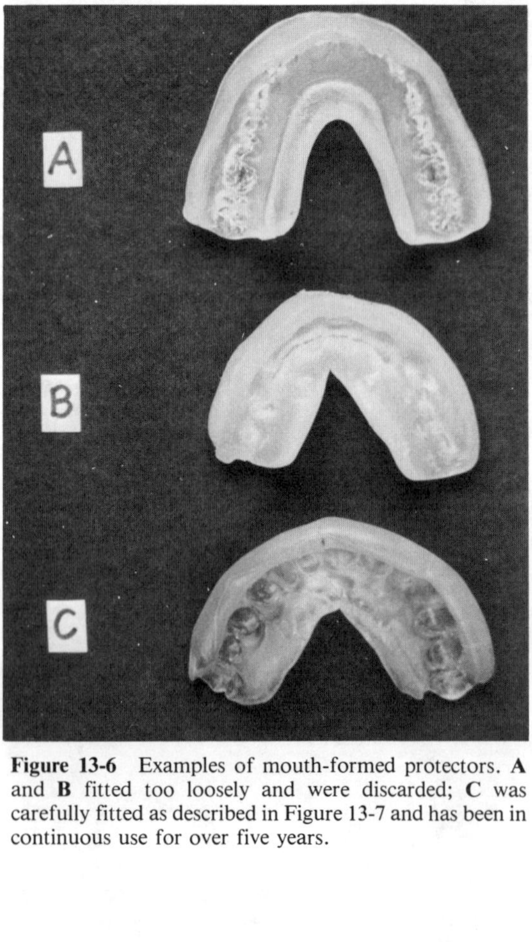

Figure 13-6 Examples of mouth-formed protectors. **A** and **B** fitted too loosely and were discarded; **C** was carefully fitted as described in Figure 13-7 and has been in continuous use for over five years.

the wire mesh that permit stick penetration through openings in front of the eyes and at the periphery (Figure 13-9). On the other hand, some models are so well designed that it is almost impossible for a hockey stick to penetrate (Figure 13-10). (See Chapter 12, Eye Injuries.)

Standardization of Protective Equipment

Because of the wide differences in designs of hockey face masks, the Canadian Standards Association (CSA) and the American Society for Testing and Materials (ASTM) have recently written performance standards for hockey face protectors that ultimately all manufacturers will have to meet if the equipment is to be offered for sale to the public. In 1978 the Hockey Equipment Certification Council (HECC) was established under AHAUS for the specific purpose of evaluating performance standards with the ultimate aim of including reference to standards in the playing rules of amateur hockey in the United States. Such a responsible action on the part of an amateur athletic organization is long overdue and will undoubtedly be considered a milestone in the annals of modern sportsmedicine.

In summary, dental injuries are unique in that healing does not follow the usual repair characteristics of other parts of the body. Therefore, the final outcome of an injured tooth even if treatment has been correctly administered, may not be known for up to five years following injury. Since extensive reports from football and hockey sources have conclusively shown that properly designed facial and oral protective equipment can almost completely eliminate dental injuries, it seems logical

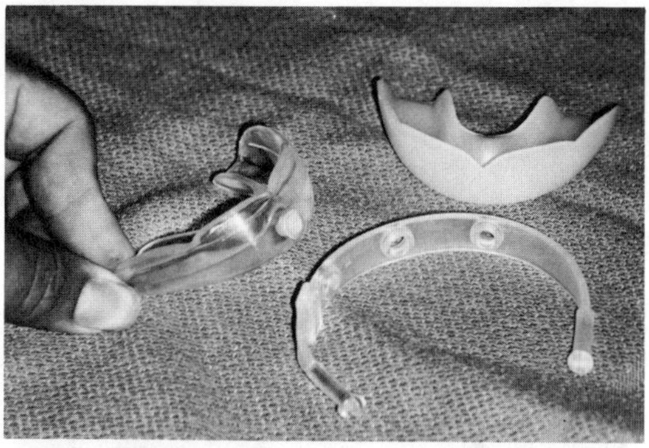

A

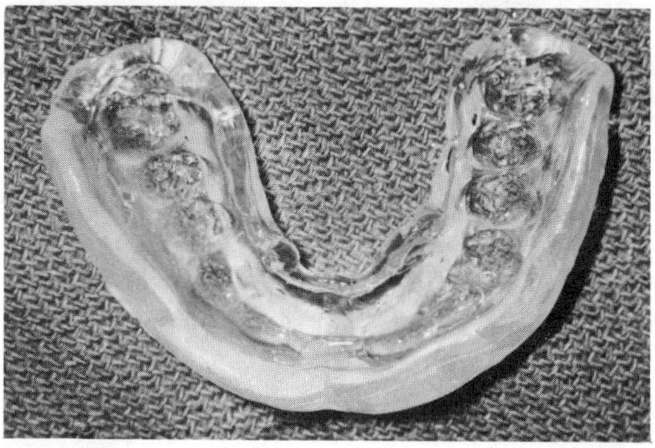

B

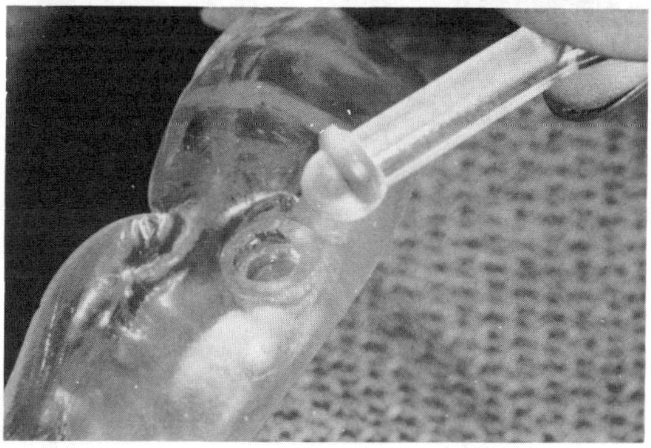

C

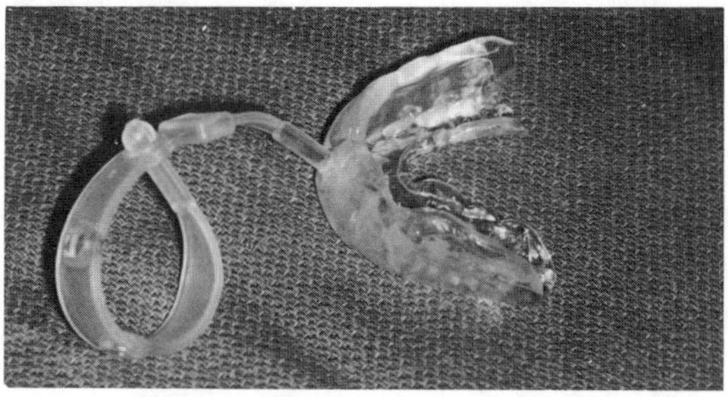

D

Figure 13-7 Technique for the Right Gard BSG 301 mouth-formed protector. **A** Technique involves three parts: a clear plastic stock mouth protector with anterior "button," a fail-safe connecting strap, and a white, hard plastic form for carrying the heated clear plastic to the mouth and compressing it against the teeth. **B** The clear plastic protector just after being removed from the mouth where it was mouth formed while in a heat-softened state; if the edges are rough, uneven, or too thick, the material may be gently reheated outside the mouth with a cigarette lighter, repositioned in the mouth, and pressed into closer adaptation to the gum or palate by the fingers. **C** The plastic button is removed and replaced by the fail-safe attachment strap for use in football or hockey when a face guard is worn. **D** Finished protector is ready for use.

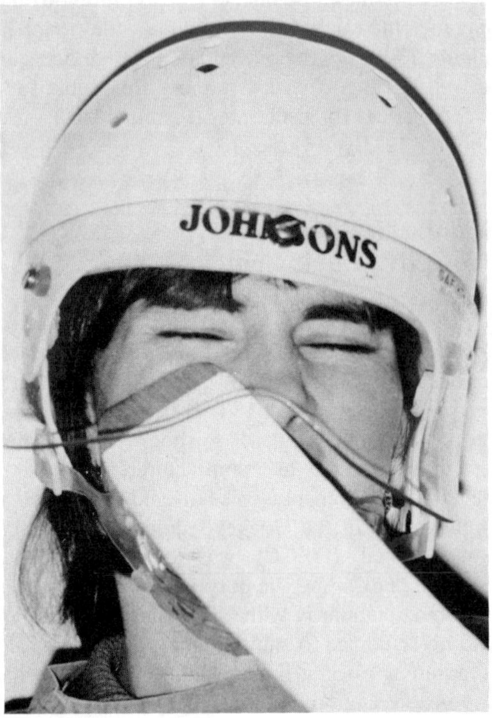

A

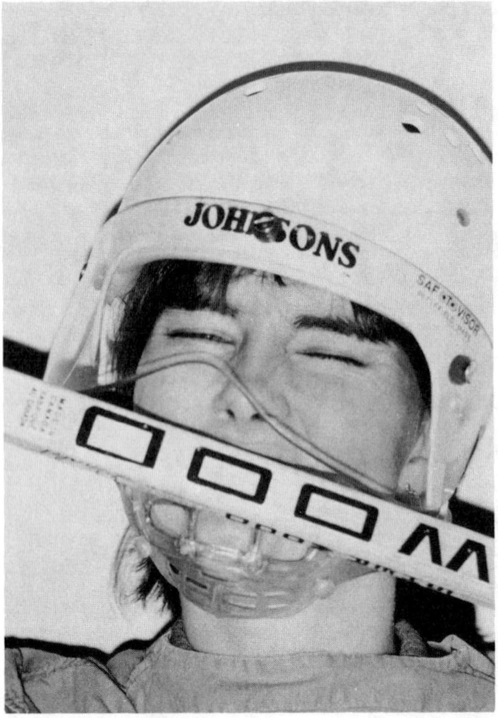

B

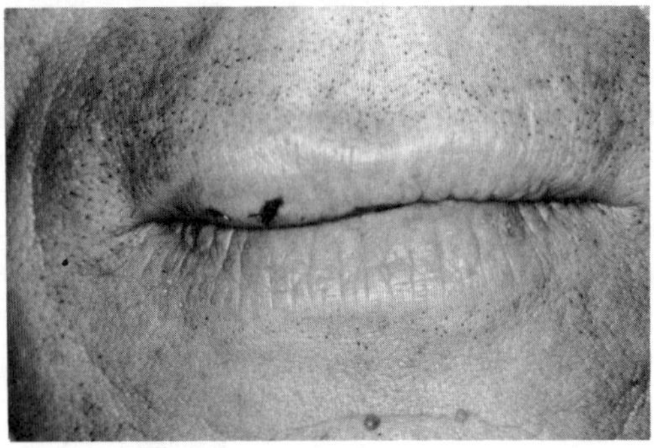

C

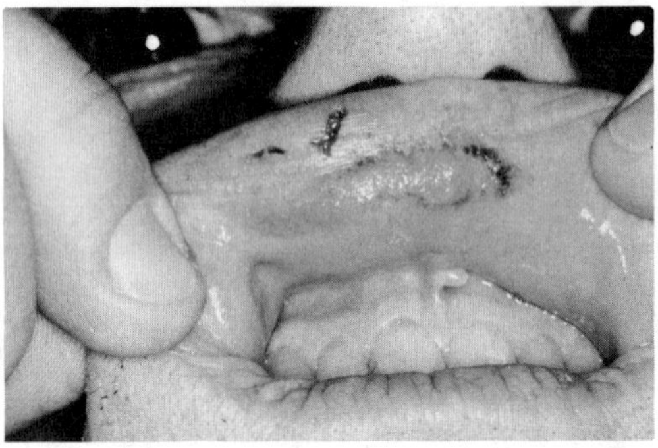

D

Figure 13-8 Clear plastic half-face shield used in ice hockey. **A** The stick blade is able to penetrate beneath the shield. **B** Injuries to the lower part of the face can still occur when a player is cross checked by an opponent's stick. **C** Example of intraoral laceration caused by cross check injury seen in **B. D** Swollen lip one day after injury seen in **B** and **C:** The player was wearing a clear plastic face shield and external mouth protector as seen in **B** and also an internal mouth guard as in Figure 13-7B.

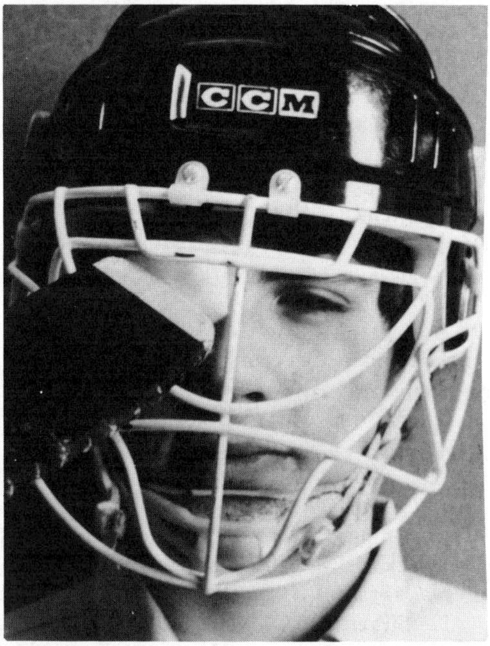

A

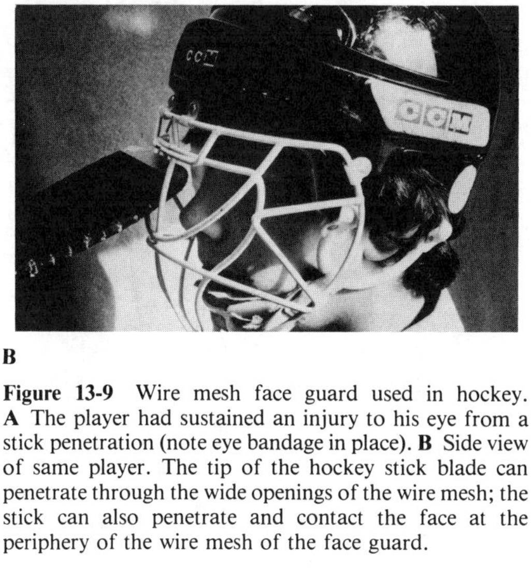

B

Figure 13-9 Wire mesh face guard used in hockey. **A** The player had sustained an injury to his eye from a stick penetration (note eye bandage in place). **B** Side view of same player. The tip of the hockey stick blade can penetrate through the wide openings of the wire mesh; the stick can also penetrate and contact the face at the periphery of the wire mesh of the face guard.

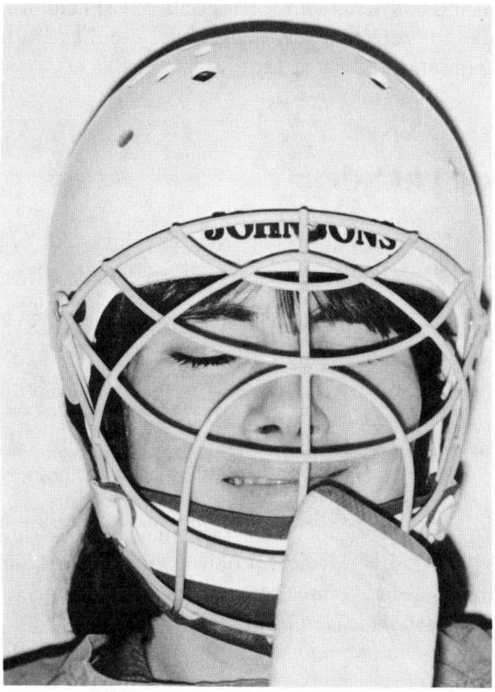

A

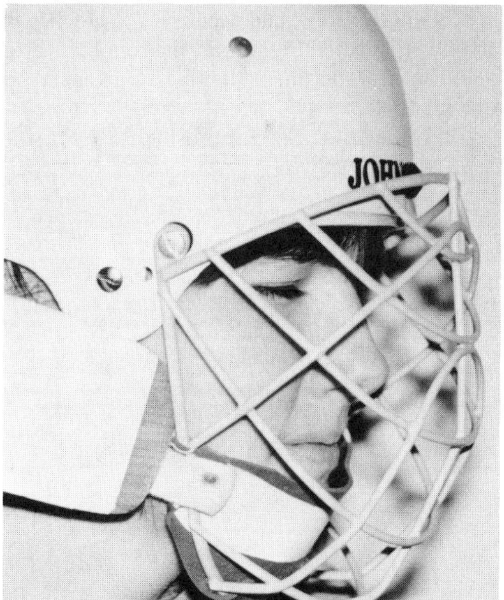

B

Figure 13-10 Wire face guard used in hockey. **A** Mesh does not permit penetration of stick blade. **B** Stick cannot penetrate at periphery of face mask.

that all body contact sports should have mandatory rules to protect players against injury to the mouth, teeth, and associated facial structures.

REFERENCES

1. Blyth, C.S., and Mueller, F.O. An epidemiologic study of high school football injuries in North Carolina – 1968–1972. US Consumer Product Safety Commission, Washington, DC: US Government Printing Office, 1974.

2. Pashby, T.J., Pashby, R.C., Chisholm, L.D.J. et al. Eye injuries in Canadian hockey. *Can Med Assoc J.* 113:663, 1975.

3. Vinger, P.F. Ocular injuries in hockey. *Arch Ophthalmol.* 94:74, 1976.

4. Rovere, G.D., Gristina, A.G., and Nicastro, J.F. Medical problems of a professional hockey team: a three-season experience. *Physician and Sportsmedicine* 6:59, 1978.

5. Marchant, L., Roy, E., and Warshawski, J.R. Sports safety research, 1973–74. Ottawa, Canada: Department of National Health and Welfare, 1974.

6. Reeves, J.G., and Mendryk, S. Hockey injury study, greater Edmonton metropolitan area, 1969–70. Edmonton, Alberta: University of Alberta, 1970.

7. Nadeau, J. Special prosthesis. *J Prosthet Dent.* 20:62, 1968.

8. Park, R.D., and Castaldi, C.R. Injuries in junior ice hockey. *Physician and Sportsmedicine* 8:81, 1980.

9. Hickey, J.C., Morris, A.L., Carlson, L.D. et al. The relation of mouth protectors to cranial pressure and deformation. *J Am Dent Assoc.* 74:735, 1967.

10. Stenger, J.M., Lawson, E.A., Wright, J.M. et al. Mouthguards: protection against shock to head, neck and teeth. *J Am Dent Assoc.* 69:273, 1964.

11. Cvek, M., Granath, L.E., and Hollender, L. Variations of occurrence of ankylosis of reimplanted teeth with duration of extra-alveolar period and storage environment. *Odontol Revy.* 25:43, 1974.

12. Castaldi, C.R. Mouth guards in contact sports. *J Conn State Dent Assoc.* 48:233, 1974.

13. Kramer, L.R. Accidents occurring in high school athletics with special reference to dental injuries. *J Am Dent Assoc.* 28:1351, 1941.

14. Stevens, O.O. Mouthprotectors: evaluation of twelve types–second year. *J Dent Child.* 32:137, 1965.

15. Cohen, A., and Borish, A.L. Mouth protector project for football players in Philadelphia high schools. *J Am Dent Assoc.* 56:863, 1958.

16. Fagan, C.B. Mouth protectors for football players. *J Am Dent Assoc.* 66:354, 1963.

17. Hayes, D. Effects of intraoral mouthguards on ventilation. *Physician Sports Med.* 5:61 Jan. 1977.

CHAPTER 14
Cardiopulmonary System—Physiological and Pathological Evaluation

Arthur J. Siegel, MD

A sequence of physiological alterations known as the training effect occurs in the cardiovascular system in response to regular exercise. The capacity to increase exercise performance can be assessed by measuring the highest oxygen uptake level that an individual can achieve during sustained physical activity of the aerobic type. The improvement in maximal oxygen uptake (VO_2 max) which occurs with endurance training results from central adaptations in cardiovascular performance and from peripheral changes in skeletal muscle. This section will deal with the components of this oxygen transport process during training and its derangement in disease.

RELEVANCE OF MAXIMAL AEROBIC POWER

Maximal oxygen uptake or maximal aerobic capacity (VO_2) for an individual defines the upper limit of oxygen transport from ambient air to working tissues of skeletal muscle. This process is schematically represented in Figure 14-1, which illustrates the conversion of oxygen in air to energy for physical work in the mitochondria of exercising skeletal muscle tissues.[1] During exercise, oxygen is consumed (VO_2) and CO_2 is produced as a by-product of cellular metabolism. The quality is determined by the intensity and duration of exercise and by the efficiency of muscle activity. The interconnecting gears in Figure 14-1 depict the coupling of ventilation (lung faction) to circulation (the cardiovascular system) for the final delivery to working skeletal muscle.

The training effect, or increase in VO_2 max with regular exercise, defines the increase in efficiency of this oxygen delivery system. Figure 14-2 shows the effects of age and training on VO_2 max from data obtained several decades ago and still valid today. There is a steady decline in maximal oxygen uptake with age in both men and women, as a correlate of the progressive decrease with age in the maximal attainable heart rate. Comparing the sedentary to trained performance for any individual, there is an improvement in maximal oxygen uptake, ranging from 10% to 30%, at all ages. Both cardiac and skeletal muscle adaptations contribute to this improved capacity with training as will be delineated in subsequent sections. The magnitude of increase in maximal oxygen uptake from sedentary to trained condition represents an important dimension of athletic performance dependent upon both central and peripheral adaptive responses.

The relevance of aerobic capacity to exercise performance in various sports is summarized in Table 14-1.[3] This capacity is highly relevant for measuring performance in isotonic sports activity based upon a sustained high intensity effort over time. It is less useful as a measurement of skill for isometric activities such as weight lifting and racket sports, or for precision events such as shooting. The levels of VO_2 max reported for international athletes in a world class caliber are shown in Table 14-2 as units of oxygen uptake per unit time.[3] Elite world class cross country skiers and long distance runners at the top of the scale show roughly twice the aerobic capacity of untrained individuals matched for age and sex, with a variety of less intense sports falling in an intermediate zone.

Sequential measurement of VO_2 max in a given athlete during training for a competitive season may be useful in quantifying this training effect as during recovery from injury. It must be stressed that maximal aerobic capacity is only one aspect or dimension of sports performance and is not by itself a reliable indicator of competitive advantage. VO_2 max takes the "oxygen pulse" of the athlete as defined by Wasserman and Whipp,[4] representing the amount of oxygen extraction by the individual with each heart beat during exercise as a barometer of total fitness (Figure 14-3). The oxygen pulse measures the quantity of oxygen extracted from the

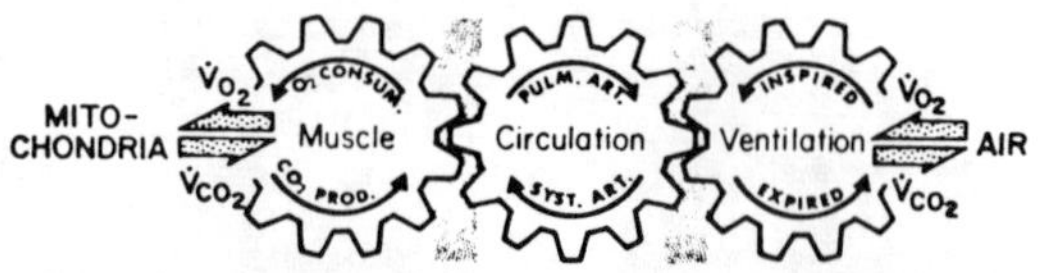

Figure 14-1 Schematic representation of the essential elements in gas exchange between the cell mitochondria and external environment. During exercise, the quantity of O_2 consumed ($\dot{V}O_2$) and CO_2 produced ($\dot{V}CO_2$) is determined by the amount of muscle activity. The interconnecting gears connote the coupling of the physiologic responses of blood flow and ventilation to metabolism. From Wasserman, K. Breathing during exercise. *N Engl J Med* 298:780, 1978 with permission.

circulation per heart beat at a given level of training. Training results in an improved capacity for consuming oxygen, which in turn enhances sports performance.

MEASUREMENT OF MAXIMAL OXYGEN UPTAKE

Precise measurement of maximal oxygen uptake involves quantification of actual gas exchange, or oxygen consumed from inspired air during progressive physical effort. This concept is illustrated in Figure 14-4, by the linear relationship between work expenditure and oxygen consumption.[2] Stroke volume and heart rate combine to increase cardiac output, which bears a linear relation to heart rate in the normal cardiovascular system. The arteriovenous oxygen difference also increases, as more oxygen is delivered to exercising muscle reflecting the increased capacity of muscle to consume O_2 in

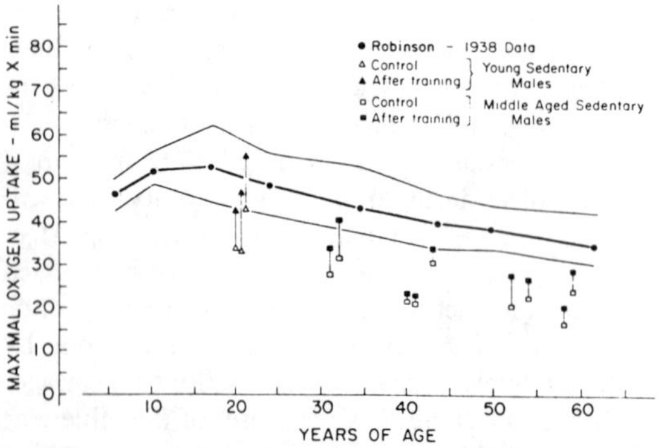

Figure 14-2 Effect of age and training on the maximal oxygen uptake in males. From Mitchell, J., and Blomquist, G. Maximal oxygen uptake. *N Engl J Med* 284:1018, 1971.

Table 14-1
Relevance of Aerobic Capacity to Exercise Performance in Various Sports

Highly relevant	Relevant	Of little relevance
Track (400 m to marathon)	Alpine skiing	Jumping and throwing
Orienteering	Judo	Diving
Swimming (100 m and upwards)	Most team sports	Weightlifting
Cross country skiing	Figure skating	Shooting
Rowing	Gymnastics	Archery
Canoeing (flat water)	Canoeing (white water)	Sailing
Cycling	Racquet Sports	Bobsledding
Speed skating		Curling
Boxing –		
Wrestling		

From Thoden, J.S., Wilson, B.A., and Macdougall, J.D. Testing aerobic power. Edited by J.D. Macdougall, H.A. Wenger, and H.J. Green. In *Physiological Testing of the Elite Athlete.* Ithaca, NY, 1982, Mouvement Publications, Inc., with permission.

Table 14-2
Levels of VO_2 max Reported for International Athletes in a World Class Caliber

	Range	
Sport	Males	Females
Nordic skiing	65–95	56–74
Middle distance running	70–86	
Distance running	65–80	55–72
Rowing	58–74	48–68
Cycling	56–72	
Swimming	54–70	48–68
Soccer	50–70	
Figure skating		42–54
Wrestling	50–70	
Gymnastics	48–74	38–48
Hockey	45–65	
Field hockey	39–49	
Basketball	45–65	42–54
Football	40–60	
Baseball	40–60	
Untrained	38–52	30–46

Adapted from the National Coaching Certification Program, Level III.
From Thoden, J.S., Wilson, B.A., Macdougall, J.D. Testing aerobic power. Edited by J.D. Macdougall, H.A. Wenger, and H.J. Green. In *Physiological Testing of the Elite Athlete.* Ithaca, NY, 1982, Mouvement Publications, Inc., 1982, with permission.

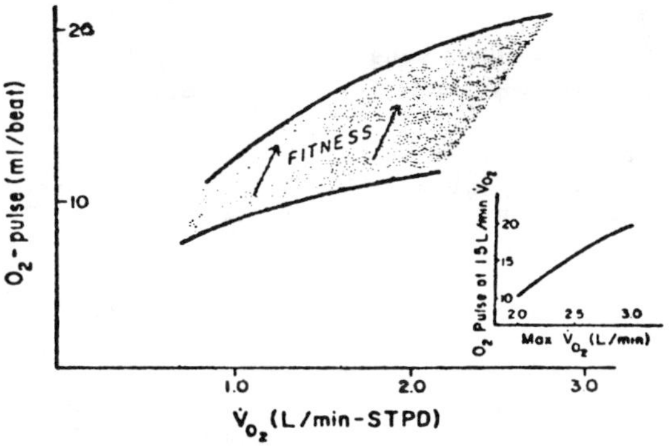

Figure 14-3 From Wasserman, K., and Whipp B., Exercise physiology in health and disease. *Am Rev Resp Dis* 112:227, 1975 with permission.

this process. With progressively increasing exercise loads there is a continued close relationship in the normal individual between heart rate and oxygen uptake. As illustrated in Figure 14-1, maintenance of arterial oxygen tension during heavy exercise depends upon a normal pulmonary system, which is not a rate limiting factor in oxygen transport in normal subjects.[1]

As work intensity increases, there is a slow rise in blood lactate as shown on the right side of Figure 14-4, which defines the ceiling or maximal workload. Continued exercise results in systemic acidosis, fatigue and cessation of exercise.

In sports activity of the aerobic type, the ability to sustain exercise at a high percentage of maximal oxygen uptake is the second major index

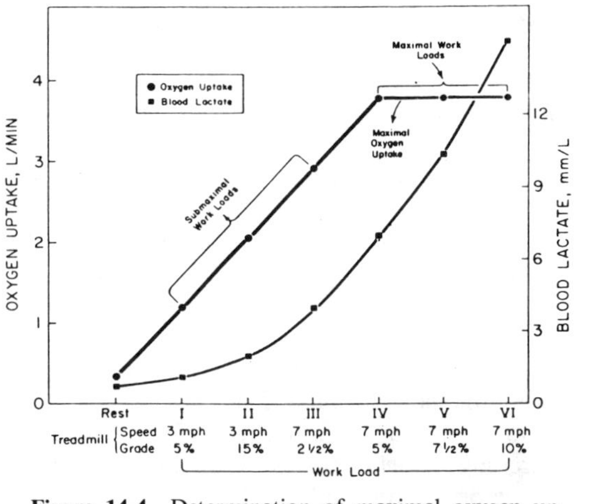

Figure 14-4 Determination of maximal oxygen uptake on a treadmill. From Mitchell, J., Blomquist, G. Maximal oxygen uptake. *N Engl J Med* 284:1018, 1971.

of competitive potential. This is measured physiologically as the anaerobic threshold, or the percentage of maximal oxygen uptake which can be sustained over time.[1,4] When exercise intensity exceeds this zone, oxygen supply can no longer meet the metabolic requirements of muscle, lactic acid builds up in the exercising tissue and leads to an increase in blood lactate. The anaerobic threshold also shifts as part of a training effect. Intensity of training rather than total time in endurance activity leads to enhancement of the anaerobic threshold.[1]

Measurement of anaerobic threshold may be especially relevant to athletes such as marathon runners and cross country skiers, where muscle glycogen depletion is the limiting factor in performance. The anaerobic threshold is the total body barometer for the energy metabolism of the exercising muscle, just as VO_2 max is the barometer for the cardiac output. Combined assessment of VO_2 max and anaerobic threshold represent corollary aspects of central and peripheral adaptations during exercise training. The maximal oxygen uptake reflects the greatest amount of oxygen that the athlete can process during peak physical work while the anaerobic threshold represents the percentage of this peak effort which the muscle can handle without showing the metabolic signs of fatigue.

Measurement of maximal oxygen uptake can be performed in the laboratory with precise assays of gas exchange during motor driven treadmill or bicycle ergomotor exercise. In the normal individual, there is a direct relationship between pulse rate and cardiac output which allows extrapolation of gas exchange from measurement of heart rate at submaximal and maximal work loads. Valid methods for estimating maximal oxygen uptake have been adapted from initial data in military personnel to the general public, according to the 12-minute test as popularized by Kenneth Cooper.[5] This simple method allows an individual to test his or her specific baseline capacity with a step wise program for exercise designed to improve endurance.

The point system of Dr. Cooper and guidelines from the American College of Sports Medicine stress the inter-relationship between frequency, intensity and duration of exercise in promoting an increase in aerobic capacity. Minimal requirements are for 20 to 30 minutes of sustained repetitive isotonic exercise 3 to 4 times per week at mild to moderate intensity. Increments in time, frequency and intensity result in augmentation of the training response but create risks for musculo-skeletal injuries. With a progressive training effect, a given level of work produces a lower heart rate, thus allowing the individual to increase work output at a given heart rate. This results in more performance per unit at the same level of perceived exertion, which is simply a restatement in training terminology of the increase in oxygen pulse as defined by the physiologist.[4]

CARDIOVASCULAR ADAPTATIONS TO ENDURANCE TRAINING

The cardiac adaptations to endurance training include central and peripheral factors as previously outlined. The training effect involves augmentation of cardiac output during exercise with improvements up to 25% as measured in estimates of VO_2 max.[2] This increase in cardiac output occurs because of an increase in stroke volume at submaximal workloads and with a lowering of heart rate for given submaximal levels of exertion. The augmented performance involves an increase in intrinsic myocardial contractility and may, over time, lead to actual hypertrophy of heart muscle as defined with electrocardiographic techniques.[6]

While strength training sports such as isometric exercise lead to a predominant increase in wall thickness, isotonic or endurance sports lead to relative cardiac dilatation with an increase in chamber size and a lesser degree in wall thickness.[6] Such characteristics define aspects of the "athletic heart syndrome" in which the dimensions of the heart may resemble findings in various pathologic states but are associated in the athlete with a super-normal exercise capacity. Table 14-3 indicates the peripheral or skeletal muscle contribution to an increase in maximal oxygen uptake with training.[7] This consists of an increase in capillary-fiber ratio for delivery of greater blood flow, an increase in oxidative capacity through induction of myoglobin, and a specific increase in oxidative enzymes involved in substrate utilization. Skeletal muscle becomes more efficient in burning or utilizing carbohydrate and free fatty acids such as fuels for oxidation.[8,9] The oxidative enzyme systems are in fact a reliable biochemical index of the increase in exercise capacity defined for the athlete's performance as a whole.

Much investigation and controversy surrounds the issue of the distribution of specific fiber types in exercise performance. Type I or high oxidated fibers are known to predominate in elite endurance athletes such as long distance runners.[10] The fiber

Table 14-3
Cardiovascular Changes During Endurance Training

Central		
1. Increased intrinsic contractility	Increased stroke volume ↘	
2. Myocardial hypertrophy		
3. Cardiac dilatation		Increased maximal oxygen uptake
Peripheral		
1. Increased oxidative capacity in skeletal muscle	Increased oxygen extraction ↗	
2. Decreased vascular resistance in skeletal muscle		

Adapted from Ross, J., and Fogoros, R. The long distance runner. *Medical Challenge* December:29–38, 1978.

type distribution was formerly felt to be a genetic profile which was part of the hereditary endowment of an individual. More recent research in fiber typing indicates a change in patterns with training from type II or anaerobic fibers to the high oxidative fibers.[11] The relationship between exercise training and fiber type specificity will occupy the attention of exercise physiologists over the coming years, perhaps with new concepts of skeletal muscle responses to specific exercise stress.

RESPIRATORY ADAPTATION TO TRAINING

During exercise, minute ventilation, or the volume of gas expired per unit time, and rate of oxygen uptake increase with work capacity. The rates of ventilation and circulation are functionally coupled to metabolic activity of the body as reflected in arterial blood, CO_2 and various lactate levels. Breathing capacity must keep pace with increasing oxygen demand during progressive workloads to permit re-oxygenation of venous blood. Expiration of excess carbon dioxide preserves the hydrogen-ion balance, which is upset if lactate levels build up.

The ventilatory control of breathing occurs at a central nervous system level and keeps arterial carbon dioxide tension and hydrogen-ion concentration constant until lactic acid produced by exercising skeletal muscle exceed the limit of respiratory compensation. The key factor is that ventilation is geared to the metabolic requirements of exercise in a step-wise fashion.

Table 14-4
Comparison of the Physiologic Characteristics of the athlete's Heart with the Pathologic Findings in the Diseased Heart

	Physiologic LVH	Pathologic LVH
Exercise testing	No ischemic response	Ischemic response probable
Indices of cardiac contraction	Normal or supranormal	Depressed
ECG	Voltage for LVH	Voltage plus ST changes, axis shift, etc
Etiology	Physical training	Aortic stenosis, hypertension, cardiomyopathy, etc

Adapted from Ross, J., and Fogoros, R. The long distance runner. *Medical Challenge* December:29–38, 1978.

The respiratory system in normal individuals is not a rate-limiting factor in maximal exercise performance. The ventilatory response to lactate production in exercise is an increase in minute ventilation. The ventilatory response to progressive exercise provides the key to the percent of maximal oxygen uptake which an individual can sustain without succumbing to fatigue. The anaerobic threshold, defined by the respiratory physiologist as the step-up from linearity in minute ventilation during progressive exercise, is the limit of steady state exercise which the athlete can sustain in training.[1,4]

PATHOPHYSIOLOGIC VARIATIONS IN MAXIMAL OXYGEN UPTAKE

Previous sections have discussed central and peripheral adaptations to endurance training in normal individuals. These include cardiac alterations which can be identical to findings in various disease states. The "athletes heart syndrome" is a term used to describe the aberrant characteristics such as cardiomegaly, characteristic of high performance athletes. Table 14-4 summarizes the distinction between physiologic characteristics of the athlete's heart and pathologic findings in disease states.[7] The athlete shows super-normal performance characteristics in contrast to the subnormal or compromised function in cardiac illness. To further confuse the issue, electrocardiographic findings in athletes may show multiple abnormalities such as sinus bradycardia, prolongation of the PR interval, junctional rhythms, and frequent ventricular ectopic beats, all of which may be features of disease in patients with cardial dysfunction.

Assessment of functional cardiac capacity by standard exercise testing is possible for patients with heart disease as with athletes. Bruce has defined parameters allowing for assessment of functional aerobic impairment as defined by exercise capacity specific for age.[12] The functional cardiac impairment is the difference between the functional limit of the patient compared to a healthy aged match person as extrapolated from normative values. Symptom-limited maximal exercise testing becomes a powerful tool in the assessment of patients with cardiovascular disease similar to assessment of recovery parameters in athletes after musculoskeletal injury.

The difficulty in distinguishing between physiologic and pathologic cardiac states is further complicated by the finding of abnormal cardiac enzymes in asymptomatic marathon runners after competition.[13] The MB isoenzyme fraction of creatine kinase is widely regarded as a sensitive and specific marker for myocardial damage. Normal heart scans in marathon runners after competition[13,14] and increased levels of CK-MB in trained skeletal muscle suggest a release from skeletal muscle altered by training during the stress of marathon competition.[15,16] For this reason, elevations of "cardiac" enzymes in endurance athletes should not be assumed to indicate myocardial damage without additional clinical evidence. Radionuclide myocardial perfusion imaging is useful to identify "false positive" isoenzymes in runners seen as patients with over-exertion.

The isoenzyme changes in skeletal muscle of marathon runners may relate to the regenerative response of skeletal muscle tissue to focal injury during strenuous training.[17,18] Recent investigations point to focal myofibrillar injury and repair as the morphologic basis for the "No pain, No gain!" adage used to sustain effort in training by athletes. This would point to the importance of rest and recovery as part of the training cycle, now documented with a scientific basis! Principles of training, clinical medicine and exercise physiology continue to deliver new insights related to athletic performance.

SUMMARY

This discussion of cardiopulmonary adaptations to exercise reviews the central and peripheral adaptations to exercise training. The improvement in maximal oxygen capacity is attributed to augmentation of cardiac function and to specific changes in exercising skeletal muscle that facilitate oxygen uptake and utilization. Performance of the system can be assessed by measuring maximal oxygen uptake as a reflection of central changes in cardiac output, and by the anaerobic threshold, which is a measure of the ability of skeletal muscle to sustain work without fatigue. Endurance training provides an increase in VO_2 max while increases in training intensity raise the anaerobic threshold.

REFERENCES

1. Wasserman, K. Breathing during exercise. *N Engl J Med.* 298:780–785, 1978.

2. Mitchell, J., and Blomquist, G. Maximal oxygen uptake. *N Engl J Med.* 284:1018, 1971.

3. Thoden, J.S., Wilson, B.A. and MacDougall, J.D. Testing aerobic power. Edited by J.D. MacDougall, H.A. Wenger, H.J. Green. In *Physiological Testing of the Elite Athlete.* Ithaca, NY: Mouvement Publications, Inc., 1982.

4. Wasserman, K., and Whipp, B. Exercise physiology in health and disease. *Am Rev Resp Dis* 112:219, 1975.

5. Cooper, K.H. *The Aerobic Way.* New York, NY: MA Evans and Co, Inc, 1977.

6. Morganroth, J., et al. Comparative left ventricular dimensions in trained athletes. *Annals Int Med.* 82:521, 1975.

7. Ross, J., and Fogoros, R. The long distance runner. *Medical Challenge* December:29–38, 1978.

8. Felig, P., and Wahren, J. Fuel homeostasis in exercise. *N Engl J Med.* November 20:1078, 1975.

9. Holloszy, J. Adaptations of muscular tissue to training. *Prog Cardiovascular Disease.* 618, 1976.

10. Costill, D.L., Fink, W.J., and Pollock, M.L. Muscle fiber composition and enzyme activities of elite distance runners. *Med Sci in Sports.* 8:96–100, 1976.

11. Pette, D., and Dolken, G. Some aspects of regulation of enzyme levels in muscle energy-supplying metabolism. Edited by G. Weber. In *Advances in Enzyme Regulation,* vol 13. New York: Pergamon Press, 1975.

12. Bruce, R. Assessment of functional cardiac capacity by standard exercise testing. *Prac Cardiol.* January:77–85, 1977.

13. Siegel, A.J., Silverman, L.M., and Holman, B.L. Elevated creatine kinase MB isoenzyme levels in marathon runners: normal myocardial scintigrams suggest non-cardiac source. *JAMA.* 246:2049–51, 1981.

14. Ohman, E.M., Teo, K.K., Johnson, A.H., et al. Abnormal cardiac enzyme responses after strenuous exercise: alternative diagnostic aids. *Brit Med J.* 285:1523–28, 1982.

15. Siegel, A.J., Silverman, I.M., and Evans, W.J. Elevated skeletal muscle creatine kinase MB isoenzyme levels in marathon runners. *JAMA.* 250:2835–37, 1983.

16. Apple, F.S., Rogers, M.A., Sherman, W.M., et al. Profile of creatine kinase isoenzymes in skeletal muscles of marathon runners. *Clin Chem.* 30:413–416, 1984.

17. Hikida, R.S., Staron, R.S., Hagerman, F.C., et al. Muscle fiber necrosis associated with human marathon runners. *J Neurol Sci* 59: 185–203, 1983.

18. Warhol, M.J., Siegel, A.J., Evans, W.J., et al. Focal muscle fiber injury and repair in marathon runners after competition. *Am J Pathol* 118: 331–339, 1985.

CHAPTER 15

Injuries Involving the Abdomen, Viscera, and Genitourinary System

Ashby C. Moncure, MD
Earle W. Wilkins, Jr, MD

In any sport, particularly those involving contact, the nature and localization of an injury is not always initially apparent. Therefore, immediate assessment for major abdominal trauma is not different from those for head, thoracic, or orthopedic injuries. As with the other injuries, assessment must be orderly, thoughtful, and thorough to identify the most serious potential injuries.

The essential components in the management of the victim of serious trauma are airway, breathing, and circulation, often called the ABCs of resuscitation.[1] In the athlete who has received a forceful blow to the epigastrium (the solar plexus) and who may be breathless or seemingly unconscious, it is mandatory that these components be considered.

1. AIRWAY. Is there an open passage by which inspired air (oxygen) can reach the lungs? Has the victim "swallowed" his tongue? Has he aspirated gum or a mouth guard? Is there any other kind of foreign body obstructing the airway? Has the larynx been fractured from a baseball, a hockey puck, a lacrosse stick?

2. BREATHING. Can the athlete respond by taking in a deep breath? Does the chest wall move, ie, ribs rise and fall, with respiration? Is that movement even, equal bilaterally? If he is unconscious, is he breathing at all? Is there evidence, front or back, of a penetrating chest injury? Is there a flail segment of ribs with paradoxical motion in breathing, ie, retraction of a segment while the rest of the rib cage expands, and vice versa?

3. CIRCULATION. Is there good pink color of face, conjunctival sacs, fingernails? Is he cyanotic? Can one feel peripheral arterial pulses: the radial at the wrist, the carotid in the neck, the femoral in the groin? Can one see, feel, or hear an actual precordial heart beat?

All of these questions should be answered by the well-trained physician, therapist, or other attendant in thorough orderly fashion in a very brief time span, perhaps 30 seconds. It is almost axiomatic in medicine that the one consideration omitted will contain the abnormality in question, or prevent appropriate, logical diagnosis.

Treatment of any abnormality encountered in assessing the ABCs requires experience in cardiopulmonary resuscitation. It is essential not only that a physician be in attendance at contact sport contests, but that he be expert in the procedure. Anticipation of possible emergencies is another requisite. This involves not only readiness of physician and trainer, but planning and availability of appropriate transportation. It includes movement of the victim from playing surface to medical room, and also from field or room to the hospital. A hand-carried stretcher should be available nearby. Not knowing whether there is associated spine injury, the attendants should move the patient to the stretcher without any flexion of the torso or neck. A cervical collar of the Philadelphia or similar type should be available. Transfer is best accomplished by a so-called scoop. If not available, simultaneous lifting with three pairs of hands and arms can be carried out as the stretcher is slid under the victim.

Transport to a hospital should be by ambulance. Immediate availability of such a vehicle depends on the statistical likelihood of serious injury. It is good to have one ready for football games, for instance. In other circumstances it is wise to know the accessibility of an ambulance, including emergency telephone number, the distance of location from the event, and the appropriate hospital destination for transfer. Emergency medical technicians manning ambulances (EMT-As) or paramedics are trained for resuscitation as well as for transport procedures.

FIRST AID

First aid is different for open and closed injuries. Wounds that involve openings of the skin, even if definitely superficial, are cleansed of dirt and debris with sterile soap, and covered with an occlusive sterile dressing. For abrasions, a nonadherent dressing may be helpful. For lacerations, decision regarding suture is paramount; this is a physician's prerogative. Puncture or penetrating wounds require transfer to hospital and investigation.

For blunt injuries involving only the abdominal wall, or subcutaneous-musculofascial contusions, primary first aid involves removal of the player from the field, examination for the possibility of peritoneal or visceral injury, and application of ice for minimizing tissue bleeding and hematoma formation. This should be applied for approximately 30 minutes. A compression dressing applied over a wadded gauze or sponge rubber pad is then useful if it can be readily applied with elastic bandage taping without inappropriate restriction of function. If pain increases during postinjury observation, if pallor or diaphoresis (sweating) ensues, or if the recorded pulse rate increases substantially, the injured player should be transferred to the hospital.

In general, there are some don'ts in first aid of abdominal injuries. Injections of local anesthetics (procaine, lidocaine), steroids, or other medications are contraindicated. Medications for pain should be withheld as long as observing the severity of pain is important. Local use of ointments, particularly antibiotics, for open wounds probably is ineffective. Return to play is solely the decision of physician or paramedical personnel (not the coach, or player), and should not be permitted unless the injury can be proved to be minor and nonthreatening.

Equipment for Initial Treatment

A first aid bag for the physician or trainer should be available, well stocked, and regularly checked. It should contain ammonia ampules, sterile gauze pads, tape of various sizes, roller gauze bandages and elastic bandages of different widths, cold packs, splints for fingers or arms (large ones for legs are usually stocked separately), cloth slings, and oral airways. A stretcher should be available close by. The use of ethyl chloride for local spray of contusions is of questionable value.

Oxygen is essential. This should be available for mask administration with an Ambu attachment for positive-pressure resuscitation if necessary. An ideal is the availability of a laryngoscope and endotracheal tubes for physician use if indicated.

The medical room is stocked more completely, the extent determined largely by the physician's role and the nature of the sport. For contact sports involving professional, college, or other amateur teams, a physician should have a medical room stocked for his possible use with sterile equipment (local anesthetics, needles, and syringes; suture material, absorbable and nonabsorbable; suturing instruments, scalpels, and blades), diagnostic instruments (stethoscope, sphygmomanometer, otoscope-ophthalmoscope) and limited nonnarcotic medications. A cricothyrotomy kit should be available for *physician* use. The variation in sport, professionalism, and accessibility to hospital units makes details to specify.

PREVENTION

The ideal in all sports is to prevent injuries rather than to have to treat them. In general, prevention of injuries is possible 1) with utilization of appropriate, well-conceived and constructed equipment, 2) with good physical conditioning and coaching, 3) with proper medical supervision to insure preseason fitness and readiness for a player returning to play after injury, and 4) with intelligent consideration of rules of play. These guidelines are probably of less importance for abdominal injuries than for facial, eye, or other specific organ trauma. In football, the quarterback with his arm upraised and poised for passing, or the receiver leaping with outstretched arms, are most vulnerable to neck, chest, and abdominal injuries from helmet, shoulder pads, or forearms of the tackler. A reasonable rule would be the requirement for below-the-waist tackling. In hockey improper use of the stick (spearing) can lead to visceral organ damage, and is outlawed with severe penalty assessment.

Prior abdominal injury is usually not a contraindication to participation in contact sports. A splenectomy does not increase the likelihood of future injury. Liver rupture, however, may, and the player probably is best advised to stay out of higher-risk contact sports. Loss of one of paired visceral organs is a controversial consideration. From a purely medical view, loss of one kidney or testis (or congenital presence of only one) is a potent argument for restriction from contact sports.

INJURIES TO THE ABDOMINAL WALL

Serious injury to the abdominal wall is uncommon in most major sports. This is because of several factors. The abdomen is largely protected as it is on the flexion side of the torso. The abdominal wall is soft in contrast to the spinous portion of the back, or the joints of the extremities, and therefore permits some give when struck. For players who are targets of thrown or propelled objects (goalies, catchers, fencers, etc), protective padding is generally well conceived, designed, and fitted. Nevertheless, the abdominal wall is the site of many minor injuries. It is important that all be checked out by an appropriate trainer or therapist, and any unusual ones referred to a physician for evaluation.

Injuries to the abdominal wall can be categorized in several ways: 1) the level of injury (skin, subcutaneous tissue, muscle layers); 2) blunt or penetrating; and 3) individually contracted (strains, twisting injuries) or the result of contact with another player or an immovable object. The last consideration is potentially the more serious. Injuries to muscles are more incapacitating and slower to respond than more superficial trauma. Penetrating injuries tend to be more serious than blunt ones, although the latter always have the potential for abdominal visceral rupture. Injuries individually contracted have far less potential for significant injury than those sustained in running into other participants or fixed structures. Ice hockey has a particular likelihood for such injuries because of the retaining boards, goal posts, and the unusually hard playing surface.

Skin

Injuries at this level tend to be minor. Abrasions are usually the result of friction burns from contact with the ground in sliding, or from ill-fitting equipment. They are best handled by careful cleansing to rid the surface of adherent dirt and debris, and covering with a light occlusive, nonadhering dressing. Petrolatum impregnated in fine mesh gauze is simple and effective.

Superficial lacerations are not common in the abdominal wall and usually can be cared for in the medical facility of a team's dressing quarters. The subcutaneous fat is less resistant to bacterial infection than the skin of the head and face where there is little fat. Therefore attention must carefully be directed to removal of foreign bodies (bits of clothing, dirt, etc) and aseptic suturing technique. Prior tetanus immunization is essential for all athletes. Perforating injuries from nails or other sharp objects, should not be sutured and must be seen by a physician. Any question of a deeper laceration into abdominal wall muscle is an indication for hospital referral. Dressings on lacerations should be minimal, used primarily for protection from clothing or equipment. Ointments are generally to be avoided.

There is an unusual potential for foreign bodies on the skin surface, including the abdomen, to be abraded into the epithelium by friction of equipment. An example is the fiberglass of hockey stick blades which, if it gets on the skin surface under rubbing equipment, can cause a painful or itching rash or skin irritation. Players should be cautioned to avoid shaving or planing their sticks when undressed.

Subcutaneous Tissue

The only significant injury at this level is hematoma, the result of arteriolar or venous bleeding into the fatty layer from blunt trauma. It is best treated by minimizing its extent with early application of ice, and avoidance of local heat for 48 hours or more. Subcutaneous hematoma rarely requires additional treatment. Aspiration can be attempted if a fluctuant collection results. Open evacuation is to be avoided except on the decision of a surgeon.

The athlete who demonstrates a penchant for developing subcutaneous hematomas should be investigated for an underlying blood dyscrasia. The more common abnormalities encountered in young athletes are leukemia and idiopathic thrombocytopenic purpura. It is reasonable to require a routine preseason complete blood count including platelets for all players involved in organized sports, especially those involving contact.

Muscle

The muscles of the abdominal wall are the two rectus muscles running parallel from costal margins to pubis, the external and internal oblique muscles, and the transversus abdominis muscle that lies closest to the peritoneal membrane. Others of smaller size and extent, and of less liability to injury include the pyramidalis muscles and the cremaster muscles that envelop the spermatic cords.

The types of muscle injuries are blunt trauma, strains, and occasionally penetrating trauma. Much has been written about the diagnosis and treatment of penetrating injuries of the abdominal wall. They can occur from faulty protection against an épée, from the sharp end of a broken stick, or from the point of a skate. They should always be seen by a physician, preferably in the hospital setting. Surgical exploration under local anesthesia for appropriate hemostasis, debridement, and suture is generally advisable. If the peritoneal membrane has been pierced, complete abdominal exploration is necessary to look for and treat visceral injury. Antibiotics are likely to be necessary.

The most serious blunt trauma injury of abdominal wall muscle is rupture of the deep epigastric vessels, arteries or veins, which causes an increasing deep hematoma within the rectus muscle sheath until self-tamponading occurs. In healthy athletes, particularly the young, this phenomenon is not likely to occur, making exploration, vessel ligation, and evacuation of hematoma necessary. Older athletes are not likely to be involved in contact sports. Persons on anticoagulant medication should not be involved in any activity where blunt abdominal trauma can possibly occur.

Muscle strains of the abdominal wall result from overstretching of a bundle of muscle fibers, usually when the torso is twisted or hyperextended in contact with other players or immovable objects, forcing the fibers to be stretched beyond their normal tensile capability. Strains can also occur when musculotendinous insertions are pulled away from bone, such as the iliac crest, or when muscle fibers are pulled away from aponeurotic sheaths or lines. This type of injury tends not to be initially incapacitating. After a variable interval, usually a matter of hours, local tenderness develops, sometimes with a small nodular swelling indicative of minihematoma. A nagging soreness ensues, especially when the involved muscle is contracted. Depending on the extent of involvement, the player may be inactivated.

Initial therapy involves application of ice to minimize secondary tissue damage from bleeding. Little can actually be done to promote recovery except to avoid reinjury and allow normal healing. After 48 hours, local heat can be applied to improve arteriolar blood supply necessary for healing. The efficacy of diathermy and ultrasound is not yet established. Local injection of anesthetic solutions and steroids is contraindicated in acute strains. However, occasionally, an acute strain becomes chronic, usually in the insertion tear, resulting in persistent local inflammation (as distinct from hemorrhage). This persistence can sometimes be helped by the injection of 50 mg of hydrocortisone or its equivalent, directly into the point of maximum tenderness. This should always be a physician's decision and treatment. Anti-inflammatory medications (phenylbutazone, indomethacin, ibuprofen, etc) may occasionally be worthy of trial, always under strict physician supervision with appropriate consideration of risk and contraindications.

INJURIES TO THE INTRAABDOMINAL CONTENTS

The patient who has sustained blunt abdominal trauma frequently has simultaneously sustained injury to another anatomic area. Therefore he must be evaluated for injuries to the head, thorax, and extremities. Failure to recognize an associated injury may lead to severe morbidity and loss of life. Diagnostic and therapeutic procedures in many instances must proceed simultaneously, each giving way to the other under appropriate circumstances, in particular, in management of airway compromise and hypovolemic shock.

Although it is usual to subdivide the category of abdominal injury into blunt and penetrating trauma, in considering athletic injuries it is perhaps appropriate in view of the overwhelming predominance of blunt trauma, to think of the problem as either immediately life-threatening, or potentially, but not immediately, life-threatening. Unlike most other anatomic areas, the abdominal cavity may be quite difficult to evaluate, the early abdominal signs of an injured intraabdominal structure frequently being quite subtle and only becoming apparent as time elapses. X-ray examination of the abdominal cavity may give little early evidence that a major injury has been sustained. It is important that the overall responsibility for management of an injured person be delegated to one person, and all those caring for the patient must clearly know whom to consult for decisions relating to priority of therapeutic and diagnostic measures.

A history of the mechanism of the injury together with a thorough physical examination should allow the physician to come to a working diagnosis promptly. Laboratory tests and roentgenograms may allow refinement of the diagnosis. Physical examination should begin with careful evaluation of the vital signs including the blood pressure, and the character and rate of the pulse and respirations. At any point the examiner should be prepared to establish an adequate airway, start blood replacement, or both, before continuing with the evaluation.

If the abdominal cavity or retroperitoneum seems to be the source of difficulty further attention should be focused on this area. The most reliable physical finding indicating peritoneal irritation is the presence of voluntary or involuntary spasm, or both. Spasm can only be determined accurately by gently placing the palm of the hand on an abdominal quadrant over the rectus muscle, asking the patient to breathe deeply, and gently depressing the examining hand with the other hand. Voluntary spasm of the rectus muscle will disappear as the patient exhales, whereas involuntary spasm will not. In the latter instance the muscle will feel tense and boardlike. The exact area of tenderness should be noted by gentle palpation. with one finger. This may suggest the viscus affected by the intraabdominal process. On removal of the hand pressing near the tender area, rebound tenderness may be felt in the primary site of pain, providing further evidence of peritoneal irritation. The flanks should be carefully palpated along the lower part of the chest wall. Examination for masses, hepatic and splenic enlargement, and free fluid within the abdominal cavity should be done. If dullness and tenderness coincide on gentle percussion, a mass should be sought in this location. Unfortunately, the character of peristalsis in the presence of acute abdominal injury is generally not helpful, as audible normal peristalsis does not exclude the possibility of intraabdominal difficulty. Examination of the groins, and pelvic and rectal examinations must be carried out to evaluate the abdomen and retroperitoneum completely.

Diagnostic needle paracentesis is frequently an appropriate procedure in evaluation of patients having sustained blunt abdominal trauma. If nonclotting blood is recovered from the peritoneal cavity, the accuracy of this procedure has been reported as high as 95% in predicting intraabdominal injury. The chance of obtaining positive results with a tap is directly related to the amount of blood in the peritoneal cavity. Paracentesis is a simple and quick procedure with relatively few complications. Although abdominal paracentesis is accurate if results are positive, no information is gained if the result is negative. The major objection to the use of the test is the high percentage of false-negative results.

An alternative to paracentesis is peritoneal lavage.[2] In the absence of previous multiple abdominal operative procedures or a penetrating abdominal injury, after decompression of the urinary bladder, a skin wheal is raised with 1% lidocaine, in the lower midline approximately one-third of the distance between the umbilicus and the pubic symphysis. The skin is incised and a standard peritoneal dialysis catheter is inserted, the trocar being advanced carefully until it just penetrates the peritoneum. It is thereafter removed, and the catheter advanced toward the pelvis. If nonclotting blood is aspirated, the diagnosis of hemoperitoneum is confirmed. If no fluid or blood is aspirated, a liter of Ringer lactate balanced salt solution is rapidly infused into the peritoneal cavity, and the patient is turned from side to side in the absence of major bony fracture. Fluid is then siphoned out of the peritoneal cavity. The presence in the aspirated fluid of more than 100,000 red blood cells per cubic millimeter, more than 500 white blood cells per cubic millimeter, an elevated amylase level, or bile or bacteria, are indications for prompt laparotomy. One may expect approximately a 3.5% false-positive, and a 3.1% false-negative rate. The major complications of this procedure are punctures of the small and large bowel, mesentery vessels, and retroperitoneal hematoma.

If a penetrating injury to the abdominal wall has occurred, the wound should be extended under local anesthesia to determine its depth. If the patient's condition is stable and the wound involves only the abdominal wall, local management and follow-up are indicated. If the peritoneum appears to have been penetrated, the abdomen should be explored.

SPECIFIC ORGAN INJURIES

Spleen

The abdominal organ most frequently injured by blunt trauma is the spleen.[3] Its injury is suggested by history of trauma to the left upper abdominal quadrant or left lower portion of the rib cage, frequently associated with a neighboring fractured rib. Abdominal pain may be surprisingly minor. Occasionally left shoulder discomfort may be produced by irritation of the adjacent left diaphragm. If hemorrhage has been substantial, hypovolemic shock may be present, requiring urgent volume replacement and emergency surgery. Left upper abdominal, left lower chest wall, and/or left flank tenderness, are the usual physical findings. Radiologic indications of splenic trauma include depression of the splenic flexure of the colon, elevation of the diaphragm, obliteration of the splenic shadow, and prominent gastric rugae. These signs, however, are frequently absent.

In those patients in whom the diagnosis is suspected but uncertain, a radionuclide scan should be obtained first. If unequivocally normal, or if injury is revealed, further studies are unnecessary. If, however, findings are equivocal, selective splenic arteriography should be performed. It is an accurate method of establishing diagnosis and of assessing the degree of injury.

Angiographic findings include leakage of contrast medium into the splenic pulp; a large, avascular area with spreading of the intrasplenic branches; irregularities in the opacified spleen in the region of a hematoma; loss of the continuous splenic contour; simultaneous visualization of the splenic artery and vein; and an increased distance between the spleen and left flank. The spleen may be displaced medially, and the kidney inferiorly.[4]

Further management is governed by evidence of the presence or absence of ongoing hemorrhage and the apparent magnitude of the injury. In that loss of the spleen may be associated with later appearance of overwhelming infection, particularly in the pediatric age population, an effort should be made to avoid splenectomy. If the patient is hemodynamically stable, observation in the hospital over a period of time (10 days) is indicated, if the splenic injury is not severe, as judged by scan and/or angiogram. If the patient, however, is hemodynamically unstable, prompt operation should be undertaken, and, if possible, repair of the spleen accomplished. If not possible, splenectomy should be done and immunization to pneumococci induced.[5]

Occasionally, a subcapsular splenic hematoma may rupture days to weeks after the traumatic event. The history of previous trauma and evidence of intraabdominal hemorrhage should suggest the diagnosis.

Liver

The liver is the second most commonly injured organ in blunt trauma.[3] Injury is suggested by a blow to the right lower rib cage or right upper abdominal quadrant. Injury to the liver is frequently associated with significant blood loss, progressive signs of peritoneal irritation beginning in the right upper quadrant, and frequently with the development of a right upper quadrant abdominal mass. The presence of hypovolemic shock mandates immediate surgery.[6] The presence of a mass associated with a stable hypovolemic state that can be maintained with transfusion, should be further investigated by arteriography at which point one may directly assess the vascular anatomy of the liver prior to exploratory laparotomy. Control may involve resection of the injured portion of the liver,[7] opening the hematoma cavity with suture ligation of vascular and biliary structures within the cavity, or ligation of the right or left hepatic artery when bleeding cannot be controlled or when resection is of such magnitude to present a major threat of loss of life. Appropriate drainage of the area and postoperative nutritional support are most important in achieving a satisfactory result.

Jejunum and Ileum

The majority of small intestinal disruptions distal to the duodenum, secondary to blunt trauma, are found in the proximal half of the jejunum or the distal ileum.[3] The mechanism responsible probably involves direct impingement of the bowel against the vertebral column or a tearing or shearing force in areas of the bowel where either the bowel or mesentery is relatively fixed, ie, at the ligament of Treitz or the ileocecal valve. Careful serial abdominal examination will eventually reveal evidence of peritoneal irritation, but early abdominal signs may be lacking or surprisingly mild, because of the nearly neutral pH of succus entericus and low number of bacteria in the small intestine. Progression of epigastric pain and evolution of signs of peritoneal irritation elicited upon serial abdominal examination confirm diagnosis. Surprisingly, free air may not be present within the abdominal cavity, presumably because there is little gas present in the small bowel in the resting state.

Mesentery

The mesentery of the small bowel and colon may be torn by the tearing or shearing force of blunt abdominal trauma. This injury may be evident early because of major hemorrhage. Its presence can also become manifest some days after injury when the bowel supplied by the vessels that have been disrupted in the injured mesentery becomes progressively more ischemic and ultimately loses viability, producing signs of peritoneal irritation and, ultimately, perforation of the viscus involved.

Pancreas

Blunt injury to the pancreas usually occurs at the junction of the body and head where the pancreas overlies the vertebral column near the superior mesenteric artery. Physical findings may be few at first because of the retroperitoneal location of the pancreas deep in the abdominal cavity, but signs of peritoneal irritation gradually develop. The serum amylase level is usually elevated.[8] Abdominal exploration should be performed when the condition is strongly suspected, even if there are few indications other than evolving peritoneal signs. Resection of the distal pancreas with oversewing of pancreatic duct and closure of the pancreatic capsule is the usual operative procedure. An alternative in a fractured pancreas is placement of a Roux-en-Y loop of bowel to the transected end of pancreas.

Duodenum

Blunt injury to the abdomen may produce isolated retroperitoneal rupture of the duodenum. It has been suggested that the blow must be unexpected and the abdominal muscles relaxed at the time. A fall upon the back has also been indicated as cause of this injury. At the time of a blow air within the duodenum may be trapped between the closed pylorus and the sharply angulated duodenojejunal junction, making it vulnerable to blast rupture or laceration. Its presence immediately anterior to the vertebral column may produce crush injury from a blow anteriorly. This injury can easily be overlooked because of the retroperitoneal position of the duodenum, and abdominal signs may be minimal initially. Coincidental injury to liver, spleen, ribs, and spine may also detract attention from an injured duodenum. Severe or mild injury to the adjacent pancreas may also be present. A history of persistent abdominal pain and progression of abdominal signs should lead one to suspect this injury.

Diagnostic studies, including lavage, presence of free air on roentgenographs of the abdomen, and serum amylase studies are frequently unreliable, but a gastrografin swallow may demonstrate duodenal disruption. If duodenal injury is suspected,[9] careful exploration of the retroperitoneal portion should be undertaken, the injured duodenum either repaired or resected, and gastrointestinal continuity restored.

Intramural hematoma of the duodenum, an uncommon lesion resulting from blunt abdominal trauma, is usually manifested as an obstruction high in the small intestine. Diagnosis is made on contrast examination of the upper gastrointestinal tract, revealing obstruction at the third portion of the duodenum. Treatment consists of nasogastric aspiration with intravenous replacement of fluid and electrolytes, and elective evacuation of the hematoma.

Stomach

Blunt injury to the stomach is unusual but may result from a direct blow to the epigastrium. Blood is usually present in the nasogastric aspirate and signs of peritoneal irritation develop early because of its acid content. Free air may also be evident on a plain roentgenogram of the abdomen. Prompt abdominal exploration and repair of the injury are indicated.

Large Bowel

Blunt injury to the large intestine is usually associated with massive peritoneal contamination, and usually occurs in association with other abdominal organ injury. The rectum is rarely injured, even in severe pelvic fractures. Surprisingly, when perforation of the colon occurs and large numbers of bacteria escape into the peritoneal cavity, signs of peritoneal irritation do not appear until infection is established. Thus, injury to colon may not be appreciated early unless suspected. Prompt operation is necessary to treat this injury and its management may involve colon resection with or without colostomy.

Diaphragm

Most traumatic ruptures of the diaphragm occur as a consequence of blunt abdominal trauma. They usually occur on the left and generally are posterocentral in position. A traumatic opening may be quite large, permitting intrathoracic displacement of abdominal contents with consequent respiratory distress by collapse of the left lung. The diagnosis may be delayed revealed only by serial films showing migration of abdominal viscera into the hemithorax. Operative repair should be undertaken as promptly as the circumstances permit.[10]

INJURIES TO THE GENITOURINARY SYSTEM

Kidney

Even though the kidneys are relatively well protected in the upper retroperitoneum under the rib cage, they may be injured by direct trauma to the flank or by a contrecoup injury in which they are thrown forward when the athlete stops abruptly. Commonly there is pain and tenderness in the flank and adjacent anatomic areas. If thrombus is formed in the collecting system, and obstructs the ureter, renal colic may be present. When there is severe hemorrhage from the kidney, an expanding flank mass may be found and hypovolemic shock may be present. Hematuria may be gross or microscopic. Plain films of the abdomen may show asymmetry or loss of renal outline, fractures of adjacent ribs and vertebrae, blurring or obliteration of psoas shadow, and elevation of the diaphragm or atelectasis. Infusion intravenous urography combined with nephrotomography allows accurate assessment of kidneys as well as outlining the ureters and bladder, and can be accomplished in nonfasting, hydrated patients.

While immediate surgical intervention may be necessary to save life or kidney or both, a delay may prevent significant morbidity and possible loss of kidney, and also may decrease the risk of operation itself particularly in the presence of frequently associated other injuries.[11] Thus it is essential to enlist the aid of a skilled genitourinary surgeon to render judgment that the renal injury requires immediate surgery because of injury to the renal pedicle, or threatened exsanguination from continued bleeding from the injured kidney; requires delayed intervention because of transcortical transcapsular lacerations with evidence of perirenal extravasation; or requires no intervention, as in the case of contusion or cortical laceration without extravasation, or intrarenal laceration without evidence of disruption of the renal capsule. Chronically diseased kidneys are more likely to be damaged than normal kidneys, so it is reasonable to advise those with renal disease to avoid contact sports.

Ureters

Ureteral injuries are most unusual as a consequence of blunt abdominal trauma. The ureter may be avulsed or damaged by fractures of the pelvis or vertebrae. Injury is usually not suspected until complications or urinary extravasation occur.

Bladder

The urinary bladder may be contused, or rupture as a consequence of lower abdominal blunt trauma. Rupture is more likely when the bladder is full, the distended bladder and overlying peritoneum splitting posteriorly with extravasation into the peritoneal cavity. Retroperitoneal ruptures may be seen with fractures of the pubic rami leading to extraperitoneal extravasation. The contused bladder may be evidenced by microscopic or gross hematuria. A ruptured bladder with urine extravasation causes lower abdominal pain and tenderness. Evaluation should include urinalysis, urethrogram, and cystography, as well as evaluation of the upper tracts by intravenous pyelography. Rupture with extravasation should be managed with exploration and repair, whereas bleeding from a contused bladder is usually successfully managed with Foley catheter drainage.

Urethra

The male urethra is divided into the anterior urethra (that portion distal to the fixed triangular ligament), which is mobile and thus rarely injured, and the posterior urethra consisting of the membranous urethra located within the triangular ligament and the prostatic urethra. Blunt posterior urethral injuries are usually caused by pelvic fractures. Mild to moderate trauma may produce hemorrhage that may result in obstruction and inability to void. Severe trauma may cause tissue destruction, hematoma formation, and extravasation of urine. The site of injury is demonstrated by urethrography and panendoscopy, best directed by a genitourinary surgeon who can determine management.[12]

Because the female urethra is short and not fixed posteriorly, injuries are rare and usually less severe than those seen in men. Blunt trauma, often from gymnastics and cycling, results in lacerations and contusions of the distal urethra. Actual urethral disruption is very rare.

Scrotum and Contents

In its exposed location this anatomic area must be carefully protected by appropriate equipment in all contact sports. Blunt injury is usually manifest by contusion that usually can be managed with ice and elevation. Occasionally exploration is indicated by the presence of continued bleeding. The presence of a single gonad should lead to careful thought prior to recommending that a young man pursue contact sports.

REFERENCES

1. Roberts, J.T., and Hayes, H.R. Cardiopulmonary resuscitation. Edited by E.W. Wilkins, Jr, A.C. Moncure, J.J. Dineen, and P.L. Gross. In *MGH Textbook of Emergency Medicine.* Baltimore: Williams and Wilkins, 1983, pp 25–38.

2. Perry, J.E., DeMeules, J.E., and Root, H.D. Diagnostic peritoneal lavage in blunt abdominal trauma. *Surg Gynecol Obstet.* 131: 742–743, 1970.

3. Davis, J.J., Cohn, I., and Nance, F.C. Diagnosis and management of blunt abdominal trauma. *Ann Surg.* 183:672–677, 1976.

4. Abrams, H.L. (Ed.) Splenic arteriography. In *Angiography.* Boston: Little, Brown and Co., 1971, p 103.

5. King, D.R., Lobe, T.E., Haase, G.M., et al. Selective management of injured spleen. *Surg.* 90:677–682, 1981.

6. Madding, G.F., and Kennedy, P.A. *Trauma to the Liver.* Philadelphia: W.B. Saunders, 1971.

7. Trunkey, D.D., Shires, G.T., and McClelland, R. Management of liver trauma in 811 consecutive patients. *Ann Surg.* 179:722–728, 1974.

8. Jones, R.C., and Shires, G.T. The management of pancreatic injuries. *Arch Surg.* 90:502–507, 1965.

9. Roman, E., Silva, Y.J., and Lucas, C. Management of blunt duodenal injury. *Surg Gynecol Obstet.* 132:7–14, 1971.

10. Ebert, P.A., Gaertner, R.A., and Zuidema, G.D. Traumatic diaphragmatic hernia. *Surg Gynecol Obstet.* 125:59–65, 1967.

11. Karmi, S.A., Young, J.D., and Soderstrom, C. Classification of renal injuries as a guide to therapy. *Surg Gynecol Obstet.* 148:161–167, 1979.

12. Persky, L., and Hoch, W.H. Genitourinary tract trauma. Monograph, *Curr Probl Surg.* September:1–64, 1972.

ADDENDUM

Injuries to the Chest

Earl F. Hoerner, MD

The chest is, in general, well protected by using proper safety equipment during athletic participation. This does not, however, rule out the possibility of injury to this area that houses the vital heart and lungs. Injuries can occur to the boney structures including the ribs, sternum, and vertebrae. Injuries can also occur to the underlying and overlying soft tissues, including the muscles, subcutaneous tissues, lungs, and heart. The most common chest injuries that occur during athletic participation include chest contusions, rib fractures, pneumothorax, costochondral separation, and myocardial contusion. They will be covered in this section.

Chest Contusions

Contusions to the chest occur more frequently than other types of thoracic injuries. Bruising of the skin and subcutaneous tissue, pectoralis major, latissimus dorsi, erector spinae, serratus anterior, intercostal muscles, or underlying ribs is most often the outcome of a severe blow to the chest. Severe pain, tenderness, muscle spasm and pain on deep inspiration are seen with this injury.

A severe contusion to the ribs and one to the soft tissue must be differentiated from one another. Examination of the injured site will reveal an area of tenderness. If the periosteum is involved, tenderness will be on the rib itself, whereas if the skin or muscle is involved the tenderness will be more superficial. In order to distinguish a rib contusion from a soft tissue one, the skin overlying the injury can be slid up or down over the ribs. If the tenderness persists over the bone, regardless of the location of the overlying skin, damage is to the bone. If the tenderness remains constant over the skin, damage is to the underlying soft tissue. If injury to a rib is suspected, a chest radiograph should be obtained to rule out a fracture.

Contusion to the chest wall does not usually require extensive treatment. The involved area should be iced and anti-inflammatory medication administered as necessary. A rib belt can be used for comfort. Padding should be applied over the contused area if the athlete is involved in contact sports.

Rib Fractures

A severe blow to the chest can produce fractures of the underlying ribs. Pain and tenderness at the site of fracture, pain on deep inspiration, splinting of adjacent muscles, and shallow, labored breathing are often seen with this injury. Crepitation along the chest wall may also be seen, particularly if more than one rib is fractured at more than one site. An attempt should be made to discern whether the injury is a fracture or simply a contusion (see section on Chest Contusion). If a fracture is suspected, a chest radiograph should be obtained as soon as possible.

Treatment of an uncomplicated rib fracture is mainly symptomatic. A rib belt or taping of the affected side is often adequate. Application of ice to the site of injury and anti-inflammatory medications may help to decrease swelling and pain. Athletes should not be permitted to return to play until the fractures have completely healed. This usually takes three to four weeks. A displaced fractured rib can pierce the pleura or adjacent lung tissue and cause pneumothorax, or tear underlying blood vessels and cause hemothorax. Both of these complications should be suspected when the athlete experiences severe shortness of breath, signs of shock, or cyanosis. This is a life-threatening situation, the athlete should be transported to the hospital immediately. Pneumothorax and hemothorax are treated by the insertion of chest tubes.

Pneumothorax

Pneumothorax occurs when air at atmospheric pressure enters the pleural space and collapses the underlying lung. This is most likely to occur in an athlete who has sustained a crushing blow to the chest and fractured several ribs as a result. The broken and unstable ends of the fractured ribs can tear the pleura and cause pneumothorax. Spontaneous pneumothorax is also possible following a severe impact. Classic signs of a pneumothorax include progressive shortness of breath, hyperresonance to percussion, absence of breath sounds, shift of the trachea and mediastinum away from the side of collapse, and cyanosis. A chest radiograph is essential in confirming a diagnosis of pneumothorax.

Emergency treatment of the athlete who has sustained a pneumothorax should be the immediate administration of oxygen and transfer to a hospital. This is a life-threatening situation requiring treatment with chest tubes and respiratory support. An athlete should not return to play following injury until the lung has been completely reexpanded and the fractured ribs completely healed.

Costochondral Separation

Costochondral separation most frequently involves a separation of the anterior end of the rib from its site of attachment to the lateral sternum. This type of injury can occur when the rib cage is squeezed or when the arm is pulled to the side causing a stretch of the costochondral junction. The athlete may report a popping sensation at the time of injury. Tenderness in this injury is usually localized to the site of dislocation. Pain on deep inspiration may accompany this injury. If the dislocation is complete, the ribs may become offset and ride up in front of the costocartilage. This can be easily palpated. In some cases it may be possible to elicit a clicking sound as alternating pressure is applied to the sternum and to the tip of the involved rib. An incomplete separation may not be palpable, and the athlete may simply complain of anterior chest wall pain, particularly when coughing, sneezing and deep breathing. A chest radiograph is rarely helpful in diagnosing this problem but should be taken in order to rule out the possibility of fractured ribs.

If no click or demonstrable deformation is seen, one may assume that some of the ligaments are still intact and can direct therapy at reducing pain and swelling and preventing further injury. The chest should be strapped in order to prevent wide excursion of the rib cage. If the ribs have been displaced, it is necessary to manipulate them back into proper position. This can often be done manually or by means of circumferential taping. Costochondral union can be slow, and six to eight weeks should be allowed for complete healing.

Myocardial Contusion

Contusions to the heart can result from a severe blow to the anterior chest. This injury can be life threatening and may accompany other severe thoracic injuries. An athlete with this injury will often complain of retrosternal pain; palpitations and tachycardia are frequently seen. Intramuscular bruising and petechial hemorrhages may cause pericardial effusion or the catastrophic cardiac tamponade. This condition may be confirmed by muffled heart sounds, engorgement of the neck veins, decreased blood pressure, and a pulse that disappears on inspiration.

This injury can be life threatening. The athlete should be observed for signs of shock and transported immediately to the hospital.

CHAPTER 16
Sports-related Skin Problems

Merrill G. Liteplo, MD

The skin problems of athletes are those of the general population, but they often assume interesting variations related to specific activities. It is important for those interested in sports medicine to be aware of how a variety of physical phenomena, infectious agents, and other creatures impact on the skin. The dermatologic diseases commonly found in athletes are organized from a pathophysiologic perspective, with reference to specific athletic activities when possible. Needless to say there is a great deal of morbidity associated with skin diseases that can severely limit one's participation in sports. The implications of some diseases go beyond the individual, however, and can affect teammates, partners, and opponents.

INJURIES CAUSED BY PHYSICAL FACTORS

Mechanical Factors

Calcaneal petechiae, also called "black heel" or posttraumatic punctate hemorrhage of the skin, is a traumatically induced condition characterized by an area of speckled, flat, bluish black pigmentation that represents accumulation of coagulated blood in the superficial dermis and overlying epidermis. It is thought to be the result of either sudden shearing forces,[1] or repeated minor trauma associated with sudden stops,[2] or a pinching trauma of the skin.[3] While most often localized at the periphery of the heel, it may also appear on fingers and toes.[4] The condition has been encountered in many sports: basketball, football, jogging, tennis, volleyball, weight lifting, and chinning, to name a few. It may be more likely to occur in athletes who play on hard wooden floors.

The condition is painless, leads to no complications, and resolves spontaneously within a few months. It is important to recognize the problem and avoid unnecessary surgery, since conditions such as plantar warts, flat moles, and even melanomas may resemble calcaneal petechiae.

The appearance of this problem on the heel may be prevented by inserting a piece of felt inside the heel of the shoe.[2] Shoes should obviously fit well, and wearing thicker socks may provide adequate protection as well.

Tennis toe is characterized by painful splinterlike hemorrhages beneath the toenails. The toe affected is the one that extends furthest. In 25% of people this is the second toe, in another 25% it is the first toe, and in the remainder of individuals both first and second toes are equally long.[5] Appearance of these hemorrhages has been explained as resulting from the toe being propelled against the tip of the shoe during the frequent abrupt stopping that occurs in tennis. It is further suggested that upward shearing forces upon the distal nail plate may be contributory.[1]

M. Pugliese (personal communication) noted in several tennis players not only the subungual hemorrhage but also the appearance of transverse ridging of the nail plate and some onycholysis.

It seems likely that in sports other than tennis where frequent abrupt stopping is the rule, a participant is at risk for developing tennis toe if he or she is wearing improperly fitted shoes. The condition should resolve spontaneously with either cessation of activity or obtaining appropriately fitted shoes.

Striae distensae, or stretch marks, have an unknown etiology. It seems likely that in athletes, mechanical stresses that stretch or distend the skin are the cause. The adolescent (aged 10 to 19) may be the most likely individual to develop striae, and girls are two and one-half times more likely to develop them than boys.[6]

Striae are usually readily recognized as shallow linear or crescentic depressions of the skin; they are initially red or dusky red blue but this color fades in time. The epidermis overlying striae is atrophic. They may occur in any area of the body where the skin is subjected to stretching. These lesions frequently develop in weight lifters and gymnasts, mostly over the anterior shoulders, lower back, and thighs, perpendicular to the direction of skin tension.[1]

Striae can result from the excessive use of topical steroids, especially in intertriginous or occluded sites such as the groin. Excessive systemic levels of glucocorticoids seen in Cushing's disease can also cause them. There is no treatment for striae, but avoidance of extreme tension may prevent some from developing.

Blisters represent accumulation of fluid within intraepidermal slits that form primarily from horizontal shearing forces acting upon the skin.[7] The slits develop secondary to prickle-cell necrosis, and fill with fluid from the dermis. Blisters are easily recognized. While usually caused solely by friction, their pattern of appearance may suggest an underlying genetic predisposition, as seen in the Weber-Cockayne syndrome, or in epidermolysis bullosa simplex. Frictional forces are reduced if the skin is dry, greasy, or very wet, but increased if it is moist. These factors primarily influence the degree of friction required to cause blister formation.[8]

Prevention of blisters is possible for athletes, and some of the following points are self-evident. Shoes should fit perfectly; thick socks interfere with such a fit. Vaseline may be useful when applied to the feet or to sites in the shoe that rub against the skin. Talc is the oldest agent in general use for reducing skin friction. Placing plain adhesive tape over an anticipated blister site also results in decreased frictional forces.

When blisters do develop it has been shown that preservation of the blister top and multiple aspirations or drainage of fluid during the first 24 hours, results in the least discomfort, and protects the blister base from secondary infection.[9] Applying adhesive tape over a drained blister will often enable the individual to resume previous activity.

Calluses are acquired areas of thickened skin, the result of hyperkeratosis, that arise from repeated or prolonged friction or pressure to the skin. Although the process of callus formation is not well understood, they are universally recognizable as occurring in weight-bearing sites, or as unique occupational or athletic marks. Calluses are usually asymptomatic but may be painful with pressure. They can easily be distinguished from corns or warts; on paring a callus the normal papillary line pattern of the skin will be seen to remain intact.

Treatment of calluses is fairly straightforward. The area should be pared with a #15 Bard-Parker blade. A piece of 40% salicylic acid plaster can be cut slightly larger than the lesion, applied sticky side down, and secured with adhesive tape. This plaster can be left on overnight or for as long as five to seven days. When it is removed the whitened, soft, and macerated skin can be removed with a pumice stone or callus file.

Obviously treatment of a callus does nothing to identify the cause. While it may be the pride of many sports veterans, it may be a constant source of discomfort for others. Care must be taken to identify poorly fitting shoes, anatomic malformations, or other factors. Referral to a podiatrist or orthopedic surgeon may be indicated in difficult cases.

Corns or clavi, like calluses, are acquired areas of thickened skin that appear at points of chronic pressure or friction. Unlike calluses, corns are usually painful, especially with pressure, and occur almost exclusively on the foot. Those occurring on the plantar surface of the foot are usually located under the metatarsal arch, and are usually the result of poorly fitting shoes. "Soft" corns are found most often in the fourth interdigital web space and result from pressure of the head of the proximal phalanx of the fifth toe on the base of the proximal phalanx of the fourth toe.

Corns can easily be distinguished from calluses and warts. After paring the lesion a central translucent core that interrupts the normal papillary line pattern becomes obvious, and no blood vessels are seen.

Treatment of a corn should begin with paring, with a view to removing the entire central core (anesthesia may be necessary). As described for calluses, 40% salicylic acid plasters may be used for additional intermittent debridement. Every effort must be made to prevent recurrences by identifying and relieving the source of pressure. Simple ring (doughnut) pads, shoe pads, and metatarsal bars may be effective. Surgical removal of bony spurs or exostoses, or correction of underlying bone or muscle problems may be indicated.

Traumatic alopecia defines that pattern of hair loss that is secondary to physical stress. It is usually recognized as a traction alopecia, the result of prolonged tension in the hair shaft that occurs with the use of hair curlers or with some hair styles (eg, ponytail, braids, tight bun). A short report has described balance beam alopecia.[10] A young gymnast had hair loss from the frontal scalp to the occiput in a linear distribution along either side of the vertex. This was presumed secondary to repeated head stands and rollovers performed on the balance beam.

An abrasion is an injury in which some skin is scraped off, usually in some superficial fashion, and secondary to mechanical trauma. The cause of most abrasions is self-evident; others, such as the abrasion over the midtibia that results from forward leaning in a rigid ski boot, or the mat burns sustained by wrestlers, may be specific for the sport in question.[11]

Superficial abrasions are easily treatable. The wounds should be washed thoroughly with either water or hydrogen peroxide. An antibiotic ointment may be applied and covered with a dry gauze bandage. Washing a wound with alcohol will irritate the skin. Dressings or bandages should be removed for at least part of each day to allow the wound to dry out.

Deep abrasions may need to be cleaned under local anesthesia and in some instances a tetanus shot may be necessary. In such cases a physician should be consulted.

Obviously, the use of protective equipment appropriate for the sport in question will prevent some abrasions. This is especially important in sports where falls are common.

Cold-induced Diseases

Cold-induced injuries can be expected to increase in prevalence in view of the popularity of such winter sports as alpine and cross-country skiing, snowshoeing, mountain climbing, winter backpacking, ice fishing, and snowmobiling. The terminology of these conditions reflects more the circumstances leading to cold injury rather than the underlying pathologic process, since all of them are caused by some combination of cold and wetness.

Pernio represents the mildest form of cold injury and is characterized by the appearance of red to bluish discoloration, edema, nodule formation, and occasionally bullae and ulcerations. It occurs on the hands or feet, and at times on the face, and calves of the legs in a symmetrical fashion. There is pruritus and burning especially upon rewarming, and the nodules may be tender. While the cause is not entirely known, both cold and dampness are necessary for perniones to appear. Shoe boots made of a waterproof outer covering and insulated lining appear to be responsible for cases when the lining becomes wet and cold.[12] As both a preventive and therapeutic measure, the patient should be kept warm, clothing ought to be appropriate for the environment, and footwear needs to be kept dry. Bed rest, elevation of the involved extremities, and suitable topical therapy are indicated for active lesions.

Frostnip, the most common injury seen on the ski slopes, is very early superficial frostbite that may occur on exposed areas of the face, nose, cheek, chin, and ears. For this to occur, temperatures must drop below freezing in the presence of a significant windchill factor.[13] White patches that are numb and insensitive characterize the condition. Rapid rewarming of the area is advised, and is best accomplished by going indoors. The application of protective facial creams prior to skiing or use of a ski mask should prevent frostnip.

Frostbite is severe cold injury that occurs in tissues after freezing from exposure to temperatures below $-2°C$. After thawing, marked inflammation, tissue ischemia, and sometimes gangrene develop. It has been noted that in subfreezing weather, the duration of exposure, wind velocity, and adequacy of protective clothing are important determinants in development and severity of frostbite.[14] Fatigue, injury, immobilization or dependency of an extremity, general body cooling, dehydration, and poor nutrition are also predisposing factors.[14]

Most physicians today classify frostbite as superficial or deep, and treat all cases in an identical fashion since it has been found impossible to predict the final outcome. Evacuation to a treatment facility should be promptly carried out. Rewarming of the frostbitten parts should not be started until the patient can be maintained in a warm environment. Normal use of the affected body parts should be avoided especially if partial thawing has occurred. Smoking and alcohol are absolutely contraindicated. The actual thawing process should be carried out rapidly in a water bath kept at between 40° and 44°C, and the affected areas kept there until the frozen tissues flush a bright pink color. Strong analgesia will be required during this process. After rapid rewarming, the frostbitten area must be protected from trauma and infection. In deep frostbite with no supervening infection, dry gangrene will result in demarcation and autoamputation with little need for surgical intervention. If infection is present wet gangrene will ensue and antibiotics and surgical intervention may be necessary.

Immersion foot develops from prolonged exposure to water insufficient to freeze tissues, usually between 0° and 15°C. It has been called "trench foot" and "seaboot foot"; a shipwrecked sailor, or one who has been adrift in a boat or raft with feet immersed in cold water for long periods of time is the individual most at risk for developing this type of cold injury. The three phases of immersion foot and principles of treatment have been outlined.[15]

Ski cheilitis is a lip disorder resulting not only from cold, but from a combination of cold, wind, and sun.[11] Skiers should protect their lips with a lipstick containing sunscreens.

Heat-induced Disorders

The heat-induced disorders that prove particularly troublesome for athletes are those that relate primarily to eccrine or sweat gland function and dysfunction. It must be kept in mind that sweating results in evaporative heat loss, which is a normal thermoregulatory function. It is the exaggeration of this normal process often coupled with pathologic states of sweat glands themselves, that creates the problems.

Hyperhidrosis is an increase above normal in sweat production. While excessive sweating is often a subjective impression and often only a cause of social embarrassment, hyperhidrosis may be a significant factor in the development of several cutaneous bacterial and fungal diseases, and contact dermatitis. Localized hyperhidrosis of the palms probably represents the most troublesome problem for athletes; it can obviously interfere with the normal performance of all racket sports, baseball, golf, and so forth. In most instances palmar hyperhidrosis and the associated plantar and axillary hyperhidrosis are the result of emotional stress and not in response to heat. The emotional stress may be the normal consequence of participation in competitive sports or may reflect underlying mental strain. For some, the simple use of a variety of grip-aids or gloves will satisfactorily solve the problem. However treatment with aluminum salts will be necessary in the more severe cases. A 20% aluminum chloride in 80% absolute anhydrous alcohol solution is applied to absolutely dry skin, covered with a plastic wrap, and left in place for six to eight hours. It may be necessary to do this daily for several days until the desired degree of anhidrosis is achieved. Thereafter, repeat treatments at intervals of three to five days may be adequate to control the problem. Systemic anticholinergic and sedative drugs are of limited value, primarily because of their unpleasant and undesirable side effects.

Anhidrosis (absence of sweating) **and hyphidrosis** (reduction below the normal level of sweating) are caused by a variety of neuropathic, congenital, and acquired sweat gland disturbances, and miscellaneous idiopathic disease states. Consideration of these conditions is beyond the scope of this chapter. However, it is important to make note of one common cause of anhidrosis/hyphidrosis, which can be life-threatening, that is very applicable to summer athletes: that is dehydration. An individual who exercises or exerts himself in hot, and especially hot and humid weather, can sweat profusely and become profoundly dehydrated. Simple heat exhaustion may result from this fluid loss, and depending on the degree of anhidrosis that is present body temperature will rise accordingly. If body temperature rises too high (eg, 110°F) heat stroke will result. Both heat exhaustion and heat stroke are easily preventable by appropriate fluid replacement and limiting exercise during periods of extreme heat.

Miliaria, or heat rash, designates that group of disorders that results from the trapping of sweat at some point in the skin. Miliaria crystallina occurs when sweat is trapped within the stratum corneum, the uppermost portion of the epidermis. Miliaria rubra, or prickly heat, results when sweat blockage occurs within the viable portion of the epidermis, and miliaria profunda is the result of sweat blockage within the upper dermis.

Miliaria crystallina is generally asymptomatic and is commonly seen after a mild sunburn, when the subsequent outpouring of sweat secondary to activity is blocked by the mild damage that has resulted to the stratum corneum. The vesicles that result appear most commonly on exposed areas and subside rapidly when sweating ceases and/or the damaged stratum corneum sloughs off.

Miliaria rubra is seen in both hot humid, and hot dry climates; in both settings the lesions are located on areas of the body covered by clothing. The rash is characterized by erythematous papulovesicles, and occasionally pustules. They are nonfollicular in distribution and usually cause stinging, burning, or itching (prickly sensations). The lesions fade after several days if there have not been renewed episodes of excessive sweating.

Miliaria profunda is seen almost exclusively in hot tropical climates and invariably after recurrent episodes of miliaria rubra. The lesion is a whitish papule giving the appearance of gooseflesh, and is asymptomatic. Patients usually develop a state of heat intolerance termed tropical anhidrotic asthenia.

The key to treatment of miliaria is placing the individual in a cool environment. In this setting the keratinous plugs blocking the sweat ducts are eventually shed, and the lesion will remit. Excessive sweating must cease; adequate ventilation and lightweight clothing are helpful; an air conditioned environment is ideal. It is generally felt that topical therapy is of little benefit, but powders and lotions such as calamine lotion may absorb some of the sweat and afford symptomatic relief.

Erythema ab igne is characterized by a persistent reticulated erythema in association with hyperpigmentation and venular telangiectasis. Traditionally the condition occurs in people who habitually warm their legs in front of an open fire (a problem perhaps for the "après skier"). Similar changes may result from the use of an electric heating pad or hot water bottle used to treat painful joints or muscles. Prolonged exposure to intense local heat is necessary for the process to develop, but once changes are noted they are usually irreversible.

Sun-induced Disorders

With the increased interest in sports and outdoor recreation in recent years, it is indeed fortunate that people have finally come to recognize more fully the potential hazards of chronic and excessive sun exposure. This may even be more relevant a concern in the near future, if the amount of ultraviolet radiation reaching the earth's surface increases because of changes in the ozone layer.

The UV (ultraviolet) spectrum of light extends from wavelengths of 200 nm (nanometers) to wavelengths of 400 nm. This spectrum is divided into three bands: UVA (320 to 400 nm), UVB (280 to 320 nm), and UVC (200 to 280 nm). UVA is responsible for most photosensitivity eruptions; UVB causes sunburn, tanning, and, after chronic exposure, aging of skin; UVC is absorbed by the ozone layer but can cause sunburn.

While sunburn is caused primarily by excessive exposure to UVB, UVA may assist in causing this effect. Sunburn may clearly vary in severity from just slight redness of the skin with tenderness to touch and a feeling of warmth, to a severe blistering reaction with intense pain and constitutional symptoms. The severity of a sunburn depends on several variables, mainly, the amount and intensity of UV light, and the amount of protective pigment in a person's skin. Nearness to the equator, the season of the year, and elevation above sea level are obvious variables. However, it should be noted that UVB is not filtered out by thin clouds on overcast days, and that snow, sand, and water each reflect UV light to a varying extent thus enhancing exposure. Wind can also intensify sun exposure. Smoke and smog around large cities partially diminish the amount of incident UVB, and window glass fully absorbs UVB. Those people with less melanin pigment in their skin, including blue-eyed persons, redheads, blondes, and frecklers, are in general more easily burned. However, even darkly pigmented individuals can sunburn with prolonged and intense exposure to UV light.

Prevention of sunburn is easy if one pays attention to all of the variables, follows some common sense rules, and uses sunscreen and/or sunshade agents. Clothing is only partially protective, and hats and umbrellas provide only moderate protection. If one can acquire a tan, it should be done gradually. The increased pigment will ultimately be protective. For those who do not tan, the use of sunscreens and sunshades is mandatory.

Sunscreen agents are chemicals that absorb UV light and sunshade agents reflect UV light. The most useful group of sunscreens are those that absorb UVB radiation; this will prevent sunburn but allow tanning to occur. The most effective of these UVB screens contain PABA (paraaminobenzoic acid) or PABA esters. Five percent PABA in alcohol is more effective than 5% PABA esters, but the latter do not stain clothing and do not wash off the skin as easily with swimming or sweating. Benzophenone compounds absorb UVB and UVA but are less effective than PABA compounds in the UVB range. Many newer products contain combinations of PABA esters and benzophenones and provide a suitable alternative to 5% PABA in alcohol for most people. Individuals who are sensitive or allergic to PABA-containing products can more than adequately protect themselves with preparations containing cinnamates and benzophenones. Sunshades usually contain titanium dioxide or zinc oxide powders; they are very effective but cosmetically unattractive and impractical to use over the entire body. Lipstick sunscreens give best protection in the UVB range.

Treatment of sunburn depends partly on its severity. Mild sunburn can be treated with cool tapwater compresses, emollients, and topical corticosteroid sprays, lotions, or creams. Topical anesthetic preparations, especially those containing benzocaine or antihistamines should not be used because of the hazard of developing sensitization to these drugs. Treatment of severe sunburn should include the above measures as well as consideration of a short course of systemic steroids (eg, prednisone, 40 to 60 mg daily for 3 days) and analgesics for pain. Aspirin if administered immediately after an excessive amount of sun exposure and used for the first 24 hours, may actually decrease the severity of the anticipated sunburn, as well as provide sufficient analgesia.

While sunburn is of immediate relevance to most athletes, we cannot ignore the chronic cumulative effects of UV light on the skin. These effects are obviously of greater concern to fair-skinned individuals. Aging of the skin is accelerated by chronic and excessive sun exposure. Sun-induced freckling (solar lentigo) as well as sun-induced pigment loss (idiopathic guttate hypomelanosis) are features of sun-damaged skin as much as the dry, wrinkled atrophic telangiectatic appearance. Of somewhat greater concern is the development of rough, red, scaly lesions called actinic keratoses. While these lesions are not serious in themselves, and are easily treatable, some one-eighth of patients with actinic keratoses will have one or more of these lesions develop into a squamous cell carcinoma. The most common type of skin cancer, the basal cell carcinoma, arises de novo from sun-damaged skin. Fortunately both basal cell carcinomas and sun-induced squamous cell carcinomas rarely metastasize and as such are easily curable by any one of several surgical modalities (eg, cryosurgery, electrosurgery, "cold steel" excision), or by radiation therapy. Regular use by people at risk of a UVB and UVA sunscreen can be expected to minimize most of these developments.

Photosensitivity reactions result from the interaction of UV light, usually UVA, with some drug or chemical present in the skin at the time of sun exposure. The drug may be acquired either systemically or topically. In either case people with the problem will show an exaggerated response to sun exposure developing a rash that may have a variety of clinical presentations. An athlete is at risk only if he or she is exposed to sun while taking one of these photosensitizing drugs or having contact with some photosensitizing chemical. The list of agents that may cause photosensitivity is long and can be found in standard reference textbooks of dermatology. It includes antibiotics, artificial sweeteners, oral diabetic medications, diuretics, plant oils, heart medications, sunscreens, tranquilizers, and coal tars. Any individual who develops a sun sensitivity should consult a dermatologist.

INFECTIONS

Bacterial Infections

Sports activities may contribute to the development of specific bacterial infections, but the contagious nature of some routine infections should also be of concern to supervisors and athletes. Contact sports, especially wrestling, present the greatest opportunity for development of epidemic bacterial infections. Early identification and treatment, as well as temporary removal from active participation, are mandatory. The last precaution pertains primarily to individuals with impetigo and certain forms of folliculitis (eg, sycosis barbae) and is less relevant when some other infections are considered.

Impetigo may be caused by either group A beta-hemolytic streptococci or coagulase-positive *Staphylococcus aureus*. Streptococcal impetigo is very contagious among young people but less so in adults. The initial lesion is a small blister that fills with pus and rapidly breaks leaving a red, oozing erosion surmounted by a thick honey or golden yellow crust. Staphylococcal impetigo begins as a flaccid blister that becomes cloudy and is rapidly replaced by a thin varnishlike crust. Factors such as warm climate, poor personal hygiene, and other antecedent skin conditions such as scabies, eczema, or contact dermatitis may contribute to the development of either type of impetigo. Both streptococcal and staphylococcal impetigo should be treated with systemic antibiotics and the advice of a physician should be sought. In most instances either penicillin, a penicillinase-resistant penicillin, or erythromycin will be used.

Folliculitis is a staphylococcal infection of the hair follicle that may be superficial or deep. Frictional trauma, maceration of the skin, occlusive clothing, and poor hygiene are some factors that predispose to folliculitis. A lesion begins as a pustule around the follicular opening; frequently a hair can be seen piercing the pustule and with time a crust replaces the pustule. If the infection is deep, a furuncle or boil can result, and occasionally a local cellulitis will develop. In most instances superficial folliculitis may be treated with an antimicrobial cleanser and topical antibiotics. Folliculitis of the male beard area, so-called sycosis barbae, or an extensive or deep folliculitis, should be treated with systemic antibiotics, either a semi-synthetic penicillin or erythromycin. Furuncles may need surgical incision and drainage. Compresses with moist heat may encourage pointing to occur, and facilitate treatment.

Erythrasma is a superficial infection of intertriginous areas—toe webs, axillae, groin, inframammary and intergluteal folds—that is caused by *Corynebacterium minutissimum.* It is seen more commonly in the tropics, and local moisture factors clearly predispose to infection. The eruption is characterized by sharply demarcated, dry, finely scaling, slightly erythematous-to-brownish skin. Diagnosis can often be confirmed by the demonstration of a coral pink to orange red fluorescence on examination of the affected area by a Wood light in a darkened room. The fluorescence of lesions may be diminished after bathing or washing with an antimicrobial soap. Wearing loose clothing, keeping as dry as possible, and washing with an antimicrobial soap may prevent infection. Once established, the infection may be treated with keratolytic agents such as 3% sulfur and salicylic acid ointment, but the treatment of choice is oral erythromycin, 1 gm per day, for one to two weeks.

Pitted keratolysis, an asymptomatic non-inflammatory bacterial infection of the stratum corneum caused by a *Corynebacterium,* is characterized by the appearance of discrete pits or craters in the stratum corneum of the soles and occasionally the palms. The tan to brown pits may coalesce to form large areas of erosion in which soil or mud may accumulate, giving the feet a dirty appearance. Pressure areas are more affected and excessive hydration from either hyperhidrosis, occlusive footwear, or water immersion predisposes to and accentuates the problem. The condition may spontaneously regress with elimination of moisture; topical application of a 5% formalin solution or oral erythromycin is effective in clearing the problem.

Erysipeloid, *Mycobacterium marinum* infection, and tularemia are less commonly encountered but nonetheless deserve mention. Erysipeloid is found in fishermen who handle fish or shellfish infected with *Erysipelothrix rhusiopathiae,* a gram-positive bacillus. The skin lesion is found on the hands as a red or purplish urticarial plaque that may become arciform or annular. Fever, malaise, and regional adenopathy may be present. The majority of cases probably resolve spontaneously in two to three weeks. Penicillin is the drug of choice when the diagnosis is made. Gloves should be worn when preparing fish, to prevent inoculation of the bacterium.

Mycobacterium marinum infection is commonly called "swimming pool granuloma." It results from the cutaneous inoculation of a variety of atypical mycobacteria that may be present not only in swimming pools but also in salt, brackish, or fresh water, including home aquariums. The skin lesions appear within two to six weeks and occur at points of trauma, most frequently the elbow or knee, but occasionally on the dorsal aspect of hands and feet. They present as erythematous or violaceous nodules that infrequently ulcerate or become verrucous. The lesions are asymptomatic and there are no systemic reactions. Confirmation of the diagnosis requires culturing the organism from a suspected lesion since the histology is not specific. Spontaneous resolution occurs after a variable time period which may be as long as two to three years. The organism is resistant to antituberculous medicine but tetracycline, 2 gm daily, administered for two to four months, has been reportedly successful.[16] Surgical excision of small lesions is probably the simplest and most expeditious therapy. Adequate chlorination of swimming pools is satisfactory for control of the bacterium in that setting.

Tularemia is usually acquired by hunters who handle or skin infected cottontail rabbits, but the infection may be acquired from arthropod bites (eg, ticks) or from eating inadequately cooked, infected rabbit meat. The disease is caused by a gram-negative bacillus *Francisella tularensis.* The skin lesion is nonspecific and consists of a small, indurated, ulcer with surrounding erythema and cellulitis. There may be a variety of systemic signs and symptoms. (A more complete discussion of tularemia can be found in standard medical textbooks.)

Swimmer's ear constitutes an acute diffuse external otitis. The classic symptoms are itching progressing to severe pain, tenderness of the ear canal, a blocked feeling of the ear, and pain on chewing. There is edema, tenderness of the canal and of the antauricular and subauricular area, and the presence of a thin greenish secretion. Fever may be present with associated fatigue and malaise. The etiology of this condition is obscure, but most likely represents a bacterial infection caused by the macerating effect of water and failure to dry the ear properly after swimming. The organism most frequently associated with swimmer's ear has been *Pseudomonas* but streptococci and staphylococci are also found. A combination of polymyxin B, colistin, and neomycin is used topically in the treatment of this condition but consultation with an ear-nose-throat physician is recommended.

Fungal Infections

Among the dermatophyte (or ringworm) fungi and the yeastlike fungus *Candida albicans* several patterns of infection are particularly common in athletes.

Dermatophyte infections include athlete's foot and jock itch of the feet and groin respectively. Dermatophyte fungi can be found in the soil and on animals. Some species only infect humans and cannot survive in other hosts. Dermatophyte fungi live in the superficial layers of the epidermis, in hair, and in nails and the spectrum of clinical infection is broad. Tinea pedis and tinea cruris are particularly common in athletes since heat, friction, maceration, and occlusive footwear are all predisposing factors. The causative fungi may be found in shoes, flooring, and clothing, often in the latter location many months after laundering. Tinea cruris and pedis frequently coexist and the patient who has the former should be examined for evidence of the latter.

Many infections are asymptomatic but pruritus, if present, is the most common symptom. Tinea cruris affects both the groin and upper inner thigh, is often symmetrical, and almost always spares the penis and scrotum. The eruption may be erythematous and scaly with evidence of an active margin, or in acute cases vesicular, weeping, and excoriated. Adjacent areas may ultimately become involved. Tinea pedis has three distinctive presentations that at times blend into one another. Interdigital toe web infection is characterized by maceration, fissuring, and scaling, most often between the fourth and fifth toes. The vesiculobullous variety involves the instep and is frequently associated with an acute inflammation resembling cellulitis. The hyperkeratotic infection involves the entire sole, with redness, scaling, and thickening of the horny layer, the stratum corneum. Fungal infection of the toenails, onychomycosis, is frequently found in association with tinea pedis.

Good treatment of fungal infections should include prophylactic preventive measures as well as local antifungal therapy. Good hygiene, thorough drying of intertriginous areas after bathing, loose, clean clothing, well-fitting nonocclusive footwear, absorbant cotton socks, and liberal use of talcum powder or an antifungal powder are some measures one can take to prevent development of fungal infections. For most infections, topical therapy with clotrimazole, miconazole, or tolnaftate, twice or three times daily for two to four weeks will be adequate to clear the infection. Hyperkeratotic infections of the soles of the feet often require concomitant keratolytic therapy, and vesiculobullous infections require astringent compresses. Extensive body infections may require treatment with griseofulvin, a systemic antifungal antibiotic. Onychomycosis is almost never cured by topical measures, and long-term administration of griseofulvin coupled with surgical avulsion of the involved toenails offers the only reasonable chance of cure. Consultation with a dermatologist should be sought.

The yeastlike fungus *Candida albicans* normally inhabits the skin, mucous membranes, and gastrointestinal tract. Under certain circumstances it can become pathogenic and cause a variety of cutaneous or mucous membrane diseases. A candidal intertrigo would likely be the most common clinical expression of infection in the active athlete. The same circumstances that predispose to infection with dermatophyte predispose to candidal infection, ie, moisture, warmth, maceration, and/or occlusion. The inframammary, axillary, groin, perianal, and interdigital areas can be involved. The lesions are red and moist ("beefy red"), macerated in the folds, with scaling or peeling at the margins, and often surrounded by satellite erythematous papules or pustules.

Treatment of intertriginous candidal infections consists of both eliminating conditions leading to moisture and maceration, and drying the areas involved. Warm light bulbs, breeze from a fan, or air conditioning all will promote drying; cool compresses with water or Burow solution are also helpful. Specific anticandidal creams or lotions such as clotrimazole or nystatin should be applied three to four times daily. In especially inflammatory infections these may be used in conjunction with 1% hydrocortisone creams or lotions. Nystatin powder is useful prophylactically but it should be noted that tolnaftate and griseofulvin are ineffective.

Tinea versicolor is a chronic, superficial, asymptomatic fungal infection of the skin, located most commonly on the trunk. It consists of white to pink to tan, scaly, macular patches that may coalesce. Examination with a Wood light may reveal a gold-to-orange fluorescence. Tinea versicolor may be treated in several ways. The most commonly used agents are Tinver lotion, applied twice daily for several weeks, and selenium sulfide suspensions, applied to the areas for 15 to 30 minutes daily for one week. Retreatment is frequently necessary.

Sporotrichosis is a deep fungal infection that results from the traumatic inoculation of the causative organism, *Sporotrichum schenckii,* into the skin. An ulcerated, painless nodule develops at the inoculation site to be followed by the appearance of one or more painless nodules along a local lymphatic vessel. While typically seen in farmers, gardeners, and miners, the hunter, hiker, rock climber, and fisherman are clearly at risk. The treatment of choice remains a saturated solution of potassium iodide (SSKI).

Viral Infections

Herpes simplex infections of the skin are by far the most common and potentially the most serious of cutaneous viral infections. Herpes simplex infections can be either primary in nature, the type seen in individuals who have had no past exposure or contact with the herpes simplex virus, or recurrent, the pattern most of us recognize as cold sores or fever blisters. Approximately 85% to 90% of people will have had a primary infection by the end of their adolescence. Recurrent herpes simplex infection represents reactivation or recrudescence of an established latent infection, the recurrence appearing usually at the site of the primary infection. Approximately 75% of people previously infected with herpes will at some time have a recurrent episode. It is important to note that people who have recurrent herpes simplex can reacquire the virus, that is to say, can develop a new primary infection. This is usually secondary to cutaneous inoculation of the virus. The clinical manifestations of this new primary infection are usually mild and indistinguishable from a typical recurrent episode. Thereafter such individuals may have recurrent infection at more than one site.

The entire spectrum of clinical manifestations in primary herpes simplex infections is too broad a subject to cover in this chapter. Suffice to say, the primary infection can be severe with extensive cutaneous lesions, pain, fever, toxicity, and tender adenopathy. On the other hand, recurrent infections are usually mild, localized, and not associated with fever or significant adenopathy. There may, of course, be pain and tenderness and a prodrome consisting of a burning or tingling sensation at the site of the recurrence. The severity of primary inoculation type herpes simplex in the previously exposed individual depends partly on the level of acquired immunity, and partly on the quantity of the viral inoculum.

Consideration of the preceding remarks is important for an understanding of the spectrum of clinical infections in the athlete. Recurrent herpes simplex of the lip (herpes labialis, cold sore), for example, can be precipitated not only by fever and other viral infections, but also by sunlight. For athletes in noncontact sports such as track and field, skiing, hiking, and baseball, ultraviolet-induced recurrences of herpes simplex constitute the worst problem. Athletes who participate in contact sports such as wrestling or rugby are at risk for acquiring primary inoculation herpes simplex.

The clinical picture of herpetic infections in the early states is typical and easily recognizable. There is a clustering of small, often erythematous vesicles arising from skin. The vesicles are initially clear but they rapidly become cloudy, purulent, and then dry and crust usually over a period of seven to ten days. The lesions may become bacterially superinfected, and at times multiple small vesicles may coalesce and evolve into a single erosion. Any area of the body can be involved. For the wrestler with inoculation infection, this is usually the cheek or the inside of the arm that contacts the face. In rugby players the major site is the scalp; in basketball players sites are the knees, elbows, and shoulders. Herpetic infections of the eyes are especially troublesome. Individuals with a history of atopic dermatitis, regardless of whether or not their eczema is active, risk developing a generalized infection.

It is clearly imperative to identify athletes with active herpetic infections and remove them from team or contact competition. Since the individual is contagious for the first five days (120 hours) after the vesicles arise, an athlete should be removed for at least that length of time and perhaps even until the disease heals. Except for individuals with sun-induced herpes, there are no preventive or prophylactic measures of proven merit. The use of lipstick sunscreens will help to prevent recurrent herpes labialis, and the broader use of sunscreen lotions on the skin may prevent sun-induced infections of other skin sites.

There are as yet no proven topical or systemic medications that predictably alter the course of herpes simplex infections. Drying of lesions in the vesicular stage can be accomplished with astringent compresses (eg, Burow solution). After a crust appears, application of an antibiotic ointment will both soften a crust, making it somewhat less painful to smile, for example, and prevent bacterial superinfection. Ocular infections should be seen and treated by an ophthalmologist but the antiviral antibiotics (idoxuridine, adenine arabinoside) effective for herpes simplex keratitis are largely ineffective when used on the skin except when combined with DMSO, a preparation unavailable in the United States.

Molluscum contagiosum is a viral tumor of man caused by a DNA-containing pox virus. The lesions are characterized by the formation of discrete, flesh-colored or pearly white papules, 1 to 5 mm in diameter, with a central dimple on the surface. There may be few or many lesions. The face, trunk, lower abdomen, pubis, inner thighs, and genitals may be involved. The contagious nature of the disease has been supported by numerous reports concerning direct human contact. The disease has been noted in wrestlers, masseurs, and those who frequent Turkish baths and gymnasiums. Molluscum lesions can be treated either with liquid nitrogen, curettage, or application of cantharidin.

Warts are also virally induced growths of the skin caused by a DNA virus of the papova group. Common warts, plantar warts, flat, and filiform warts are easily recognizable lesions that induce few symptoms unless because of their size and/or location they become painful or awkward. The wart virus can be transmitted by direct or indirect contact as well as by autoinoculation, but transmission among athletes does not appear to be a recognizable problem as it is for the molluscum virus. The primary problem for athletes is the interference with optimal performance that can be caused by a painful wart (eg, plantar) or by a wart in some disadvantageous position (eg, fingers or hands). There are many therapeutic modalities available for the treatment of warts and to a large extent treatments need to be individualized. In general, cryosurgery with liquid nitrogen is the best therapy for common warts of the fingers and hands, but keratolytic therapy with salicylic and lactic acid paints can be equally successful. Plantar warts are best treated conservatively since electrosurgery and sharp scalpel excision often lead to the development of a painful scar. Cryosurgery is acceptable therapy but very uncomfortable during the actual application of liquid nitrogen. Often the best approach, and this is especially true for large mosaic plantar warts, is the application of 80% tri- or monochloroacetic acid and 40% salicylic acid plasters following surgical paring of the lesions. This treatment can be repeated every two to three weeks until the warts resolve.

INJURIES ACQUIRED FROM LIVING CREATURES

This section will highlight man's encounter with the living world of arthropods, a variety of aquatic life, and reptiles. It is in no way a comprehensive treatment of the subject but rather will focus on those disorders with broader epidemiologic importance for athletes involved in team and contact sports. The intent is not to minimize the importance or seriousness of any one individual's contact with these animals; the implications of many of these encounters, however, transcends the cutaneous barrier and calls for the knowledge and expertise of a variety of medical and nonmedical specialists.

Arthropods

There are two classes of arthropods with which man frequently interacts—the arachnids and insects. Arachnids of medical importance include scorpions, spiders, ticks, and mites; the insects of importance are flies, mosquitos, bees, wasps, ants, lice, and fleas.

Scorpions capable of causing death to man are found only in tropical or subtropical desert areas, and infants are by far at greatest risk. Few people over the age of 15 perish from scorpion bites. Scorpions inject a hemolytic venom that can produce a severe local reaction as well as systemic symptoms. In severe cases an antiscorpion venom administered early can significantly improve chances of survival.

Two genera of spiders, *Latrodectus* and *Loxosceles,* are responsible for most of the serious spider bites in the United States. Spider bites can result in allergic or toxic reactions, but by far the most serious reaction encountered is a toxic one caused by a species of *Latrodectus,* the black widow spider. The brown recluse spider is a member of the *Loxosceles* genus, and it too, can produce a severe local and systemic reaction. The local clinical picture following the bite of a brown recluse is more impressive than that following the bite of a black widow. The latter often shows just slight redness or edema while the former results in a gangrenous slough of skin that may require grafting. Identification of the spider that caused the bite is important because treatment of the systemic reaction differs. Brown recluse reactions are treated with systemic steroids. Black widow reactions require injection of an antivenom prepared in horses.

Ticks are large relatives of mites whose bite is painless; they are noticed often only after they have become engorged from sucking blood or when mild pruritus develops. The risk from tick bites includes the acquisition of rickettsial infections (eg, Rocky Mountain spotted fever), and erythema chronicum migrans (Lyme arthritis syndrome). Local tick bite granulomas can occur. The tick should not be forcibly plucked off but should be coaxed to release itself by applying chloroform, mineral oil, or gasoline. In some instances complete removal will be possible using a pair of forceps. Touching the body of the tick with a hot nail or a just extinguished matchhead may also cause it to release itself but at the risk of accidentally burning the individual. Protection against tick infestation is best accomplished by applying the insect repellant diethyltoluamide to clothing.

Infestations with the itch mite *Sarcoptes scabiei,* var. *hominis,* produces the extremely pruritic condition we call scabies. Scabies is highly communicable and is acquired principally through close personal contact, but it may be transmitted by fomites such as clothing, linens, and towels in which the female mite may survive for one or two days. Miniepidemics can easily occur. Scabies constitutes a significant risk not only for athletes involved in such sports as wrestling, rugby, basketball, and football but also for team members sharing locker facilities, uniforms, towels, etc. The primary symptom is pruritus, which seems to become more marked after the individual goes to bed (nocturnal pruritus). The principal finding is the scabietic burrow, a thin, threadlike, S-shaped ridge or line 5 to 20 mm long; more commonly one will find only papules, vesicles, excoriations, and nonspecific eczematous patches. The lesions are located in the interdigital webs of the hands, the wrists, elbows, nipples, umbilicus, lower abdomen, genitalia, and gluteal cleft. Erythematous nodules on the glans penis and scrotum are common. The diagnosis of scabies can be confirmed by demonstration of the mite from scrapings taken from a burrow, papule, or vesicle and examined under a microscope. Eggs and fecal material are also diagnostic but in the absence of positive identification the clinical picture suffices for a correct diagnosis in most cases.

Scabies is most commonly treated with gamma benzene hexachloride lotion applied to the entire body from the neck down and left on for 12 to 24 hours at which time it is washed off. The treatment is repeated in one week in order to destroy any recently hatched larvae or nymphs. Antihistamines and topical steroids are useful in relieving some of the pruritus and hastening resolution of the allergic, eczematous component. Family, close friends, sexual contacts, and team members all should be considered for treatment to prevent reinfection and miniepidemics. Clothing and linens of affected individuals may be specially hot-washed or dry cleaned, but no specific insecticidal measures are necessary for furniture, rugs, bathrooms, and so forth.

Most of us need little introduction to the world of stinging and biting insects, for it is likely that few if any have failed to be visited by one of these creatures. In general, the local reactions to these bites and stings are well recognized. Flea bites appear as pruritic, grouped urticarial papules, some with central punctum, often on the legs. Fly bites vary in morphology depending on genus and species, but are generally painful or pruritic papules, nodules, or vesicles that may last for weeks to months. Mosquito bites result in pruritic wheals. Stings from bees and wasps result in immediate burning and pain followed by swelling and itching. Fire ants produce a more severe local reaction with hemorrhage, vesiculation, crusting, and scar formation. Lice also parasitize humans. However, the vast majority of serious reactions to insects that bite and sting are not local, but those that result in anaphylaxis because of an acquired hypersensitivity. Over twice as many people die yearly from bee or wasp stings in this country, as die from rattlesnake bites. Prompt treatment for people with such hypersensitivity reactions is mandatory, preferably in a hospital equipped to handle acute respiratory and cardiovascular emergencies. (Medical texts contain discussions of treatment of anaphylaxis and anaphylactic shock.)

Prophylaxis against stinging insects is the best medicine. Insect repellants containing diethyltoluamide are effective against mosquitos, flies, and fleas, but need to be reapplied frequently in hot, windy weather and to all exposed areas. Clothing can also be treated as can nets, tents, and sleeping bags. Unfortunately, no insect repellant will protect against wasps, hornets, bees, and yellow jackets. Anyone who has ever experienced a severe local reaction or developed urticaria and respiratory symptoms from the sting of one of these insects, should have with him at all times during the bee/wasp season, an emergency epinephrine injection kit. The individual should probably also carry some epinephrine inhalation spray, ephedrine tablets, and antihistamines. Sensitive individuals should also see an allergist for evaluation and consideration of desensitization. A pure venom extract product for immunotherapy has now been FDA-approved and is sold under the trade name Pharmalgen. These venom injections are not curative, but 70% of individuals who undergo therapy will show complete protection, and 30% partial protection, against future stinging insect reactions.

Blood-sucking lice parasitize man in three forms: the head louse *(Pediculus humanus),* the body louse *(Pediculus humanus,* var. *corporis),* and the pubic or "crab" louse *(Phthirus pubis).* The head louse is transmitted through shared clothing and brushes; the body louse by bedding and clothing; and the pubic louse by personal contact and occasionally by fomites such as clothing, bedding, or towels. The epidemiologic implications already discussed for scabies are applicable to lice infestations. Miniepidemics can easily occur.

The main symptom of lice infestation is pruritus. The skin findings are often meager when dealing with the head or body louse, since these lice are rarely present on the body and often impossible to find on the scalp because of the small number usually present. Nits are present on the hair shaft and there may be secondary infection from chronic scratching. The skin manifestations of the body louse are rather nonspecific as well. Excoriations, eczematous changes, hives, and persistent papules are present at times. The findings with pubic lice are usually more striking, with numerous nits and readily demonstrable adult organisms. Body and axillary hair, as well as the eyelashes, may be infested.

The treatment of pubic lice is identical to that described for scabies except that the gamma benzene hexachloride lotion need be applied only to infested and adjacent areas. Clothing, linens, and towels should be washed in very hot water or dry cleaned. Lice on eyelashes can be treated with physostigmine ophthalmic ointment. Head lice should be treated with gamma benzene hexachloride shampoo; with body lice it is usually necessary only to treat the infested clothing and the skin washed with soap and water. In cases of head and pubic lice, nits should be removed from the hair with a fine-toothed comb. Contacts of affected individuals should also be considered for treatment.

Aquatic Life

The sea offers unpleasant surprises to those swimmers, scuba divers, surfers, fishermen, and beachcombers unfortunate enough to encounter one of a number of venomous marine animals. Coelenterata (including the jellyfish, man-of-war, sea anemone, and coral), sea urchins, sponges, cone shells, stonefish, stingrays, and catfish are just some examples of marine life capable of producing severe local dermatitis as well as fatal systemic reactions. Fortunately the number of fatalities from encounters with these animals is extremely small in comparison to the number of fatalities due to bee and wasp stings. It will not be possible to discuss each of these animals and the diseases they produce in this chapter. For those interested in pursuing this subject, a recently published atlas covers this subject matter in a well-illustrated and comprehensive fashion.[17]

There are two disorders not caused by venomous creatures that should be mentioned. One is swimmer's itch, a schistosomal cercarial dermatitis characterized by pruritic papules resulting from the inflammatory reaction to cercariae at their point of entry into the skin. It is acquired from swimming in fresh water, especially the small lakes of the Midwest. The course is self-limited and only symptomatic treatment is necessary.

The other disorder is sea-bather's eruption. This condition results from salt-water swimming off Florida and in the Caribbean. It is clinically similar to swimmer's itch, but not traceable to cercarial penetration. It too, is self-limited and requires only symptomatic treatment.

Reptiles

Gila monsters, rattlesnakes, water moccasins, copperheads, and coral snakes are the only venomous reptiles in the United States. The rattlesnake is by far the most commonly encountered. It is a pit viper that injects a hemolytic toxin responsible for both the local and systemic manifestations of the snakebite. Water moccasins and copperheads are also pit vipers; the coral snake and Gila monster secrete a neurotoxin. First aid measures should be instituted promptly. Immobilize the bitten part; make an incision over the fang marks and apply suction from a rubber cup; get the victim to a hospital as soon as possible.

CONTACT DERMATITIS

People involved in athletic activities are exposed to a wide variety of potential irritants and sensitizers. These materials can cause two types of reaction patterns in the skin: primary irritant contact dermatitis and allergic contact dermatitis.

The primary irritant contact dermatitis is a nonallergic reaction of the skin caused by exposure to irritating substances. In general, any substance can act as an irritant provided the concentration and duration of contact are sufficient. An allergic contact dermatitis implies that sensitization has occurred, and exposure to the offending contact allergen will result in a reaction only in such sensitized individuals.

Irritant dermatitis is encountered far more frequently than allergic dermatitis. In both instances, however, the skin reaction takes the form of an eczematous dermatitis. There may be erythema, vesiculation, oozing, crusting in the acute stages of both types of reactions; in the chronic phases of an irritant reaction one is likely to find dry, scaly, thickened, fissured skin. The distinguishing features of an irritant or allergic dermatitis, however, are not in the morphology of lesions but in their distribution and configuration. The eruption is confined to the areas of contact and may have a bizarre or artificial pattern with, for example, straight margins or acute angles.

The items that commonly cause allergic contact dermatitis in athletes are plants, topical medicaments, rubber and leather products, grip aids, and clothing.[1] Plants causing contact dermatitis include poison ivy, poison oak, and poison sumac. Topical medications include antibiotics, anesthetics, antiseptics, liniments and "rubbing" compounds, and moisturizers. Rubber articles such as straps, pads, bands, shoes, hand grips, adhesive tapes, kneepads, swimming equipment, and rubber balls can cause allergic contact dermatitis as can leather articles such as gloves, shoes, jackets, headbands, chin straps, and balls. Grip aids include rosin, beeswax, and tincture of benzoin. A primary irritant dermatitis frequently is due to repeated or prolonged contact with soaps, detergents, and solvents, and not infrequently is the result of excessive hygienic measures.

Since successful treatment of contact dermatitis involves avoidance of the offending contactant, assessment of patients should involve careful and detailed questioning about the individual's total environment and personal habits. In some instances patch testing will be necessary for specific identification of the allergen. For an acute dermatitis treatment should include Burow compresses or soaks and application of topical steroid creams. In severe cases, a course of systemic steroids may be necessary; prednisone, at an initial dose of 60 mg daily, can be instituted and tapered over two to three weeks. Chronic dermatitis requires frequent use of lubricants in addition to topical steroid ointments. As with many other skin problems of athletes, it is frequently necessary to eliminate or minimize the effects of heat, humidity, friction, and maceration.

EXACERBATION OF EXISTING SKIN PROBLEMS

Many preexisting cutaneous problems can be exacerbated by athletic activities. The following sections make note of the most important of these conditions.

Physical Urticarias

Several types of physical urticaria including cold, cholinergic, dermatographism and pressure, and solar urticaria are found more frequently in athletes. It has been reported[18] that 14% of sportsmen with chronic urticaria of all types had a physical urticaria, compared to a 2.4% incidence in a group of general dermatology patients with chronic urticaria. Of the various types, cold-induced urticaria was found most frequently. Treatment of physical urticarias must be tailored to the clinical type present. In general, therapy is difficult and disappointing.

Raynaud Disease and Phenomenon

Raynaud disease is an idiopathic hypersensitivity to cold; Raynaud phenomenon represents the identical cold hypersensitivity but secondary to a number of diseases such as scleroderma, lupus erythematosus, and cryoglobulinemia. It may occur occasionally as a sequela of frostbite. In both instances, a triphasic reaction of pallor, cyanosis, and hyperemia develops symmetrically, involving fingers and/or toes. There is initial numbness and pain, and later there is tingling and burning. The reaction as noted is usually precipitated by cold but can be brought on by emotional stress. Treatment of Raynaud disease and phenomenon consists of protection from cold, sedation if stress is a factor, and cessation of smoking, which often causes vasoconstriction.

Dry Skin or Xerosis

Skin is dry not because it lacks grease or skin oils, but because it lacks water. It is a condition that is found more frequently among the elderly but can be associated with a number of hereditary or acquired skin conditions. It is found more frequently during the winter when decreased relative humidity and cold dry winds lead to enhanced water loss from the skin. Repeated exposure to solvents, soaps, and disinfectants will remove skin oils and allow for increased water loss. Athletes who are forced to bathe very often may experience dry skin problems. Such individuals should arrange their athletic activities so that they will bathe but once a day. Frequent use of emollients, especially after bathing when the skin is still moist, is to be encouraged. The severity of dry skin will determine whether a lotion or some thicker cream or ointment is necessary.

Acne

Acne is a condition that requires little definition for the teenager, the majority of whom suffer from it at some time or other. It is a problem that for some, unfortunately continues well into adulthood. Acne can be exaggerated by perspiration, heat, friction, pressure, or occlusion. It occurs particularly commonly in football players on the chin secondary to chin straps, a condition termed "football acne."[19] The same phenomenon can occur, however, under backpacks, life jackets, headbands, and helmets of all kinds.[1] Ideally, treatment would mandate removal of the exacerbating items, something not always possible or reasonable. The usual acne treatment regimens should be instituted without delay.

Atopic Dermatitis

Atopic dermatitis is a pattern of eczema that frequently occurs on a hereditary basis, often in association with asthma and hay fever. Severe, easily triggered itching is the hallmark of the atopic patient. All age groups can be affected. Sweating, friction, irritation, temperature changes, occlusive clothing (especially wool), solvents, and detergents are all capable of triggering pruritus and a flare of eczema. As with dry skin, bathing only once daily and frequent use of emollients are indicated. Topical corticosteroids represent the mainstay of therapy, however, and antihistamines may need to be used orally to assist further in suppression of itch. Potent fluorinated topical steroids should be used initially with a switch to 1% hydrocortisone for maintenance therapy, or when treating the face, genitals, axillae, and groin.

Dyshidrotic Eczema (Dyshidrosis)

Dyshidrosis is a recurrent blistering disorder of the hands and feet. It may be simply a unique presentation of atopic dermatitis, but continues to be classified separately by most dermatologists. The disease when active, can interfere for obvious reasons, with athletic activities. Many of the same factors that exacerbate atopic dermatitis apply to this pattern of eczema as well. Treatment differs mainly in the need to address its blistering phase with wet soaks or dressings using Burow solution. Topical steroids clearly are necessary in the acute phases.

Miscellaneous

An article on swimming and the skin makes reference to three phenomena that should be briefly mentioned in this section.[20]

Salabrasion manifests itself as abraded denuded skin in areas where swimsuits are tight. It occurs only in salt water and is the result of friction and the abrasive action of salt. Time spent in the water is clearly an important factor, and one would not expect to find this problem in the casual ocean swimmer.

Excessive amounts of chlorine in swimming pools and prolonged sun exposure combine to produce blonding of hair. This is presumably due to the bleaching effects of chlorine.

"Green hair" is seen quite often in blonds who swim in pools where the levels of chemicals have not been properly adjusted. Shampooing after swimming prevents the problem.

REFERENCES

1. Houston, S.D., and Knox, J.M. Skin problems related to sports and recreational activities. *Cutis* 19:487, 1977.
2. Ayres, S., Jr., and Mihan, R. Calcaneal petechiae. *Arch Dermatol.* 106:262, 1972.
3. Verbov, J. Calcaneal petechiae. *Arch Dermatol.* 107:918, 1973.
4. Nabai, H., and Mehregan, A.H. Black heel. *Cutis* 6:751, 1970.
5. Gibbs, R. Tennis toe. *Arch Dermatol.* 107:918, 1973.
6. Freeman, R.G., and Knox, J.M. Striae. Edited by D.J. Demis, R.L. Dobson, and J. McGuire. In *Clinical Dermatology*. Hagerstown, Md: Harper and Row, 1979.
7. Moschella, S.L. Physically induced blisters. Edited by S.L. Moschella, D.M. Pillsbury, and H.J. Hurley. In *Dermatology*. Philadelphia: W.B. Saunders, 1975.
8. Wilkinson, D.S. Cutaneous reactions to mechanical and thermal injury. Edited by A. Rook, D.S. Wilkinson, and F.J.G. Ebling. In *Textbook of Dermatology*. Oxford: Blackwell Scientific Publications, 1972.
9. Cortese, T.A., Jr., Fukuyama, K., Epstein, N. et al. Treatment of friction blisters: experimental study. *Arch Dermatol.* 97:717, 1968.
10. Ely, P.H. Balance beam alopecia. *Arch Dermatol.* 114:968, 1978.
11. Spoor, H.J. Sports identification marks. *Cutis* 19:453, 1977.
12. Short, J.M. Pernio. Edited by D.J. Demis, R.L. Dobson, and J. McGuire. In *Clinical Dermatology*. Hagerstown, Md: Harper and Row, 1979.
13. D'Ambrosia, R.D. Cold injuries encountered in a winter resort. *Cutis* 20:365, 1977.
14. Short, J.M. Frostbite. Edited by D.J. Demis, R.L. Dobson, and J. McGuire. In *Clinical Dermatology*. Hagerstown, Md: Harper and Row, 1979.
15. Short, J.M. Immersion foot. Edited by D.J. Demis, R.L. Dobson, and J. McGuire. In *Clinical Dermatology*. Hagerstown, Md: Harper and Row, 1979.
16. Izumi, A.K., Hanke, C.W., and Higaki, M. *Mycobacterium marinum* infections treated with tetracycline. *Arch Dermatol.* 113:1067, 1977.
17. Fisher, A. *Atlas of Aquatic Dermatology*. New York: Grune and Stratton, 1978.
18. Mikhailov, P., Berova, N., and Andreev, V.C. Physical urticaria and sport. *Cutis* 20:381, 1977.
19. Farber, G.A., Burks, J.W., Hegre, A.M. et al. Football acne—an acneiform eruption. *Cutis* 20:356, 1977.
20. Hicks, J.H. Swimming and the skin. *Cutis* 19:448, 1977.

CHAPTER 17
Low Back Injuries

Robert C. Cantu, MD

At one time or another, almost everyone will experience low back pain.[1-4] A recent US Public Health Service report indicates that 70 million Americans have experienced at least one severe, incapacitating, prolonged episode of low back pain.[4] The National Center for Health Statistics states chronic and recurring back ailments form the largest single medical ailment.[4] Today, low back pain represents a major national health problem, with over 15 billion dollars expended annually on the treatment and compensation of the condition. In industry, compensation for low back problems represents a figure in excess of the cost of all other industrial injuries combined.[5]

Experience in sportsmedicine indicates that low back problems are very common ailments in the athlete and nonathlete alike.[6] The medical team for the Canadian athletes at the 1976 Olympic Games found low back pain a common problem in their highly trained athletes.[7] Many outstanding Olympic athletes tolerate it as a constantly recurring problem. In some cases the disorder has progressed to the point of neurologic involvement with the athlete still competing.

What are the causes of low back pain? Why are young, vigorous, physically fit, male and female athletes suffering the same symptoms so prevalent in the unfit, sedentary middleaged? The answer requires an understanding of the anatomy and pathology of low back pain.

ANATOMY OF THE LOW BACK

The lower back is composed of five mobile lumbar vertebrae with cartilaginous cushions (discs) between them, and the fused bones of the sacrum and coccyx that form the back of the pelvis. There are also ligaments, thick dense tough strands of connective tissue that attach one bone to another. These ligaments hold the foundation blocks of the low back, the vertebrae, sacrum, coccyx, and pelvis together. All these ligaments have some elasticity and thus provide the back with mobility. The five major ligaments of the low back include:

1. Interspinous—These ligaments extend from one spinous process to another and limit forward bending. They relax in extension and are torn or ruptured by extremes of forward bending (flexion).
2. Intertransverse—These ligaments extend from one transverse process to another and limit sideward bending. They are torn or ruptured by extremes of sideward bending.
3. Ligamentum flavum—These form the roof of spinal canal and bind rear segments of vertebrae. They are more elastic than other ligaments and are rarely torn.
4. Anterior and posterior longitudinal—These run front (anterior) and back (posterior) along the longitudinal surface of one vertebra to another. They blend with and reinforce the annulus fibrosus. The anterior is much stronger than the posterior; the posterior disc ruptures more often then the anterior.
5. Annulus fibrosus—These are the hard outer circumferential coverings of the nucleus pulposus or disc. The radial relationship of the fibers adds strength and has been copied by industry with the radial ply tire. The annuli serve to restrict excessive motion between the vertebrae and to hold in place the nucleus pulposi (discs) with their resultant cushion effect.

The muscles of the back are responsible for both the support and movements of the back. There are four groups of muscles essential for support of the back and that play a major role in back pain. It is convenient to think of the low back as a pole held erect by four guy wire muscle groups.

The abdominal muscles, the anterior guy wires, include the rectus abdominus, internal oblique, external oblique, and transverse abdominus. These muscles extend from the rib cage to the sides and front of the pelvis where they attach by strong rough connective tissues called tendons. They support the abdominal cavity and control bending movements of the spine. When tensed, they relieve strain on the back. Investigators have demonstrated it is strong abdominal muscles that allow one to lift weights that would otherwise crush the spine.

The extensor muscles, the posterior guy wires, consist of many layers, some spanning a single vertebra, and others many, from the low back to the neck. Their tendons attach to the spine, pelvis, ribs, and head. These muscles are maximally used, and are thus injured by posterior (arching) movements of the back. They are used for pulling or pushing heavy objects.

The side muscles, the two lateral guy wires, control the sideward bending of the back by contraction of the quadratus lumborum and the psoas major (one of the body's largest muscles that runs from the side of the spine through the pelvis to attach to the anterior surface of the femur just below the hip joint).

These four groups of muscles, the abdominal, extensor, and side muscles, constitute the four guy wires to support the back.

The hips, by virtue of their relationship to the pelvis and thus the pelvis to the spine, have a very significant effect on the back. Of the four hip muscle groups, the flexors (lifts hip up), abductors (turns hip out), adductor (turns hip in), and extensors (lifts hip back), the latter are the most massive and important to the back. The hip extensor muscles as a group control lumbar lordosis, a condition which, when excessive, is called "sway back" and is a major cause of back pain. The hip extensors in combination with the hip flexors are essential in maintenance of good posture.

THE COMMON CAUSES OF LOW BACK PAIN IN THE ATHLETE

Few athletic back injuries involve a ruptured disc or spine fracture. The definitive medical treatment of these disorders is beyond the scope of this chapter, but early recognition and emergency care are vital, and will be covered later.

Almost all athletic injuries to the low back involve contusion, a bruise from a direct blow; sprain, a pulling with stretching and tearing of the muscles or their tendons; or strain, tearing of a ligament. In general, strain is most painful when the back is forced in the opposite direction, and a sprain produces pain when the affected muscle is contracted. Because of the intricate relationships of the muscles, tendons, and ligaments of the back, and the fact that most injuries involve two or all three entities, trying to separate them is academic.

The cause of most back strains and sprains in the athlete and nonathlete alike is weak muscles, especially the abdominal muscles and hip flexors; and tension or lack of flexibility, especially in the hamstring hip extensor muscles. But how could world class athletes have weak muscles? During intensive training for the specific requirements of their sport, they neglect anatomic areas (the back-abdomen-hip) that do not seem to require development. At the 1976 Olympics, the Canadian medical team found abdominal muscles underdeveloped in many world class athletes.[3] Some of Canada's top athletes had trouble executing more than one or two bent-knee sit-ups. In general, athletes have strong extensor muscles of the back and hip, but the flexor muscles in one or both regions are frequently underdeveloped.

Mechanism of Back Strain and Sprain

Most strains and sprains develop in one of two ways. The first is by a sudden, abrupt, violent extension contraction on an overloaded, unprepared, or underdeveloped spine, especially when there is some rotation in the attempted movement. This can result in degrees of injury from stretching a few fibers, to complete tears, to avulsion fracture of a spinous or transverse process.

The second mechanism involves a chronic strain, often with associated poor posture, excessive lumbar lordosis, or sway back. Here there is a continuation of the underlying disease, with recurring injury to the original and/or adjacent sites.

Through the repetition of training, many sports predispose to low back pain. Most sports involve either strong back extension as opposed to flexion movements, or else external forces that produce extension. Track athletes run in forced extension. The discus thrower, shot putter, or weight lifter all propel heavy weights with the back extended. Gymnasts repeatedly dismount with a hyperextended low back as their feet hit the mat. So, too, the diver hits the water in extension with foot-entry dives.

EXAMINATION OF BACK INJURIES

Acute

For back examination of an acutely injured athlete seen on the athletic field, the essential medical equipment includes ice and/or ethylene chloride freezing spray, and a fracture board or rigid stretcher.

When an athlete is stricken with a back injury during competition, initial examination should be on the spot. Although unstable fractures and fracture dislocation with and without neurologic involvement are uncommon in the low back, a careful examination to eliminate their presence is essential, as suspicion alone dictates great care in transport. When one arrives at the side of the conscious injured athlete, the first question asked is, where does it hurt. For the back-injured athlete, even before examination, the next question is whether any loss of feeling, numbness, or weakness is appreciated in the lower extremities. The spinal cord ends at the lower border of the first lumbar vertebra in most adults. Injury to the spinal cord usually implies a fracture dislocation or dislocation of the vertebra at the instant of impact with spontaneous relocation. Both should be considered unstable, and the athlete is transported off the field to a hospital on a fracture board.

Injury to the spinal cord may produce either complete or incomplete loss of function of the nervous system below the level of the lesion. In a complete lesion sensation, motor power, and reflexes in the legs are lost, as well as bowel and bladder control. In an incomplete lesion, varying degrees of these functions are retained. The seriousness of either a complete or incomplete lesion of the spinal cord renders essential an immediate neurologic evaluation of sensation, movement, and knee and ankle reflexes. If any neurologic deficit is recorded, the patient must be transported from the field on a fracture board.

Fortunately, few back injuries have neurologic impairment. Having determined there is none, the back muscles themselves should be examined. Palpation of the back should start in the midline with a thumb pressing over each spinous process. Exquisite pain over one spinous process suggests a possible fracture or tear of interspinous ligaments. Such a fracture rarely has associated vertebral instability. Pain described as deep in the back with localized tenderness either over one, or in between two spinous processes, raises suspicion of compression fracture of a vertebra. Most compression fractures involve either the 11th or 12th dorsal vertebra or the first two lumbar vertebrae. While most compression fractures, like spinous or transverse process fractures, are stable, if one is suspected because of focal midline tenderness on palpation, it is wisest to transport the athlete on a fracture board until such time as x-rays clearly establish that the fracture is stable. Definitive treatment of these fractures and their complications is beyond the intent of this chapter.

Having eliminated the most worrisome back injuries as will usually be the case, one should continue to palpate the back paraspinal muscles, around the abdominal wall, being certain to include the side flexor and rotator muscles. Areas of focal tenderness may be found that indicate local spasm. If a large swelling is present, this usually represents a contusion with hemorrhage into the muscle. A slight swelling could indicate contusion, strain, sprain, or any combination thereof. Immediate treatment is application of cold to the trigger point, either by an ice pack or freezing spray. Later treatment involves heat, rest, pain and antiinflammatory medication. In virtually all of these injuries, the athlete can safely walk from the field under his own power.

Nonacute

A small percentage of athletes with low back problems will not only have low back pain, but also pain that radiates from the back into the buttock and/or down one or both legs. Coughing, sneezing, straining to pass urine or at bowel movement usually makes the leg pain worse. Numbness may also be felt, usually in the foot either over the medial half or along the lateral side. This pattern of pain is called sciatica and suggests a ruptured disc is pressing on a nerve root. Discs are the fibrocartilaginous cushions between the vertebrae. As the body ages, they lose fluid content, becoming slightly narrower, and thus cause the body to shrink slightly in height. The outer, more fibrous capsule of the disc, called the annulus fibrosus, may also tear allowing the disc to rupture posteriorly out of the disc space, and compress the nerve root as it exits from the spine. Most simple ruptures can be treated successfully with a period of bedrest, muscle relaxants, antiinflammatory medicines, analgesics and, later, exercises. A minor percentage with neurologic deficit, ie, reflex absence at knee or ankle, weakness of ankle or great toe extension, or persistent pain and numbness, will require surgical excision of the ruptured disc. With careful selection, the success of such surgery should exceed 90%. Following surgery, the athlete should adhere to the exercises and advice given by his physician and should be able to resume competition.

A third group of athletes with low back problems suffer from mechanical malalignment of the vertebrae, spondylolisthesis. This diagnosis is established by x-ray. If there is instability documented by further malalignment as the back is placed through flexion and extension maneuvers, a surgical procedure of lumbar fusion may be indicated.[8,9] An abnormal lateral curvature of the spine called scoliosis, is yet another cause of low back pain. If severe in children, this may require surgical correction, a very extensive and time-consuming procedure. Severe scoliosis renders athletic excellence very remote. The mild form seen in some athletes can be pain-free if exercises are followed. Only a physician, especially an orthopedist or neurosurgeon, is properly qualified to evaluate and treat the athlete's low back problem.

Exercises

The exercises and advice in this chapter are primarily directed at the athlete with low back pain but without neurologic deficit, or who has already had concern for a ruptured disc or spinal instability eliminated by appropriate medical consultation.

The vast majority of athletes with low back pain will have no neurologic symptoms, deficits, or spinal instability. Palpation, as with the acute injury, of the paraspinal, side flexor and rotator, and abdominal muscles, usually reveals segmental spasm, tenderness, or an area of point tenderness.

Athletes are usually thin, quite physically fit, but have an accentuated lumbar lordosis when walking. The posterior erector spinal muscles are strong, but the abdominal (flexor) muscles, although flat, in comparison are quite weak. A good test of abdominal muscle strength is a slow bent-knee sit-up. An athlete should be able to do 20 or more, but some Olympic class athletes with back problems had trouble doing one.[7] The back extensor muscles are tested with the athlete on his abdomen with a pillow under the hips. To test the upper back, with the hands behind the head, raise elbows, chin, and trunk off the floor as long as possible (Figure 17-1). Low back strength is tested by keeping the head down with hands behind, while both legs held together with knees straight, are raised off the floor (Figure 17-2). In both exercises, 20 seconds indicates strong muscles and under 10 weak.

Frequently, back rotation is weak. When the overdeveloped extensors are tight, both flexion and rotation are compromised. In some athletes, the hip flexor and hamstring muscles will be tight. In such cases, one cannot touch the floor with fingertips with the knees straight (Figure 17-3). Ideally, the hamstring muscles should be at least 60% to 80% as strong as the quadriceps; the closer to 80%, the fewer back problems encountered. To test the strength of the hip flexor muscles, have the athlete lie on his back, legs extended, hands clasped behind the head. With legs touching, have him lift his feet about 10 inches off the floor and hold this position for as long as possible. Over 20 seconds indicates strong, under 10 quite weak hip flexor muscles (Figure 17-4).

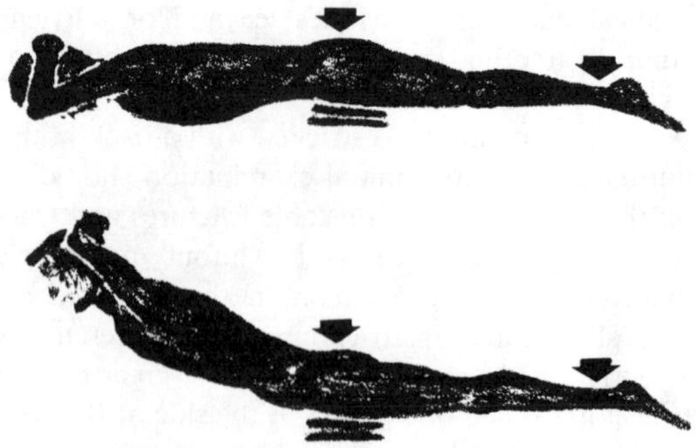

Figure 17-1 Test for upper back strength.

TREATMENT

The successful treatment of low back pain in athletes involves a three-step program. First is relief of pain and spasm; second, adoption of an appropriate exercise program that includes both stretching and strengthening exercises; third, an educational program that takes into consideration one's training program and is tailored to preventing future injuries.

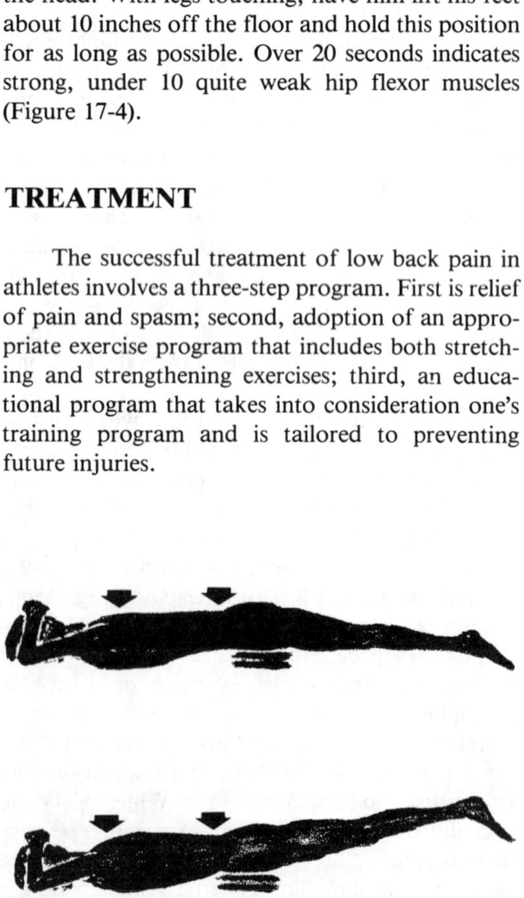

Figure 17-2 Test for lower back strength.

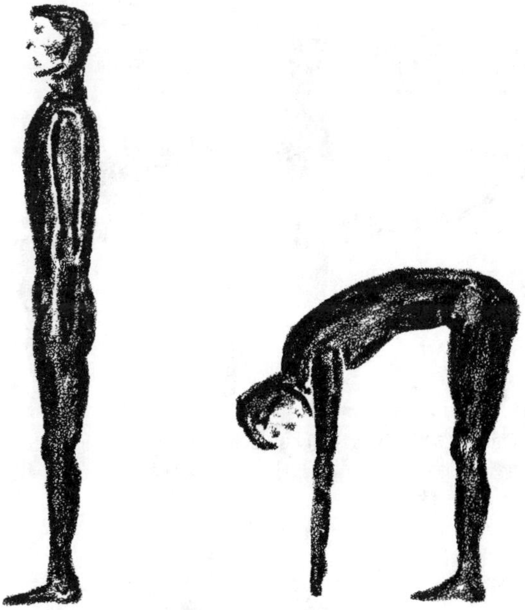

Figure 17-3 Test for tight hip flexor and hamstring muscles.

Relief of Pain and Spasm

Ice, analgesics, muscle relaxants, antiinflammatory agents, and rest, are used in acute stages. Heat, muscle stimulation, and/or ultrasound, physical therapy, and the same pharmacologic agents are used 12 or more hours after injury. Ultrasound and gentle muscle stimulation seem more rapidly to dissipate muscle spasm, point tenderness, and general soreness. This is probably due to enhanced muscle circulation and exchange at the cellular level of prescribed pharmacologic agents, plus elimination of toxic cellular products.[7]

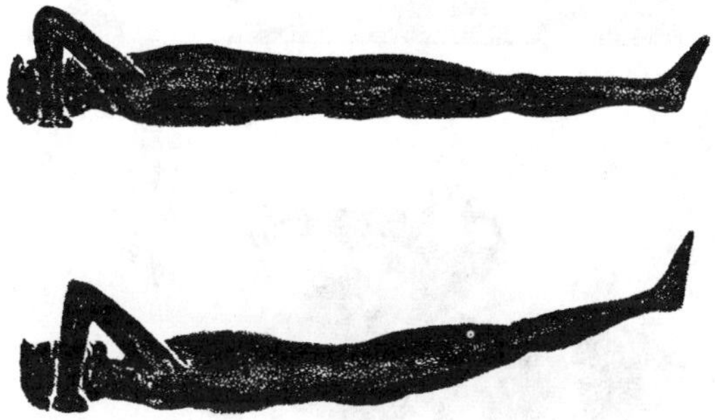

Figure 17-4 Test for hip flexor strength.

Actually, while modes of pain relief exist, no one treatment has been clearly demonstrated to accelerate actual tissue healing.

Stretching and Strengthening Exercises

Medications, manipulations, massage, ultrasound, and hot and cold applications do not strengthen a weakened or compromised part of the body. Low back pain is usually because of muscles that are weak, tense, fatigued, or all three. Once the healing process has occurred, it is essential to embark on an exercise program to rebuild the back and abdominal musculature.

Before the strengthening exercises are commenced, it is important first to have executed specific stretching exercises for the lumbar extensor and pelvic rotator, hip flexor, and hamstring and hip extensor muscles.

Stretching Athletes can stretch their lower back muscles by lying on their backs on a mat and bringing their feet and legs up over their faces to touch extended toes to the floor beyond their heads (Figure 17-5). It is important that these movements are executed fluidly with no sudden jerking. A good exercise to stretch the hip flexor muscles is shown in Figure 17-6. The athlete lies on his back, knees bent under the buttocks. Then the arms reach as far toward the knees as possible as the back arches and the hips are maximally extended. The straight leg raise (Figure 17-7) and standard one leg on waist-high table, nose-toe touch (Figure 17-8) are good flexibility exercises for the hamstrings; while the single knee raise and double knee hug (Figures 17-9, 17-10) stretch the hamstrings, low back, and hip extensors. The athlete must work daily on flexibility exercises to maintain a good range of motion. They should become a routine part of his daily warm-up and cooling-off exercises.

Strengthening Exercises that strengthen the low back and abdominal muscles include some of the same exercises that stretch the hamstring and hip flexor muscles. Ten such exercises are presented. They should be carried out on a hard, flat surface with adequate padding. A tumbling mat is ideal, but a thick rug with underpadding may suffice. For those exercises done supine, most find a small pillow placed under the neck will provide more comfort. One should wear loose, unrestrictive clothing. As mentioned previously, the exercises must always be initiated slowly to

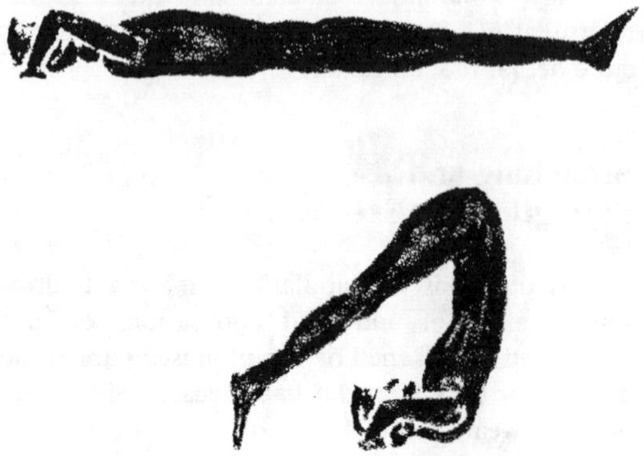

Figure 17-5 Exercise for stretching lower back muscles.

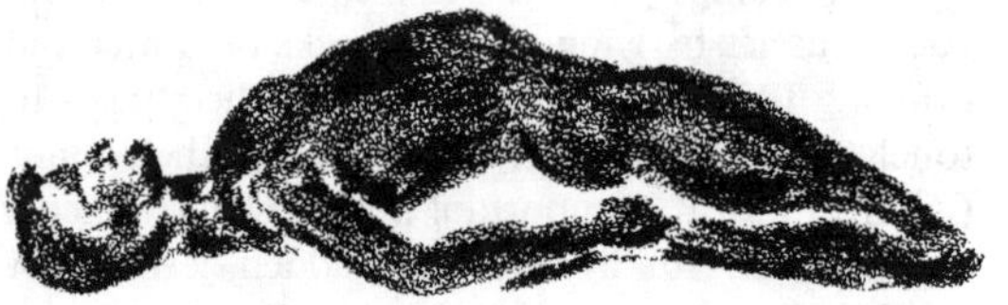

Figure 17-6 Exercise for stretching hip flexor muscles.

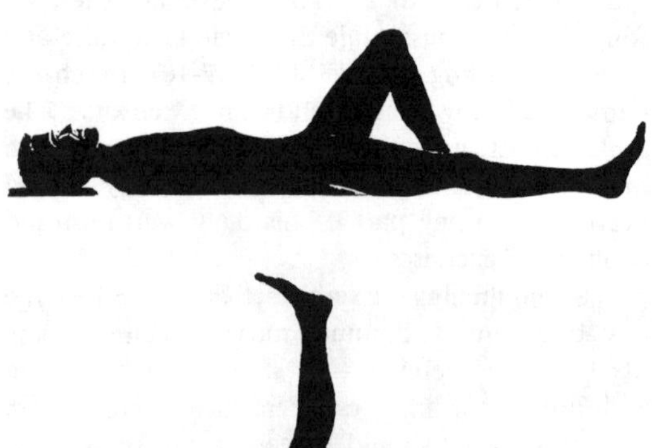

Figure 17-7 Straight-leg raise for flexing the hamstring muscle.

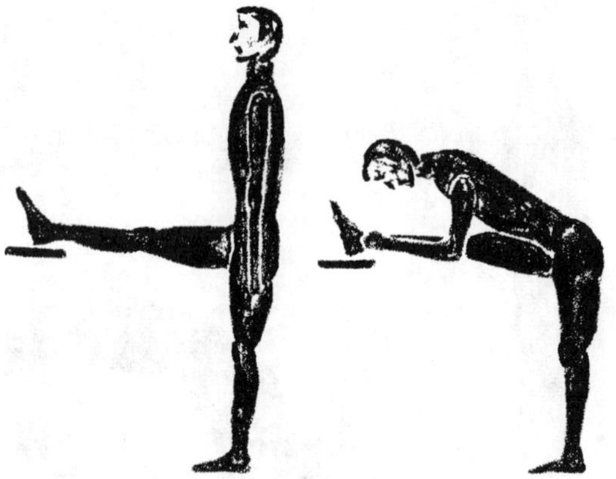

Figure 17-8 Exercise for stretching the hamstring muscle.

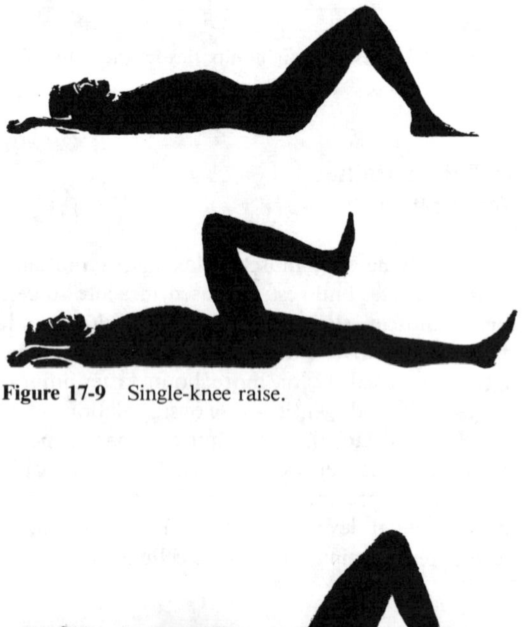

Figure 17-9 Single-knee raise.

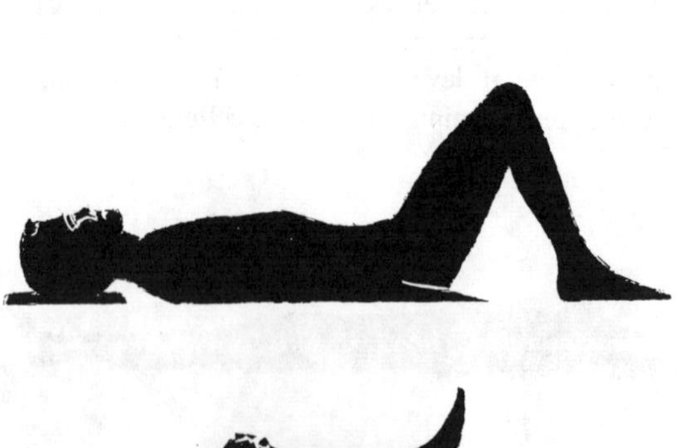

Figure 17-10 Double-knee hug.

allow muscles to loosen up gradually. At no time should one employ jerking or snapping movements. Most find relaxing before exercising beneficial, and that heat treatment to the low back aids in loosening tight muscles. Slight discomfort may occur as the exercises are performed, but if frank pain is experienced, the exercise period should be terminated. They should be done daily, ideally twice a day in the beginning. Each athlete should progress at his own pace. Initially, five repetitions will suffice; then add a repetition or two daily to each exercise that can be accomplished with relative ease. If one or more of the exercises results in appreciable discomfort, then it should be abandoned while the remainder are continued. Only resume an exercise when it can be done without discomfort.

1. The back flattener (Figure 17-11) is to strengthen gluteal (buttock) and abdominal muscles and flatten the low back, lumbar lordosis. Lie on the back on a padded floor with knees well bent. Relax with arms above head. A small pillow may be placed under the head if desired. Squeeze buttocks together as if trying to hold a piece of paper between them. At the same time, suck in and tighten the muscles of the abdomen. The back should flatten against the floor. This is the flat back position. Hold this position for a count of ten (10 seconds), relax and repeat the exercise three times in the beginning. Gradually attempt to increase to 20 repetitions.

After the basic exercise has been done for a week or more, additional flattening can be achieved by doing the exercise with the buttocks slightly raised (1 to 2 inches) off the floor at the time the buttocks are squeezed and abdomen tensed. Hold for the count of ten, relax, and repeat.

After several weeks of the basic exercise, gradually do the exercise with the knees less and less bent, until the exercise is executed with legs straight. The buttock raise need not be combined with this modification.

2. Single-knee raise (Figure 17-9) is to stretch the low back, hip flexor, and hamstring (posterior thigh) muscles. Lie on back on a padded floor with arms above head and knees bent. Tighten buttocks and abdominal muscles as in exercise number 1. Then raise one knee over chest toward chin as far as possible, hold for 10 seconds, return to starting position, and relax a few seconds before repeating with the opposite leg. Start with three repetitions of each knee, gradually advancing to ten.

3. The single-knee hug (Figure 17-12) has the same purpose and is essentially the same exercise as the single-knee raise, except the hands are not placed above the head, but rather are placed around the knee to be raised. The arms are used to pull (raise) the knee higher over the chest than was possible in exercise number 2. This produces greater stretching of the low back and hamstrings. The same 10-second hold, number of repetitions, and advanced modification pertain as with the single-knee raise.

4. The double-knee hug (Figure 17-10) stretches the low back and hanstring muscles, and strengthens abdominal and hip flexing muscles. Lie on back on a covered floor with knees bent, arms at sides, and a pillow under the head if desired. Tighten buttocks and abdominal muscles so that low back is flat against the floor. Grasp both knees

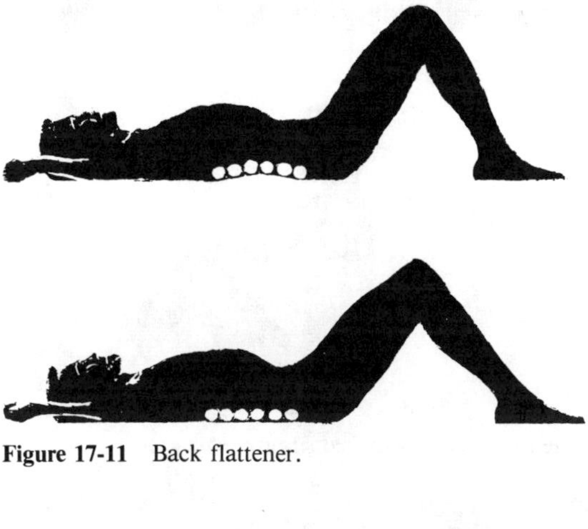

Figure 17-11 Back flattener.

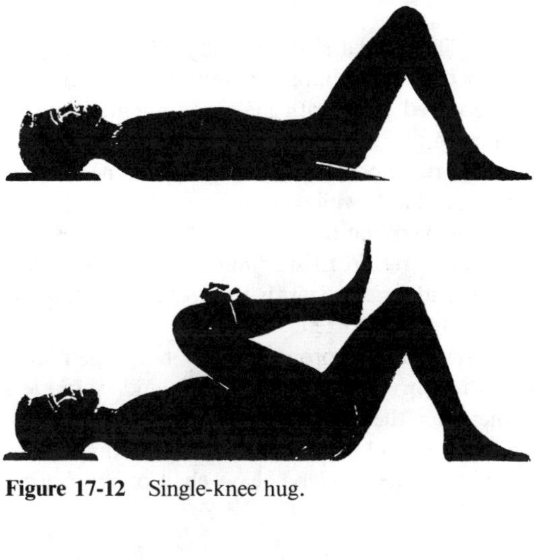

Figure 17-12 Single-knee hug.

with hands and raise them slowly over chest as far as possible. Hold 10 seconds, return to starting position, relax a few seconds, then repeat. Start with three repetitions and gradually build to ten.

After a month or more of the basic exercise, attempt the double-knee hug starting with both legs extended straight. Tense buttocks and abdomen and then taking care to keep the back flat, bend both knees, grasp knees with hands and raise over chest, hold 10 seconds, and return to starting position to relax before repeating. The low back tends to arch when lifting and lowering the knee. If this cannot be done with the back against the floor, the athlete is not ready for this modification and should resume the basic knees-bent position. This extended-leg starting position strengthens both the hip flexing and abdominal muscles.

5. The single-leg raise (Figure 17-7) also stretches the low back and hamstring muscles, and strengthens abdominal and hip-flexing muscles. Lie on back on a covered floor with one knee bent and one leg straight, arms at sides and a pillow under the head if desired. Tighten buttock and abdominal muscles, then slowly raise the straight leg, keeping it straight and the back flat. Raise the leg as far as comfortably possible, then slowly lower the leg to the floor, keeping it straight and the back flat. Relax a few seconds and then repeat with the other leg. Start with three repetitions of each leg and gradually increase to ten.

After a month or more, attempt the single-leg raise starting with both legs extended straight. Tense buttocks and low back and with back flat and legs out straight, raise one leg up as far as possible. As the leg is raised, the back may not remain flat. Check by using hand to see if back lifts from the floor when the leg is lifted and lowered. If it does, resume the basic exercise with one knee bent.

6. The partial sit-up (Figure 17-13) strengthens low back and abdominal muscles. Lie on back on a covered floor with knees well bent. Squeeze buttocks and tighten abdominal muscles; with low back on the floor, slowly raise head, neck, and lastly shoulders while extending arms to knees. Keep low back flat on the floor. Hold this position 10 seconds, return to starting position, rest a few seconds and repeat. Start with three repetitions and progress to at least ten.

After having progressed to ten repetitions, begin to progressively lift head and shoulders farther from the floor. The back will now lift off of the floor. Keep knees bent. In the begining, it may help to place feet under a heavy chair or some other

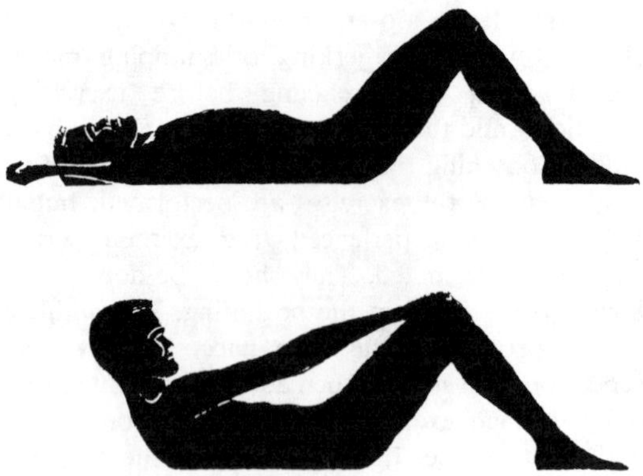

Figure 17-13 Partial sit-up.

restraint. Once abdominal muscles are strong enough, this should not be necessary and should not be done, as this action actually allows legs to help the abdomen in raising the body. The motion should be a gentle, smooth curling and uncurling. Never jerk to achieve greater height or an additional repetition and never strain or exert beyond reasonable comfort. Again, start with three repetitions and progress to at least ten.

7. The advanced sit-up (Figure 17-14) is used to maximally strengthen low back and abdominal muscles. Lie on back on a covered floor with knees well bent. Squeeze buttocks and tighten abdominal muscles. Start with arms folded over waist and lift head, shoulders, and back smoothly up to the posi-

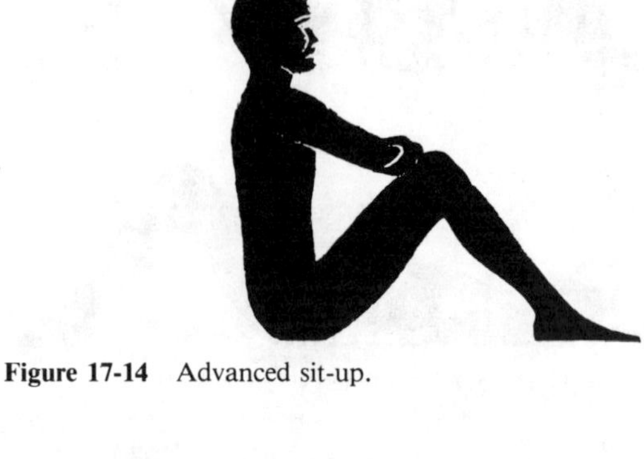

Figure 17-14 Advanced sit-up.

tion of arms touching knees. Hold 10 seconds, return to the starting position, relax a few seconds, and repeat. Again, start with three repetitions and progress to at least ten.

Progress gradually until ten of the basic advanced sit-ups can be easily and comfortably executed. Then try folding the arms in front of face instead of waist. Curl up to knees, hold 10 seconds, then return to the starting position, relax a few seconds and repeat. Start with three repetitions. When this modified version can be accomplished ten times, a sit-up with hands clasped behind the head can be attempted. When this version can also be done ten times, attempt the most maximal version of a sit-up. This involves lying on the back on a padded inclined surface (ie, a tilt board with the foot end elevated). Knees should be bent as always, then with hands clasped behind neck, slowly and carefully execute the sit-up, hold 10 seconds, slowly uncurl to the starting position, relax, and repeat. This last version is clearly optional. The more inclined the board, the greater strength and effort will be required of the back and abdomen to accomplish the sit-up.

8. The sitting bend (Figure 17-15) strengthens the low back while stretching the low back and hamstring muscles. Sit on a hard chair, feet flat on the floor, knees not more than 12 inches apart, arms folded loosely in the lap. Squeeze buttocks and tighten abdominal muscles so that your back goes flat against the chair. Bend over, letting head go between knees with hands reaching for the floor. Bend as far as is comfortable, hold for a count of five, then slowly pull body back to the flat back sitting starting position. Relax a few seconds, repeat initially three times, gradually increasing to ten repetitions.

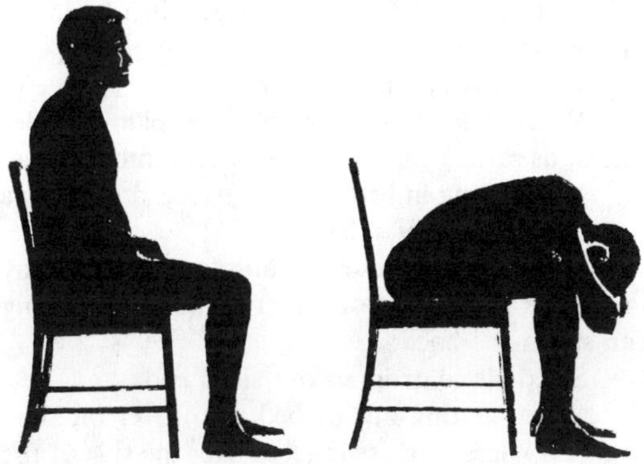

Figure 17-15 Sitting bend.

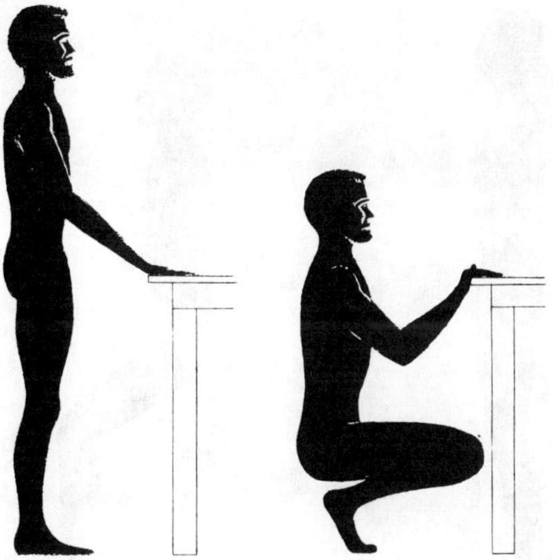

Figure 17-16 Deep-knee bend.

9. The deep-knee bend (Figure 17-16) strengthens hamstring and quadriceps muscles. Do not begin this exercise until it has been confirmed by a viewer that a good back flattener (number 1) has been accomplished. Most should not attempt this exercise until a month into this exercise program. Discontinue this exercise if there is considerable lasting discomfort in knees or hips.

Stand behind a sofa, desk, heavy chair, or similar structure holding onto it for balance. Squeeze and tighten buttocks and abdomen. Slowly bend knees and with a flat back, squat down as far as is reasonably comfortable, stop, stand up using only legs, and not arms. Relax for a second or two and repeat initially three times, gradually building up to ten repetitions.

10. The posture check (Figure 17-17) helps correct standing and walking. It also determines if the exercise program is accomplishing its goals.

Stand with back to the wall pressing heels, buttocks, shoulders, and head against the wall. There should be no space between the low back and the wall; if there is, the back is too arched and not flat. Move feet forward, bending knees so back slides a few inches down the wall. Now again, squeeze buttocks and tighten abdominal muscles, flattening lower back against the wall. While holding this position, walk feet back so as to slide up the wall. Standing straight, walk away from the wall and around the room. Return to the wall and back up to it to ascertain that the proper posture was kept.

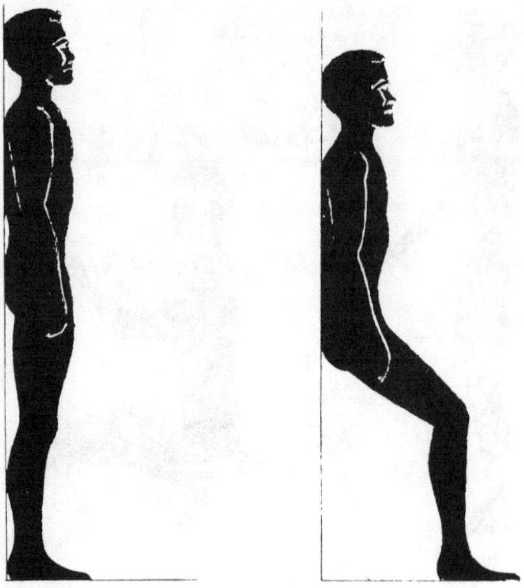

Figure 17-17 Posture check.

Educational Program

The final link in the low back pain elimination triangle involves educating the athlete how to avoid back problems, both in training and in daily life. As previously mentioned, good posture is achieved by rotating the top of the pelvis backward, which flattens the curve in the low back. Common everyday tips to avoid the occurrence of low back pain include the following.

Standing and walking Stand with low back erect and as flat as possible. By squeezing buttocks and sucking in and tensing abdomen, the lower back is straightened. Walk, stand, and sit as tall as possible.

Bend knees when leaning, as when over a wash basin. Avoid leaning whenever possible, instead squat with a straight lower back.

Avoid high heeled shoes. They shorten the Achilles tendons and increase lordosis.

Avoid standing for long periods of time, but if it is necessary, alternate leaning on the left foot and right foot, and if possible use the bent knee position as on a stool. This flattens the lower back.

When standing, do not lean back and support the body with the hands. Keep hands in front of body and lean forward slightly.

When turning to walk from a standing position, move feet first and then the body.

Open doors wide enough to walk through comfortably.

Carefully judge the height of curbs before stepping up or down.

Sitting Sit so that lower back is flat or slightly rounded outward, never with a forward curve.

Sit so that knees are higher than hips; this may require a small footstool for a short person in a high chair.

Hard seat backs that begin contact with back 4 to 6 inches above the seat and provide a flat support throughout the entire lumbar area are preferable.

Do not sit in a soft, or overstuffed chair or sofa.

Avoid sitting in swivel chairs or chairs on rollers.

Do not sit with legs out straight on an ottoman or footstool.

Never sit in the same position for prolonged periods, get up and move around.

Driving Push front seat forward so that knees will be higher than hips and the pedals are easily reached without stretching.

Sit back with back flat, do not lean forward, sit tall.

Add a flat back rest if car seat is soft or if travelling a long distance.

If on a long trip, stop every 30 to 60 minutes, get out of car and walk about, tensing buttocks and abdomen to flatten the back for several minutes.

Always fasten seatbelt and shoulder harness.

Be sure car seat has a properly adjusted headrest.

Bedrest Sleep or rest only on a flat firm mattress. If one is not available, place a bedboard of no less than three-quarter inch plywood under the mattress. A board of less thickness will sag, preventing proper spine alignment.

When sleeping, the preferred position is on the side, both arms in front, and knees slightly drawn up toward chin.

Do not sleep on stomach.

When lying on back, place a pillow under knees, as raising the legs flattens the lumbar curve.

When lying in bed, do not extend arms above head, relax them at sides.

If the doctor prescribes absolute bedrest, stay in bed. Raising the body or twisting and turning can strain the back.

Sleep alone or in an oversized bed.

When getting out of bed, turn over on side, draw up knees, then swing legs over the side of the bed.

Lifting When lifting, let the legs do the work, using the large muscles of the thighs instead of the small muscles of the back.

Do not twist the body, face the object.

Never lift with legs straight.

Do not lift heavy objects from car trunks.

Do not lift from a bending forward position.

Do not reach over furniture to open and close windows.

Tuck in the buttocks and pull in the abdomen when lifting.

Only lift holding the object close to body.

Lift a heavy load no higher than the waist, and a light load no higher than the shoulders, as greater height increases lumbar lordosis.

To turn while lifting, pivot feet turning the whole body at one time.

In training, to minimize back injuries, the athlete should always warm up slowly and cool down after the main workout. Both the warm-up and cooling-off periods should include back-stretching exercises. Calisthenics that involve hyperextension of the back such as back bends, straight leg sit-ups, or straight leg raises should be avoided when possible.

By faithfully carrying out a daily program of back exercise, the athlete can pursue a variety of potentially hazardous sports with minimal risk of back injury.

SPORTS MOST HAZARDOUS TO THE BACK

As discussed previously, most back injuries are sustained by acute hyperextension of the back. Football is felt by some to be legalized assault, often between physical unequals. It is one of the most hazardous sports to the body, and to the back in particular. This is especially true for the interior linemen (defensive ends, guards, tackles, and centers). A report from a major university with a recent number one national ranking, cited the fact that during one year, 50% of interior linemen sought medical attention for low back pain.[10] This report postulated biomechanics of the back injury. As the lineman drives forward attempting to push the opponent backward, the lumbar spine is extended and this converts more of the force to a shearing force that can lead to pars interarticularis injury. It concluded that the high incidence of spondylolysis and spondylolisthesis seen in interior linemen is the result of repeated forces being transmitted to the pars interarticularis while players are in the lumbar extended posture.

Weight-lifting is another high-risk back-injury sport. This is especially true for the overhead military press, and clean and jerk. Severe lordotic postures are also assumed when spiking a volley ball, hitting a twist serve or deep overhead in tennis, putting the shot, throwing the discus and hammer, or even stretching for the tape in track. Extreme backward arching movements are required by the gymnast (especially in dismounts), diver, trampolinist, and squash, soccer, handball, and racquetball enthusiasts. Also sledding, downhill skiing, and snow and water ski-jumping can result in excessive stresses to the low back. Both the hang glider and pole vaulter occasionally have precipitous descents in awkward postures that can result in back strain or even compression fractures.

Sports that are less likely to result in back injury include baseball, basketball, bowling, golf, figure skating, softball, ping-pong, water skiing, canoeing, rowing, fencing, cross-country skiing, badminton, and archery. Sports least likely to result in back injury include bicycling, hiking, swimming, fishing, curling, darts, skindiving, boccie, billiards, pool, and sailing.

As emphatically repeated throughout this chapter, the athlete can best prevent back injuries by daily execution of appropriate back and abdominal muscle stretching and strengthening exercises. For any sport, the athlete should always warm up slowly and include back stretching exercises. In some sports, the most hazardous maneuvers, those carried out with the low back in extension, can be modified. The serve and overhead are the two tennis strokes most strenuous to the back. By tossing the serve slightly forward, less back extension is required and, thus, less back strain. For those who play a serve and volley game, it will also aid in gaining forward momentum toward the net. When hitting the overhead, go up to the ball hitting it slightly in front of the body. When trying for a low ball, whether tennis, handball, volley ball, softball, or baseball, whenever possible bend the knees rather than the back. Most gymnastic sports, including diving, stress good posture. The athlete at all times should sit and stand as tall as possible. The runner, equestrian, diver, and gymnast alike should keep their low backs flat by tensing their buttocks and abdominal muscles whenever possible.

Thus, intelligently pursued, with adequate preparation, a variety of sports potentially hazardous to the low back with little risk of back injury can be played. There is no substitution for the faithful daily back exercise program. The ultimate responsibility for eliminating the risk of back injury, therefore, lies with the athlete.

REFERENCES

1. Friedmann, L.W., and Galton, L. *Freedom from Backaches.* New York: Pocket Books, 1973.

2. Jones, L. *The Postural Complex.* Springfield, Ill: Charles C Thomas, 1955.

3. Kraus, H. *Backache Stress and Tension.* New York: Simon and Schuster, 1965.

4. Root, L., and Kiernan, T. *Oh, My Aching Back.* New York: New American Library, 1975.

5. Akeson, W.H., and Murphy, R.W. Editorial. *Clin Orthop.* 129:2–3, 1977.

6. Harris, W.D. Low back pain in sports medicine. *J Arkansas Med Soc.* 74:377–379, 1978.

7. Smith, C.F. Physical management of muscular low back pain in the athlete. *Can Med Assoc J.* 177:632–635, 1977.

8. Wiltse, L.L. Etiology of spondylolisthesis. *Clin Orthop.* 10:48–60, 1957.

9. Wiltse, L.L. Spondylolisthesis: classification and etiology. In *American Academy of Orthopaedic Surgeons Symposium on the Spine.* St Louis: C.V. Mosby, 1969.

10. Ferguson, R.J. Low back pain in college football linemen. *J Sports Med.* 2:63–80, 1974.

CHAPTER 18
Injuries of the Upper Extremities

Arthur M. Pappas, MD

The upper extremity is important in all athletic events, sometimes in the form of active participation, sometimes in the form of a kinesiologic balance mechanism. In the events where its role is active, ie, throwing, the action is seen as originating in the shoulder girdle and extending onward to the distal portion of the upper extremity. In the majority of instances, this is an appropriate sequence in which to consider relative incidence of injury. However, when analyzing the function of this area in any athletic event, one must not consider it in isolation from the remainder of the body. The upper extremity is observed as a critical end organ in the act of throwing; the remainder of the body, its coordination and balance, influence the process of throwing.

The characteristic pattern of throwing demonstrated by a skilled baseball pitcher is initiated by the push off and rotational thrust from the ipsilateral foot. The contralateral leg-kicking phase is the next sequence, and the body momentum is thrust forward. Associated with this force transfer is rotation of the trunk while the arm is being abducted and externally rotated to the cocking phase. The upper extremity is moving in the opposite direction from the remainder of the body. As the contralateral kicking foot lands and the trunk is brought forward, the upper extremity starts its sudden forward acceleration and derotation through the shoulder. The final sequence includes the ultimate direction of the throwing motion to the elbow, wrist, hand, and finger contribution and release of the ball (Figure 18-1).

It is important to review the biomechanics of the entire process to comprehend the physical demands of the event, throwing or hitting, and not limit the entire examination to the end organ of delivery. For example, if a baseball pitcher or golfer is suffering from an inflamed great toe, Achilles tendinitis, or lower back pain, his entire body muscular rhythm and throwing biomechanics will be changed. The role of the upper extremity in such sport events as running and skating is both power and kinesiologic balance. A painful area in the shoulder will result in a significant negative influence on performance. Thus, when analyzing the problem of pain or decreased performance in the upper extremity of an athlete, one should not necessarily assume the entire source of a problem to be within that area.

A major principle that must be underscored in the care of the injured athlete, is that the demands of the event or performance frequently determine treatment and subsequent expectations following injury. Injuries to the upper extremity are frequently related to the demands of the athletic act. The demands of the baseball pitcher on the coordinated function of the shoulder girdle, elbow, wrist, and hand are considerably different from those of the football offensive interior lineman. Also, the patterns of injury observed in the pitcher and lineman are different as to anatomic involvement and effect on participation. Thus, a comprehensive understanding of the demands of the event and the mechanism the athlete has developed to meet these demands must be understood for the comprehensive analysis of each injury and determination of an appropriate treatment program.

In general there are two major categories of athletic injury: those associated with a single major abrupt force, and the chronic injury or complaint of pain associated with repetitive stresses such as overuse, overdemand, or attrition. At times the problem is obvious; at other times it requires careful observation of the athlete during the performance to identify causative factors or combination of factors. For example, when a football player reports that his shoulder popped anteriorly while he was making an arm tackle, there is a high likelihood of there having been an anterior subluxation or dislocation of the glenohumeral joint. This single-force acute trauma as the probable mechanism of injury provides a rapid characterization of the injury process and related anatomic consequences, implying certain steps in the treatment process.

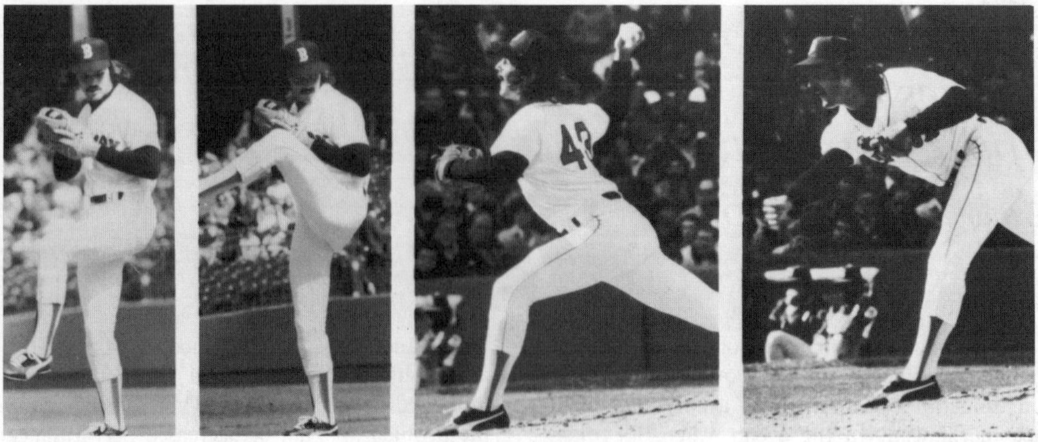

Figure 18-1 Coordinated phases of baseball pitching motions.

When a baseball pitcher first complains of ill-defined shoulder pain that is only present after he attempts to throw at maximum speed and in certain styles of delivery for 10 to 15 minutes, analysis of the factors is much more complex. Etiology of this form of overuse syndrome associated with high-demand repetitive stresses is more difficult to determine. In some instances, the demand of repetitive action will result in one small focal area of damage and/or inflammation. This degree of insult will gradually result in one muscle and/or group of muscles becoming slightly weaker and unable to perform in the usual fashion. A minor muscle imbalance in a high-demand performance will result in a pattern of muscle substitution. This in turn will result in a negative change of function, subsequent loss of effectiveness, and continued pain.

The anatomy of the shoulder girdle, and the coordinated function of the shoulder girdle and the glenohumeral joint, are more complex than is generally appreciated. When analyzing the throwing motion in careful radiographic, photographic, and electromyographic studies, information has been recorded, computerized, analyzed, and the various sequences of the throwing act carefully described. There is a very specific dynamic rhythm for scapulohumeral function. The rhythm starts at the level of muscle groups associated with the cervicothoracic spine and the scapula. As the wave of muscle action extends across the scapulothoracic areas, another group of muscles interacts to initiate and stabilize the motion of the glenohumeral area. Observing what would appear to be 180° of shoulder motion, approximately one-third of that motion is scapulothoracic, and two-thirds is glenohumeral. The contribution of pelvic-trunk rotation and vertebral flexion and extension have not been carefully evaluated.

Although there are many tools for analysis of medical problems of athletes, there are still areas in which clinical experience is the primary diagnostic tool. When analyzing the levels of highest athletic performance, it is difficult to separate the integrated roles of changing rapid motions, and overall multiple neuromuscular skeletal coordination of early performance. It is in this area that the greatest need for continued research becomes most obvious to the physician dealing with sports performance and injury. It is also in this area where one appreciates the greatest difficulty in translating clinical judgment acquired from experience to the treatment of an injury.

In analyzing injuries of the upper extremity, one is generally confronted either with an obvious deformity or pain. When there is an obvious deformity present, in most instances there is a specific mechanism and time of injury that can be identified and associated with the problem. Such would be the instance of an injury to an acromioclavicular joint or an acute glenohumeral dislocation. In the instance of chronic shoulder pain, the examiner must spend more time eliciting the history, and performing a comprehensive examination of the area of complaint and related anatomic structures. For example, the anatomy of the shoulder joint and its relationship with the cervical spine are well known to any professional involved in caring for athletes. All too frequently, however, one fails to consider a previous head or neck injury and its possible relation to a current complaint of shoulder pain. A

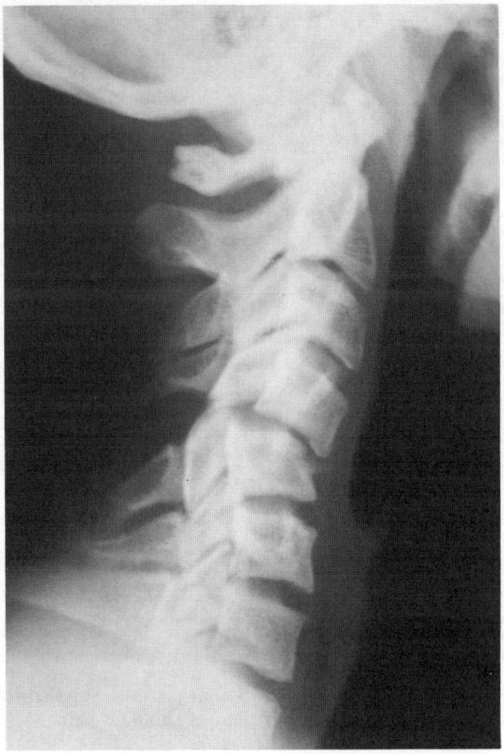

Figure 18-2 Residual spine deformity with shoulder pain.

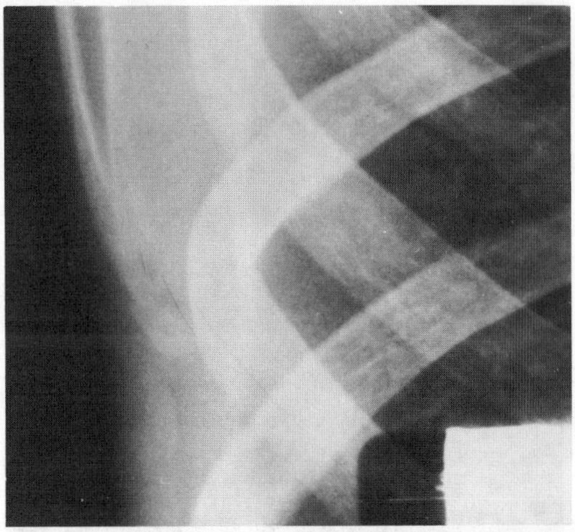

Figure 18-3 Avulsion fracture of inferior pole of scapula, attachment of latissimus dorsi in adolescent tennis player.

previous cervical spine injury may have resulted in vertebral malalignment, nerve root irritation, or brachial plexopathy (Figure 18-2). Thus, in considering all aspects of shoulder pain, we must have a complete understanding of the mechanics of that individual's performance in athletics; in analyzing the anatomic contributors to shoulder pain, the cervical spine must be an integral part of examination, including past history, physical, and radiographic examinations. If any of these aspects results in positive findings, further diagnostic steps and consultations may be indicated.

ACUTE SHOULDER INJURIES

The broad spectrum of shoulder pain is presented in two categories: single direct acute trauma resulting in sudden pain and/or deformity, and chronic discomfort usually associated with dynamic imbalance and overuse stresses of repetitive action.

Acute injuries about the shoulder girdle can be generally categorized as sprains, dislocations, and fractures. These injuries are usually the product of a single, abrupt, forceful injury associated with subsequent apparent clinical deformity readily confirmed by radiographs in two planes at 90° to each other. At times, it will be necessary to take other radiographic views to ascertain the details of the injury. For example, in fractures of the body of the scapula or avulsions of muscle groups from the scapula, various oblique views will be necessary to identify the site of injury (Figures 18-3 and 18-4). In certain subluxations without dislocations of the shoulder, or uncommon fractures about the shoulder, oblique views of the glenoid in different positions are necessary to appreciate the relationship of the humeral head to the glenoid and associated structures (Figure 18-5). In some instances, even if the plain radiographs appear normal, the athlete's complaints and/or the examiner's clinical experience will direct the examination to specialized radiographic techniques for more comprehensive information, eg, arthrography, tomography, arthrotomography, and nuclear scans (Figure 18-6).

The treatment for most fractures about the shoulder is well outlined in the majority of texts and does not warrant extensive discussion in this chapter. Sprains, subluxations (partial dislocations), and dislocations are basically part of a continuum of the same process: a variable degree of injury to the ligaments and other soft tissues that normally

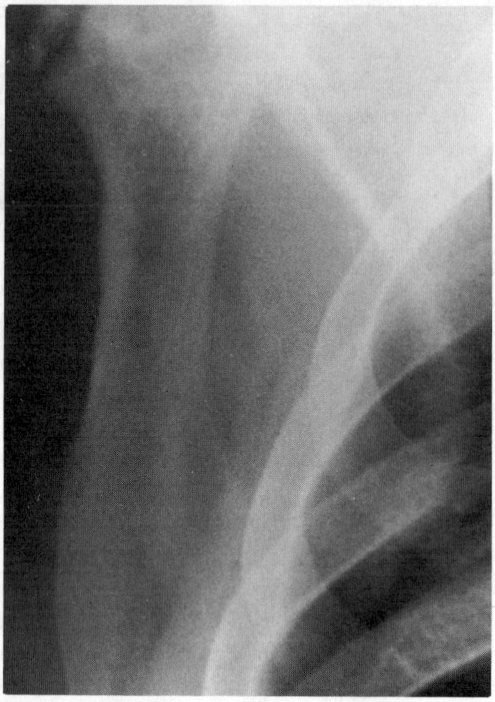

Figure 18-4 Avulsion fragment of inferior posterior margin of glenoid causing persistent pain with throwing.

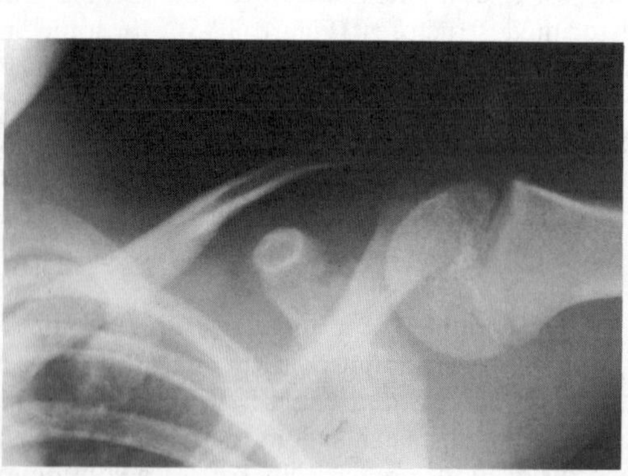

Figure 18-5 Fracture of coracoid in young football player.

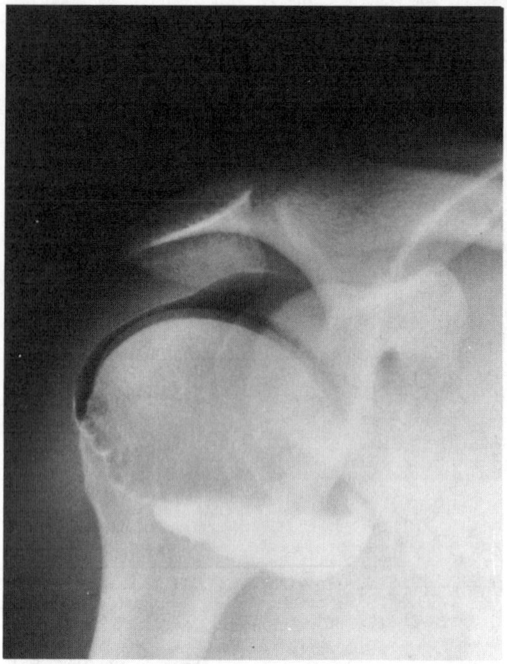

Figure 18-6 Shoulder arthrogram provides supplemental information on the evolution of shoulder pain.

provide the integrity of a joint. In general, the milder injury results in a sprain, the moderate injury in a subluxation, and the severe injury in a dislocation. These injuries are frequently identified as class I, sprain; class II, subluxation; and class III, dislocation.

The class I injury results in stretching and/or minimal tearing and disruption of ligamentous structures that provide integrity of the joint. There is no major displacement between the two sides of the joint. There is moderate local sensitivity to palpation over the injured area. Rest and appropriate strapping of the area for one to three weeks are usually necessary prior to return to athletics. During the entire treatment period, from injury to return to participation, there must be a complementary program for continued general conditioning, and progressive reconditioning of the injured area.

In class II injury of the joint there has been a partial tear and disruption of the ligamentous structures. One would estimate between 25% to 75% disruption of the ligamentous support. There would be a similar percentage of abnormal relationship between the joint surfaces. Examination would identify swelling and sensitivity over the injured area. The treatment for this degree of injury includes rest and support, continued general conditioning, progressive reconditioning, and the use of appropriate strapping, padding, and support prior to resumption of athletic activity.

In the class III injury there has been a near complete or complete (75% to 100%) tear of the ligamentous and associated soft tissue structures. The examiner should anticipate a major malposition or lack of contact of the joint surface. When the forces have resulted in a severe disruption, there are usually other evident locations of injury. In some joints it will probably include other aspects of the joint capsule or related musculotendinous structures. When the injury results in such severe soft tissue disruptions, there is a greater need to consider surgical intervention.

There is a poor correlation between the time when an athlete returns to full participation and rate of healing determined by cytologic, histochemical, and tensiometric criteria. The class I injury is characterized more by clinical discomfort than it is by either ligamentous disruption (0% to 25%), or obvious joint deformation (other than mild, local swelling, and/or effusion). These injuries provide reasonable criteria for gradual return to activity and necessary rehabilitative progression for the entire involved area. It is usually necessary to prescribe or design equipment modification for protection of the injured area, both for comfort and prevention of additional injury. In temporal terms, return to participation is usually 7 to 21 days.

Class III injury is characterized by severe discomfort, major (75% to 100%) ligamentous disruption, and obvious significant joint deformity and laxity. If the goal of treatment is to provide the best anatomic and functional result, the athlete should not return to participation earlier than three months postinjury, and then with major supplemental protective measures. If the objective is not to return until there has been near complete healing by classic laboratory criteria, one should probably defer competitive athletics for at least six months. At time of return the athlete should use supplemental protective measures.

The class II injury is the most difficult one for which to predict accurately the rate of recovery and return to competitive participation. This degree of injury is characterized by moderate (25% to 75%) ligamentous disruption and associated joint deformity and laxity. Clinical follow-up examinations indicate a decline in discomfort long before there has been commensurate healing to the point of allowing a safe return to participation. It is the class II injury, with resultant moderate joint laxity, that requires surgical consideration in the athlete who must return to competition. The hazard of too early a return to participation (usually recommended because of decreased pain and an encouraging clinical examination) is a recurrence of injury, or worse, conversion to a class III injury. Thus judgment should be based on clinical examinations, assessment of injury, knowledge of the basic science of tissue healing, demands of the sport on the involved area, and the possibility of adequate protection to the involved area. When a positive judgment is made on the basis of these criteria, the athlete should first return to participation of the basic, least physically demanding skills and movements. Only after these have been achieved without discomfort and up to expected performance levels, should one consider gradual return to more competitive participation. Return cannot be gradual in degrees of competition, only in the time allowed to compete; all athletes understand the immense stress differential between practice and full-scale competition. Most will have difficulty accepting prolonged absence from activity when they are generally feeling healthy and, in their opionion, ready to return.

Sprains, subluxations, and dislocations in the shoulder area are most frequently identified at three sites: acromioclavicular, glenohumeral, and sternoclavicular joints. The acromioclavicular joint usually provides minimal motion but it is extremely important in articulation of the upper extremity to the axial skeleton. Because of its location and limited degree of motion, it is susceptible to frequent injury. This joint is maintained in its customary anatomic position by ligaments about the joint as well as by two major ligaments, acromioclavicular and coracoclavicular. Diagnosis of injury is readily made from understanding the mechanisms of injury, complaints of the injured athlete, examination of the area, and radiographic appearance. These injuries are usually secondary to a direct fall on the elbow or outstretched hand, resulting in a directed force along the extremity to the acromioclavicular joint. This same directed force in an older individual would perhaps result in a fracture or in injuries to the tendinous anatomy about the shoulder.

Acromioclavicular Injuries

Injuries to the acromioclavicular joint are generally classified in three groups: first degree (mild) sprain, second degree (moderate) subluxation, and third degree (severe) dislocation. Obviously, the extent of injury will be closely paralleled by the sensitivity to palpation over the joint and deformity. The more severe the injury, the greater the degree of ligamentous disruption, and the greater the degree of step-off placement between the acromion and the distal end of the clavicle. It is important to corroborate clinical findings and possible associated fracture by anteroposterior radiographic films, with the patient standing with his arm at his side, and holding a weight in the hand on the injured extremity to distract the joint maximally. Treatment of these injuries is generally related to their classification.

Treatment Initial treatment in first and second degree groups is use of a sling shoulder immobilizer with an appropriate compressive padded dressing across the outer end of the clavicle and under the proximal ulna, providing a compressive force on the dislocated outer clavicle. It is the outer clavicle that is riding high in relationship to the acromion and thus, the forces should be made to equalize the superior margin of both the acromion and the clavicle. The previously described splinting mechanism accomplishes this goal.

In class III injuries the initial treatment is the same as for class I and class II injuries. In a severe dislocation there is probably a tear of the ligaments about the acromioclavicular joint as well as the two major supporting ligaments, the acromioclavicular and coracoclavicular. There continues to be significant variation in the minds of many orthopedic surgeons as to whether primary surgical repair is the treatment of choice, and whether or not it offers the best long-term results. Some prefer nonsurgical treatment in the early stages and various types of arthroplasties and resections at a later stage. In class III injuries it is suggested that appropriate consultation be sought with full awareness of the controversy regarding surgical vs nonsurgical treatment (Figure 18-7).

In some instances, if an athlete has experienced repetitive although generally mild acromioclavicular injuries, it is possible that early degenerative changes will occur within the articular surfaces of the joint (Figure 18-8). In such an event, one is dealing with local degenerative arthritis. Treatment considerations would range from the use of oral antiinflammatory medications to operative intervention and resection of the distal end of the clavicle.

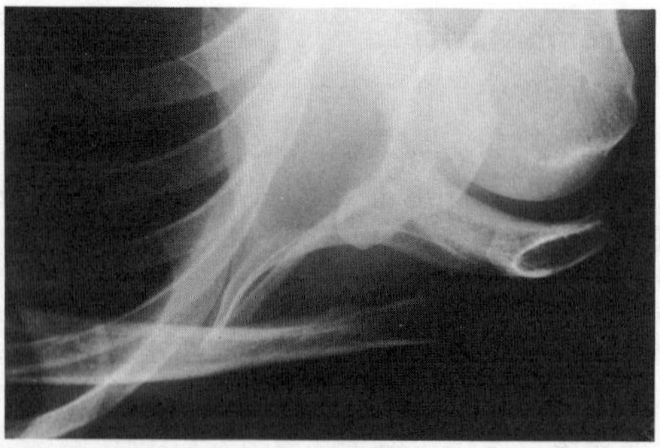

Figure 18-7 An acute severe acromioclavicular injury (class III).

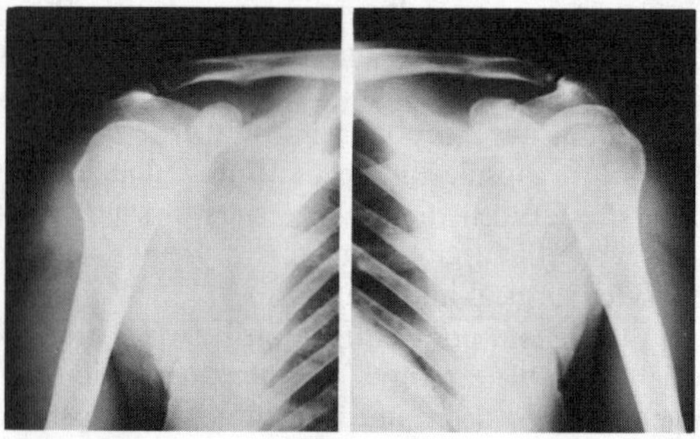

Figure 18-8 Comparative views of acromioclavicular joints in college-age football player who had experienced multiple "shoulder separations" on his left side.

After completing treatment of the acute phase of acromioclavicular injury, one must gradually pursue reconditioning of muscles about the shoulder, motion of the entire shoulder girdle, and finally possible modification of equipment necessary to permit continued participation in sports. As these injuries are very common in football, it is usually necessary to repad the shoulder pads to provide a redistribution of force anterior, posterior, and lateral to the joint, thus minimizing the likelihood of a recurrent direct blow and reinjury.

Glenohumeral Injuries

Injuries to the shoulder (glenohumeral) joint are generally related to its anterior portion. It is estimated that in acute injuries to the shoulder joint, 98% to 99% are to the anterior portion and 1% to 2% to the posterior portion, although recent reports are indicating more posterior anatomical findings. The cause for this distribution is partly because of anatomy, in that the glenoid does have a slight canter to provide less support anteriorly than it does posteriorly. Also, the majority of injuries resulting in glenohumeral problems are associated with the arm in the abducted and externally rotated positions, which place greater stress across the anterior portion of the joint. If the arm is being adducted and internally rotated in moderate forward flexion, the forces are directed to the posterior joint. It is important to document whether the injury is anterior or posterior, as it is frequently assumed that a shoulder problem is anterior. If treatment is determined for an anterior dislocation when the problem is actually posterior, the anatomic and healing situations will be made worse. Radiographic confirmation is required to ascertain whether the pathology is anterior or posterior.

The categorization of glenohumeral injuries is the same as for those of the acromioclavicular joint: class I, sprain; class II, subluxation; and class III, dislocation. The most frequent mechanism of injury is depicted by the football arm tackle or the entrapped skipole and moving skier. Since the anterior capsule is not a strong stabilizing force, a major contributor to the support for containment of the humeral head within the glenoid is from the overlying soft tissue structures, particularly the subscapularis tendon. If there is an abnormality in the formation and excessive anteversion of the glenoid or injury to the glenoid labrum, or if there is attenuation or inherent laxity of the capsule and/or subscapularis, a minimal force in the described planes will sublux or dislocate the shoulder. When the glenohumeral joint is dislocated anteriorly, the normal muscle forces will adduct the humeral head toward the midline and it will appear as if it is under coracoid. Thus, on clinical examination there will be an apparent defect in the deltoid mass at the subacromion level and the humeral head will be palpated beneath the coracoid. Radiographically, the humeral head will be out of normal relationship to the glenoid, and adducted to a position inferior to the coracoid.

If the shoulder does not frankly dislocate and the athlete describes a pop forward and snap back, that would be termed a subluxation. If it does not really pop or come forth but the injury results in moderate discomfort, it would most likely be a sprain. It should also be noted that in individual athletes, soft tissue characteristics will be important in assessing the likelihood of recurrent glenohumeral subluxation or dislocation. The individual with lax ligaments and less muscle bulk is much more likely to experience frequent dislocations than the tightly muscled individual. It is possible that the latter, against similar forces, is more likely to experience either a subluxation or a tear of the glenoid labrum and will present a history similar to a meniscal injury with snapping, locking, and clicking of the shoulder on the motions of abduction and external rotation. Injuries of the glenoid labrum may cause functional glenohumeral instability.

Treatment Initial examination of the shoulder dislocation should include evaluation of the remainder of the extremity to assess associated deformity, abnormal function, and neurovascular impairment. Once this is complete, making the patient comfortable prior to relocation is most important. The methods for achieving satisfactory reduction of the dislocated shoulder are well described and illustrated in a number of classic textbooks. Before reduction, if possible, it is important to obtain satisfactory x-rays to be certain there are not associated skeletal injuries. There should also be a postreduction radiograph to ascertain complete reduction of the joint as well as review the status of associated skeletal tissues regarding the possibility of other injuries.

Treatments for sprain and subluxation are quite similar. One must immobilize the shoulder to provide relief of pain from the ligamentous stretching, possible tendinous stretching, and secondary synovitis. This is usually accomplished by using a commercially available shoulder immobilizer, or a sling and swathe with elasticized bandages for 7 to 14 days.

Postreduction treatment following the first shoulder dislocation is somewhat controversial. Some physicians feel that the customary treatment of immobilization in a sling and swathe for three weeks followed by progressive reconditioning, is the appropriate sequence. Statistics on 15- to 25-year-old individuals treated in this pattern demonstrate a high incidence of subsequent recurrent dislocations. Thus, some feel that if the injured person is a highly competitive athlete, the likelihood of recurrent dislocations is so great that they will consider a primary soft tissue reconstruction following the initial dislocation. Others feel that a longer period, six weeks, of immobilization in a sling and swathe followed by a supervised reconditioning program, will result in a lower incidence of recurrent dislocations. Therefore, fewer individuals will require surgery.

In general, it appears currently that the majority of physicians prescribe three to four weeks of shoulder immobilization followed by a progressive reconditioning program prior to returning to full competition. If subsequent dislocations occur, surgical reconstruction is recommended. It is important to be aware that controversy regarding dif-

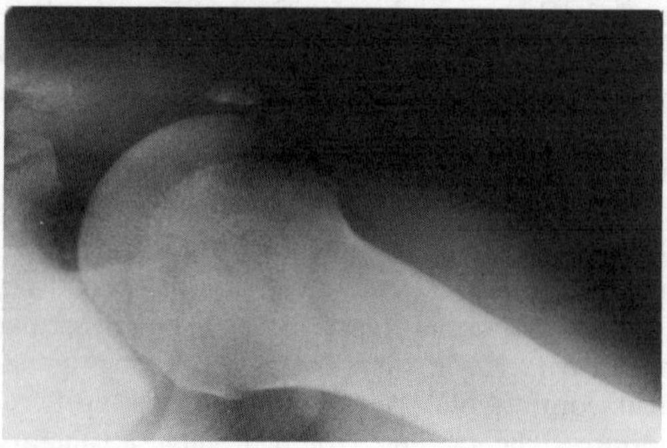

Figure 18-9 Axillary view of shoulder demonstrating intraarticular osteocartilaginous loose fragment in football player with recurrent dislocated shoulder.

ferent treatment methods persists. Whenever a high school or college athlete has a history of recurrent subluxations or dislocations and is unable to participate in his sport with a customary holding device, surgical intervention is recommended.

A number of different surgical procedures are available for the repair of a recurrent subluxating or dislocating shoulder. In the majority of instances, most of these procedures competently performed should achieve a 95% or better likelihood of correction. Whatever procedure is performed, it should include arthrotomy and examination of the intraarticular aspects of the glenohumeral joint for tears in the labrum, loose cartilaginous fragments, or osteocartilaginous irregularities in either the humeral head or the glenoid (Figure 18-9). Once this inspection and the necessary action have been completed, reconstruction of the capsule and tendons will be determined by the surgeon's findings and influenced by the anticipated demands of the athlete. If he requires maximum throwing or overhead swinging ability, such as a baseball pitcher, football quarterback, or tennis player, the surgeon must be aware that many of the customary procedures will limit external rotation and thereby limit the ability of the individual to perform. Thus, modification in surgical technique will be required and particular attention directed to the freedom of motion of the anterior portion of the shoulder joint. Following surgical reconstruction the shoulder should be immobilized for approximately four weeks, after which a gentle, progressive reconditioning program should be undertaken. It is unwise for an athlete to return to competitive athletics for at least three months after such surgery. A period of six months will assure a more advanced state of healing, greater range of motion, and greater strength of the associated controlling musculature of the joint.

There is an increasing use of shoulder arthrography for the diagnosis and treatment of intraarticular glenohumeral pathology. Labral fragments can become interposed between the articulating surfaces resulting in functional glenohumeral instability. Such instability can also be caused by fragments of biceps tendon and rotator cuff as well as intraarticular chondral and osteochondral fragments. In patients with suggestive symptomatology, we are finding arthroscopy capable of detecting these abnormalities and of removing them in some cases.

Sternoclavicular Injuries

Injuries to the sternoclavicular joint are generally caused by forces that drive the shoulder and shoulder girdle forward and consequently drive the clavicle toward the sternum. The integrity of the sternoclavicular joint is provided by the ligamentous structures between the clavicle and the sternal manubrium as well as between the clavicle and the first rib. Within the articulation between the clavicle and the sternal manubrium is a fibrocartilaginous disc. This may be torn as part of a severe injury and result in symptoms of intraarticular derangement. Most frequently, the disruptive force carries the clavicle portion of the sternoclavicular joint anteriorly. On occasion it does dislocate posteriorly and if it is a severe dislocation, one must be aware of the underlying vascular structures and the possibility of an associated major complication.

The injuries for this joint are classified in the categories of the other joints about the shoulder: first degree, sprain; second degree, subluxation; and third degree, dislocation with associated ligamentous disruption. In first and second degree injuries, the usual treatment is with a sling until sensitivity subsides and a gradual rehabilitation program can be instituted. In the third degree, there are frequently associated tears of both the sternoclavicular and costoclavicular ligaments, and the intraarticular meniscus. An attempt at closed reduction is recommended; however, if this fails either because of extensive disruption of the ligaments or malposition of the fibrocartilaginous disc, early open reduction is indicated. One is cautioned to be aware of the proximity of the major vascular structures when considering open repair of this joint injury. In some instances when there is a long-standing chronic recurrent dislocation of the sternoclavicular joint, one must determine whether it is better to accept the disability or to attempt a secondary repair. If a late secondary repair is to be attempted, the author's experience is it is probable that one will require a supplemental tissue transfer to achieve satisfactory stabilization. This is frequently indicated because damage to the ligament is so extensive that it is impossible to achieve satisfactory apposition of the attenuated structures. In such instances satisfactory results can be achieved using a transfer of autogenous fascia lata as a supplement to the repair.

Whenever an individual has had major injury to the sternoclavicular joint it is important that he be carefully advised as to return to activity. Once again, initial healing time for the preliminary stage of ligamentous healing is a minimum of three weeks, and if there has been a major disruption, one should realistically look to a six-week period prior to returning to competitive athletics. The determination of a satisfactory healing period prior to return is critical for this injury, as there is no way of realistically providing support by way of holding devices or taping.

RECURRENT SHOULDER PAIN

Recurrent shoulder pain is a frequent complaint from athletes who use their upper extremities in repetitive, high frequency, high velocity motion such as baseball pitching. Although many athletic events place great demands on the structures about the shoulder, a baseball pitcher must be considered the prime example of physiologic overuse and overload. Thus, it seems reasonable to use the example of the throwing motion of the baseball pitcher as a model for discussion of various chronic, soft tissue complaints about the shoulder. The enormous force required to complete one pitch at greater than 90 mph is a phenomenon in its own right. However, the feat is more astonishing when one realizes that a baseball pitcher must perform this act up to 200 times every four or five days for seven months a year. That the anatomy of any human being is able to tolerate this repetitive motion with its associated tremendous forces, without more frequent complaints of discomfort or evidence of degeneration, is remarkable.

The act of throwing requires total body coordination with the ultimate force being directed through the shoulder girdle and along the upper extremity. Throwing is customarily divided into the phases of cocking, acceleration, and follow-through. The cocking motion is responsible for directing the shoulder and shoulder girdle into a position of hyperabduction, hyperextension, and extreme external rotation through the glenohumeral joint. This position places great stress at the acromion, humeral interphase, and across all of the supportive structures of the anterior capsule of the shoulder joint. Extreme hyperabduction and external rotation may result in squeezing or impingement of the tendons of the anterior rotator cuff between the humeral head and the acromion. These forces result in a stretching and in a compressive, potential irritation of many of these structures. In such instances specific tendinitis or an impingement syndrome may be diagnosed.

The next phase of pitching, acceleration, delivers the shoulder forward and derotates the glenohumeral joint. To achieve this motion there is a sudden contraction of all the muscles across the anterior shoulder joint, particularly the internal rotators. Thus, release and stabilization of the joint in addition to individual stress contractions may result in focal areas of damage or inflammation. The acceleration phase also results in initiation of enormous stresses through the elbow, because of the whipping action that results in a valgus force to the elbow, resulting in medial stretch and lateral compression.

The follow-through phase of pitching is the primary deceleration phase and it places great stress through the posterior shoulder, on the basis of eccentric action of the muscles of the posterior shoulder area. The rhythm of throwing and the resultant relaxation of the posterior muscles in the final phase may result in excessive stretching of the capsule and tendinous portions.

Although we are able to define the phases of throwing and specifically identify the interaction of muscle groups at different stages of the action, we are unable to account for the forces generated within each muscle group and the coordination of these forces that is required to achieve excellence in throwing.

From the knowledge we have on throwing and complaints regarding shoulder pain, there seems to be a general way of classifying recurrent shoulder pain: anterior, superior, and posterior. Anterior discomfort is most frequently associated with inflammation of the tendinous portion of the long head of the biceps. On occasion there will be associated discomfort in other tendinous groups of the anterior shoulder joint.

Complaints of the superior regions seem to be more related to a combination of the intraarticular portion of the biceps tendon; anterior portion of the rotator cuff, particularly the supraspinatus tendon; and mechanical impingement of the abducted and rotating humeral head in the glenoid and against the acromion. This entire process is closely related to the flexibility or loss of flexibility of the glenohumeral capsular and ligamentous anatomy.

The most frequent discomfort posteriorly is associated with either the medial head of the triceps or the insertion of the teres minor. The problem may be an isolated true bursitis secondary to injury in some contact sport, or from repetitive abduction of the shoulder by an individual who has not adequately trained for such activity. In other instances, bursitis may be the presenting symptom for other shoulder abnormalities, such as injuries to the rotator cuff or subluxation. It is unusual to see major rotator cuff disruptions in young athletes, however. Episodes of inflammation and focal injury are common in athletes who perform the throwing or overhead swinging act on a repetitive basis. The degrees of abnormalities identified in these problems of tendinitis and bursitis range from the focal area of trauma resulting in hemorrhage and inflammation, to partial tear or complete disruption. Again, these three distinctions of injury are frequently defined as class I, class II, or class III tendinous injuries of the shoulder.

Treatment Once the source of discomfort is identified, the first stage of immediate treatment is rest, with avoidance of throwing motion for a minimum of one week. If there is acute sensitivity, the use of oral antiinflammatory agents is appropriate. Steroid injections should be avoided as a first line of treatment, as it is well documented that the deposition of steroid directly into tendon substance can result in areas of focal necrosis and further tendon injury. If the pain has not diminished in a period of seven to ten days on a course of rest and oral antiinflammatory medications, judiciously utilized local anesthetic and steroid may be considered. Again, the potential hazard of repetitive steroid injections and increasing risk of additional tendinous injury must be emphasized. After use of injectable steroids for treatment of the tendinitis or bursitis, there must be a continuing objective of complete rehabilitation prior to returning to competition. When sensitivity has diminished, an attempt should be made toward achieving and maintaining a full range of painless motion. Only after this objective has been achieved should strengthening the weakened muscle groups begin.

Rehabilitation

In the author's experience, the most common error in delay of recovery from shoulder injury and pain is lack or inadequate supervision of a rehabilitation program. In general, if one major muscle is one unit weaker than it was prior to injury or pain, it will fatigue more quickly and will result in a change in the method of performance that will restrict the athlete in returning to a previous level of performance. For the majority of athletes this is usually loss of control, recurrence of pain either in the same or other areas of the shoulder complex, and a loss of velocity. All result in worsening performance. Thus, it cannot be over-emphasized that one must completely rehabilitate the shoulder to complete motion and strength prior to permitting an athlete to return to the strenuous and competitive demands of participation and competition.

An isokinetic machine is recommended for both testing and rehabilitative phases of upper extremity injuries. The machine permits an athlete to recondition the impaired muscle group without progressive discomfort and damage. In the testing phase, force units generated in the different ranges of shoulder motion are compared for dominant and nondominant sides. It is detrimental to permit anyone to return to competition until the rating for the injured dominant side equals the strength of the nondominant side.

Thus, as we analyze the reason for shoulder pain injury in most throwing athletes, it must be concluded that demands on the upper extremity are truly anomalous to what the upper extremity was anatomically designed to perform. With each attempt to throw forcefully, the athlete is essentially separating his upper extremity from his trunk without major osseous connections, but with only the attachment of certain critical tendons and ligaments. The repetitive demands on these soft tissue structures and possible compression and mechanical influences of joint motion on tendon structures, result in inflammation about some of the tendons (and occasionally in small areas of focal necrosis within the tendons), and areas of inflammation and bursitis between them. Any one of the pathologic phases may later result in progressive tendon deterioration, weakening of the upper extremity, and compromising of the person's potential.

Although it is impossible to avoid some of these demands when participating in certain activities, the athlete should be advised of the need for a comprehensive preconditioning program before the season, and a continued conditioning program throughout the season. The vital aspects of any such program, whether it be for the upper extremity or other areas of the body, include maximum flexibility, strength, and endurance.

THE ELBOW

The forces moving through the shoulder in the act of throwing or other athletic action, are extended distally through the arm to the elbow area. The final phases of throwing, acceleration and follow-through, place enormous stress on the elbow, with the valgus stress across the elbow joint resulting in stretching on the medial side of the elbow, rotary compression through the lateral side of the elbow, and finally, compression of the olecranon and the humerus in the ultimate act of elbow extension. The final motion results in compressive forces both in the concavity of the olecranon as well as its tip from the pull of the triceps tendon. Pathologic processes have been identified in all of these sites in athletes who perform repetitive throwing motions.

The most common problems identified on the medial side of the elbow joint include bony avulsions, injuries within the flexor mass, ulnar nerve inflammation secondary to repetitive stretch and/or subluxation in the ulnar groove, and spurs on the medial edge of the olecranon. If the area of complaint focuses on the medial side of the elbow, one must consider all possibilities. In the younger athlete, there may be a frank avulsion of the entire medial epicondyle or major portions of the medial epicondyle (Figure 18-10). A single-force injury should first direct one to consider traumatic avulsion from the medial epicondyle or a tear within the body of the flexor group. If the complaint is related to chronic stresses, the anatomic problem is more likely to involve medial olecranon traction spurs. These may cause chronic discomfort or become fractured, and be the sources of acute pain (Figure 18-11).

The forces on the lateral aspect of the joint are mostly related to repetitive compressive forces between the radial head and the capitellum in a combination of forces that includes both direct compression and rotation of the head of the radius against the capitellum. This combination results in

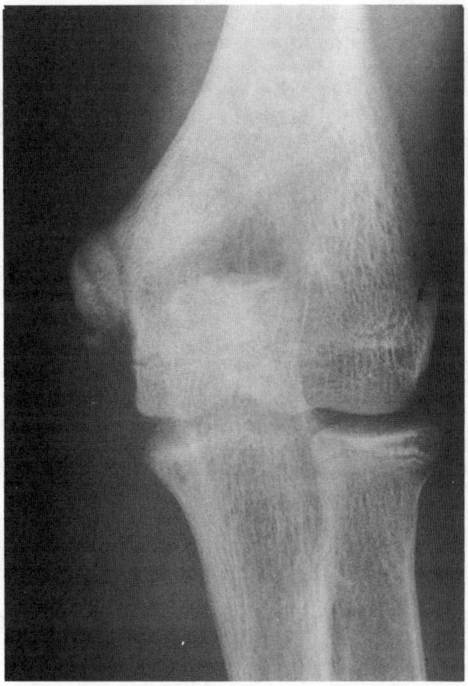

Figure 18-10 Avulsion fracture of medial epicondyle in adolescent baseball pitcher, origin of flexor muscle group.

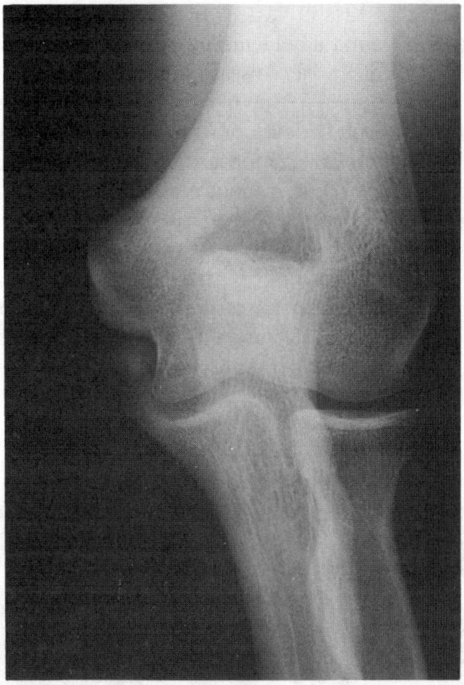

Figure 18-11 Fracture of traction exostosis on medial edge of olecranon in professional baseball pitcher.

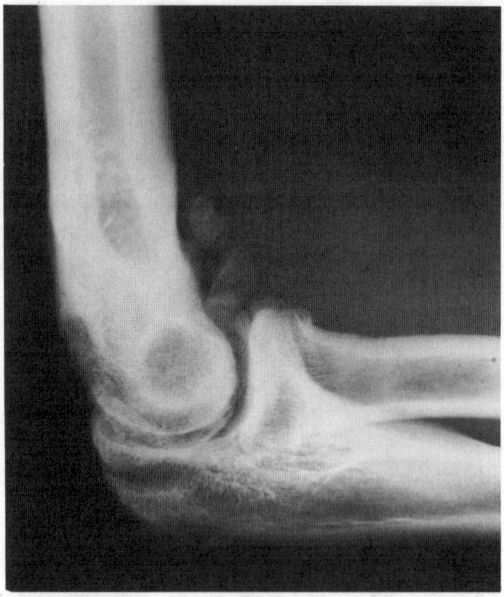

Figure 18-12 Multiple osteocartilaginous fragments in elbow of professional baseball player.

a shearing action on the radiohumeral joint. On occasion, the result is damage to the articular surfaces with progressive fragmentation of the articular cartilage and formation of intraarticular loose bodies (Figures 18-12 and 18-13). In the younger athlete this may be initially identified as a focal avascular area, called Panner disease (Figure 18-14). The whipping motion in the final stages of elbow extension may result in development of articular damage in the humeral olecranon articulation in both the concavity of the olecranon, and posteriorly at the tip of the olecranon, even an avulsion of the triceps insertion (Figure 18-15).

The traction pull of the triceps and intraarticular compression force of the tip of the olecranon against the olecranon fossa of the humerus may result in articular damage, fragmentation, and ectopic bone formation (Figure 18-16). Although these areas of involvement are primarily for the skeletally mature athlete, they can be involved in the growing athlete with resultant abnormalities of growth, premature degeneration, and long-term intraarticular deformity (Figure 18-17). It should be emphasized that the young athlete who continues to have open epiphyses, thus demonstrating active growth potential, should be advised of the same

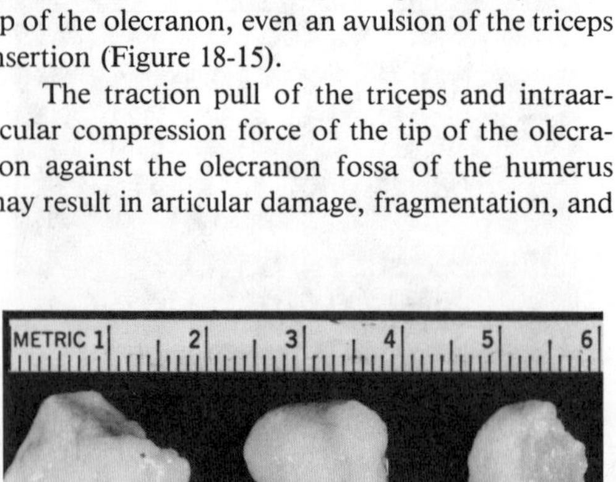

Figure 18-13 Appearance of size of osteocartilaginous fragments after surgical removal.

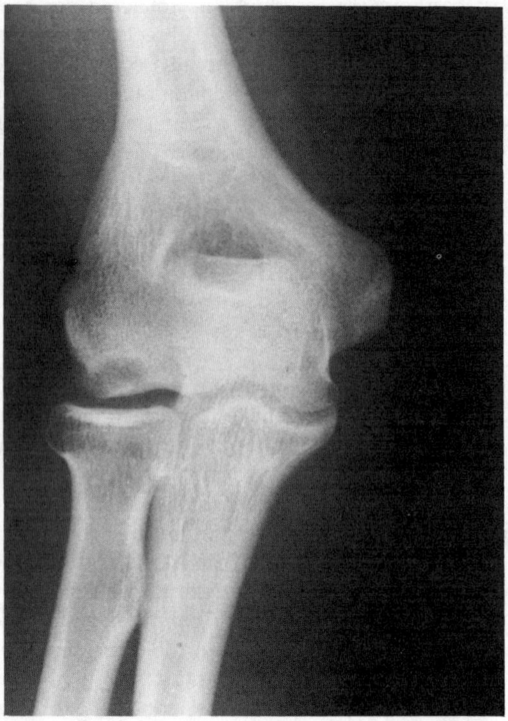

Figure 18-14 Osteochondrosis of capitellum (Panner lesion) in adolescent athlete.

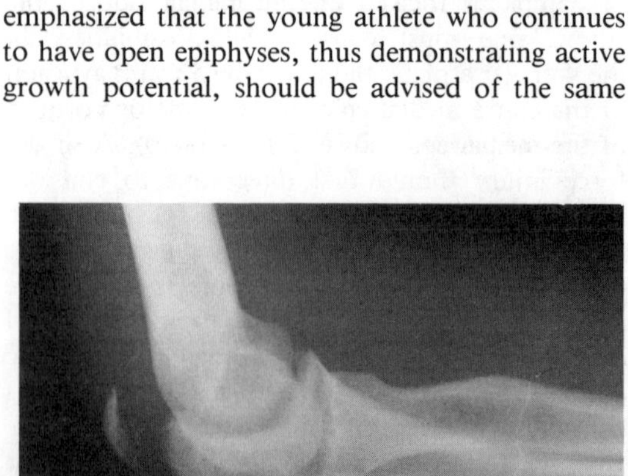

Figure 18-15 Avulsion of triceps tendon insertion in adolescent football player.

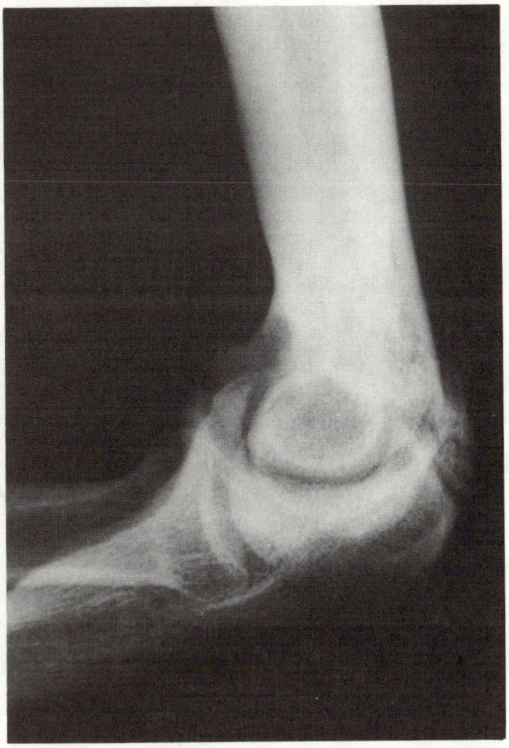

Figure 18-16 Ectopic bone development in insertion of triceps tendon limiting elbow extension by 60°, in retired baseball pitcher.

restrictions for limited pitching as recommended by the Little League regulations. It is impossible to define chronologic age limits as to when one should and should not pitch; they are related to the individual player's skeletal development and maturation. The greater the number of innings pitched by a child with open epiphyses, the greater the likelihood of some anatomic impairment and, ultimately, restriction of the athletic career.

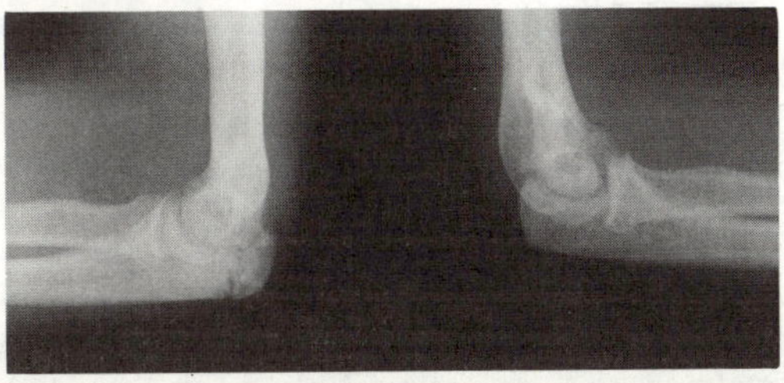

Figure 18-17 Persistent elbow pain in adolescent baseball pitcher secondary to failure of normal closure of olecranon epiphysis. Comparative lateral view of both elbows.

Tennis El

The
in athl
sourc
mus
ob
mation
carpi radial
most likely mech
related to overuse and
lack of appropriate precondi

Obviously, the first phase of t be prevention and appropriate advice conditioning. If the athlete presents with dis fort in the characteristic anatomic location, primary treatment should be rest, application of cold packs, and prescribed oral antiinflammatory medications. If symptoms persist, local injection with a combination of local anesthetic and steroid may be used. In chronic situations, use of an elbow brace or a nonelastic band distal to the elbow area decreasing the excursion and stress on the extensor origin, may be helpful. In some instances, recommended treatments for an acute or chronic tennis elbow fail. In these situations surgical intervention should be considered and may prove successful. However, one should not look to surgery as the primary cure-all without a carefully advised and supervised postoperative rehabilitation program.

A rehabilitation program includes necessary flexibility exercises to assure a full range of motion for the elbow, forearm, wrist, and fingers; and isotonic and isometric exercises to assure maximum strength of the forearm musculature. In addition, specific attention should be directed toward equipment, such as the size and weight of the racquet, tension of the racquet strings, and circumference of the handle grip.

Other injuries of the arm and elbow are most frequently related to soft tissue contusions, well-described fractures, and lacerations. An associated chronic condition that may result from any of the acute injuries is myositis ossificans (Figure 18-18). This is a significant complication of injuries of the arm and elbow that raises questions as to treatment and return to participation. A guideline for treatment is rest until the sensitivity subsides, and gradual increase of motion. Once motion and strength have improved without sensitivity and without extension of the ossification process proved by sequential radiographs, it is reasonable for the athlete to return to participation. Appropriate padding should be placed over the affected

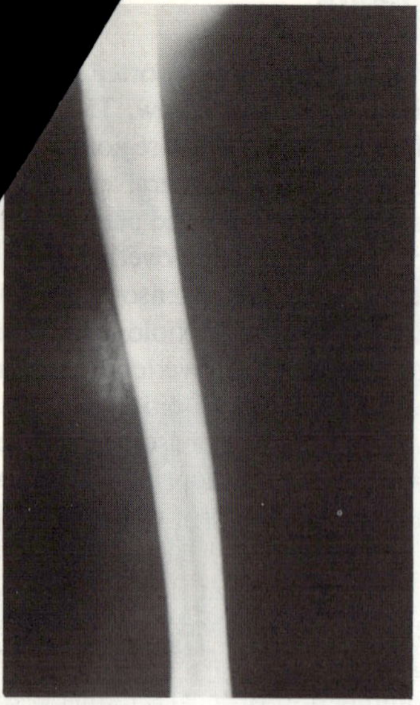

Figure 18-18 Myositis ossificans of arm in high school interior lineman. Affected area was at impact of improperly fitted shoulder pads.

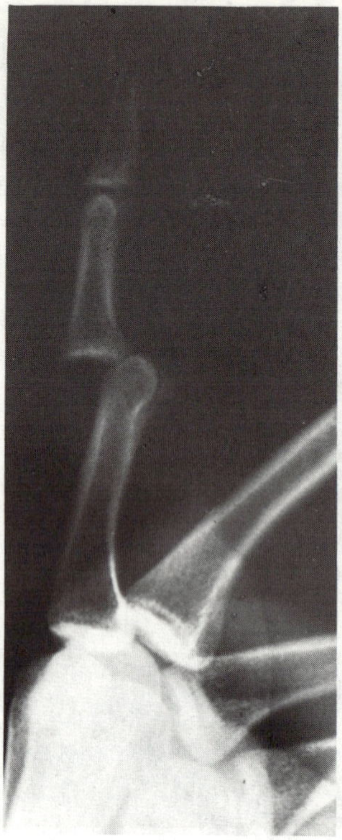

Figure 18-19 Proximal interphalangeal dislocation without fracture in baseball pitcher.

area to prevent repetitive contusion and the possible extension of the myositis ossificans process.

INJURIES OF THE WRIST, HAND, AND FINGERS

Injuries of the wrist, hand, and fingers are common in all sports. The clinical result following a wrist or hand injury may have a profound influence on an athlete's return to participation. A closed dislocated interphalangeal joint is a common injury for football interior linemen. Frequently, it is reduced on the field or at the sideline with immediate return to participation. The dislocation is reduced and two fingers are taped together. However, a similar interphalangeal dislocation of the index finger of the dominant hand of a baseball pitcher results in an extended period away from participation and possible significant influence on the remainder of his career (Figure 18-19).

Injuries to the wrist range from mild ligamentous injuries to dislocations that frequently require surgical reduction, and major tendon injuries that may terminate careers. The biomechanical demands through the wrist joint and the intercarpal joints are greatest in the activities that require a wrist snap and/or turnover intercarpal rotation. These motions are most important in events that require the swinging of an object, as in baseball, tennis, golf, lacrosse, or in events that require the release of an object with sudden wrist action as in bowling, weight lifting, and certain track and field events. These forces can result in subluxation of tendons of the wrist, straining of ligaments at the wrist and intercarpal joints, dislocation, and carpal fractures. It is to prevent such injuries that athletes frequently wear various tape or leather supports on their wrists. Accurate diagnosis of wrist injuries can be one of the most challenging and trying areas in sportsmedicine. Frequently it is necessary to obtain comparative radiographic views of both extremities, and additional fluoroscopic and tomographic examinations.

Wrist injuries occur as the result of acute single trauma and of repetitive force overload. Single trauma injuries include sprains, fractures, and dislocations of the wrist joint and at all the intercarpal levels. The most frequent acute carpal fracture is to the carpal navicular joint. Frequently this fracture is not identified on the first series of radiographs. If an area of local sensitivity persists seven to ten days after a presumed sprain of the

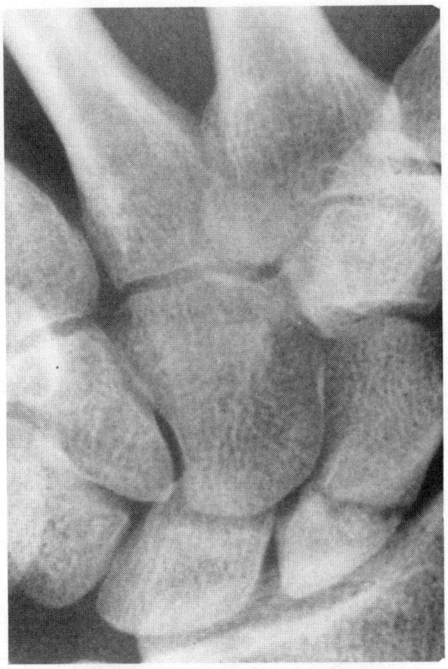

Figure 18-20 Delayed union of a carpal navicular fracture.

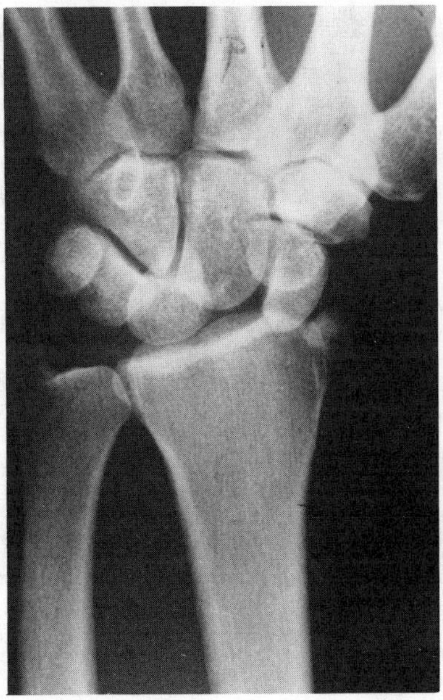

Figure 18-21 Posteroanterior view of wrist demonstrating transnavicular fracture and perilunate dislocation.

carpal navicular, additional x-rays should be taken. The radiologist should be advised of the suspected location of the injury and specific views should be taken to cover the area. Chronic discomfort from a malunited or ununited carpal navicular injury frequently requires surgical intervention for realignment and bone grafting (Figure 18-20).

Some of the most difficult fractures to identify and treat are fractures of the hook of the hamate. These frequently require various radiographic techniques for identification and may ultimately require surgical treatment (Figures 18-21 and 18-22). Chronic discomfort following repetitive stresses to the wrist area may also include areas of focal avascular necrosis, particularly of the carpal lunate (Kienbock syndrome), as well as instability of various intercarpal ligaments, and therefore the pain of subluxation associated with swinging a baseball bat, tennis racket, golf club, lacrosse stick, or hockey stick (Figure 18-23).

The most frequent injuries of the hand and fingers include fractures, sprains, and dislocations. Most fractures of the hand and fingers are closed and appear relatively innocuous. This may prove to be deceiving as the tendency towards malalignment and malrotation of digital fractures is of significant potential disability. Lack of early fracture reduction is also a major concern. In closed treatment of a closed fracture of the hand and fingers, one must pay particular attention to achieving satisfactory alignment and rotational position, and subsequently maintaining the reduction. If this is not possible, early open reduction and pin fixation are to be considered.

One of the most common injuries of a finger in athletes is a combination of tendon injury and fracture, the mallet finger. The injury is on the dorsal aspect of the distal phalanx at the distal interphalangeal joint. The mechanism of injury is usually a direct blow on the tip of the extended finger resulting in either a rupture of the tendon at its insertion, or the avulsion of the tendon with a fragment

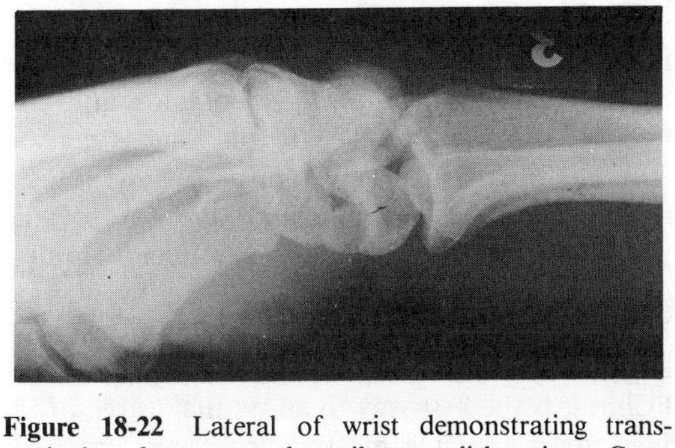

Figure 18-22 Lateral of wrist demonstrating transnavicular fracture and perilunate dislocation. Comparative views of contralateral wrist assist in questionable diagnosis.

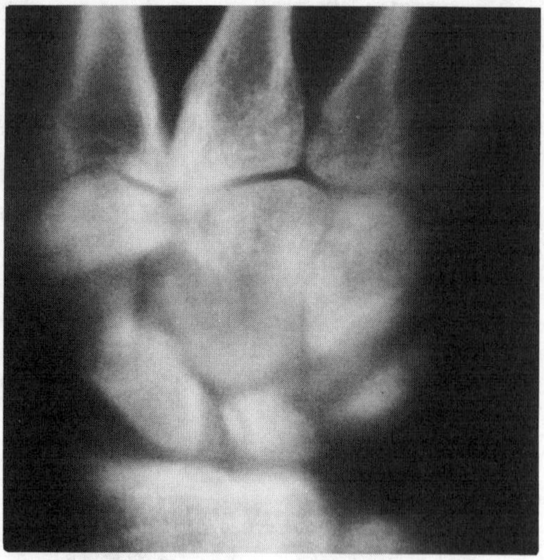

Figure 18-23 Tomographic demonstration of articular fracture of lunate not visualized on anteroposterior or oblique radiographs.

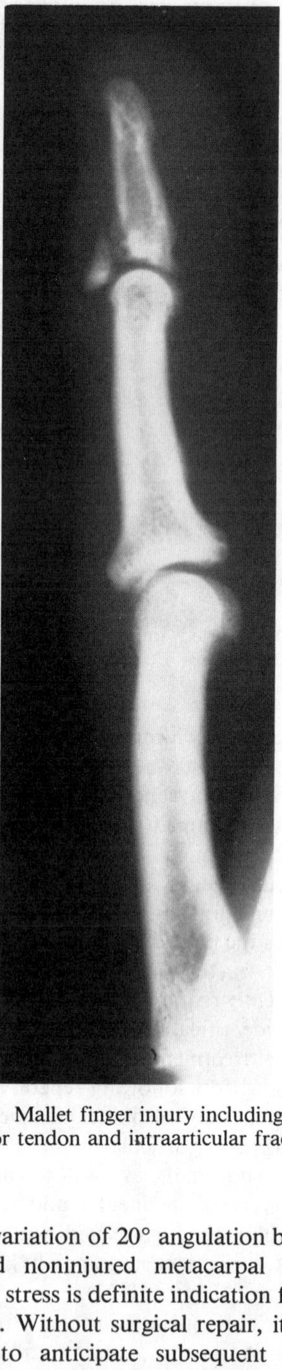

Figure 18-24 Mallet finger injury including insertion of distal extensor tendon and intraarticular fracture.

of bone. It is imperative to obtain early radiographic confirmation of the presence of bone fragments (Figure 18-24). The bone fragment usually involves a portion of the articular surface of the distal phalanx. Selection of closed vs open treatment, frequently depends on the size of the articular fragment and degree of separation from the body of the phalanx. The objectives of treatment are twofold: first, to maintain satisfactory function of the extensor tendon on the distal interphalangeal joint; and second, to maintain satisfactory articular function of the distal interphalangeal joint.

Sprains and dislocations of the hand and fingers generally receive primary treatment at the site of participation. Unfortunately, they are frequently forgotten until there is a residual chronic problem associated with the injury. This is best exemplified by an injury of the ulnar collateral ligament of the metacarpophalangeal joint of the thumb (Figure 18-25). This is a common injury in many sports. The stability of this joint is derived from the ulnar collateral ligament and the related musculotendinous insertion into the base of the proximal phalanx. This injury is frequently underestimated because there is usually only moderate local discomfort and no major deformity. However, the stability of the thumb under stress on this ligament is the best way to assess the degree of injury. As is true for most radiographic stress examinations, it is frequently necessary to block the nerves to prevent muscle spasm interference with the test. A variation of 20° angulation between the injured and noninjured metacarpal phalangeal joints under stress is definite indication for surgical intervention. Without surgical repair, it would be reasonable to anticipate subsequent instability, compromise of pinch strength, and probably early degenerative arthritis. Most other sprains are quite evident from examination and do not carry the potentially severe residual compromise of performance and function as the thumb metacarpophalangeal joint ulnar collateral injury.

Frank dislocations of metacarpophalangeal

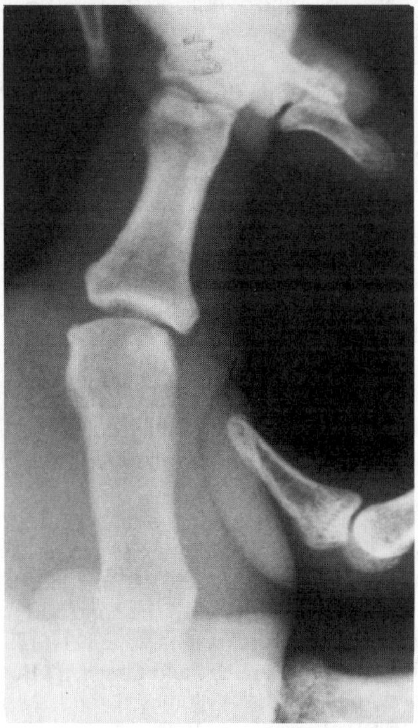

Figure 18-25 Stress test demonstrating incompetence of ulnar collateral ligament of thumb metacarpophalangeal joint.

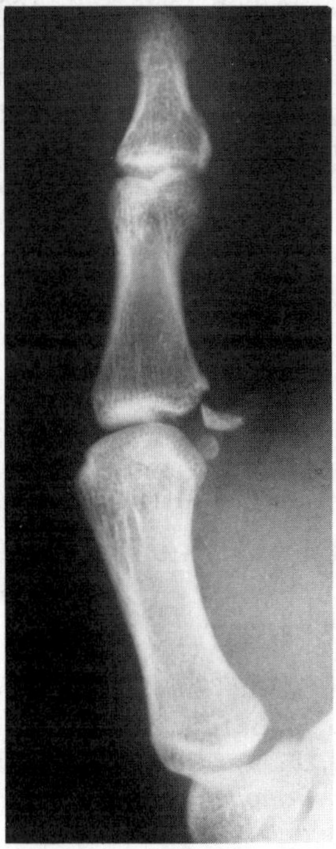

Figure 18-26 Avulsion fracture of base of proximal phalanx thumb, attachment of ulnar collateral ligament.

joints are frequently difficult to reduce by closed manipulation because of entrapment of the volar plate and the collateral ligaments. In such instances, open reduction is required to achieve a satisfactory reduction and repair of the injured soft tissues. A particular note of caution is directed to the treatment of all digital and hand dislocations: radiographs should always be part of the diagnosis and treatment (Figure 18-26). Although reduction of the dislocation may be readily achieved at the site of injury, it does not rule out the possibility of associated ligamentous avulsion fracture, which in the intraarticular region, could result in a major compromise of future function.

An unusual fracture dislocation is the Bennett fracture, which is intraarticular, with dislocation including an avulsion injury. Again, reduction of the articular fragments must be perfect to provide satisfactory long-term function. In some instances this can be achieved by closed reduction, but it frequently requires open reduction (Figure 18-27). Other acute closed injuries of the hand include ruptures or avulsions of various tendons.

In certain sports where there is continued pressure in one digital nerve area, such as bowling, baseball, or swinging any object for contact with another object, there is the possibility of compressive force resulting in neuroma formation. Such neuromata may respond to short-term rest and steroid instillation; the preferential treatment is prolonged rest. If they have not improved

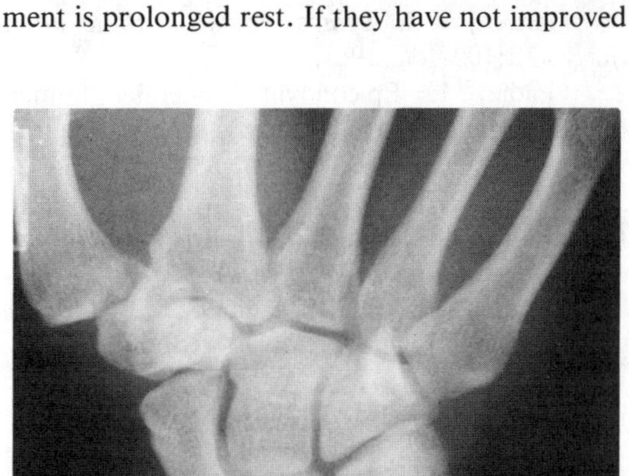

Figure 18-27 Bennett fracture in adolescent football player.

at later reexamination, there may be consideration for surgical intervention. The athlete should be advised of the unknown etiology of neuromas and that some individuals possess a greater propensity for neuromatous formation. Thus, there is the possibility of a recurrent neuroma following resection. Treatment of these problems should be in the domain of experienced hand and/or neurosurgeons.

SUGGESTED READINGS

Basmajian, J.V. *Muscles Alive: Their Functions Revealed by Electromyography.* Baltimore: Williams and Wilkins, 1974.

Basmajian, J.V. (Ed.) *Therapeutic Exercise,* 3rd Ed. Baltimore: Williams and Wilkins, 1978.

Bateman, J.E. Cuff tears in athletes. *Orthop Clin North Am.* 4:721–745, 1973.

Bateman, J.E. *The Shoulder and Neck.* Philadelphia: W.B. Saunders, 1972.

Behling, F. Treatment of acromioclavicular separations. *Orthop Clin North Am.* 4:747–757, 1973.

Bennett, G.E. Shoulder and elbow lesions of the professional baseball pitcher. *JAMA.* 117: 510–514, 1941.

Burton, R.I., and Eaton, R.G. Common hand injuries in the athlete. *Orthop Clin North Am.* 4:809–838, 1973.

Froimson, A.I. Treatment of tennis elbow with forearm support band. *J Bone Joint Surg.* 53A:183–184, 1971.

Garden, R.S. Tennis elbow. *J Bone Joint Surg.* 43B:100–106, 1961.

Goldie, I. Epicondylitis lateralis humeri (epicondylalgia or tennis elbow), a pathogenetical study. *Acta Chir Scand [suppl].* 339:1+, 1964.

Inman, V.T., Saunders, J.P., Dec, M. et al. Observations on the function of the shoulder joint. *J Bone Joint Surg.* 26:1–30, 1944.

Klafs, C.E., and Arnheim, D.D. *Modern Principles of Athletic Training,* 4th Ed. St Louis: C.V. Mosby, 1977.

Linscheid, R.L., Dobyns, J.H., Beabout, J.W. et al. Traumatic instability of the wrist: diagnosis, classification and pathomechanics. *J Bone Joint Surg.* 54A:1612–1632, 1972.

Neer, C.S., and Welsh, R.P. The shoulder in sports. *Orthop Clin North Am.* 8:583–591, 1977.

Nelson, C.L. The use of arthrography in athletic injuries of the shoulder. *Orthop Clin North Am.* 4:775–785, 1973.

Nirschl, R.P. Tennis elbow. *Orthop Clin North Am.* 4:787–800, 1973.

O'Donoghue, D.H. *Treatment of Injuries to Athletes,* 3rd Ed. Philadelphia: W.B. Saunders, 1976.

Pappas, A.M. Elbow problems associated with baseball during childhood and adolescence. *Clin Orthop.* 164:30–41, 1982.

Pappas, A.M., Goss, T.P., Kleinman, P.K. Symptomatic shoulder instability due to lesions of the glenoid labrum. *Am J Sports Med.* 11:279–288, 1983.

Perry, J. Anatomy and biomechanics of the shoulder in throwing, swimming, gymnastics and tennis. *Clin Sports Med.* 2:247–270, 1983.

Posner, M.A. Injuries to the hand and wrist in athletes. *Orthop Clin North Am.* 8:593–618, 1977.

Rockwood, C.A., Jr, and Green, D.P. (Eds.) *Fractures in Adults*, Volumes 1 and 2. Philadelphia: J.B. Lippincott, 1984.

Rockwood, C.A., Jr., Wilkins, K.E., and King, R.E. (Eds.) *Fractures in Children*, Volume 3. Philadelphia: J.B. Lippincott, 1984.

Rokous, J.R., Feagin, J.A., and Abbott, H.G. Modified axillary roentgenogram. A useful adjunct in the diagnosis of recurrent instability of the shoulder. *Clin Orthop.* 82:84–86, 1972.

Rowe, C.E. Acute and recurrent dislocations of the shoulder. *J Bone Joint Surg.* 44A:998–1008, 1962.

Tullos, H.S., and King, J.W. Lesions of the pitching arm in adolescents. *JAMA.* 220:264–271, 1972.

Tullos, H.S., and King, J.W. Throwing mechanism in sports. *Orthop Clin North Am.* 4:709–720, 1973.

Weaver, J.K., and Dunn, H.K. Treatment of acromioclavicular injuries, especially complete acromioclavicular separation. *J Bone Joint Surg.* 54A:1187–1194, 1972.

Wilson, J.C., and McKeever, F.M. Traumatic posterior (retroglenoid) dislocation of the humerus. *J Bone Joint Surg.* 31A:160–172, 1949.

CHAPTER 19
Injuries of the Lower Extremities

Thomas E. Hoerner, MD

What are the common athletic injuries to the lower extremity, hip, groin, thigh, knee and calf? How are they recognized? How are they treated? How can they be prevented? The injuries that are involved are contusions, sprains, subluxations, dislocations, fractures, hematomas, open wounds, and compartment syndromes. They may be acute or chronic.

CONTUSIONS

A contusion is a bruising of the skin or underlying tissue caused by a direct blow to the body. Capillary rupture and infiltrative effusion followed by edema and inflammation result in local swelling, tenderness, pain, heat, and vasomotor changes. The swelling may be superficial or deep.

Treatment The first principle is to limit bleeding by resting and elevating the attached extremity and applying ice and compression (RICE). After a period of 48 to 72 hours, heat, mobilization, activity, protection and a process of physical restoration are instituted.

STRAINS AND SPRAINS

A strain is a stretching injury to a muscle, tendon, or the tendomuscular junction of a muscle unit. Sprains occur in ligaments and are produced by the same mechanisms. Strains and sprains are classified as first, second, and third degree, or mild, moderate and severe.

Mild or first degree strains occur in the weakest point in the tendomuscular unit and involve a stretching of less than 25% of the muscle fibers. They can be caused by rapid accumulation and dispersion of a high amount of energy, or by overuse and tissue fatigue where continued force function results in local spasm. This is followed by inflammation and ischemia with resulting irritation in the muscle (myositis), tendon (tendinitis), or tendon sheath (tenosynovitis). Although these appear to be entirely different conditions, the etiology and progression are similar and treatment follows the same principles as for contusions.

A second or moderate degree of strain occurs when there is actual loss of function because of stretching of 25% to 75% of the fibers. There is more pain and swelling than in a first degree strain, and further decrease in the range of motion. Physical restoration can take two to three weeks.

Third degree or severe strains involve over 75% of the muscle fibers in the area of damage. Surgery is usually the mode of treatment if restoration of the tissue and its function is anticipated.

OTHER INJURIES

A *dislocation* is the complete disarticulation of a joint. A subluxation is a partial displacement with some remaining contact between the articular surfaces of the bones forming the joint.

Fractures occur in all sport activities, and are treated as any fracture in the general population.

A *hematoma* is a collection of pooled blood within a relatively constricted area that does not infiltrate within the tissue planes. The treatment includes initially controlling the bleeding tissue using the principles of RICE followed by protection while physical restoration occurs.

Myositis ossificans occurs as a complication of soft tissue injury such as a contusion, or hematoma. It appears to occur more often in young adults after chronic irritation. This is probably because of increased osteogenic capacity of young athletes and the increased incidence of tissue irritation from contact sports and overuse syndromes.

Open lacerations, punctures, and abrasions are treated with first aid and the usual emergency care procedures and techniques.

Compartment syndromes occur when the pressure within a closed fascial compartment exceeds the physiologic tolerance of the tissue within. The inciting event may be ischemia, crush injury, fractures, contusion or an overuse syndrome. The syndrome may be insidious in nature and must be suspected or the diagnosis will be missed. The diagnosis is made through the measurement of compartment pressures. Treatment ranges from rest and observation to surgical release.

HIP AND PELVIS

The pelvis is a uniquely designed mechanism that is constructed to transfer the body weight of the trunk from a single weight-bearing axis to the bipolar lower extremity supports. The spine attaches to the pelvis by the single connections at the sacrum and, to establish stability, anteriorly, posteriorly, and in the transverse, sagittal, and frontal planes. Through the pelvis, the weight of the upper trunk and spine is transferred from the spinal column to the lower extremities. The primary function of the pelvis, including the bones, joints, ligaments and muscles is the mechanical transfer of weight. The secondary function is to prevent injury to the abdominal viscera. Injuries to the pelvis are relatively unusual. Injuries to the hip joint are also rare in athletes. The hip is an intrinsically stable ball and socket joint encased in a thick capsule and surrounded by large muscles making fracture or dislocation rare with the energy achieved in nonvehicular sports.

Pelvic disorders include: sacroilitis, iliac apophysitis, osteitis pubis and ischial avulsions. All may be treated conservatively once infections and neoplastic etiologies have been ruled out (Figure 19-1). Athletes in the 11 to 12 year range may complain of hip, thigh or knee pain. These athletes should be evaluated for slipped capital femoral epiphyses. The examination demonstrates a Trendelenburg gait and a lack of internal rotation. The frog lateral hip x-ray demonstrates the pathology (Figure 19-2).

Differential diagnosis of hip pain also involves trochanteric bursitis and gluteus medius tendinitis (Figure 19-3). The patients should be carefully evaluated by history, physical examination and radiographic studies. The examination should localize tenderness, assess strength and muscle bulk, compare leg lengths and appraise iliotibial band tightness. Treatment includes rest, ice, heat, ultrasound, electrical stimulation, anti-inflammatory medication, local injections of steroids, leg length balancing and stretching exercises. Surgical treatment is reserved for those rare cases where conservative measures fail.

THIGH AND LEG

Hamstring strains, groin pulls and adductor strains are the most common injuries of the thigh area. Acute treatment in all of these cases is to apply the techniques of RICE. After initial immobilization of two to three days, range of motion exercises are initiated within the limits of comfort. Running in a straight line is begun when the patient has a full and comfortable range of motion. During this program, protective strapping, wrapping or a well-fitted support should be used.

The tendency of the hamstrings in their daily function is to shorten and contract. Therefore, as a compensatory mechanism, stretching the hamstrings to their full length is necessary on a daily basis. The exercises performed by an athlete should be set up specifically for his individual problems. Techniques should be varied to obtain the same end result—elasticity of the hamstring muscles (Figures 19-4 to 19-9).

Some athletes strain muscles frequently, some rarely, and others not at all. The individual predisposition to these injuries seems to be related to the degree of extremity laxity or suppleness with tight-jointed athletes being more at risk for strains.

Myositis ossificans occurs most commonly in thighs of young athletes and may complicate any of the above injuries. Stress fractures of the femur have now been reported in runners and may also account for thigh pain.

Calf pain may have a variety of etiologies. History and physical examination will make the diagnosis in most cases. The differential diagnosis should include a gastrocnemius-soleus strain including achilles tendon rupture, peroneal tendinitis and plantaris tendon rupture. A complete loss of the integrity of the achilles tendon gives a positive Thompson test, in addition to edema, ecchymosis and a palpable defect. Surgery must be strongly considered. The incidence of phlebitis is rare to the point of nonexistence in the active athlete.

Anterior leg pain is commonly referred to as shin splints. A variety of conditions may cause pain in this area. They include:

1. anterior tibial tenosynovitis
2. tibia stress fracture
3. compartment syndromes
4. periostitis
5. interosseous membrane tears
6. anterior compartment muscle strain.

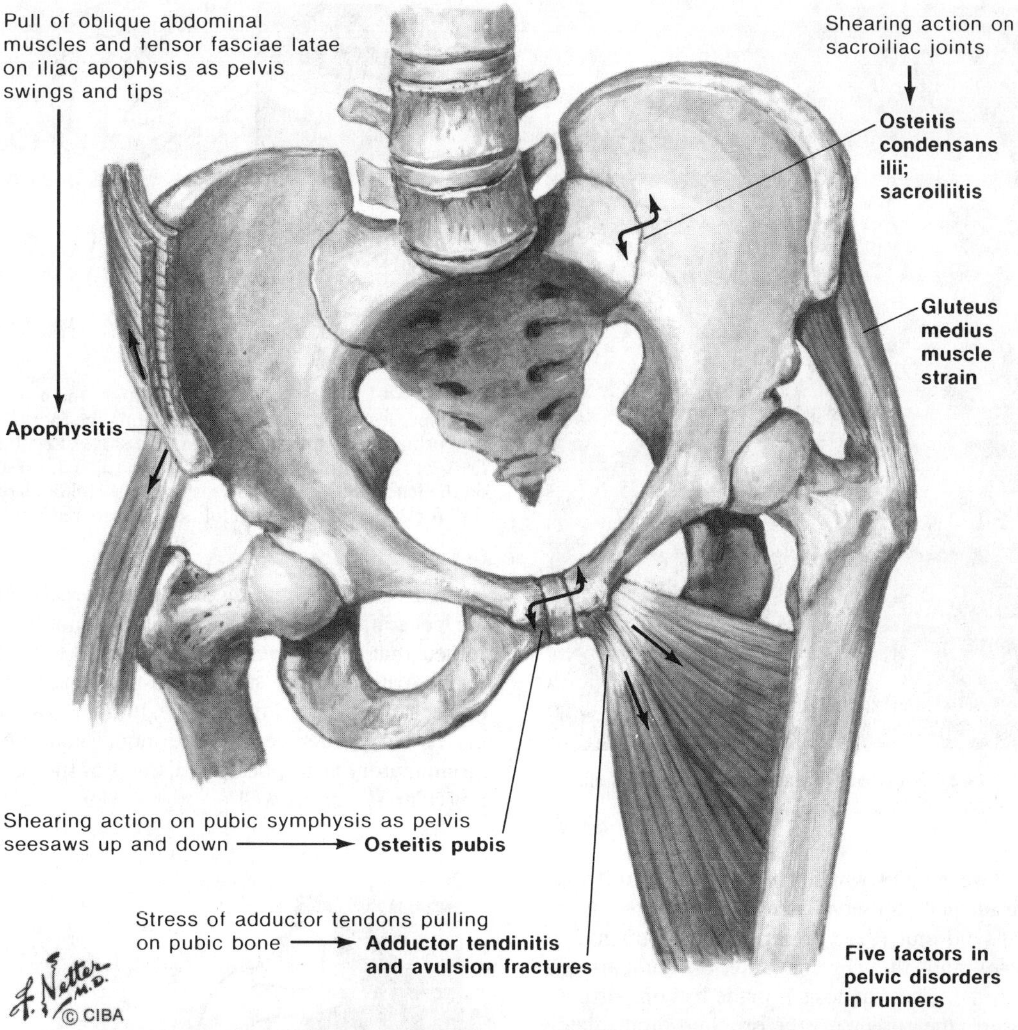

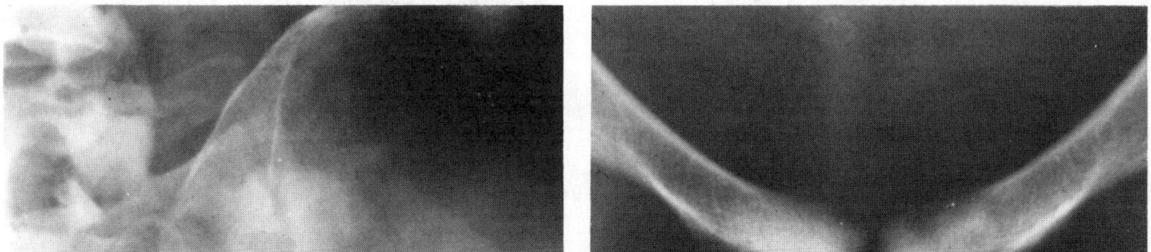

Sacroiliitis: x-ray showing sclerosis and irregularity of sacroiliac joint (appears late)

Osteitis pubis: sclerosis on both sides of pubic symphysis seen on x-ray (appears late)

Figure 19-1 Stress fractures and related disorders of the pelvis. Copyright © 1980 Ciba Pharmaceutical Company, Division of CIBA-GEIGY Corporation. Reproduced with permission from *Clinical Symposia*, illustrated by Frank H. Netter, MD. All rights reserved.

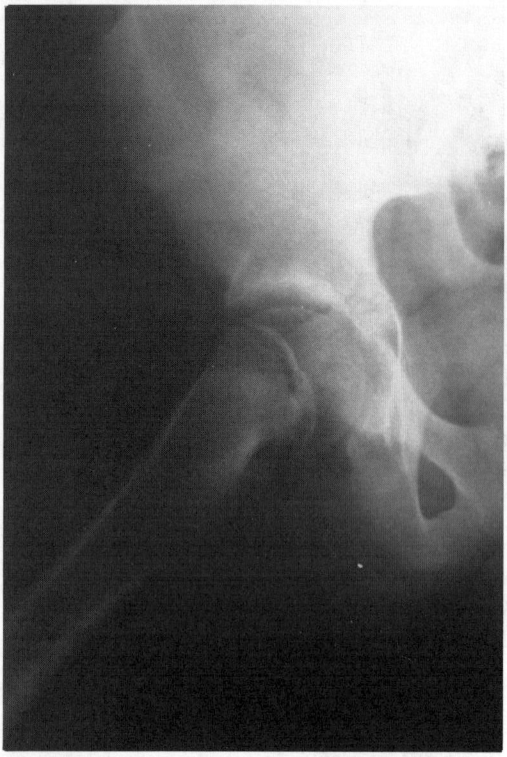

Figure 19-2 X-ray of frog demonstrates lateral slipped capital femoral epiphysis.

Two entities which may become chronic despite adequate conservative programs are the medial tibial syndrome (deep posterior compartment syndrome) and the chronic anterior compartment syndrome. The diagnosis is made by compartment pressure measurements before and immediately after exercise and the treatment is selective surgical fasciotomy.

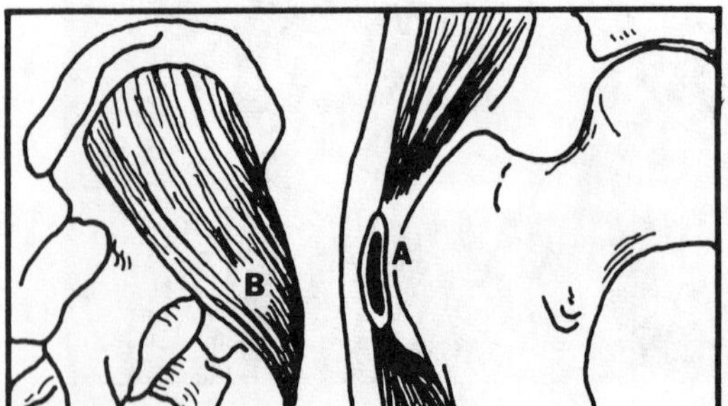

Figure 19-3 Injuries of the hip: (a) trochanteric bursitis, (b) gluteus medius tendinitis.

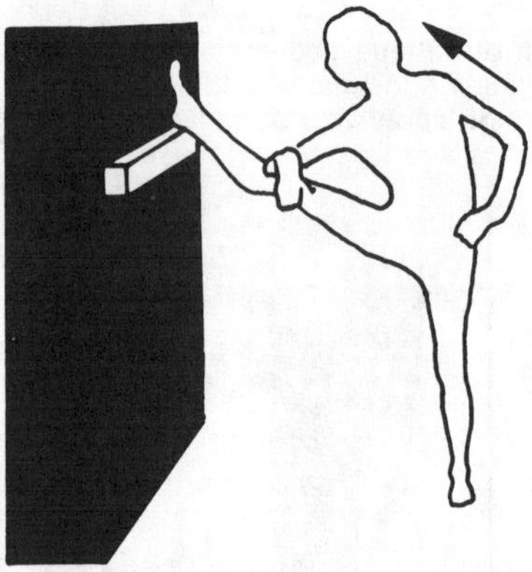

Figure 19-4 Using this raised-leg position, the inside of the upper leg can be stretched by pointing the foot of the supporting leg to the side. Look in the same direction as the foot is pointing. Bend sideways toward the leg resting on the fence until you feel an easy stretch. Hold this position for 20 seconds. Be careful not to overstretch.

Athletes are not immune to problems affecting the general population and it should not be assumed that all complaints are referable to an injury. Athletes may develop osteomyelitis, soft tissue sarcomas, primary bone tumors, vascular insufficiency, metabolic or hormonal conditions, inflammatory arthritides and diseases of the neuromuscular system as well as others. Only a careful

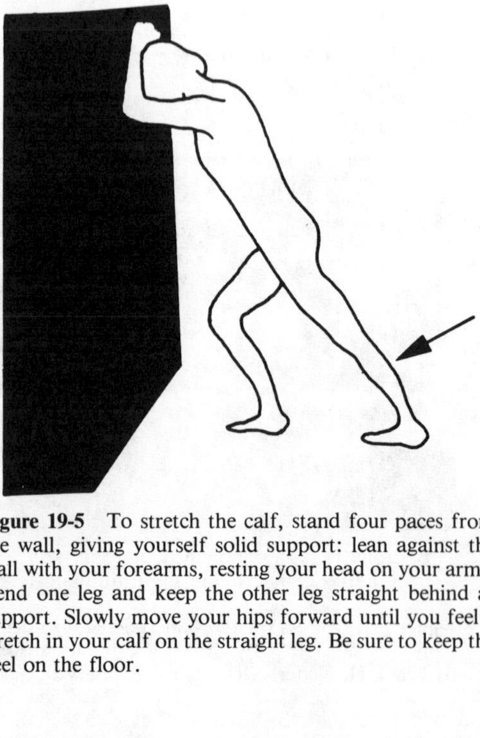

Figure 19-5 To stretch the calf, stand four paces from the wall, giving yourself solid support: lean against the wall with your forearms, resting your head on your arms. Bend one leg and keep the other leg straight behind as support. Slowly move your hips forward until you feel a stretch in your calf on the straight leg. Be sure to keep the heel on the floor.

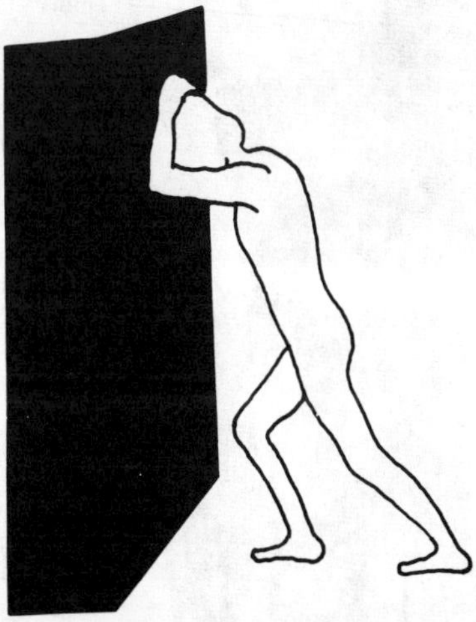

Figure 19-6 To stretch the soleus and Achilles tendon, slightly bend the back knee from the position in Figure 19-5, keeping the straight foot flat. This gives a much lower stretch that is good for maintaining or regaining ankle flexibility. Do both the stretch in Figure 19-5 and this one for 15 seconds on each leg. Do not bounce.

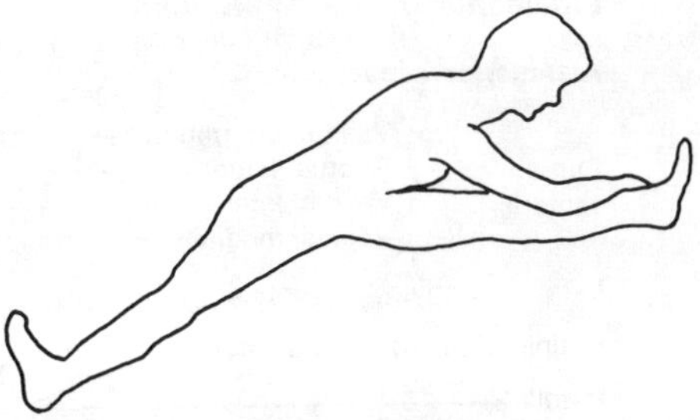

Figure 19-8 For stretching the left hamstrings and the right side of the back, slowly bend forward from the hips toward the foot of the left leg from a sitting position with the legs spread. Keep the head forward and the back straight. Hold the stretch for 20 seconds. With repetitions, the stretch will become easier. Repeat the stretch with the opposite leg.

history, thorough physical examination and a suspicious mind supported by other studies will allow the early diagnosis and treatment of these less common, but frequently more threatening entities.

Abnormal x-ray findings can occur in various anatomic sites. If osteolytic or osteoblastic reaction is identified, a bone tumor must be considered. A stress fracture may mimic Ewings sarcoma, myositis ossificans may mimic a parosteal osteosarcoma. The site of the pathology and history helps in the differential diagnosis of the clinical pathology.

Preventive sports medicine is necessary to limit the frequency and severity of athletic injuries. The prevention process demands the evaluation of all aspects of the biophysical profile—flexibility, agility, strength, power, speed, extensibility, endurance, reaction and reflex times, elasticity, and range in the involved anatomic areas.

KNEES

Disorders of the knee may be mechanical or inflammatory, intra-articular or extra-articular. In order to properly evaluate the knee, the comprehen-

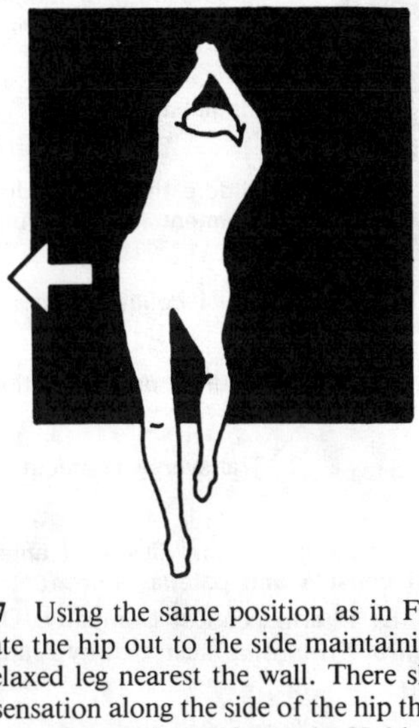

Figure 19-7 Using the same position as in Figure 19-5, slowly rotate the hip out to the side maintaining support with the relaxed leg nearest the wall. There should be a stretching sensation along the side of the hip that is not as striking a sensation as the calf stretch. Hold 15 seconds on each side of hips.

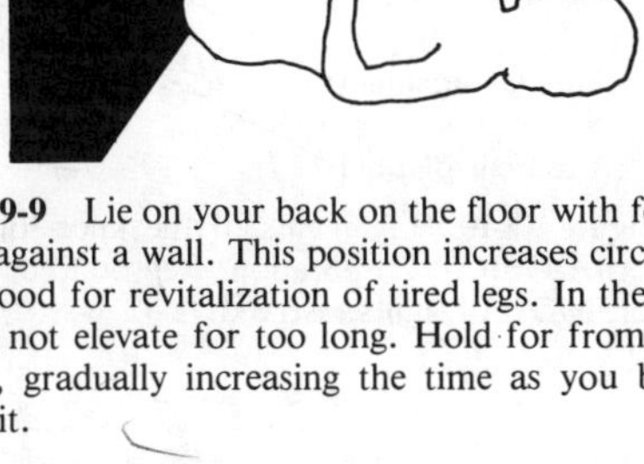

Figure 19-9 Lie on your back on the floor with feet and legs up against a wall. This position increases circulation and is good for revitalization of tired legs. In the beginning do not elevate for too long. Hold for from 1 to 5 minutes, gradually increasing the time as you become used to it.

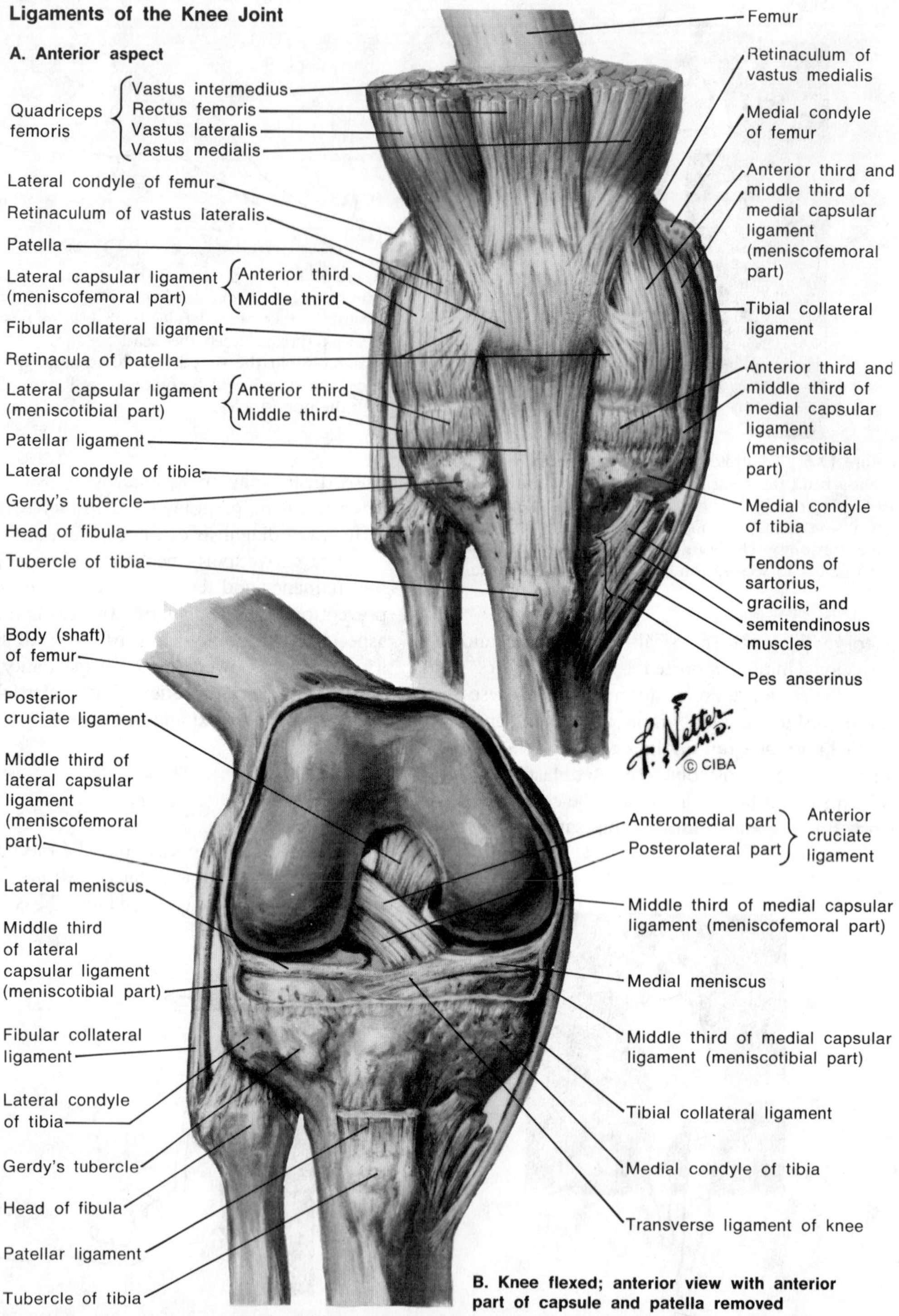

Figure 19-10 Ligaments of the knee joint. Copyright © 1977 Ciba Pharmaceutical Company, Division of CIBA-GEIGY Corporation. Reproduced with permission from *Clinical Symposia*, illustrated by Frank H. Netter, MD.

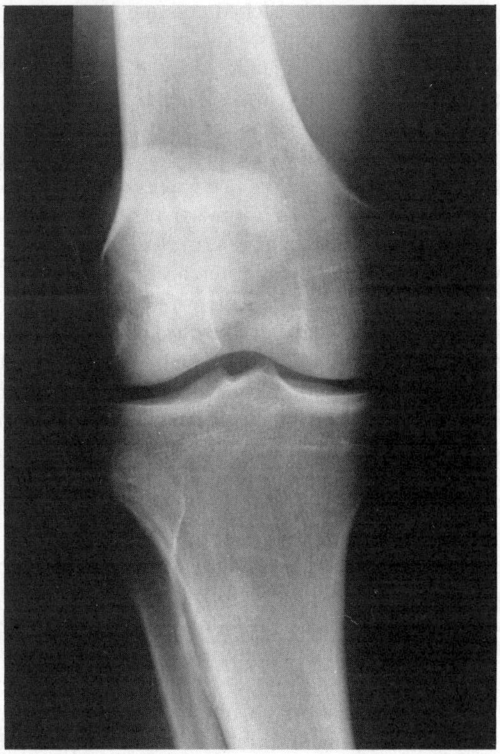

Figure 19-11 Roentgenograph of the knee, anterior view.

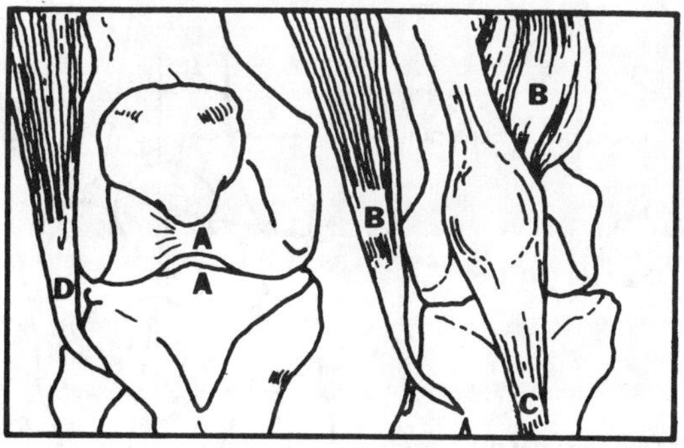

Figure 19-12A Injuries of the knee: (a) chondomalacia, (b) patellar compression syndrome, (c) patellar tendinitis, (d) iliotibial band friction syndrome.

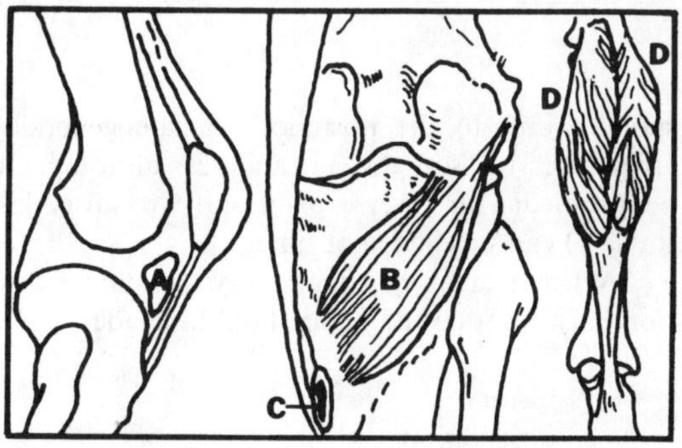

Figure 19-12B (a) Fat pad inflammation, (b) popliteus tendinitis, (c) pes asernine bursitis, (d) medial and lateral gastrocnemius tendinitis.

sive history and physical examination must be performed, supported by radiographic and, when appropriate, laboratory studies. At times, arthroscopy is useful as a diagnostic tool which also has the capacity for treatment.

The most common causes of disorders of the knee are: 1) a torn medial meniscus; 2) patella malalignment syndromes; and 3) strains of the medial collateral, lateral collateral, and anterior cruciate ligaments (Figures 19-10–19-12). The menisci (semilunar cartilages) are structures that aid in the transfer of force from the femoral condyles to the tibial plateau. They move from anteriorly to posteriorly, particularly the lateral meniscus during flexion and aid in stability. When torn so that a portion becomes unstable, the menicus may cause mechanical instability, synovitis and pain.

Patella malalignment refers to a condition wherein the patella does not track centrally in the trochlear groove. With lateral posture of the patella on full extension, hypermobility of the patella, dysplasia or atonia of the vastus medialis, high riding patella, hypertrophy of the vastus lateralis or an increased Q angle, the patella has a tendency to sublux laterally (Figure 19-13). This may cause chondromalacia patella and much less commonly, a tendency to frank dislocation.

The four major ligaments of the knee are the medial and fibular collateral ligaments, and the anterior and posterior cruciate ligaments. The collateral ligaments protect against valgus (abduction) and varus (adduction) stresses to the knee and severe strains to either of these ligaments leads to opening of the joints as in the opening of a book.

Complete rupture of the anterior cruciate ligament generally leads to anterolateral, posterolateral or posteromedial rotatory instability. The description of the instability describes the translational motion of the tibial plateau relative to the femoral condyles.

The posterior cruciate is the strongest of the knee ligaments. Its orientation is most nearly vertical and it defines the central axis of knee motion. A larger amount of energy is required to rupture this ligament than usually occurs in nonvehicular

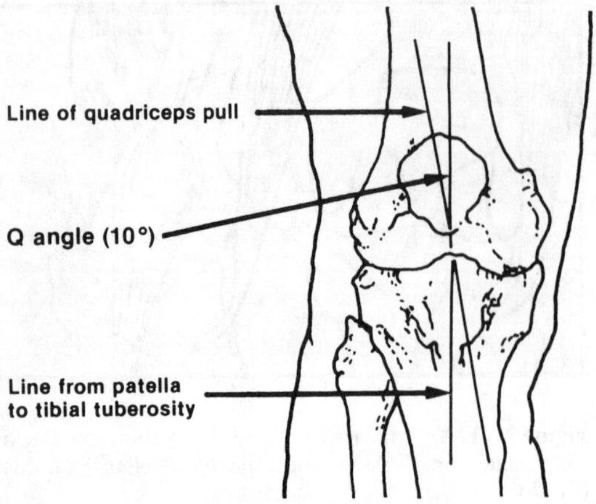

Figure 19-13 Normal Q angle.

sport. Injury to the posterior cruciate generally gives rise to straight instabilities although a posteromedial or reverse pivot shift (rotatory instability) can be elicited at times.

When evaluating a joint, a systematic evaluation must be followed. This should include:

1. history
2. observation
3. anthropometric measurements
4. palpation
5. active movements
6. passive movements
7. specific tests
8. functional tests
9. a review of the peripheral vascular and neurologic status
10. a review of related joints.

The history is of extreme importance. In traumatic injuries the athlete should attempt to relate the mechanism of injury and the location of pain. This information gives clues to which anatomic structures are at risk. Whether the athlete was able to locomote independently or with assistance from the playing surface may give an indication of the severity of injury. Time elapsed from injury to apparent swelling suggests whether a hemarthrosis or effusion is present and its probable source. An audible "pop" at the time of injury may be a helpful clue.

In the evaluation of subacute or chronically malfunctioning knees, several points must be examined. Is the primary difficulty instability, swelling, locking or pain? A history of popping or clicking is frequently elicited and may be caused by a variety of conditions. Instability is usually described as buckling, giving way or the sensation that the knee may give way. When this buckling exists it usually represents a serious intra-articular mechanical abnormality such as a displaced meniscus or rotatory instability. Impending giving way may be secondary to intra-articular malfunction such as patella malalignment or extra-articular as in weakness of the dynamic stabilizers.

The majority of patients with chronic rotatory instabilities ambulate into the physician's office and generally are without pain. Their disability occurs entirely during periods of activity when they are attempting to run, cut, or pivot. True locking is a mechanical block with unimpaired flexion. It usually represents a displaced meniscal tear. Loose bodies, hamstring spasm, posterior capsulitis and joint effusions may all limit extension.

A pain history reveals the character, location, intensity, temporal variation and activities which aggravate or alleviate this symptom. Complaints of bilateral knee pain usually relate to malalignment syndromes.

It is unusual not to obtain a history of knee swelling following an injury. The examiner should be specific regarding the location, amount and time to its detection as well as its response to rest and activity. Acute hemarthrosis occurring within two hours following an injury are usually secondary to anterior cruciate ruptures, but may be caused by intra-articular fractures. Swelling appearing a day or more post-inury are usually hydroarthrosis. Arthrocentesis is rarely indicated acutely for swollen knees that are clearly post-traumatic.

Chronic synovitis and its attendant effusion by definition represents intra-articular inflammation. In athletes this usually is caused by a meniscus tear, rotatory instability, loose bodies or advanced chondromalacia patellae. Examiners must remind themselves that athletes are not immune to leukemia, pigmented villonodular synovitis, rheumatologic disease, joint sepsis, crystalline arthropathy, osteochondritis dissecans and other causes of synovitis.

Examination through observation is appropriate as many biomechanical faults and malalignment syndromes can be seen and evaluated through inspection. These biophysical faults include: pes planus; pes cavus; bowleg (genu varum); internal tibial torsion; knocked knees (genu valgus) squinting patella; and femur-upper leg abnormalities. The bowlegged individual and athletes with internal tibial torsion have a tendency to produce degenerative joint disease of the medial compartment of the knee. Internal tibial torsion causes the patellae to turn in, while external tibia torsion causes the patellae to turn out. If the patellae point straight ahead, the position of the feet should be noted. Are they normal (7° to 10° turned out), pointed in or in the position known as sloth-footed? Difficulty will certainly occur if the examiner attempts to correct or treat something occurring within the knee when in reality the fault lies above or below the knee.

Further examination should assess the status of the vastus medialis muscle. It is best to examine this muscle with the athlete seated, although functional hyperextension of the knee can only be evaluated in the standing position. The patient is seated on an examining table and the muscle is evaluated for volume, shape, mass, thickening, or elongation, and how it is developed. Estimate the *Q* angle. Is the tendon thickened, does it show swelling, or does it lack bulk?

The examiner then reviews the shape and size of the patellae. Are they lying high, or do they fan in or out? Are the patellae tilted in or out? What is the congruity between the patella and femoral condyles?

The examination continues through the inspection-palpation process. The patient is requested to slowly and then rapidly flex and extend the knee. Patella motion is observed, as well as the dynamic function of the entire quadriceps mechanism and the inferior patella tendon. During leg extension against gravity, the last 15° to 20° of full extension activates the vastus medialis oblique muscle. Its function is to carry out terminal extension and to aid in control of the patella as it glides over the femur condyles. If the vastus medialis muscle is atrophied, atonic, or weak, full knee extension does not occur. With vastus medialis pathology, there is diminished force stabilizing the medial aspect of the patella to act as an antagonist to the powerful lateral extensor retinaculum. This abnormality in the vastus medialis muscle can constitute a major role in patello-femoral malalignment syndromes.

Further examination is performed with full extension of the knee. Palpate the thickness of the quadriceps superior tendon insertion. Is there a balance between the lateral and medial components? Does a concavity occur in the tendon insertion and muscle component of the vastus medialis?

The condition classified as hypertrophied fat pad (Figure 19-12B) continues to be diagnostic and in many circumstances causes pain and swelling on the lateral aspect of the knee. An increase in size of this tissue is usually related to a biomechanical fault, chronic stress, or irritation of the anatomic area.

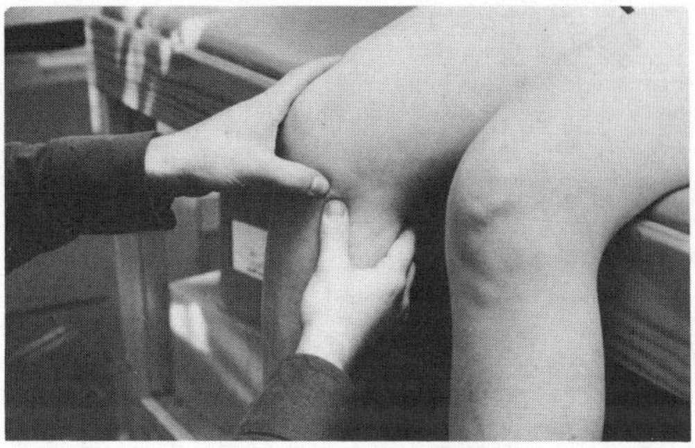

Figure 19-14 Palpation of the pes asernine insertion and bursa can identify insertional strain or bursitis.

The condition termed jumper's knee or runner's knee is the synonym for inflammation of the inferior patella tendon and should be diagnosed as patella tendinitis (Figure 19-12A). Palpation of this tendon will elicit tenderness and pain within the tendon and its insertion on the distal end of the patella. This pathologic entity is usually associated with atrophy or atonia of the quadriceps group of muscles. However, it may also be a result of a biomechanical fault as in the individual with pes planus or hyperpronation of the foot in dynamic function with its resultant increase in the medial rotation of the femur.

Pes anserine ligament and concomitant bursitis (Figure 19-14) is also related to the same causative factors as for inferior patella tendinitis.

Palpation of the patella for chondromalacia is performed with the leg in full extension relaxing the entire quadriceps mechanism. Each facet can be digitally examined for tenderness (Figure 19-15). The patella grind test is performed by placing downward pressure on the patella in extension to determine if pain can be elicited with patello-femoral pressure (Figure 19-16). Resistive knee extension with one hand on the patella will determine if crepitus or pain can be elicited. The apprehension test is performed with one thumb medially exerting lateral pressure on the patella as the knee is gradually flexed and observing the patient's face for signs of anxiety.

In the history-taking, information concerning previous tibial tubercle apophysitis or Osgood-Schlatter disease should be noted. If this has been present, calcification can occur in the inferior patella tendon causing a false joint at the tibia tubercle. This false joint may be painful.

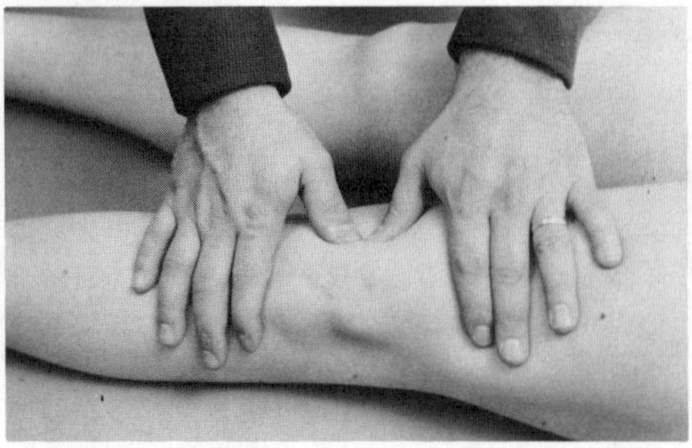

Figure 19-15 Palpation of the medial facet of the patella is helpful in identifying chondromalacia patellae.

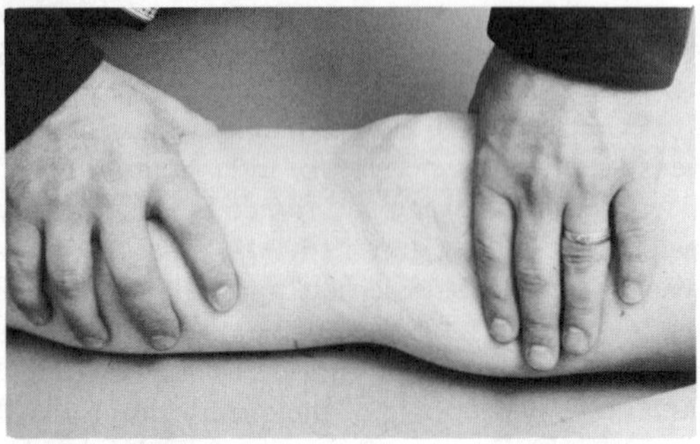

Figure 19-16 The patella femoral grinding test may elicit pain, which indicates chondromalacia patellae. This position, however, may cause false-positive results. Instead, 20° of flexion is recommended.

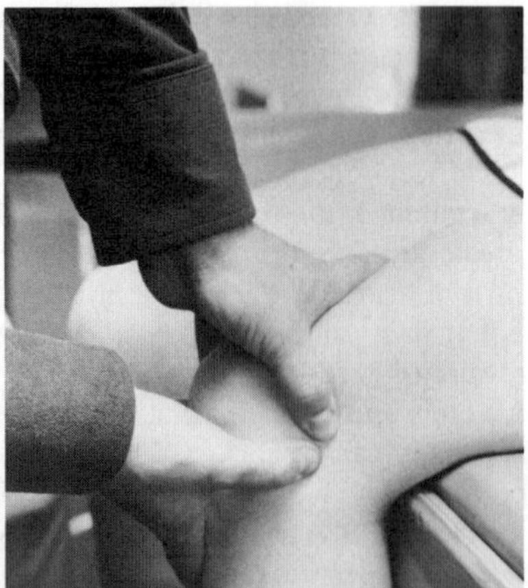

Figure 19-17 Palpation of the lateral collateral ligament tests for sprain from the proximal to distal insertions.

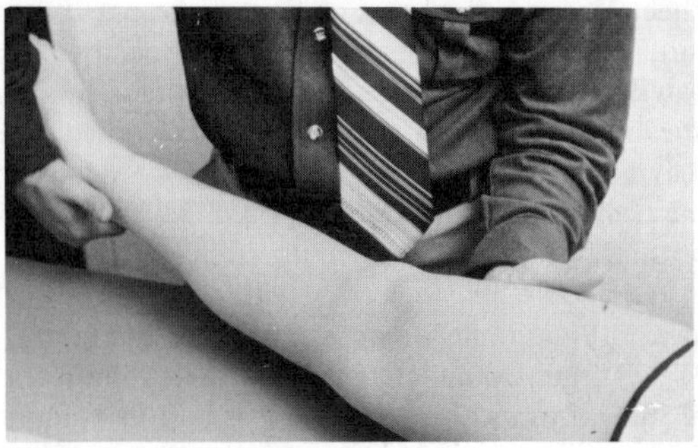

Figure 19-18 Abduction (valgus) stress test in knee extension is helpful in identifying injury to the medial or lateral compartment and posterior cruciate ligament.

The process of inspection and palpation to locate swelling and determine if it is intra-articular or extra-articular can be difficult. Prepatellar swelling can be directly anterior or toward either the lateral or medial side. Intra-articular fluid is usually superior to the patella. The swelling may be obvious because of the loss of all usual landmarks, or more subtle with an elevated patella. With the knee extended and the intra-articular fluid expressed into the suprapatella pouch, ballotement may aid in identifying the effusion.

Palpation and specific testing is performed through the complete range of motion to determine ligamentous involvement. Palpate for points of tenderness in the ligament insertions of the femur and tibia and throughout their structure (Figure 19-17).

Abduction stress tests of the injured knee are performed in terminal extension (Figure 19-18) and at 30° of flexion (Figure 19-19). By placing the knee in 30° flexion, the posterior capsule and posterior

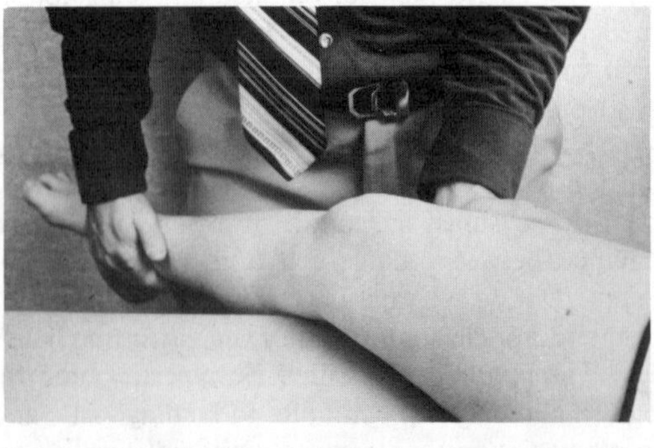

Figure 19-19 Abduction (valgus) stress test in 30° of knee flexion isolates the medial or lateral compartment structures; laxity reflects a lesion of the structures.

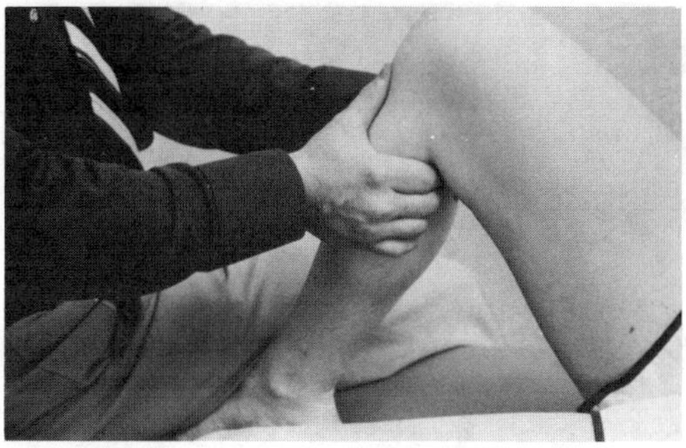

Figure 19-20 The anterior drawer test helps identify anterior subluxation of the tibia relative to the femur.

cruciate ligaments are slack and this is in contradistinction to fully extended position where these structures are tight. It is important to start this valgus-varus test with the hip and knee flexed so as to avoid a hamstring spasm. A positive abduction test in full extension is indicative of a posterior cruciate rupture.

The Lachman test is used to evaluate the anterior cruciate ligament. Although the physical examination is notoriously inaccurate in evaluating acute ruptures, the Lachman test has probably decreased the number of missed injuries. It is performed facing the patient with the lateral hand grasping the thigh and the medial hand, the tibia. With the hamstring relaxed and the knee held in 20° of flexion, an anterior translating force is exerted.

The anterior drawer test is performed with the knee flexed 90° and the examiner seated on the patient's foot to stabilize the extremity (Figure 19-20). The tibia is grasped with the thumbs below the patella along the inferior patellar tendon and across the joint line. Anterior translatory force is applied to identify anterior subluxation of the tibia relative to the femur. Rotary instabilities can be evaluated by applying rotational forces to the tibia during the draw test. Relaxation of the hamstrings is necessary for a valid test. A positive test is usually indicative of a meniscotibial ligament tear although an anterior cruciate injury augments the test.

Tests for rotational instabilities are performed by observing the movements of the tibia relative to the femur when stress is applied (Figure 19-21, 19-22). With the posterior cruciate intact, movement occurs around this ligament concentrically. For example, if the tibia is placed in a neutral position or internal rotation, and rotary stress is applied, anterolateral rotary instability is indicated if

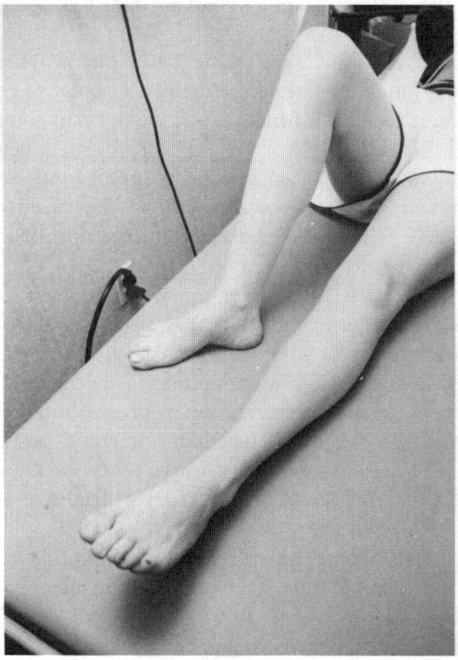

Figure 19-21 With the knee in external rotation, this rotary instability test indicates anteromedial instability with involvement of the posterior oblique ligament and the medial capsule.

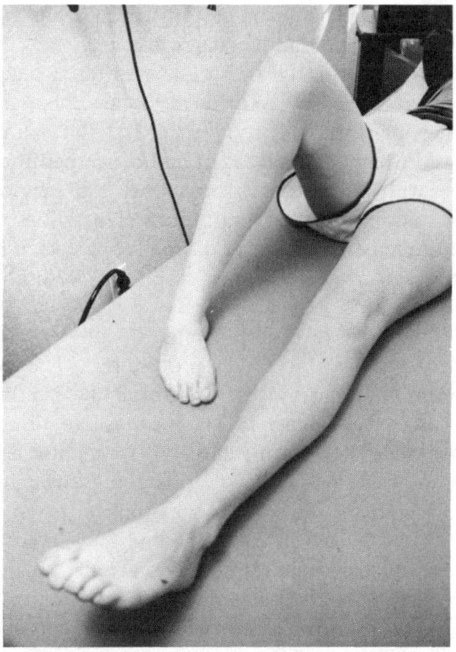

Figure 19-22 With the knee in internal rotation and anterior stress applied, this rotary test will identify anterolateral instability with involvement of the arcuate complex.

the lateral tibial plateau moves anteriorly compared to the medial tibial plateau.

A very important test to carry out in the examination is the lateral pivot shift. Usually seen in anterior cruciate injuries, a positive test may signify a disabling knee instability. The jerk and Slocum tests are variations on this test. More recently, the posteromedial or reverse pivot shift has been described. The general use and appreciation of this test has yet to be recognized.

The posterior drawer sign is performed in a similar manner to the anterior drawer sign and test procedure except a posterior translatory force is applied to the tibia. Good alignment is necessary for observation and interpretation of proper bony relationship to determine whether one has a positive anterior drawer sign, or a positive posterior drawer sign signifying laxity of the posterior ligament and posterior capsule.

With ligament involvement, swelling may not be obvious. If the synovium or capsule is not broken, the swelling will be intra-articular. If the injury is more extensive and the synovium is torn, the hematoma of the injury will be extra-articular and no intra-articular swelling will be apparent. Injuries of the posterior cruciate ligament usually do not involve a hemarthrosis. Fortunately, tenderness and minimal swelling can be palpated by the examiner in superficial ligament injuries and thus aid in establishing a definitive diagnosis.

Approximately 75% of knee-injured patients walk into the sports medicine clinic, physician's office, or emergency room unaided. The examiner must be highly suspicious of and concerned for the knee with a ligamentous sprain or tear. When walking and performing most normal activities, the athlete may not have any disability, but when running, cutting, jumping, or stopping the disability can be 100%.

Meniscus injuries, at times, can be distinguished by specific test procedures. The well-known MacMurray test is helpful in detecting a meniscus tear (Figure 19-23). It is positive if there is an audible click or an end feel of sponginess as the pathologic meniscus involved is going through the motion from flexion into complete extension. Point tenderness at the joint line may indicate a meniscus tear, or a capsular or coronary ligament sprain (Figure 19-24).

Anthropometric measurements are necessary to establish a baseline for initiating a therapeutic program and recording status of improvement or lack of response to treatment. Most textbooks advocate a girth circumference measured bilaterally from comparable sites on each knee, such as a specific centimeter from the top of the patella. However, in knee pathology, the top edge of the patella is not always in the same position. To alleviate this clinical problem and probable error, it is better to select the site of measurement as so many centimeters above the tibial tubercle of tibial

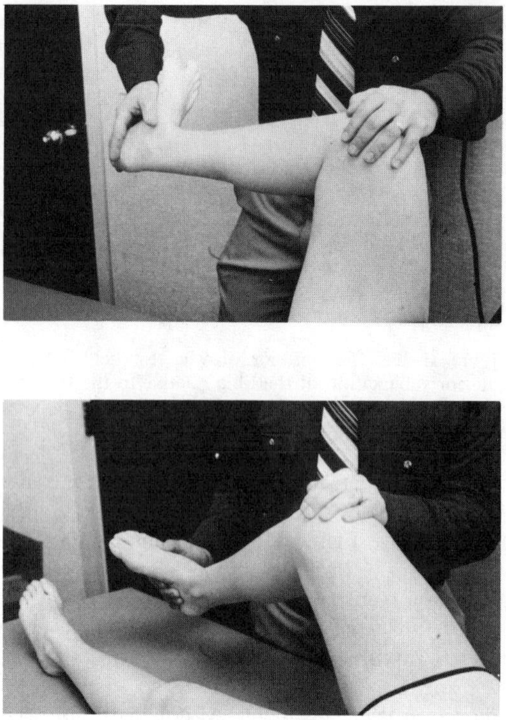

Figure 19-23 **A** and **B** McMurray test is helpful in detecting a meniscus tear, although it is not recommended for the acute knee because of pain and effusion.

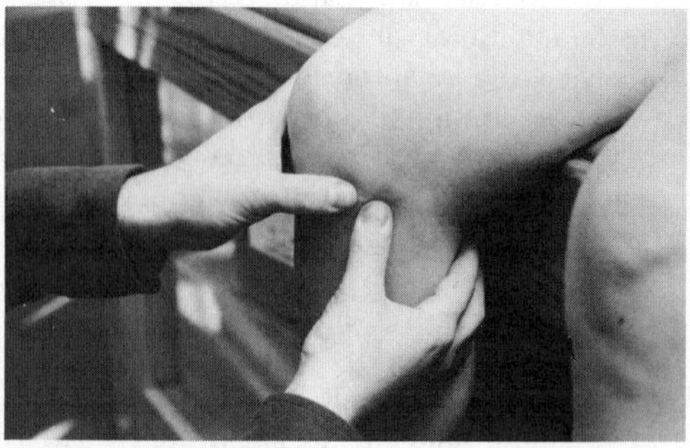

Figure 19-24 Palpation of the medial joint line may identify point tenderness, suggesting a meniscus injury, coronary ligament sprain, or both.

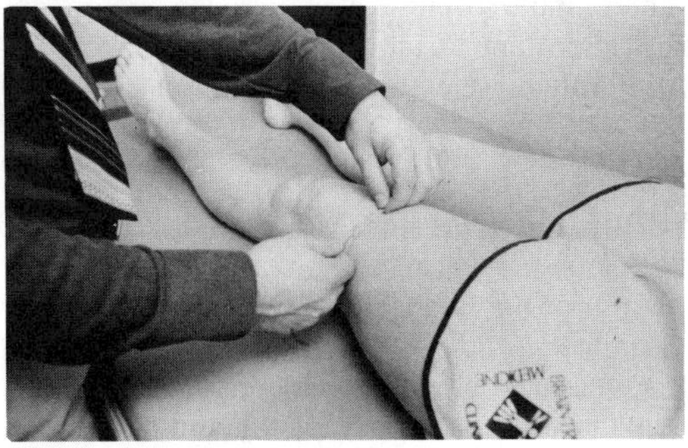

Figure 19-25 Anthropometric measurement of the quadriceps femoris is one of the five recommended measurements for comparing injured and noninjured knees.

plateau. In this manner successive measurements will be comparable having the same point of origin or basepoint. It is recommended that anthropometric measurements be taken at five different sites and recorded (Figures 19-25, 19-26). They may include:

1. joint line
2. 8 to 10 cm above the tibial plateau
3. level of tibial tubercle
4. belly of the gastrocnemius muscle measured in cm from the tibial tubercle
5. suprapatellar, 2 cm above the superior border of the patella with a recording in cm of site of measurement above the tibial tubercle, and
6. goniometer joint measurement.

Functional testing and examination, including the athlete's gait pattern, should be carried out. Watch the athlete stop, turn, step, climb, undress, and dress. Take weight bearings on both lower extremities. At some time depending on the athlete's status, take him to an open space and have him (in both internal and external rotation), squat, jump, stretch, duck walk, jog up and down stairs, run corners, hop and cut figures-of-eight clockwise and counterclockwise. Ability to perform these maneuvers will help determine the level of responses to therapy.

Pain to the knee may be referred from other joints. Hip injuries or pathology is referred to the knee joint through the obturator nerve. The lumbar spine and the lumbar and sacral plexus must always be reviewed and evaluated for related or unsuspected pathology. Their overlapping nerve myotomes and innervations can produce knee symptoms and dysfunction when in reality the lesion is in the spinal cord or lumbar-sacral area (Figures 19-27, 19-28).

Throughout the evaluation and examination process, attention should also be given to pulses, sensation, muscle function, and the presence of both normal and abnormal reflexes. (Figures 19-29, 19-30).

As an attempt at personal audit and for peer review, it is recommended that all examiners keep a log of knee examinations and patients in order to further this skill and clinical acuity. Record findings and clinical impressions. Follow the knee problems through the treatment programs, other diagnostic procedures, and if indicated, examination under anesthesia or surgery.

Through this personal clinical review, one will learn and be able to ascertain what injuries can be analyzed and prognosticated on clinical examination, what injuries are impossible to diagnose

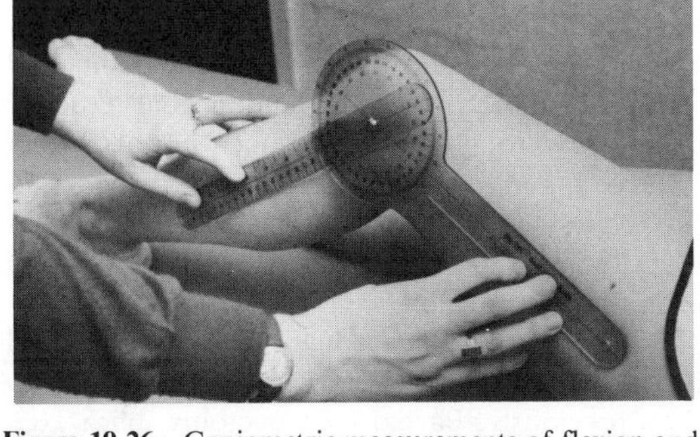

Figure 19-26 Goniometric measurements of flexion and extension are useful to establish a database for reference during therapy.

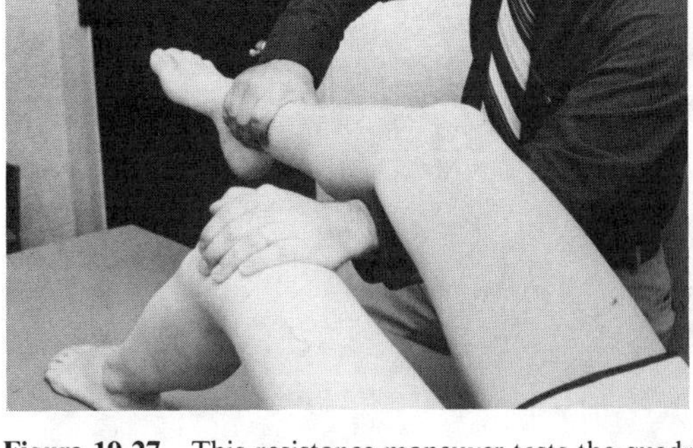

Figure 19-27 This resistance maneuver tests the quadriceps femoris group for strength and for innervation from the respective spinal cord levels.

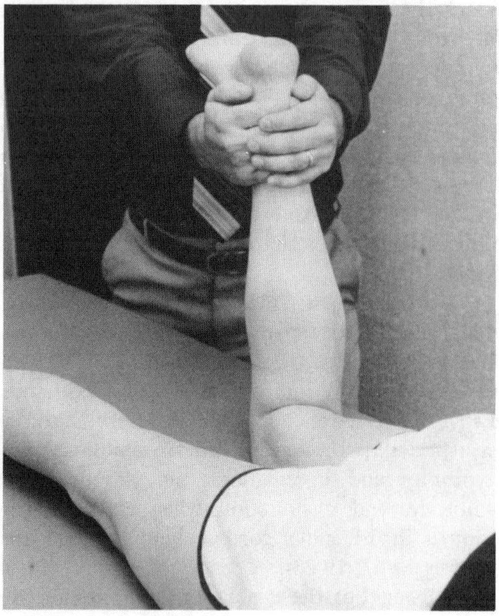

Figure 19-28 Strength and innervation of the hamstrings are tested in this resistance maneuver.

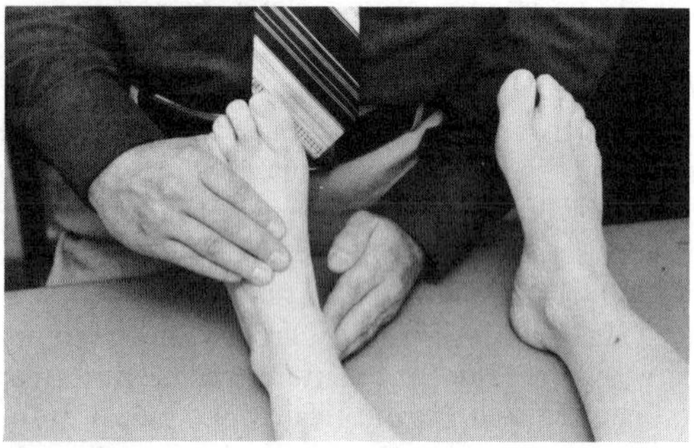

Figure 19-29 Palpation of the posterior tibial pulse is one step in assessing circulation distal to the knee.

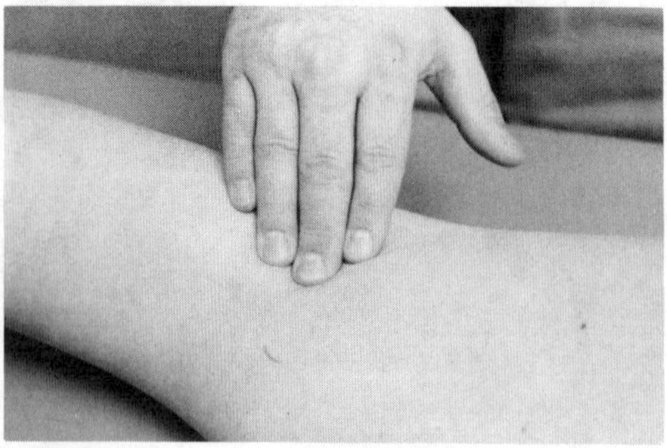

Figure 19-30 Palpation of the popliteal fossa can be used to assess circulation and to discover a Baker cyst.

without more sophisticated instrumentation and most important of all, improve one's own ability for thorough evaluation and diagnosing.

Additional Diagnostic Tests

Joint fluid analysis may be helpful in evaluating chronic effusions when they do not clearly seem to be post-traumatic. Generally, they should be evaluated for cell count and differential, glucose, crystals and culture, and sensitivity. The string test may give an early indication whether an effusion is inflammatory.

Arthrocentesis of acute hemarthroses is rarely indicated. When performed, inspection may reveal fat globules confirming an intraarticular fracture. The examiner must be reminded of the possibility of introducing an infection.

X-rays are always indicated in lower extremity injuries. The risk is small and they may suggest, metabolic abnormalities, infections or hard or soft tissue processes not previously suspected. Knee roentgenograms may reveal effusions, fractures, loose bodies, osteochondriti defects, meniscal calcification, arthritic changes, bipartite patella and a host of other findings that might otherwise have gone unappreciated.

Arthrography allows the visualization of radiolucent structures such as menisci and ligaments as well as documenting the presence of Baker's cysts. It is frequently used as a screening tool to eliminate unnecessary arthroscopy.

Arthroscopy

Arthroscopy has enjoyed a meteoric rise in popularity both as a diagnostic tool and as a means of treatment for mechanical problems within the knee. As a diagnostic tool it allows for an assessment of the synovium, the three articular compartments, menisci, popliteus tendon and cruciate ligaments through a single utility portal. When necessary, additional portals allow the introduction of probes to further examine the integrity of cruciate ligaments or menisci or biopsy forceps to sample the synovium.

Some surgical procedures may be performed through the arthroscope with far less morbidity than previously. Partial meniscectomy, plica excision and loose body removal are of proven value and may be performed under local or general anesthesia on an outpatient basis. Because only puncture wounds are necessary, rehabilitation can be initiated early in the post-operative course. Later, reconstructive procedures need not be compromised on the basis of previous incisions. In the event an arthrotomy is necessary, the incisions may be less extensive because the diagnostic arthroscopy has already permitted an extensive examination of the joint and localization of the pathology.

Arthroscopy may be helpful in assessing patello-femoral malalignment syndromes and monitoring the release of the lateral retinaculation. Cartilage debridement through various shaving techniques is of dubious value. Joint lavage is temporizing. The ultimate effectiveness of techniques for closed meniscal suturing, osteochondritic pinning and cruciate reconstruction will not be known with certainty for many years.

SUGGESTED READINGS

Brody, D.M. Running injuries. *Clin Symp*. 32:4, 1980.

Ellison, A.E. Skiing injuries. *Clin Symp*. 29:1, 1977.

Galway, R.D., Beauprey, A., and MacIntosch, D.L. Pivot shift, a clinical sign of anterior cruciate insufficiency. *J Bone Joint Surg*. 54B:763, 1972.

Hamberg, P., Gillquist, J., and Lysholm, J. Suture of new and old peripheral meniscus tears. *J Bone Joint Surg*. 65A:193, 1983.

Hsieh, H.H. and Walker, P.S. Stabilizing mechanisms of the loaded and unloaded knee joint. *J Bone Joint Surg*. 58A:87, 1976.

Hughston, J.C., Andrews, J.R., and Cross, M.J. et al. Classification of knee ligament instabilities. *J Bone Joint Surg*. 58A:173, 1976.

Joyce, M.J., and Mankin, H.J. Caveat arthroscopos: extra-articular lesions of bone simulating intra-articular pathology of the knee. *J Bone Joint Surg*. 65A:289, 1983.

Larson, R.L. Editorial: The knee—The physiological joint. *J Bone Joint Surg*. 65A:143, 1983.

Noyes, F.R., et al. The symptomatic anterior cruciate deficient knee. *J Bone Joint Surg*. 65A: 154, 1983.

Rorabeck, C.H., et al. The surgical treatment of exertional compartment syndrome in athletes. *J Bone Joint Surg*. 65A:1245, 1983.

CHAPTER 20
Foot and Ankle Injuries

Earl F. Hoerner, MD
Sheldon Langer, DPM, FACFO

The foot is a complex structure of 26 bones, numerous joints, muscles, tendons, nerves, vessels, and protective tissues. In athletic competition, it is placed under considerable stress. The functions of the foot in stance and motion are primarily stability and support, and secondarily, propulsion of body weight under varied conditions. In order to function efficiently the structures must work in intricate balance, allowing effortless support, voluntary control, and effective propulsion. If this takes place, there is no energy wasted, no friction, extra motion or inefficient protective activity. However, there are basic anatomical, physiological and sports-activity-related factors which can upset this delicate balance and untoward conditions which result in overstressing or overuse of the body.

Overuse implies that problems develop because the body is underconditioned. Each organ and tissue of the body can be conditioned to a high level of efficiency, assuming that the proper basic structural elements are present and are adaptable to specific demands of the training program. If the tissues of the body are underconditioned, overuse injuries will occur. Therefore, it is of paramount importance for the athlete to properly "train up" gradually according to a planned program. Selection of proper equipment, shoes, support taping and balancing orthotics, when necessary, will help to reduce or eliminate abnormal stress. However, conditioning is essential to success.

In discussing foot injuries, two major categories stand out: those caused by chronic or recurrent imbalance, and those caused by acute, sudden traumatic episodes. Imbalance injuries of the foot may be described in terms of the reference planes of the body, namely:

1. sagittal (forward-backward), (flexion and extension injuries) such as plantar fasciitis, Achilles tendinitis
2. frontal (side-to-side) plane problems, inversion or eversion sprains of the foot and ankle
3. transverse (rotational) problems, such as in-toe, or secondary knee and hip torsional (twisting) problems.

Each plane can be related to specific imbalance conditions within the foot and leg. Imbalance of the foot will allow either direct trauma to the body as a result of loss of balance, tripping or twisting, or the body will compensate for the imbalance with additional stress in the form of overuse, such as strain, muscle fatigue, cramps, tendinitis or stress fractures. Specific muscle and soft tissue abnormalities may also cause imbalance injuries.

Traumatic injuries to the foot may be caused by a direct blow of short duration (acute) or be the result of continuous or repetitive injury (microtrauma) over an extended time period. Both types of trauma will cause tissue destruction. However, the extent of injury depends on several factors.

1. Duration: Sudden blow vs repetitive or continuous microtrauma. An injury due to a sudden blow is more serious because it is not reversible since it creates unmitigated acute damage.
2. Type of injury: external forces vs internal instability or imbalance. External forces cause greater disability because the body has no defense against them.
3. Direction of forces: vertical vs twisting forces. Twisting (torsional) forces affect more tissues. Therefore, they tend to be more destructive.
4. Depth of injury: skin, subcutaneous connective tissue, bone. The more deeply the destructive force penetrates, the more severe is the injury.

CYCLE OF OVERUSE INJURY

Figure 20-1 describes the gradual progress of trauma through the superficial areas of skin (microtrauma) to the deep areas of subcutaneous

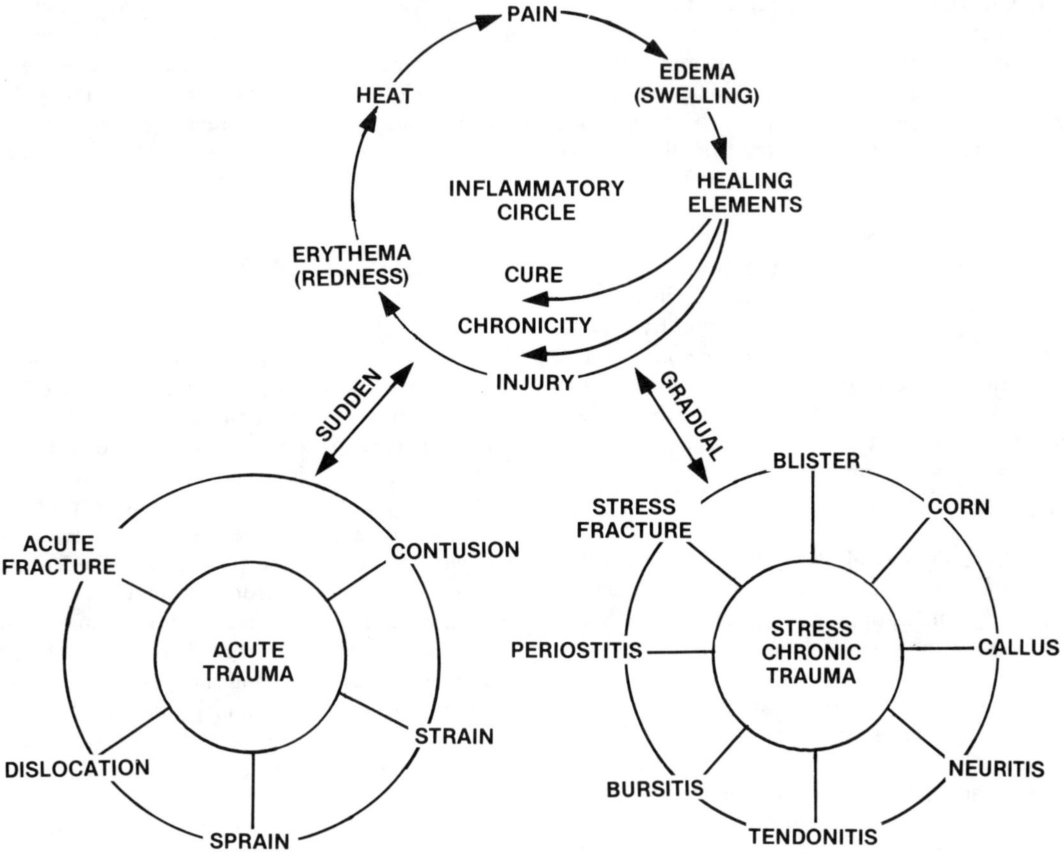

Figure 20-1 The inflammatory process.

structures including bone. While the body provides several lines of defense against injury, direct injury may transcend natural barriers, depending on severity.

The skin is sensitive to irritation from pressure, friction and temperature. Microtrauma to the skin will produce inflammation. The inflammatory process includes redness (erythema), heat, swelling, pain, loss of function and the production of healing elements. It is reversible if irritation stops. Inflammation is the body's method of warning against overuse, and it initiates the healing process. The cycle of intermittent, chronic or acute injury almost always involves some degree of inflammation. With minor microtrauma we see as one of the first indications:

Blisters which develop to separate the upper from the lower levels of the skin and create an antifriction hydraulic cushion.

Callus or specific nucleated corn which may develop as a protection to the deeper structures if microtrauma is over an extended time. A protective fat layer around the minor nerves, vessels and tendons helps to prevent damage to these structures. However, if more prolonged or chronic trauma results, the following conditions may result:

Neuritis (nerve inflammation) can occur through external injury or impingement (pinching) between other structures. This is painful and disabling. When the cause is found, treatment is successful.

Tendinitis (tendon inflammation) is actually inflammation of the tubular sheath. Since tendons have no blood supply of their own, they usually heal slowly. The most common cause is a stress microtear of the tendon. This must be treated with adequate rest or disability may be extended.

Bursitis is inflammation of a closed sac of fluid over an area subject to irritation. This is relieved quickly when the area of irritation is found. Inflammation is relieved with protection, injection or, occasionally, surgical removal of the bursal sac.

Periostitis (bone bruise) is a common injury of the foot because of its many bone prominences (Figure 20-2). In a bone bruise, the periosteum covering of the bone is separated from the bone by a clot of blood. If this is drained and the bone is protected, it heals quickly with a minimum of disability. If it is not treated, it forms an enlargement (exostosis) of the bone that produces further friction, irritation and, therefore, disability.

Stress fracture, the most common fracture in the foot, is a crack in the shaft of the bone because of overuse or excessive stress. Bone is living tissue that must be conditioned for severe stress. When alignment of the fractured bone parts is good, healing is rapid. Most common areas of stress fractures are the metatarsal and heel bones.

Acute injuries also are accompanied by inflammation but are generally caused by sudden or intense trauma as opposed to microtrauma. Some examples of these are:

Contusion to the foot or ankle is not disabling unless tendon or nerve damage occurs. Prolonged swelling in this area is destructive in that it produces pressure and ischemia (lack of blood supply) to the deeper, more critical structures.

Sprain (a tear in ligaments) may be mild, moderate or severe. Reduction of pain and pressure are good indications of healing. Ligaments, like muscles, do not regenerate, and occasionally surgical repair is necessary.

Strain (a tear in the muscle-tendon complex) may be mild or moderate. The more severe, the more scar tissue. Muscle does not regenerate.

Dislocation of bones and joints may follow severe sudden trauma and needs professional treatment. Disability varies with extent of injury.

Acute fracture of bone with or without displacement of the fragments. These must be reduced and placed into a plaster cast. Disability may be severe and prolonged.

Specific foot injuries are common to particular sports such as running, skiing, basketball, football and golf. Each athletic activity puts its own demands on the foot, leg and body. Through non-weight-bearing examination of the lower extremity, observation of stance, gait and electrodynogram (EDG) testing of function, it is possible to determine imbalance and thereby avoid overuse syndromes of the foot and leg with proper training techniques and equipment.

Proper evaluation and accurate diagnosis are essential to the understanding and treatment of foot problems. When injuries occur, they should be treated with a minimum of pain and disability. Of prime importance to the athlete is return to his sport as soon as possible. *However, treatment must be specific, complete and uncompromising.*

THE BIOMECHANICS OF RUNNING

As running is a part of most athletic endeavors, understanding and correcting abnormal foot function during running allows us to help many athletes. A knowledge of the biomechanics of the feet and legs is a prerequisite for attempting to control abnormal foot function in the runner.

The human foot is a complex structure that is designed to convert the rotations of the leg and upper extremity into forward motion. Normal locomotion places a great deal of stress on the foot as it accepts the body weight from above and attempts to adjust to varying changes in the walking surface. Jogging and running produce even greater stresses. When normal foot function is not present, overuse breakdown of the lower extremity is possible.

A normal foot is one that, during function, places no undue stress on itself or the joints proximal to it — the ankle, knee or hip joints. Normal does not mean average in as much as the average function of the foot for a given population may be abnormal. Abnormal function over a period of time may lead to soft tissue and bony deformities of the lower extremity; therefore, treatment of abnormal function is mandatory.

Kinematics of Walking

Familiarity with biomechanics of walking is a prerequisite for an appreciation of the biomechanics of running. Normal walking is comprised of the swing phase (35%), and the stance phase (65%), of a total cycle lasting from heel strike to heel strike (Figure 20-3). During the swing phase, the foot is not in contact with the ground and the opposite lower extremity is internally rotating because the swing side hip is forming an arc in a forward direction.

During the first 15%to 25% of the stance phase of gait following the time during which the heel and foot make contact with the ground, the

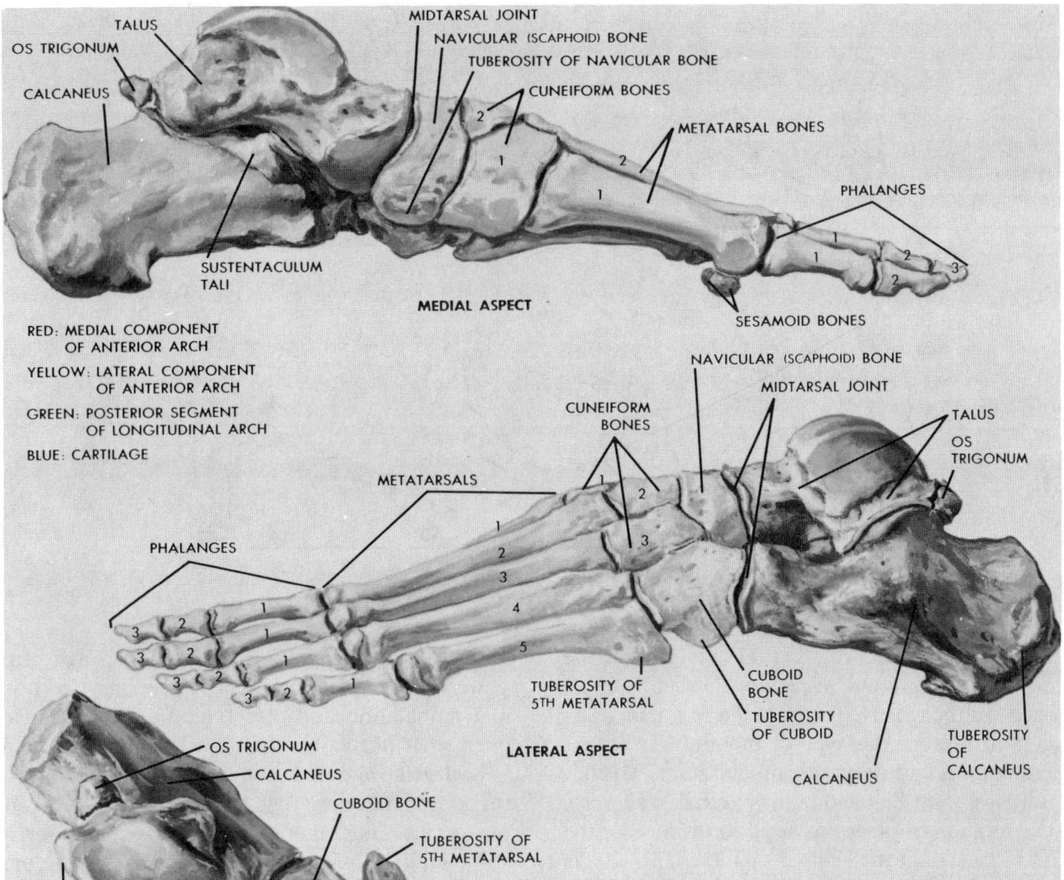

Figure 20-2 Bones of the foot and ankle. Copyright © 1965 Ciba Pharmaceutical Company, Division of CIBA-GEIGY Corporation. Reproduced, with permission, from *Clinical Symposia*, illustrated by Frank H. Netter, MD.

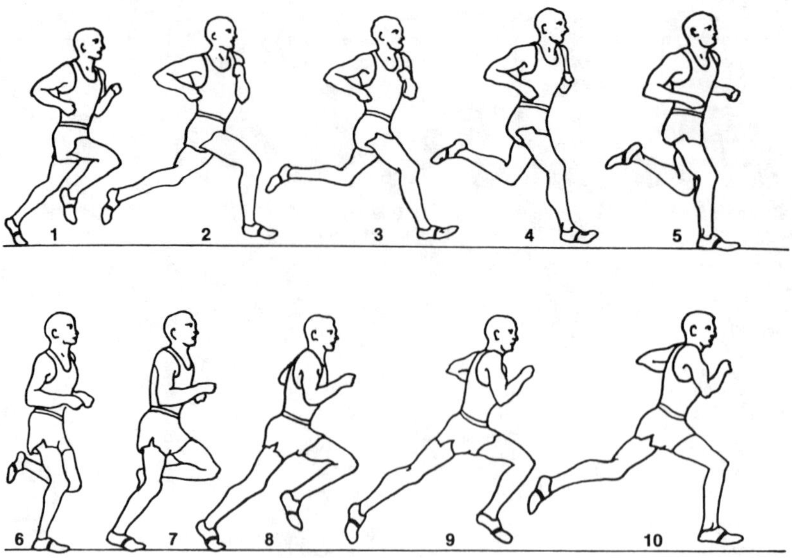

Figure 20-3 Phases in running.

limb is still internally rotating. However, once the foot is on the ground, it cannot internally rotate because of the reactive forces of the contacting surface that prevent this type of motion. Therefore, the foot is dependent on the subtalar joint, which is a universal joint that allows for internal, transverse plane rotation of the leg to occur at the level of the foot by closed kinetic chain pronation. This results in apparent rolling in of the ankle as the calcaneus everts and is accompanied by concomitant lowering of the medial longitudinal arch of the foot. This combination of first subtalar, and then, midtarsal joint pronation, results in "unlocking" of the foot. This makes it an ideal structure for ground surface adaptation.

The pronating foot functions as a mobile adaptor on uneven ground surfaces. This is a useful function for such activities as golfing, hiking, running or even walking in the sand. However, too much pronation that does not reverse itself can often cause symptoms of malfunction and overuse. Therefore, although mobility is desired during the contact phase of gait, it is undesirable during the toe-off phase.

During the midstance phase of gait the foot should stop pronating and should start to resupinate. Thus, it starts to become more rigid, and by toe-off should be a rigid lever as the leg is externally rotated. From midstance to toe-off, the foot should continue to supinate as the leg externally rotates. This results in raising the medial longitudinal arch. Since supination prepares the foot to act as a rigid lever and enables a strong, powerful toe-off to occur, it is necessary for normal ambulation and forceful propulsion. Consequently, if normal or prolonged pronation occurs at heel strike and does not correct itself in allowing the foot to become a rigid lever, proper toe-off cannot occur. Thus, there will be a loss of power in stride and various postural symptoms may occur.

Figure 20-4 demonstrates the stance phase and swing of the foot in normal ambulation. During the first 15% to 25% of the stance phase (the contact phase), the foot is acting as a mobile adaptor and the stance leg is internally rotating during this time. During the midstance phase of gait, which is the middle 35% of the stance phase, the leg starts to externally rotate and the foot is moving from the attitude of a mobile adaptor to that of a more rigid structure for acceptance of kinetic stress in preparation for toe-off. Thus, the foot should move out of pronation and into supination.

The remaining 40% of the stance phase of gait comprises the propulsive phase. This commences when the heel leaves the ground. At this time the first ray is actively being plantarflexed around its independent axis and at the same time the remainder of the foot is actively supinating and becoming a very rigid lever. This stabilizes both the medial and lateral column of the foot and allows the structures inserting into the great toe to provide a very powerful toe-off. Failure to accomplish each of these episodes on time results in deformities ranging from shear calluses underneath metatarsal

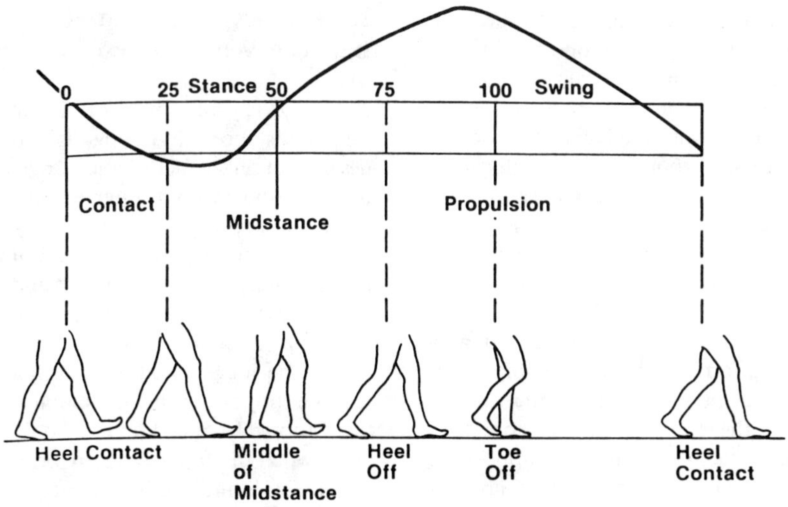

Figure 20-4 Gait cycle in walking.

heads to hallux valgus and hammer-toe deformities. In addition, it has been noted that the pronated foot at toe-off adversely affects the ankle, knee and leg, and results in many overuse symptoms in athletes.

In view of the potential for damage caused by faulty foot function, the electrodynogram (EDG) test should be used to acquire an objective analysis of the force/time relationships and the sequence of events that are occurring in the feet in order to identify the potential for injury to help reduce it and to maximize performance. Therefore, by relating the kinematics and biomechanics of walking to running, one can gain knowledge as to the importance of neutral orthotic control in running.

Kinematics of Running

Running varies from walking by the fact that there is an intervening airborne period when neither lower extremity is in contact with the supporting surface. In walking, one foot is always on the ground. Figure 20-5 demonstrates division of running into a support phase that consists of three periods: foot strike, midsupport and take-off; and a recovery phase divided into the periods of follow-through, forward swing, and foot descent. Foot strike begins when the foot first touches the running surface and continues for a brief moment during which the foot becomes firmly fixed. Midsupport starts once the foot is fixed and continues until the heel begins to rise from the running surface. Take-off begins when the heel begins to rise, and continues until the toes leave the running surface.

During the recovery phase, follow-through begins as the trailing foot leaves the ground and continues until the foot ceases its rearward motion. Forward swing begins with the beginning of forward motion of the foot and terminates when the foot reaches its most forward position, reverses direction, and descends toward the running surface in a rearward direction, and terminates with foot strike.

A review of Figure 20-5 illustrates that the phases in running are similar to those of ambulation and that the contact foot goes through similar motions. This is, of course, dependent upon the speed of running. During the support phase, high-speed sprinters have a tendency to stay on the ball

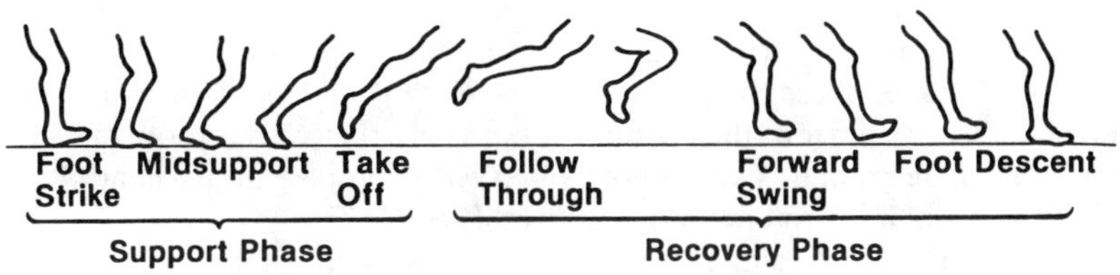

Figure 20-5 Gait cycle of running.

of a foot, although the heel may sag towards the running surface during midsupport. Middle-distance runners often momentarily contact the running surface with the heel of the foot initially and then move rapidly onto the ball of the foot. In longer distance runners, foot strike is usually at the heel with the forefoot following. Similarly, joggers usually go through a heel-midfoot-toe gait.

During the support phase, the foot must first act as a mobile adaptor and subsequently quickly convert itself into a rigid lever by supinating to allow for a powerful propulsive toe-off. At midsupport in running, one notes that the tibia of the support leg is about perpendicular to the running surface and that the foot should be close to a neutral position. Just beyond this midsupport the leg moves forward creating an angle of approximately 10° over the neutral foot. This is analogous to normal ambulation, and suggests that with tightness, shortness or lack of flexibility of the posterior muscle groups, the incidence of overuse symptoms may significantly increase.

The forward motion of the foot must be accelerated over a very short distance to keep pace with the forward velocity of the body. At foot strike the foot is moving near zero forward velocity in relation to the supporting surface to minimize the horizontal force. This smooths out the braking action on the body's center of gravity. This is not true, however, during changes of velocities such as acceleration, deceleration or change of direction during which time there are considerable horizontal components of force at foot strike. Therefore, the foot is required to be a primary dynamic shock absorber and force converter. It accomplishes these tasks through the following actions.

At the instant of right foot strike, the foot makes contact with the ground initially in a slightly supinated position. As weight is accepted, it proceeds into pronation until the forefoot is securely fixed to the running surface. The right hip is internally rotating and extending during this period. After the right forefoot is on the ground until toe-off, the right limb should be externally rotating. After toe-off, the entire right leg begins to rotate internally as soon as forward swing is intitated. Thus, we see an analogous situation between running and walking wherein pronation occurs at heel strike to the middle of midstance phase and supination occurs throughout the remainder of the period of time that the foot is on the ground. This allows the foot to convert from a mobile adaptor to a rigid lever; to accept and dissipate stress and then to lock-up to facilitate a powerful thrust at toe-off.

Kinematics – Connotations between Walking and Running

A review of slow motion films of sprinters, middle-distance, and long-distance runners suggests certain conclusions. Joggers and long-distance runners go through a heel-midfoot-toe gait in which the foot functions are very much the same as those encountered in normal ambulation. The heel strike may be quite abrupt and jarring or may be less jarring with a more rapid, shorter stride and with more foot surface contact.

Some joggers and long-distance runners contact the supporting surface initially flatfooted. This "slap-footed" contact may also be jarring, especially when the foot is already pronated (flattened) at contact. Some middle-distance runners appear to contact on the ball of the foot, have the heel sag back to contact the supporting surface, and go into a ball-of-the-foot and toe-off phase. Most sprinters contact and remain on the ball of the foot. It is further noted that sprinters coming out of starting blocks have a tendency to abduct and pronate their feet at the beginnings of their starts to allow for more secure contact of the feet with the running surface. After this initial take-off phase, they begin to point their feet in a more straight-ahead pattern and do not pronate as severely.

We have been able to correlate prolonged pronation with an abducted angle of gait and suggest that this may result in the situation of lowered efficiency in running. Some counter-clockwise track competition allows for supinating forces upon the left foot and pronating forces upon the right foot in the turns. However, this varies with the speed of the race, the radius of the curve and the bank of the track.

To reiterate, a review of the biomechanics of running and correlation with normal ambulation allows one to compare similarities and differences. Running may be divided into support and recovery phases. The running support phase consists of foot strike, midsupport, and take-off, and roughly corresponds to the contact, midstance, and propulsive phase of normal ambulation. It becomes apparent that devices (orthotics) that control a foot in normal ambulation may be specifically modified to control abnormal motion in running. Further investigation of the kinematics of running, and especially that of the foot contact, should help to provide proper foot control assessment for athletes.

It is extremely important at this point to note that new technological advances have recently been made which go beyond the optical visualization techniques employed in kinematic studies of the feet and legs in ordinary ambulation and running. The most important of these is the electrodynogram (EDG) system which facilitates the acquisition of force/time data from seven key segmental locations on the bottom of each foot.

The EDG system has the distinct advantage of being totally objective and non-influential on either walking or running patterns since the data are gathered by paper-thin flexible force sensors and are transmitted to a microprocessor which is mounted around the waist of the athlete. The athlete may walk or run in any kind of shoes, in any environment, at any place since there are no attachments to the main computer. Also, the entire system is remotely activated so that no artificial subject interference with the actual activity is encountered.

After the test data are compiled and fed into the main computer, all of the elements of the gait cycle are analyzed according to the principles of clinical electrodynography with respect to the actual times of occurrence, duration and percentages of the various phases of the gait cycle, shock, pressures and duration of forces on the foot and the normality or abnormality of the sequence of the various important stability, balance and propulsive foot episodes. Finally, human and computer logic permits data summary statements to be made which enhance the determination of treatment objectivcs and training directions.

EDG testing is objective functional testing at its best as opposed to nonweightbearing or static physical examination of the feet for such factors as ranges of motion, positions and structures. Although athletes may have ample ranges of motion, as has been conclusively demonstrated, they often perform as though they are tight or restricted in their movements. Electrodynographic testing demonstrates such actual function as opposed to static examination from which the examiner can only deduce or predict certain actions often incorrectly or incompletely.

FOOT DEFORMITIES

There are two broad classifications of foot deformities, rigid and nonrigid. Nonrigid feet may be normal or show abnormally with weight-bearing only. A nonrigid foot with a dynamic deformity may eventually become arthritic and progress to a rigidly deformed foot. These are quite painful and often prevent involvement in athletics. The time period for conversion from a nonrigid, dynamically deformed foot to a rigid, statically deformed foot is variable, individual and hard to predict. For this reason, periodic examination of nonrigid deforming feet appears to be reasonable with some documentation as to progress of deformity. One of the main goals of treatment of nonrigid (flexible), yet deformed feet, is to prevent their conversion into rigid nonflexible deformed feet.

Treatment for nonrigid dynamically deforming feet should be instituted as soon as possible and conservative treatment is generally indicated. Surgery is reserved for those cases in which conservative treatment fails or in which deformity is so severe no other alternative remains.

The nonrigid foot is considered normal when the calcaneus functions around a perpendicular to 5° valgus position in bipedal stance. When the calcaneal valgus (eversion) is between 5° and 10°, a mild to moderate flatfoot deformity is present. A calcaneal valgus beyond 10° indicates a severe flatfoot deformity (Figures 20-6 and 20-7).

In contradistinction to various types of flat feet, a high-arched foot may be present. In these feet the calcaneus is in a varus (inverted) attitude. A rearfoot varus foot is present with a calcaneal varus of about 4° to 5°. This is a structural deformity. However, if there is dynamic flexibility in the subtalar joint, the calcaneus can be pronated well beyond the perpendicular. When the calcaneus cannot be pronated beyond the perpendicular, a moderate to severe cavus deformity is present. A calcaneus which is rigidly fixed in more than 5° varus is classified as a severe cavus foot deformity.

Flexible Pronated Feet and High-Arch (Cavus) Feet

The goal of treatment of flexible deformities is to prevent the arthritic changes that occur secondary to subluxations. Subluxations are the results of joints that function beyond their normal ranges of motion. Thus subluxations may cause arthritic jamming of joints with eventual stiffness and painful motion.

The flexible flatfoot, if idiopathic and without neurologic basis, responds well to conservative treatment within certain limits. Conservative treatment consists of functional orthotics. When a forefoot varus of over 10° is present it is difficult to control the total deformity with an orthotic. This is

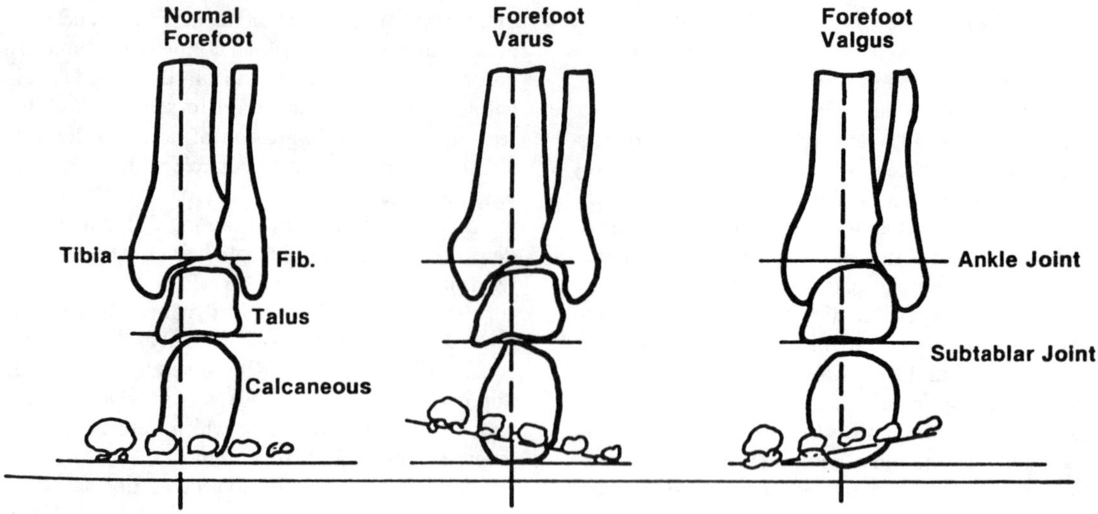

Figure 20-6 Forefoot terminology.

partly because of the difficulty of placing the neutral orthotic and the foot into a shoe.

Rearfoot Varus

The rearfoot varus feet are moderately flexible but occasionally tend to have a mildly limited total range of motion of the subtalar joint. These feet may present with a range of motion of 15° to 17° of supination with 4° to 5° of pronation. This often allows for a partially compensated rearfoot varus deformity that results in excessive strain upon the ankle, knee and hip joints (Figure 20-8). These feet tend to be mildly rigid and some firmness of the plantar foot structure is present. Besides the usual runner's bumps, chondromalacia, shin splints, plantar strains, spurs and bursitis, there is an increased tendency towards hamstring pulls and soft tissue problems around the buttocks and hip joints. This may be because of mild limitation of pronatory shock-absorbing properties. This foot type appears to be more common in distance runners.

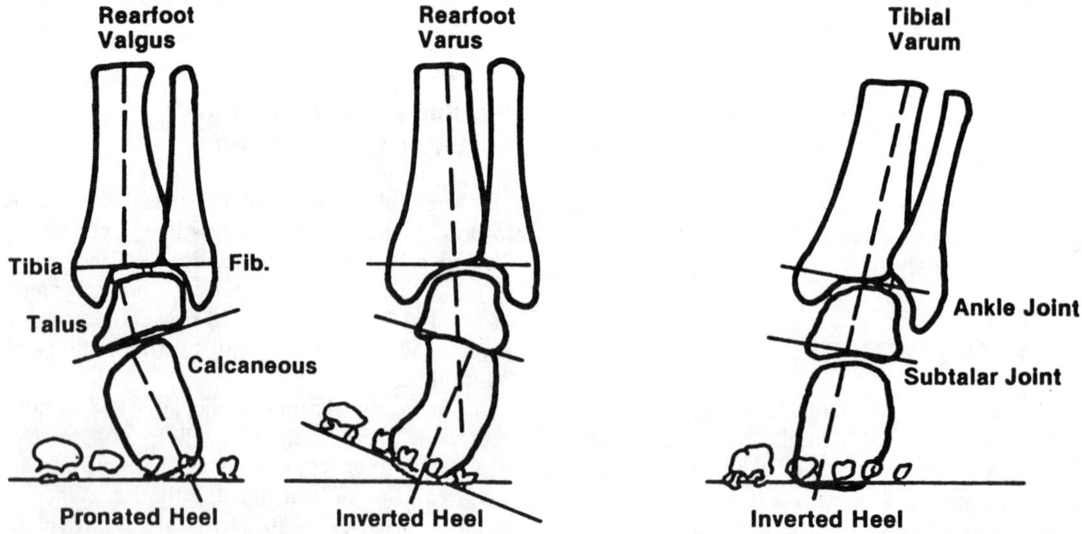

Figure 20-7 Rearfoot terminology.

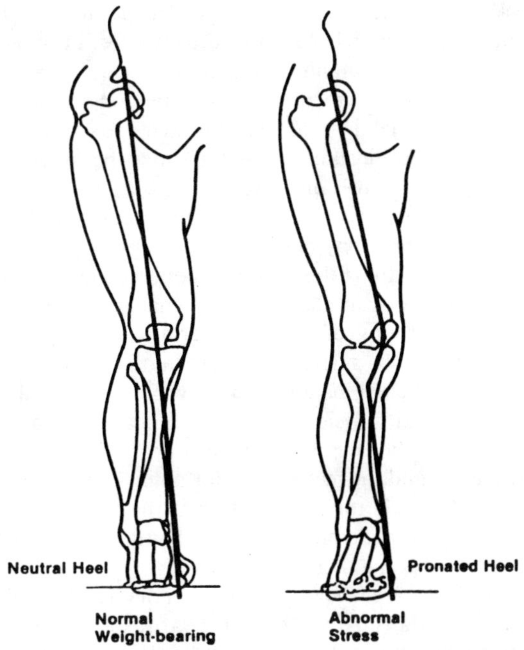

Figure 20-8 Abnormal knee stress secondary to abnormal foot function.

It is usually the stress of athletic training that results in symptoms. The nonathlete seldom develops symptoms. Many problems that are associated with it respond well to functional foot orthotics with shock-absorbing elements.

Flexible Cavus Foot

The flexible high-arch (cavus) foot is one in which the structures are very mobile. These feet appear to have a very high arch when they are dangling and not in contact with the ground. Yet, the medial longitudinal arches depress with the force of gravity on standing. The toes appear to be mildly clawed when nonweightbearing, but clawing partially disappears with full weightbearing. Often there is associated rearfoot varus. The foot is predisposed to medial calcaneal plantar process bruises. An adventitious bursa will often form under this prominent medial process and at times will develop into a traumatic fibroma. The fibroma may even progress so far as to entrap the medial calcaneal nerve branch.

Initially this foot is flexible and tends to accept the stress of running, but in time it may progress to a less flexible, flatter foot that accepts less stress and produces a jarring effect upon the body. The problem is that the time span for progression of deformities is difficult to predict. They may be congenital or occasionally secondary to neuromuscular disease. The neuromuscular diseases may be difficult to diagnose, and the patient may otherwise appear to be totally normal.

Treatment consists of orthotics to insure proper foot function and strengthening exercises to increase muscle tone.

Moderate (Semi-Rigid) Cavus Foot

The moderate cavus foot is one in which the dangling foot shows claw toes that do not entirely disappear upon weightbearing. There is a tightness and firmness of the plantar aponeurosis and the plantar intrinsic foot muscles. Therefore, this foot is more susceptible to plantar fascial strain. The metatarsal heads appear to be prominent and calluses form under the ball of the foot. The clawing toes form corns over their dorsal surfaces. The calcaneal varus is flexible enough to allow pronation to the perpendicular or mildly beyond.

Because this foot tends to have fewer shock-absorbing properties, shock is transmitted to the ankle, knee, and back, and problems in these areas are more common. Athletes with these foot problems tend to sprain their ankles frequently. This foot type may appear to have tight tendo-Achilles, and the athlete may present as a toe runner. This, however, may not be the case, inasmuch as the forefoot may be mildly plantar-flexed on the rearfoot, giving the appearance of limited ankle motion. This foot is often associated with bony limitation of dorsiflexion at the ankle joint. Talar exostoses, or spurs, are not uncommon as the talus contacts the tibia during dorsiflexion of the foot upon the leg phase of running. These talar exostoses may cause pain or go so far as to compress nerves and vessels at the ankle joint level.

When hammer-toe deformities and plantar calluses are severe enough to prevent pain-free athletic competition, surgical intervention may be indicated. This should be planned to slow down or impede progression of semi-rigid deformity to a totally rigid deformity. When symptoms are less severe, a semi-rigid functional orthotic may be utilized to help stretch out the plantar foot structures and possibly prevent such rapid progression of deformity. This foot type is often associated with a plantar-flexed first ray or forefoot valgus deformity, in which case the orthotics would utilize a forefoot valgus post.

Severe Cavus Deformity

The severe cavus foot deformity is one in which the calcaneus cannot be pronated beyond a 5° varus position. This foot is very rigid and has a high arch. There is often arthritis of the midtarsal joint, and dorsal beaking at the talar navicular joint may be present. In addition, there may be talar neck exostoses. The heel is in varus and the forefoot is in valgus position. There is clawing of all toes, and painful plantar calluses may form under the metatarsal heads. Tendency to sprained ankles is increased. This foot type is poorly suited for many sports and often requires some form of surgical intervention.

OVERUSE SYNDROMES OF THE FOOT AND LEG

During the early season of most sports, specific exercise programs are instituted to develop the athletes' physical condition, as the different muscle groups' hypertrophy, strength, agility and stamina contribute to better performances. With the increase of tone and hypertrophy of these muscle groups, adequate amounts of energy are realized because of a more efficient conversion phase.

The runner is concerned with two groups of muscles: extrinsic and intrinsic. The extrinsic muscles are those that originate proximal to the foot (Figures 20-9 and 20-10) namely: gastrocnemius, plantaris, soleus, tibialis anterior, tibialis posterior, flexor digitorum longus, flexor hallucis longus, extensor digitorum longus, peroneus longus, peroneus tertius, and peroneus brevis.

Adequate strength and resilience of these muscles are important in order to maintain the closed kinetic chain in linear projection. Unless our feet function at maximum efficiency nothing can be accomplished as anticipated. The feet can be described as two component parts functioning as one unit: the forefoot and the rearfoot.

Most sprinters' stress and activities will be borne by the forefoot. The muscular functions are centered around the muscles crossing the hips, knees and ankle joints. The intrinsic muscles that originate in the feet play a vital role in stabilization and coordination in the process of reciprocal interaction with the extrinsic muscles. Any structural imbalance of even minor degree can result in incapacitating injuries and persistent disabilities. With structural imbalance, muscle function will not be proportionately distributed to the feet in order to achieve maximum efficiency.

Another element that must be considered is the functional adaptability of muscles to structural change. For instance, the foot may be severely everted, creating considerable strain on the flexor group of muscles while their antagonistic muscles, the extensors, may have half their normal amount of work to do. If the condition comes on gradually and the foot can adapt itself to change, there will be hypertrophy of the flexor group. This hypertrophy may be sufficient to maintain normal functional muscular balance, thereby preventing joint tension and muscle strain. This functional adaptability of the muscles maintains normal balanced function and the feet are comfortable. Should there be a change in the coordination of the antagonistic muscles, functional disorder will manifest itself, thereby leading to pain.

There is a law in foot function that is attibuted to John Martin Hiss: "Comfort varies directly with function." It is well to consider the foot at the distal aspect or the end of the hip joint and the pelvic girdle. The functional arrangements of the specific muscle groups in the lower extremities have a direct interrelationship with the coordinating mechanism of locomotion. Comfort depends upon maintaining the function of this mechanism.

When an athlete is injured, progress depends primarily upon determining just how much functional improvement can be made and less upon the complete correction of abnormal structures. Minimal structural change is all that is necessary to restore comfort. Dr Hiss has stated that the fundamental factors include:

1. Support — the resistance of bone and ligaments against superimposed body weight.
2. Balance — the control of body weight over the center of gravity.
3. Locomotion — the coordination of muscles to move joints for the purpose of propelling the body through space.
4. Adaptability — the coordination of support locomotion and balance to compensate for changed position.
5. Distribution — control of contact pressure made by the sole of the foot on the ground as the weight moves through the foot during locomotion.
6. Power-action of the muscles. The

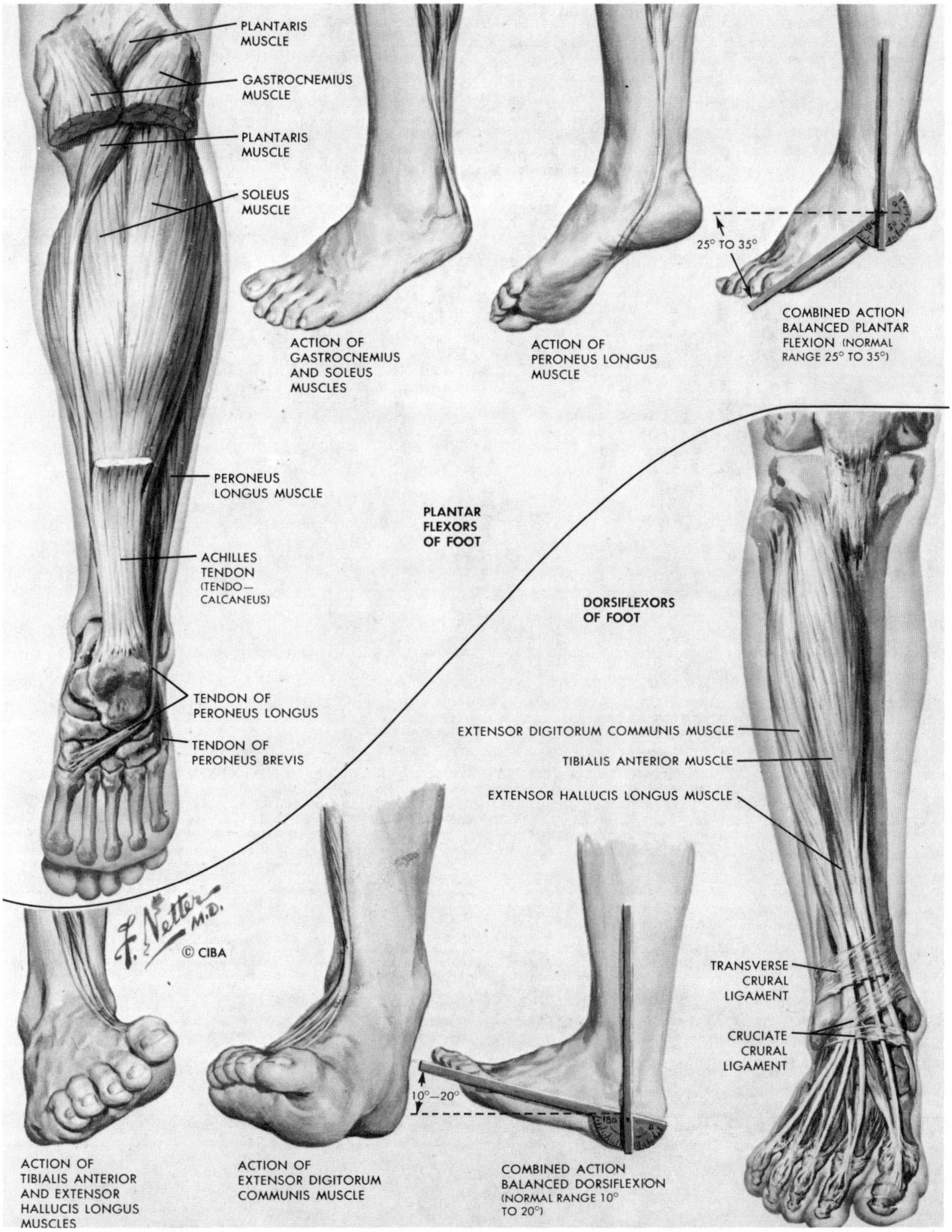

Figure 20-9 Plantar flexors and dorsiflexors of the foot. Copyright © 1965 Ciba Pharmaceutical Company, Division of CIBA-GEIGY Corporation. Reproduced, with permission from *Clinical Symposia*, illustrated by Frank H. Netter, MD.

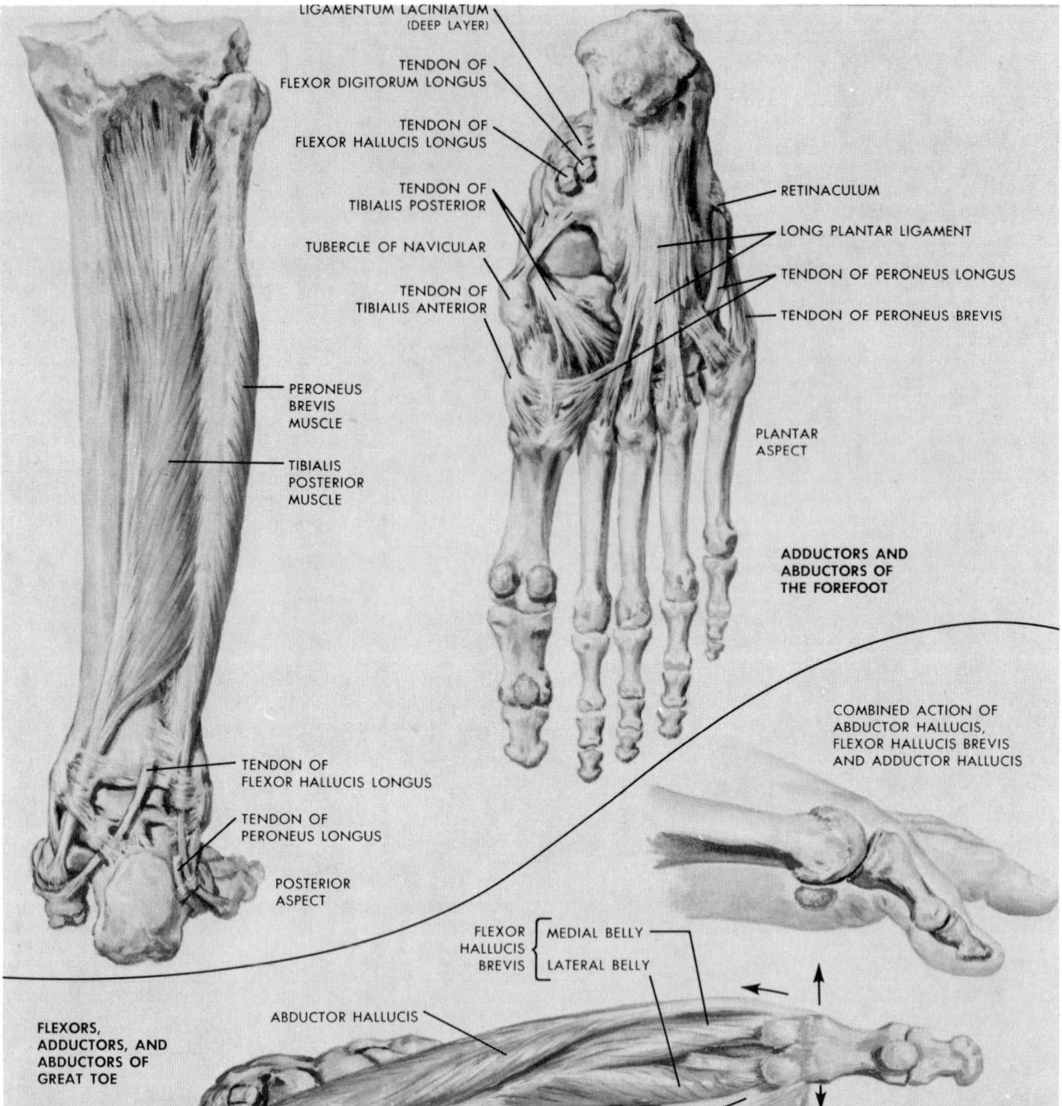

Figure 20-10 Adductors and abductors of the forefoot and great toe. Copyright © 1965 Ciba Pharmaceutical Company, Division of CIBA-GEIGY Corporation. Reproduced, with permission, from *Clinical Symposia*, illustrated by Frank H. Netter, MD. All rights reserved.

muscles are the unit of power that transform chemical energy to mechanical energy.

Principles of Treatment

Physical restoration of the athlete should never be left up to experimentation. The athlete's health is a most important asset, and a program of adequate evaluation and care should be professionally administered upon the report of any disability, irrespective of its intensity.

A properly conceived treatment plan should employ the following sequence:

1. First reduce effects of inflammation through use of: ice massage, infrared, paraffin bath, diathermy, ultrasound, whirlpool, and electrical stimulation.
2. Physical restoration of the musculoskeletal system of the lower extremities through strengthening and stretching programs.
3. Biomechanical realignment of the foot, by adequate taping and prescribing special prescription foot orthotics after the specific examination and measurements are pursued.
4. Isometric and progressive resistive exercises for the extremities for the abdominal and back extensor muscles.

Common Injuries

Stress fracture The metatarsals and fibula are particularly susceptible to stress fracture. This condition appears as aching pain, soreness and distress on function. There is usually no history of acute injury; however, examination will reveal local tenderness over the bone. Early x-rays will usually be negative. The patient is often treated for contusion or sprain. X-rays after 10 to 14 days may often reveal a crack in the bone.

The significance of stress fracture of the fibula is not as great as that of the foot since the fibula is a nonweightbearing bone. Careful rehabilitation is imperative lest the patient develop chronic muscular disability in the leg. Frequently, by the time the fracture is found, the time for immobilization will have passed, and the treatment will be local heat, ice massage and careful muscular restoration.

Fracture of the metatarsal bone In cases without displacement, partial immobilization with a zinc oxide-gelatin cast in addition to a semi-rigid sole, a rigid sole or a rigid postoperative shoe will suffice. A semi-rigid boot or rigid orthotic can also be helpful.

Anterior tibial (compression) syndrome The anterior tibial, extensor hallucis longus, and extensor digitorum longus muscles arise from the anterior compartment of the leg. This compartment is tightly roofed by the anterior fascia. In the anterior tibial syndrome, there is rapid swelling of the muscle within the compartment. This may come from active exercise of muscles that have not been previously conditioned, resulting in edema and swelling. It may also arise following direct injury in which there was hemorrhage and swelling in the space.

Treatment depends upon the extent of involvement. Early treatment should be prompt application of ice without pressure dressing. This condition is not common, but when it occurs it is an extreme emergency. Care should be taken not to mistake the condition for muscle spasm, shin splint, or cramping. Attention should focus on the unresolved boring, aching pain made more severe by function and not relieved with rest.

Tendo-Achilles bursitis This condition is caused by a subdermal enlargement immediately above the tendo-Achilles insertion, although it is not the usual site of bursae. It is caused by prolonged pressure from the upper margin of the shoe counter pressing against a prominent posterosuperior border or tuberosity of the calcaneus.

Plantar fibromatosis and/or heel spurs These can occur in either the flatfoot (pes planus) or immobile rigid foot with the high arch (pes cavus) caused by a biomechanical fault or disturbance in function. This condition usually needs realignment of the foot fault by strapping or orthotics (foot supports).

SHIN SPLINTS

The definition of shin splints varies from simple lay statements to precise medical terminology. The lay definition is expressed in terms of the shin bone and related muscular attachment to the anterior section of the lower leg. Precise medical terminology relates to: anterior tibial myotendonitis, posterior tibial myotendonitis, stress fractures, interosseus membrane tearing, anterior tibial tenosynovitis, and partial avulsions. Examination of shin splints is done by palpation, x-ray, and passive manipulation.

Anatomy of the Lower Leg

Anatomic structures are the tibia, fibula, interosseus membrane, and the structures of the longitudinal arch of the foot. Basic understanding of the origins and insertions of the tibialis posterior, flexor hallucis longus, and flexor digitorum longus muscles is necessary. These are on the posterior aspect of the fibula, tibia, the four toes, and into the arch of the foot. Also, the course and function of the tibialis anterior is important. Its origin is from the tibia lying across the anterior (front) part of the ankle, inserting into the longitudinal arch of the foot for dorsiflexion (pulling the foot up) and inversion of the foot (see Figures 20-6 and 20-7).

Symptoms

Pain is usually in the middle one third or lower one third of the tibial crest. It increases with passive dorsiflexion plus great toe hyperextension while the knee is locked. It also occurs with extreme passive plantar flexion (pushing the foot down). There is a markedly decreased range of motion of the ankle. The patient is unable to dorsiflex to 10° or plantar-flex to 45°. This creates strength imbalance and/or tension, present expecially upon dorsiflexion and indicates that a tight gastrocnemius muscle is producing excessive antagonistic muscle action with the dorsiflexor of the ankle.

Causes

The causes of shin splints are related to climate, track, running on hard surfaces, poor conditioning procedures, poor biomechanics of running, preexisting foot and arch problems, running over uneven terrain as in cross-country training, downhill running, and overexertion without proper conditioning. The problem of shin splints is not limited to any one sport.

Pain is usually precipitated when the untrained or unconditioned athlete overexerts himself, changes to a hard playing surface or changes his footwear. The stress of overexertion or overloading with constant work increases the tightness and strength of the gastrocnemius muscle group that is used in the push-off phase of gait. The anterior tibial muscle group only has to maintain ankle stability during the stance phase and produce dorsiflexion during the swing phase. Thus, the combination of actions creates an antagonistic muscle imbalance.

Heel height of shoes, such as seen on Western cowboy boots with a one-and-one-half inch heel, compared to the running shoes or spikes with no heels, reduces stress upon the tight gastrocnemius muscle group but increases stress on the anterior tibial muscle. Also, uphill running, as in cross-country running, creates the problem of a tight gastrocnemius muscle group. This is compounded with the body's forward lean for balance, increasing lower leg stress.

Posterior shin splints involve the posterior tibial, flexor hallucis longus and flexor digitorum longus muscles. Deeper structures may also be involved. Generally, the characteristic symptom is pain similar to anterior shin splints, but it occurs medial and slightly posterior to the shin bone (tibia). Since these muscles function to reduce pronation and stabilize the medial side of the foot, any activity, shoe or environment that increases pronation or causes overpronation will make the condition worse.

Another important aspect, now being studied with photography, is the relation to the degree of leaning an athlete has in running the turns of a track. Reference is made to the adduction angle of the inside leg while running a turn. Measurements are made from the anterior superior spine, perpendicular to the ground, in relation to the number of degrees from a reference line drawn from the anterior superior spine to the point of foot placement on the ground. The angle measured between the two lines indicates how far under the body the support leg is from the perpendicular line. This is referred to as the adduction angle, as seen in Figure 20-11A. Those athletes with marked posterior shin splint problems have a significantly higher adduction angle. Figure 20-11B illustrates a lesser adduction angle with those athletes who have never experienced shin splint problems.

Physical Restoration

The main concern of any treatment program is to have the athlete back in operation without losing maximum physical and physiologic function.

Immediate treatment After examination, x-ray and medication by a physician in order to

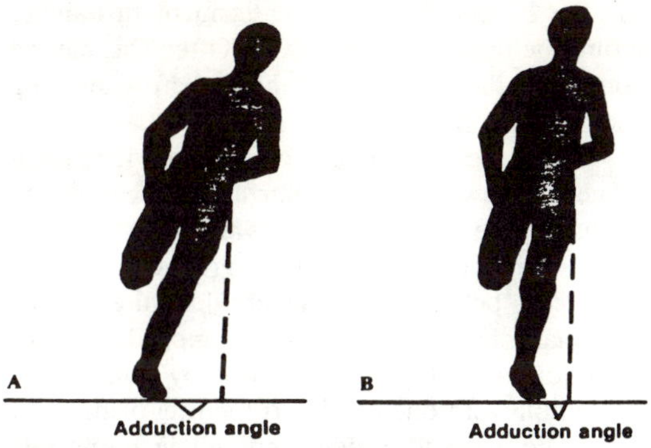

Figure 20-11 **A** High adduction angle often seen in athletes with shin splints. **B** Lesser adduction angle.

rule out the possibility of a stress fracture, apply the following treatment which was successfully carried out with 30 patients who were diagnosed as having shin splints.

1. Ice packs or ice massage should be applied to the entire tibial surface. Patients should then be given two aspirins. This should be done before workouts. The ice massage provides immediate anesthetic effect, decrease of spasticity of muscle tissue, and stimulation of the circulatory system to increase the blood flow.

A convenient method of icing the anterior tibial area is by freezing water in a Styrofoam cup, peeling away part of the Styrofoam and massaging the ice directly on the skin. Marked erythema will be noted within four to five minutes. Ice massage is continued for 10 to 12 minutes.

2. The longitudinal arch of the foot should be taped and supported with a felt pad, or a flexible orthotic should be provided.

3. Good shoes with arch supports should be emphasized for workouts. Street shoes with hard soles and normal heel height should be used for daily activities.

The above program allowed daily workouts to continue, and the patients became symptomatically pain-free within 10 to 14 days.

Exercise program The objectives of the exercise program are to increase flexibility of the plantarflexor muscle group, and to increase the strength of the dorsiflexor muscle groups. Plantarflexor flexibility is mainly achieved through stretching the Achilles tendon muscle group. Dorsiflexion strength is achieved by:

1. Dangling legs while sitting on the edge of a table. Use a weight system across the toes of both feet and dorsiflex the feet. Hold for a count of five. Repeat, increasing the number of dorsiflexions gradually.
2. Towel-gathering and marble pick-up exercises using the toes to increase the strength of the intrinsic foot muscles for arch development.
3. Isometric contraction of the dorsiflexor muscles by turning the foot inward while standing, pulling the arch up and inward to increase muscle tension.

Preventive program Prevention centers on good pre-season flexibility and a strengthening program for the leg musculature. This includes Achilles tendon stretching, dorsiflexor muscle strengthening with weights on the toes, and isometric exercises for developing arch strength. Emphasis is placed on good shoes for workout and street use. Most important, development of good training and running skills is necessary to decrease mechanical stresses. These techniques are not new in the area of exercise, but may be in their application to a specific athletic problem. Many of the exercises have been used successfully as preventive procedures, although a number of coaches have used similar stretching and strengthening techniques without emphasizing prevention of a particular problem. Organizations that have incorporated the above types of exercise into their preseason and in-season conditioning programs report that shin splints are a condition that they do not have to deal with. It is felt that strengthening and stretching the appropriate muscles have completely eliminated this problem. For those athletes in whom the problem has occurred, the program has reduced recurrence.

ANKLE INJURIES

Sprained Ankle

Why is the old adage, "A sprain is worse than a fracture," so often true? A fractured ankle is treated with integrity, care, interest, and concern; but if the x-rays are negative, the response will usually be, "Wrap it up in an Ace wrap," "take it easy," "tape it," "don't tape it," "soak it in hot water," soak it in cold water," "run on it," "don't run on it," and so forth. Then there is "cast it," and "don't cast it," if not, why not? What criteria are there for plaster immobilization? For surgical repair? Should there be stress radiography on all sprains? Is the conservative approach with plaster immobilization as effective as primary surgical repair for the torn lateral ligament? The treatment of this common problem in athletes places more responsibility on the examiner.

Treatment has two objectives: 1) To have the athlete back in action in the shortest period of time and with the least amount of game time lost; 2) To see that in the exuberance to carry this out, meticulous care and understanding are given so as not to aggravate the injured ankle further.

Nothing can be more frustrating to the trainer, coach, player and team physician than the athlete who has become a chronic problem. He is in the lineup one week, out two, back in again and so on. (This has been seen not only with ankle sprains but also with nagging groin and hamstring pulls.)

Medical authorities use terms such as first, second and third degree sprain or mild, moderate and severe. How does one differ from the other? The ankle ligament may be stretched, which is the most common type of sprain. Some fibers may be torn (partial tear), and, the most severe is a complete tear of the ligament.

Diagnosis

The difficult problem is determining what degree of injury is being confronted. Is the ligament just stretched or torn? There is really no scientific check-off list. There are principles to adhere to, but much depends on the experience and maturity of the trainer, team physician and podiatrist. There is no substitute for experience. Some criteria can be established to help formulate an overall treatment regimen, what problems to look for, and how to evaluate them.

Inversion or lateral ligament sprains are most common and troublesome. If it has been determined that the patient has a sprained ankle, it should be ascertained if he heard or felt a snap. The player should be asked to describe the exact mechanism of the injury. Before evaluating the ligament, immediately palpate the base of the fifth metatarsal and the proximal fibula. The patient will almost always feel pain over the lateral ligament, but the two above-mentioned areas are frequently fractured in severe twisting injuries.

The lateral ligament of the ankle joint is made up of the anterior and posterior talofibular ligaments and the calcaneofibular ligament with secondary lateral support from the talocalcaneal ligaments in the tarsal sinus (Figures 20-12 and 20-13). If possible, lateral ligament instability should be determined clinically. Often this can be done immediately after the injury before swelling and spasm appear.

Place the index finger on the anterior lateral corner of the superior joint surface of the talus. At the same time stress the foot in varus with the other hand. If the ankle is unstable, a groove can be felt to develop between the talus and lateral aspect of the tibial joint margin as stress is applied. Anteroposterior instability can be noted by holding the lower tibia with one hand and the heel of the foot with the other, and pushing and pulling in opposite directions. The examiner can feel the talus slip from the socket under the anterior lip of the tibia. If, clinically, there is any indication of ligamentous instability, one must consider stress radiography. If the patient is not seen immediately after the injury, then certainly the amount of swelling, spasm, and pain should be noted.

Treatment

Athletes should not be treated like the nonathletic patient. The businessman or bus driver is not treated as vigorously as the star halfback or basketball player. Naturally the severity of symptoms will affect the type of treatment used.

1. Immediate treatment should be ice, compression, and elevation. There is no substitute for ice. Together with ice, use compression.
2. Foot x-rays and standard three views of the ankle should be taken. Also note pain over the proximal fibula, and obtain x-rays accordingly.
3. Immobilization such as muff wrap, gelo cast, posterior splint, elastic wrap with foam rubber compression, tape and plaster immobilization should be used.
4. Enzymes and anti-inflammation medication should be considered.
5. Taping may be used. There is really no hard scientific proof of the effectiveness of taping. Experts disagree and debate the issue. Albert Ferguson, professor of orthopedic surgery at the University of Pittsburgh School of Medicine and orthopedic consultant for the Pittsburgh Pirates, stated, "If a taping job has been done correctly, it inhibits the motion of the subtalar joint, which acts as a safety valve for the knee." Thus, to do the job correctly, it is necessary to incorporate the heel lock to insure the locking of the subtalar joint. However, by doing this, there is no give (safety

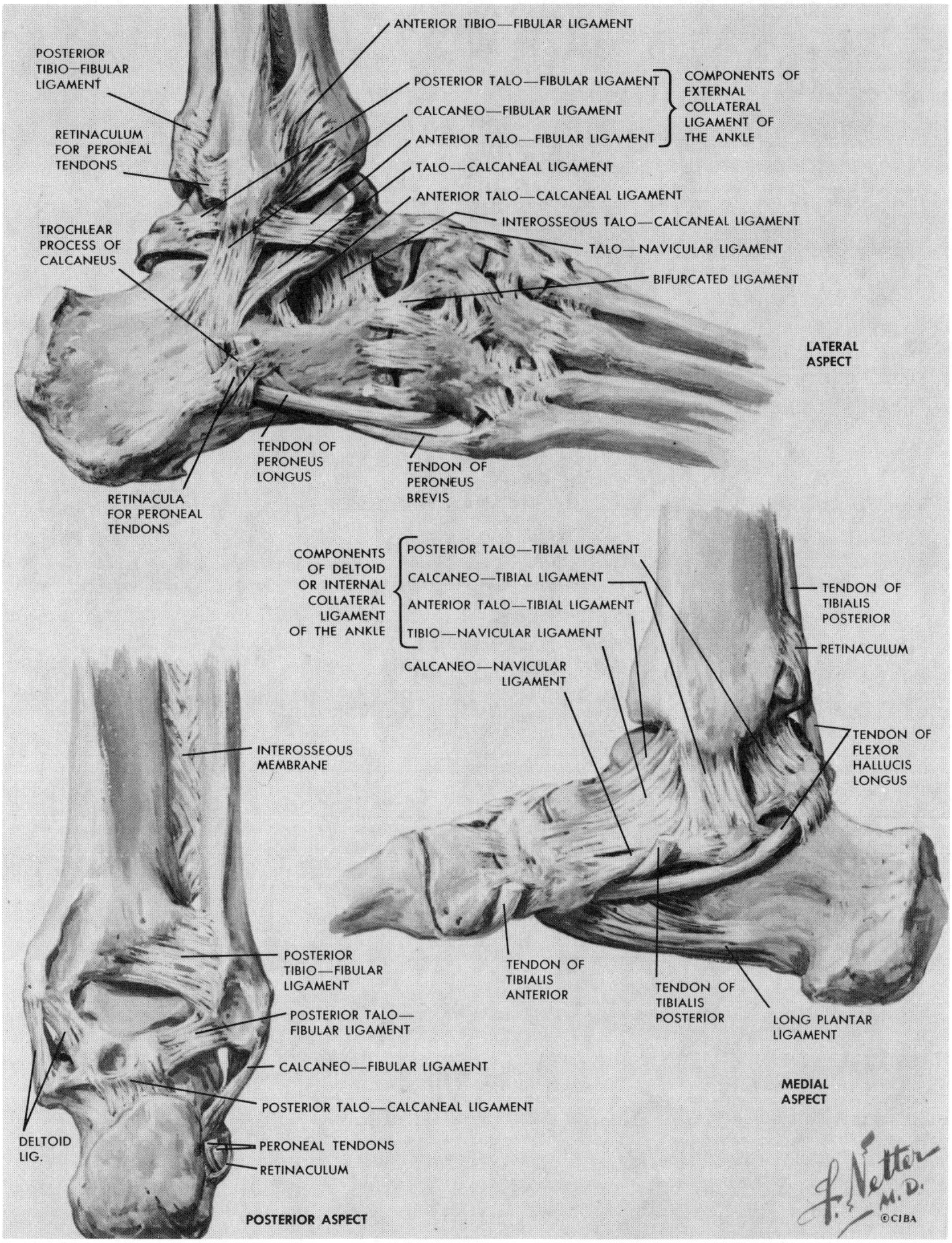

Figure 20-12 Ligaments of the ankle and foot. Copyright © 1965 Ciba Pharmaceutical Company, Division of CIBA-GEIGY Corporation. Reproduced, with permission, from *Clinical Symposia*, illustrated by Frank H. Netter, MD. All rights reserved.

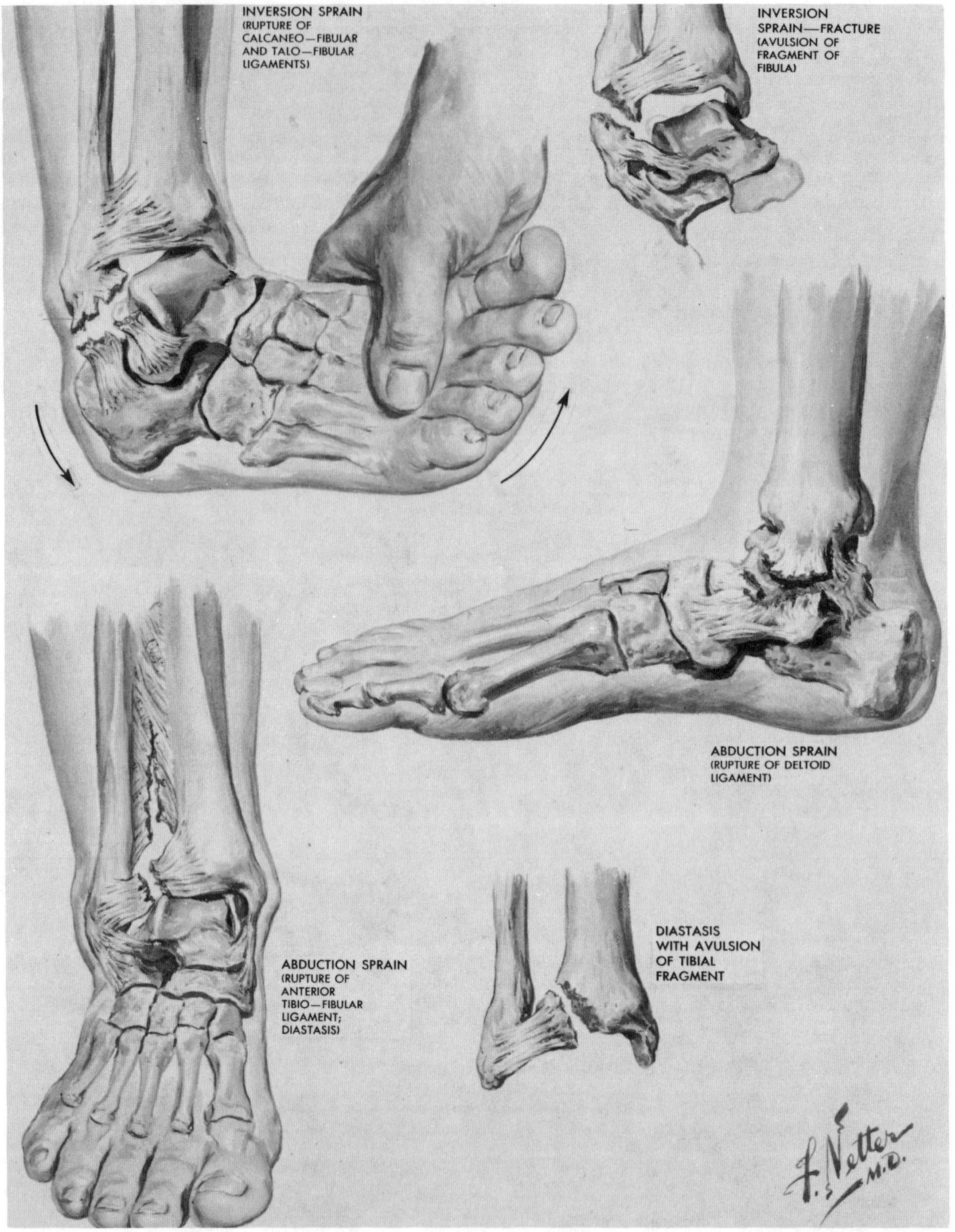

Figure 20-13 Major sprains and sprain fractures. Copyright © 1965 Ciba Pharmaceutical Company, Division of CIBA-GEIGY Corporation. Reproduced, with permission, from *Clinical Symposia*, illustrated by Frank H. Netter, MD.

valve) if the leg and/or ankle is hit in a certain way. Hence, the ankle remains stable but the knee gives. Obviously, if the taping is done incorrectly, as it often is, the tape loosens after a few minutes of activity and is practically useless. The four most common types of taping methods have been described as: a) basketweave alone, b) basketweave with stirrup, c) basketweave with stirrup and heel lock, and d) basketweave with heel lock alone.

These four conventional methods of taping were evaluated in a study. It was reported that regardless of the type used, after 10 minutes of very vigorous physical activity, 40% to 50% of the supporting strength of the strappings was lost. The most efficient strapping incorporated a basketweave, heel lock and stirrup.

The real aim in taping is to prevent the ankle joint from exceeding its physiologic limits of motion. It is still the most effective and reliable method of protection. Although it must be agreed that support is not as great as many believe, it does lessen the severity of the potential tear.

6. Sural nerve injection with a local anesthetic inhibits the autonomic nerve system at the sensory nerve ending in injured tissue, thus preventing vasodilation and effusion of fluids that in turn further stimulate these nerve endings. The advantages are: a) the technique is simple, b) it avoids the possibility of infection by not injecting the injured tissues, c) it can be used for stress radiography with less potential sequelae than the common peroneal block, d) it relieves peroneal muscle spasm and makes the patient more comfortable, particularly prior to casting, and e) it cuts down on healing time, removes pain, spasm, and swelling.

Injections are never given to relieve pain so that the athlete can return to play. Use of local anesthesia for this purpose is deplored.

7. Stress radiography. Unstable ankles are seen later on in life because of the lack of vigorous treatment at the time of injury, particularly the lack of plaster immobilization. However, stress films help to establish the need for plaster casting. To do a stress film properly, it is necessary to stress the ligament. The procedure should be carried out with caution. An advantage of stress films is that they give a permanent record, particularly in this day of malpractice problems. They are also used frequently to validate the continuance of conservative treatment. If stress films prove significant ligamentous instability and if the patient has symptoms, then surgical repair can be considered. Stress radiography is useful for the patient with a chronic history of sprain and instability from previous repeated injuries and inadequate treatment.

Stress radiography should not be done as a routine procedure in all fresh ankle sprains. In fact, it should be done only in instances of fresh sprain where clinical judgment indicates the advisability of a surgical repair. Since there is a great deal of controversy as to the relative merits of surgical repair vs cast immobilization other than in complete ruptures, stress films should be considered, but evaluation of the patient is most important before proceeding.

8. Arthroscopy, fiberoptic visualization of the interior of the ankle joint, is also of clinical value.

9. Post-sprain therapy and physical restoration. Physical therapy is a must and is the reason some athletes are back playing before others. Post-sprain therapy and physical restoration include: contrast whirlpool, ultrasound, lateral Ace with foam rubber compression, and resistant exercises.

Ankle Restoration and Strengthening

Following an injury or surgery to the ankle, this rule will hold true: When you can walk without a limp, you may jog; when you can jog without a limp, you may run and work to a sprint; when you can run and sprint, you may cut, then you may return to full activity.

While pain is something that an athlete can endure, a limp during activity will affect everything he tries to do. In contact sports, for example, an athlete who limps makes an inviting target. A basketball player who limps may find his leg, knees, and low back beginning to bother him as he compensates. In all sports, a limp will affect reaction time and quickness, and reduce the athlete's recovery and return to full participation.

Proper shoes Wear a good, well-built pair of shoes during recovery from an ankle problem. This does not include conventional sneakers, rundown loafers, sandals, and the like. A pair of lace-up boots is excellent, particularly in a more severe ankle injury.

Ankle taping The ankle should be shaved, sprayed with a good skin protector and taped with a medium-grade adhesive tape. The taping must include heel locks and a figure-of-eight. Be aware of potential tape problems such as blisters, skin irritation, swelling, coolness or discoloration of the toes because of tightness.

For three weeks after the injury, the ankle must be taped continuously. Taping should be changed daily if possible, or at least every two or three days. During the fourth through the sixth weeks, it must be taped for all practices and games. No tape, no activity.

Ankle Exercise Program

Note (Instructions to Patient): All progression in the following exercises is determined by pain tolerance. Be sensible, do not be too anxious or you may set yourself back days, even weeks. Work and progress within your pain tolerance.

Exercise 1: Warm-up With the knee and hip extended, bring toes up as far as possible. Turn soles of feet inward, then outward. Repeat 30 times.

Exercise 2: Alphabet Sitting on a table with knee straight and only ankle extended over the end of the table, print, in capital letters, the entire alphabet with foot.

Exercise 3: Pick-up Pick up marbles, a small piece of sponge rubber, or a piece of used gauze roller bandage. Alternate placing the object in the hand opposite the knee of the good leg and in the hand behind the buttocks of the injured leg. Repeat 10 to 15 times with each foot.

Exercise 4: Heel-raisers Stage 1: Stand with feet approximately one foot apart, flat on the floor. With feet toed in, rise up onto the balls of feet, hold for a few seconds, and return to starting position. Start rising on both feet and gradually work to rise just on affected foot alone. Alternate toeing in, toeing out, and pointing straight ahead. Repeat each position 20 times.

Stage 2: Place a book or a 2 × 4 under toes and balls of feet. Rise up on balls of feet, hold, return to starting position. Repeat 20 times.

Stage 3: Heel rises with weight (barbells). With the weights (50 lb and up) in hands or on shoulders, rise upward, hold, return to starting position. Toes and balls of feet should be on 2 × 4. Repeat for three sets of 10 repetitions. Universal gym: Use the leg press station, lower pedals. Begin at 80 lb, both legs. Wear a good pair of nonskid tennis shoes and place toes and balls of feet on lower half of pedals. With legs completely extended, push outward with toes and feet, hold, return to starting position. Repeat for three sets of 10 repetitions.

Stage 4: Same as Stage 3, but single-leg. When using the barbells, have someone spot until sure of balance. *Note*: When performing three sets of 10 repetitions, alternate sets between each leg until completing the series.

To progress from one stage to the next, first be able to complete fully, for five days, the beginning stage or the one currently being practiced. Do not progress until this stage is reached or until physician or therapist instructs otherwise.

Exercise 5: Isometric balance This will be one of the most difficult exercises to perform. Stand on one foot, placing the other foot to rest on the calf of the leg that is exercising. Raise arms straight out from side. Close eyes, keep foot on the floor and try to maintain balance. Count for the required number of seconds.

Progress from one time stage to the next only when this can be performed for five days, with full control, unless instructed otherwise. Do not try to skip stages, or try to go through all seven stages in as many days.

Stage 1	10 seconds,	10 times each leg
Stage 2	15 seconds,	10 times each leg
Stage 3	20 seconds,	10 times each leg
Stage 4	30 seconds,	10 times each leg
Stage 5	40 seconds,	5 times each leg
Stage 6	50 seconds,	5 times each leg
Stage 7	1 minute,	5 times each leg

This exercise is isometric. Do not be misled by its simplicity. Have someone else try it and watch the muscles of the ankle and foot as they do.

Exercise 6: Curl-up towel Sit on a chair or bench. Place a towel on a smooth floor. With foot on the towel, use toes to pull the towel (curl it up) under foot. Keep heel and towel on the floor at all times. Continue curling until one-half or more of the towel is under foot. Straighten the towel and repeat 15 times. As the exercise becomes easier to do, place books, weights, etc, on the end of the towel to give added resistance.

Exercise 7: Hopping If there has been ankle injury within the past six weeks, then this exercise is to be done with the ankle taped. Standing on the good leg, hop as high as possible. Then repeat on the injured leg. Repeat 10 times on each leg. Skip rope, alternating feet. Attempt to work up to a minute of skipping. *Note*: To progress from hopping to rope-skipping, be certain that hopping can be done in good form. This means that as you jump and come down, you are able to do it without landing hard and flat-footed. You should be able to absorb the shock of landing smoothly.

Exercise 8: Calf stretch Stand with feet hip-width apart, toes slightly pigeon-toed, weight on the outer borders of the feet. Lean against wall or fence or something immovable, the body always being kept straight. This should produce a slight stretch on the calf muscle. Lean forward by bending the elbows just far enough to increase the stretch effort mildly. Overstretching may cause the muscle to react by tightening and cramping. Keep back straight. Do not bend at the hips. Hold the stretch position for 15 seconds, push out and relax for a few seconds. Repeat this 15 times. Rushing this exercise will defeat its purpose and may cause further tightness. Slow steady stretching produces best results. *Do not bounce stretch.*

Exercise 9: Ankle PREs (progressive resistive exercises) with ankle exercise boot. Equipment needed: There are no substitutes for the equipment listed below other than more expensive clinical equipment.

1. Adult or child's aluminum boot with toe extension
2. One 18-inch aluminum bar
3. One set of aluminum collars
4. One small aluminum weight pan
5. Two 1/2-lb weights
6. Five 1-lb weights
7. Towel roll

This exercise is both difficult and time consuming, but it is one of the better exercises for rebuilding muscular power in the lower leg and ankle. Read the instructions carefully to avoid wasting time. Strap the boot to foot, place appropriate weight on weight pan and/or bar. Make sure that the boot has been tightly strapped. Sit on a table high enough so that foot with boot and weight pan attached is barely touching the floor. Place a towel roll underneath knee to act as padding and a fulcrum for exercise.

Use the standard disk weights found in any weight set available in sporting goods and department stores. Fold two towels in half lengthwise, roll them (as if rolling a bathing suit) into a single roll. Secure with tape or string.

Stabilize knee during this exercise. Lean slightly forward, grabbing the lower leg just below the knee with both hands so as to steady the lower leg. Only the ankle and foot should move during this exercise, not the leg. With experience, it may not be necessary to hold the leg. The procedure is as follows.

Part I: Attach the weight pan to the toe rod. Begin with 70% of maximal leg raise (MLR). With the weight shoe tightly strapped on, bring toes and foot up as far as possible, hold for a count of five and slowly return to the starting position. Relax. Repeat this for three sets of 10 repetitions. All movement is at the ankle and subtalar joint, not in the knee and leg.

This exercise is the exact opposite of the heel raise. The heel raise works the gastrocnemius muscle group. This exercise works the anterior tibialis muscles.

Part II: Attach the 18-inch bar to the boot. Attach a 2-lb weight on the lateral side of the bar. Begin with the sole of the boot turned inward (side with weight will be pointed downward).

Attempt to turn sole of foot outward. This movement will produce a side motion at the ankle joint, the weight will move from its initial down position upward and out, and the muscles on the side of the leg, in particular, will be felt to be working. Hold the weight at its highest point for a count of five. Return to the starting position. Relax. Repeat this procedure for three sets of 10 repetitions.

There will be a tendency for entire leg to move sideways during this exercise. Follow the same method for stabilizing leg as in Part I.

To increase resistance begin with 2 lb and increase by 3 1/2 lb every seven to ten days. Resistance may be increased in two ways. First, by adding more weight; second, by varying the length of the bar and the distance the weight is from the side of the boot. The further the weight is out on the bar, the more difficult the exercise. Vary the distance out on the bar rather than increasing the weight.

Exercise 10: Running sequence All of the following are done with the ankle taped. Taping must include stirrups, heel locks, and figure-of-eight.

Stage I: Walk. When you can walk without a limp, proceed to Stage II.

Stage II: Jog. Start out as a fast walk; progress to a jog, straight ahead only. Follow the sequence below. When you can jog without a limp, proceed to Stage III.

1. Walk 25 yards, jog 25 yards
2. Walk 25 yards, jog 50 yards
3. Walk 25 yards, jog 75 yards

Stage III: Run. Start out as a fast walk, progress to a jog and then to a sprint. When you can run straight ahead without a limp, run the following patterns:

Pattern 1: Run circles both clockwise and counterclockwise. Start out with a large circle and work down in size of diameter.

Pattern 2: Run figure-of-eights. Begin with large eights and work down until you are rapidly making cuts.

Pattern 3: Run a zig-zag course the length of the court or field.

Pattern 4: Run and quick-cut at right angles both left and right, on command.

Remember: Progress from stage to stage or from pattern to pattern, only when able to complete fully a given stage or pattern without a limp for a minimum period of two days. Without a limp means that someone else watching cannot notice limping. Do not rely on your own judgment.

SUGGESTED READINGS

Drake, E.T. Shin splints: the trainer's point of view. In *Proceedings of the 8th National Conference on the Medical Aspects of Sports.* Chicago: American Medical Association, 1967, pp. 32–34.

Elftam, H. Biomechanics of muscles with particular application to studies of gait. *J Bone Joint Surg.* 48-A(2):363–377, 1966.

Fenn, W.O. Work against gravity and work due to velocity changes in running. *Orthop Clin North Am.* 4(3):433–462, 1973.

Gray, J. Muscular activity during locomotion. *Br Med Bull.* 12(3):203–209, 1955–56.

Johnston, R.C., and Smidt, G.L. Measurement of hip joint motion during walking, evaluation of an electrogoniometric method. *J Bone Joint Surg.* 6:1083–1094, 1969.

Klein, K.K. Shin splints: prevention and rehabilitation. *Scholastic Coach*, June, 1963.

Leech, W.F., and Brower, T.W. Shin splints, their nature and causal factors. Presented at the 1970 Meeting of the American College of Sports Medicine, Nashville, Tenn, May 7, 1960.

Murray, R.A. Shin splints and fatigue fractures. In *Proceedings of the 4th National Conference on the Medical Aspects of Sports.* Chicago: American Medical Association, 1962.

CHAPTER 21
Metabolic, Hormonal, and Dietary Considerations

Edward S. Horton, MD

The effect of nutrition on physical performance has been of great interest to those involved in sports for many centuries. Specific training diets were followed by athletes in ancient Greece and the food customs and taboos of many primitive cultures are related to the relationship between diet and the capacity for physical exercise. Even today, many athletes and coaches seek at least a partial cause for success or failure in sports performance in the nutritional preparation that is undertaken, sometimes with superstitious zeal. Many questions exist regarding the most effective training diet for a particular type of competition; practices vary considerably from one individual to another. The composition, amount, and timing of the precompetition meal has taken on a special significance for many athletes, even to the point of secrecy for fear a rival will learn one's secret of success. In endurance events such as long distance running, cycle racing, or cross-country ski racing, and in certain team sports, the question of providing feedings as well as fluid and salt replacement during the competition has also received considerable attention in recent years.

In sports requiring great muscle strength and size, special diets, protein supplements, and large doses of anabolic steroids have been used widely to gain these attributes, often with little or no rational basis. This has become common among boxers, weight lifters, shot putters, and other similar groups of athletes, as well as among some women athletes in whom an increase in muscle mass and strength would provide a distinct competitive advantage.

To have a rational approach to the problem of proper nutrition and dietary strategy for maximal performance in sports it is necessary to have a basic understanding of how the body in general, and the muscles in particular, generate the energy for muscular work. Factors such as the type of exercise, duration, intensity, and effects of training are all important. In this chapter, an attempt will be made to review briefly the current knowledge in this area and apply it to a practical dietary program.

BASICS OF ENERGY METABOLISM

One can compare energy metabolism in man to the energy required to operate an automobile, a steam engine, or any mechanical device that consumes energy to perform work. The internal combustion engine is a good example. Two basic ingredients are required for operation: an oxygen supply, and a fuel to be burned, in this case, gasoline. For efficient operation these must be present in the proper mixture.

When the engine is at idle and the car stopped, no external work is being done and the rate of oxygen and gasoline consumption is low. When the car is being driven, the rate of consumption depends on the amount of work being done. This varies with the speed at which the car is driven and the load it is carrying. How long it will go depends on the amount of gasoline in the tank, the amount of work being done (speed and load) and the inherent efficiency of the engine, that is the percentage of the energy generated that is converted into useful mechanical work rather than into heat.

In man and animals, similar conditions hold. At rest a certain amount of energy is required to maintain normal body functions such as breathing, circulation of the blood, digestion, and the maintenance of a normal internal environment in the body. This is referred to as the basal metabolic rate. Any work done above this basal level will use additional energy at an efficiency of about 30% for muscular contractions.

In animals, energy is usually measured in kilocalories (kcal). In an average size person weighing 70 kg (154 lbs) the basal metabolic rate is approximately 1000 kcal/24 hr. Depending on the amount of physical activity, total energy can vary from as low as 1500 kcal/24 hr in a sedentary individual to 5000 to 6000 kcal/24 hr in one who is performing heavy work for several hours. The rate at which calories are used depends largely on the intensity of the exercise being done. For example, for a person of average size, sitting quietly requires approximately 115 kcal/hr, walking slowly requires 250 to 300 kcal/hr, and jogging requires 800 to 1000 kcal/hr. During competitive activities such as swimming or cross-country ski racing, energy utilization may be as high as 1000 to 1200 kcal/hr. Running a marathon requires a total of approximately 2400 kcal.

Where do these calories come from? There are three major substances that can be used for energy in the body: carbohydrates, fats, and proteins. These metabolic fuels are contained in the foods we eat and are present in varying amounts and forms in the body. Carbohydrates are the various sugars and starches that are consumed in the diet and usually make up to 45% to 50% of the total intake of calories. These sugars and starches are digested and absorbed into the blood stream as single sugar units; the principle one is glucose. When one speaks of the blood sugar level, one is speaking of the concentration of glucose in the blood. A limited amount of glucose can be stored in the body as a much larger chemical compound called glycogen. This occurs mainly in the liver and in muscles where stores amount to approximately 75 gm and 150 gm respectively.[1] When these stores are called on for energy production, such as during a period of fasting or during exercise, the glycogen can be broken down rapidly to glucose. The glucose produced in the liver by this reaction is released into the blood stream and is thus made available to all the glucose-requiring tissues in the body, primarily the brain, the nerves, and exercising muscles. The glucose released in muscle by the breakdown of glycogen is not released into the blood but is used directly in the muscle for energy production.

When glucose is metabolized completely to carbon dioxide and water it provides 4 kcal/gm. Since total body stores of glucose, nearly all in the form of glycogen in liver and muscle tissue, amount to about 250 gm, this will provide 1000 kcal of energy, enough for approximately 10 hours of fairly light activity or for less than 2 hours of heavy work if this were the only fuel consumed.

Fortunately, the body has a mechanism to make glucose from other compounds and thus can supplement the glucose derived from glycogen stores. This process occurs in the liver but not in the muscles. Several compounds are extracted from the blood by the liver and converted into glucose which is then returned to the blood stream. These compounds include lactate and pyruvate, which are products of glucose metabolism in muscle and other tissues; several amino acids, which are derived from the breakdown of body proteins; and glycerol, which is released from fat tissue along with fatty acids during times of increased energy requirements. As will be discussed later, the ability to maintain an adequate blood glucose concentration and an adequate supply of glycogen in the muscle for energy production is a major factor in the ability to perform endurance exercise, and failure of this system is usually associated with exhaustion.

The second major metabolic fuel is the fatty acids that are released from the breakdown of neutral fats in the body. Fats in the diet, like carbohydrates, come in a wide variety of forms. They include both oils and solid fats of either animal or vegetable origin and normally comprise 30% to 40% of total calories. Dietary fats are digested and then resynthesized into neutral fats called triglycerides that enter the blood stream and then are either taken up by the liver, are broken down into free fatty acids and glycerol for energy production, or are taken up in adipose tissue for storage as body fat. In men, the normal body fat content is 15% to 25% of body weight and in women it is 20% to 30%. Highly trained athletes usually have a somewhat lower body fat content and in trained distance runners body fat may be only 5% to 10% of body weight in men and 10% to 15% in women.

Fat is the major storehouse of energy in the body. The adipose tissue contains 70% to 80% fat and fat yields close to 9 kcal/gm. Thus, in an average 70 kg person, there will be approximately 15 kg of fat containing 135,000 kcal.

The third type of compound that is used for energy is protein. Proteins are made up of chains of amino acids and are found in virtually all living tissues. The major dietary sources for man are meats and vegetables, and proteins normally make up 15% to 20% of total energy intake. Proteins in the diet are digested in the gastrointestinal tract to their constituent amino acids that are absorbed into the body and either used to synthesize new proteins or are used for energy. Unlike carbohyrates and fat, there is no storage form for protein in the body. All proteins serve a function, either as compounds involved in specific chemical reactions or as structural components of body tissues and organs. The largest single source of protein in the body is that found in the muscles themselves.

When needed for energy, amino acids derived

from proteins in the diet or from the breakdown of body tissues can be used in small quantities directly by exercising muscles. A much larger portion, however, is taken up by the liver and converted to glucose. Thus, when glucose supplies are limited, proteins are consumed to maintain adequate blood sugar levels and to provide glucose for energy production.

The mixture of metabolic fuels that is consumed (oxidized) at any given time is influenced by a number of factors including the composition of the diet, the intensity and duration of physical exercise, and the level of physical training. As one might expect, a diet high in carbohydrates results in an increased proportion of glucose that is consumed for energy production, whereas a high-fat diet increases the amount of fat oxidized. A high-protein diet tends to act like a high-carbohydrate diet, since a large proportion of the ingested protein is converted to glucose in the body.

Within the body, the various tissues and organs have different requirements for specific metabolic fuels. For example, the brain and nerves derive nearly all of their energy from the oxidation of glucose except under conditions of chronic glucose deprivation when an adaptation to use some fat-derived fuels occurs. Muscle, on the other hand, varies its fuel requirement considerably, depending on the intensity and duration of exercise, level of training, and the antecedent diet. When the diet contains normal amounts of carbohydrates, proteins, and fats, resting muscle derives 85% to 90% of its energy requirements from the oxidation of fatty acids, about 10% from glucose, and only 1% to 2% from amino acids.[2] During exercise, the proportion of glucose that is used increases progressively as the intensity of the exercise increases so that at 85% to 90% of maximal effort, virtually all of the energy is derived from glucose. During exercise at 50% of maximal aerobic capacity, approximately one-half of the energy is derived from glucose and one-half from the oxidation of fat.[3] When the oxygen supply to muscle is adequate, a high proportion of both glucose and fatty acids is oxidized to carbon dioxide and water, releasing the maximum amount of energy available. When the intensity of exercise exceeds the maximum aerobic capacity, the oxygen supply cannot meet the demand for energy, glucose is metabolized incompletely to lactate, which then accumulates in the muscle and blood. This process releases only about 7% of the available energy in the glucose and creates a so-called oxygen debt that can be repaid later when the exercise is stopped or the intensity decreased and the accumulated lactate is oxidized to carbon dioxide and water. Obviously, this type of very high intensity exercise, which is characteristic of weight lifting or sprinting, is metabolically inefficient and cannot be sustained for more than a short time. A simple isometric contraction can be maintained for only about 30 seconds.

During less intensive exercise of long duration, the pattern of metabolic fuel utilization is somewhat different than during high-intensity aerobic exercise. For the first few minutes after the onset of exercise, there is a rapid increase in the rate of glucose oxidation, coming primarily from the breakdown of glycogen stores within the muscle. As exercise continues, the muscle takes up both glucose and fatty acids from the blood for energy production. Blood glucose levels are maintained by the release of glucose from the liver and blood fatty acids gradually rise as they are released from the fat stores. The uptake of glucose reaches a maximum after about 90 minutes of sustained exercise and then decreases slightly as fatty acids become progressively a more important source of energy. The glycogen stores in both muscle and liver are gradually consumed and, although the synthesis of new glucose in the liver increases, the total output of glucose from the liver eventually declines. When the intensity of the exercise is greater than 70% of the maximum aerobic capacity, depletion of glycogen stores and failure to maintain an adequate level of glucose in the blood are usually associated with exhaustion.

EFFECTS OF ENDURANCE TRAINING

Endurance training has a significant effect on both the capacity and pattern of metabolic fuel utilization during exercise. The maximum rate of oxygen utilization increases so that total work capacity is enhanced. This can be measured by determining the uptake of oxygen from air at progressively increasing work loads on a treadmill or stationary bicycle until the point is reached at which further increases in the work load do not result in any further increase in oxygen consumption. This is referred to as the maximum aerobic capacity or maximum rate of oxygen consumption. Average values for untrained individuals are 2 to 3.5 liter/min, depending on body size and age. In trained persons, values of 4 to 5 liter/min are common, and in highly trained endurance athletes such as cross-country ski racers, values as high as 6 liter/min may occur.

Several changes also occur in muscle tissue with training that result in an increased capacity of muscle to oxidize both glucose and fatty acids.[4] The blood flow through trained muscles is increased allowing more oxygen and metabolic fuels to enter from the circulation, and the muscle cells develop an increased capacity to oxidize both glucose and fatty acids. This results in more complete utilization of metabolic fuels and less accumulation of lactate during exercise. In addition, a shift in the fuel mixture occurs, so that at any given work load the proportion of energy derived from the oxidation of fatty acids is increased and the proportion from glucose is decreased. This has a sparing effect on the glycogen in muscle and liver, allows adequate blood glucose concentrations to be maintained for a longer time, and results in an increase in endurance.

EFFECTS OF DIET

The effect of diet on strength and endurance has been of great interest to athletes for over 2000 years and continues to attract a great deal of attention today. The practice of consuming large quantities of meat on the assumption that this would result in increased muscle mass and strength was recorded in Greek athletes as early as the fifth century BC. In more recent times, practices such as fluid restriction, periodic fasting, high-meat diets, high-carbohydrate diets, low-carbohydrate diets, and a host of dietary supplements such as protein tablets, vitamins, and anabolic steroids have all had their champions. In addition to the concern about the best training diet for maximum sports performance, the composition, quantity, and timing of the precompetition meal has taken an almost superstitious significance for many athletes as has the proper method of providing nutrients and replenishing body fluid and salt losses during long events. What is the current scientific evidence for or against any of these practices?

The Training Diet

It is now generally agreed that a well-balanced diet is best for training and that special diets providing an excess of one component or another are of no advantage and may, in fact, be detrimental. A well-balanced diet should contain 15% to 20% of the calories as protein, 30% to 40% as fats, and 45% to 50% as carbohydrates. It should contain sufficient variety to provide an adequate intake of vitamins and trace minerals and enough total calories to meet the increased energy expenditures of training and competition. A once-daily vitamin and mineral supplement may be taken if desired. There is no evidence that larger doses or megavitamin therapy are helpful.

During the initial stages of training, some loss of body weight may be desirable as unneeded fat stores are decreased. However, this loss of weight is often compensated by an increase in muscle mass, depending on the type of training, and total body weight may change only slightly or not at all. Once a steady level of training has been achieved, body weight should remain relatively stable and total caloric intake can be adjusted accordingly. A special situation exists in the younger athlete who is still growing. Here, adequate calories and protein are needed for the formation of new body tissues. A well-balanced diet is best but the total amount of calories should be sufficient to provide for both the high energy expenditure and for normal growth.

Although still widely practiced by some groups of athletes, particularly those involved in sports requiring great muscle strength, the consumption of large amounts of protein as meat or supplemental protein tablets does not increase muscle mass or strength. As noted previously, there is no storage form of protein in the body and extra protein in the diet is metabolized for energy much like carbohydrates. A normal diet provides sufficient amino acids for rebuilding proteins that are continually turning over in all body tissues and for the increase in muscle size that occurs as the result of training. Strength training, itself, is the major factor in increasing muscle size and strength, and there is no evidence that this process is enhanced by consuming extra protein in the diet.

For those athletes participating in endurance events lasting 30 minutes or more, the practice of carbohydrate loading has become common. This applies to situations where depletion of glycogen stores in muscle and liver may become significant factors in the ability to sustain a high level of energy expenditure and includes such events as long-distance running, swimming, cross-country skiing, and bicycle racing as well as some team sports such as soccer, basketball, football, and ice hockey. As described above, the more vigorous the exercise, the greater is the dependence on glucose for energy production in muscle. During endurance exercise of high intensity, muscle and liver glycogen stores become progressively depleted and when critically low levels are released, the high level of energy production can no longer be maintained and exhaustion occurs. Training has a sparing effect on glycogen stores by increasing the utilization of fat for energy and thus increases endurance. A major question now is: does the composition of the diet have any effect on this process?

Several decades ago, scientists in Scandinavia observed that the work-time to exhaustion of men performing submaximal exercise on a stationary bicycle was increased after three or more days of a diet containing large amounts of carbohydrates and was decreased after a similar time on a low-carbohydrate diet.[5] Since these early studies, a needle biopsy technique has been developed that makes it possible to sample small portions of muscle at repeated intervals in man for analysis of the content of glycogen, fats, and other chemicals involved in energy production. Using this technique, it has been discovered that diet and exercise both have effects on muscle glycogen content and that endurance at work loads of 70% or more of maximal aerobic capacity is closely related to the amount of muscle glocogen present at the beginning of exercise.[6,7] When the effect of diet alone was studied without added exercise, changes in muscle glycogen content were rather small. Several days of a low carbohydrate diet resulted in a small decrease in glycogen content, a week of starvation produced only a 30% to 40% decrease, and a high-carbohydrate diet resulted in only a very slight increase. After depletion of muscle glycogen stores with exercise, however, it was found that the composition of the diet had a marked effect on the rate of reaccumulation of glycogen stores. Both a low-carbohydrate diet and total starvation resulted in a very slow rate of recovery, normal values not being achieved for several days. A high-carbohydrate diet, on the other hand, resulted in a rapid increase in muscle glycogen content to values well above the normal resting level. The overshoot phenomenon was most pronounced following exhausting exercise in which muscle glycogen content was nearly totally depleted.

Thus, two conditions work together to achieve very high muscle glycogen levels. First, muscle glycogen stores must be reduced to a very low level by strenuous exercise and second, a diet high in carbohydrates must be eaten to allow rapid reaccumulation of glycogen to occur. It was further learned that the maximum increase in muscle glycogen could be obtained if, after depletion of muscle glycogen stores by exercise, muscle glycogen levels were kept at a low level for two to three days by eating a low-carbohydrate diet and then allowed to reaccumulate rapidly by three days of a high-carbohydrate intake. This practice has now been adopted by large numbers of athletes participating in endurance events and does appear to have a sound scientific basis. Increased stores of glycogen in muscle and liver make it possible to sustain a high intensity of muscular work for a longer period of time, help maintain normal blood glucose levels, and may provide the source of energy for the final push that is often important in winning a race.

Some note of caution regarding carbohydrate loading is needed, however. Since it will be of benefit only in those situations where nearly complete exhaustion of glycogen stores is likely to occur, there is no evidence that this dietary strategy will enhance performance in events lasting less than 30 minutes. When glycogen is deposited in tissues, water is stored along with it. This may result in a sensation of swelling and stiffness in the muscles, which is unpleasant and may hinder performance in short events such as sprinting. Carbohydrate loading may not be advisable for individuals with certain medical conditions such as diabetes mellitus or increased blood lipids, although there is little information regarding this subject at the present time.

Precompetition Feeding

Another major area of concern among athletes and coaches is the question of what to feed during the few hours before a competition. How much? What type of food? How long before the event? Although the answers to these questions are not altogether clear and will depend somewhat on the type of event (eg, endurance, sprint, or strength events) and individual preferences, certain facts are now known regarding the effects of precompetition feeding on endurance performance.

Since the rate at which muscle and liver glycogen stores become depleted during exercise affects endurance, it is beneficial to slow the rate of glycogen utilization during exercise by deriving as much energy as possible from the oxidation of fatty acids. The rate at which fatty acids are extracted from the blood and metabolized by muscle is related directly to their concentration in the blood. This, in turn, is determined by the rate at which they are released from adipose tissue. It has been demonstrated in laboratory animals that raising the blood concentration of fatty acids prior to exercise markedly increases endurance.[8] Muscle and liver glycogen levels decrease more slowly and blood glucose remains normal for a longer time suggesting that a carbohydrate-sparing effect of fatty acids is largely responsible for the increase in endurance.

The effect of feeding glucose 30 to 50 minutes before exercise has been studied in man. This results in an increase in the blood glucose concentration and in the oxidation of glucose for energy production.[9] Free fatty acid levels in the blood are decreased and correspondingly less fat is used for energy. Under these conditions, muscle and liver glycogen stores may be depleted rapidly and endurance may be decreased. In one study, the ingestion of 75 gm of glucose 30 minutes prior to an endurance test on a cycle at a work intensity of approximately 80% of maximum aerobic capacity was associated with a 19% decrease in endurance whereas similar feedings of milk or water had no effect.[10]

There is now some evidence that the ingestion of caffeine one hour prior to the onset of exercise and periodically during exercise can increase work output.[11] This is presumably related to the effect of caffeine on the adipose tissue where it increases the rate of release of fatty acids into the blood, although a central nervous system stimulating effect is also possible.

Current evidence would suggest, then, that for maximum endurance, a high-carbohydrate meal should be avoided during the hour or so before competition to avoid inhibition of the release of fatty acids from adipose tissue and their utilization for energy. A cup of coffee or other caffeine-containing beverage may enhance fatty acid mobilization and utilization, thereby decreasing glucose oxidation, sparing glycogen stores and increasing endurance. At least two to three hours should be allowed between a large meal and the onset of competitive exercise to allow adequate time for complete digestion to occur and for the body to shift back to a state in which fat can be rapidly mobilized for energy production.

Feeding During Competition

A final area of concern is the question of what to feed during competitions lasting more than one hour. Unlike the situation of precompetition feeding, small amounts of carbohydrates taken at frequent intervals during endurance events can be utilized for energy and help maintain adequate blood glucose levels and glycogen stores. The amount of glucose that can be absorbed from the gastrointestinal tract is limited, however, and for practical purposes does not exceed 50 gm per hour.[12] Since there is also a need for fluid and salt replacement during long events, the most common practice is for the athlete to drink a mixture containing a combination of glucose and various salts at 10 to 20 minute intervals. This drink should not be too concentrated or it will not be absorbed rapidly and may, in fact, drain fluid from the body into the gastrointestinal tract and temporarily increase the degree of dehydration. For best results, a flavored solution containing 5 gm of glucose per 100 ml is usually used. If salt is needed, 1.5 gm of ordinary table salt can be added to each liter.

Opinions vary widely regarding the requirements for salt and water, dependent on the type of exercise, amount of perspiration, and climatic conditions. During strenuous exercise, water is lost from the body through perspiration, through the respiratory tract and by the formation of urine. On hot days, the rate of loss may exceed 2 liters per hour and if not adequately replaced, a marked decrease in performance may result. A decrease in body water equal to 4% to 5% of body weight has been found to result in a 20% to 30% decrease in capacity for strenuous work.

In planning a program of fluid replacement during endurance exercise it is best to start in a well-hydrated state and to stay ahead by starting fluid replacement early. Small amounts should be taken every 10 to 20 minutes, but no more than one liter per hour if overdistention of the stomach is to be avoided. Since some water is released within the body from the breakdown of glycogen and the oxidation of glycogen and fatty acids, not all of the water loss needs to be replaced by fluid intake. As much as 1.5 liters of water can be derived from internal sources during exhausting endurance exercise.

Although some commercially available drinks for fluid, carbohydrate, and salt replacement contain potassium, there is no evidence that supplemental potassium is needed during endurance exercise.[6] As glycogen stores are broken down, large amounts of potassium are released into the blood. Losses of potassium in perspiration are small so that replacement during exercise is not necessary. However, during recovery of muscle and liver glycogen stores, potassium is utilized and replacement may be necessary at that time, particularly if carbohydrate loading is practiced. Normally, there is sufficient potassium in the diet to meet these needs and supplemental potassium preparations should never be taken without strict medical supervision because of the danger of over-replacement that may produce serious, even fatal, complications.

ANABOLIC STEROIDS

Unfortunately, the use of sex steroids to promote increased muscle size and strength has become a worldwide practice among athletes in the hope that this will improve performance in strength-requiring events. Often, amounts are taken regularly that far exceed those used for legitimate medical purposes and consequently little is known about the long-term effects and complications of this practice.

The major reason for the widespread use of sex steroids is the well-known growth-promoting effects of testosterone, the major sex hormone in men, during puberty and adolescence. This hormone, produced mainly in the testes but also present in small amounts in women, has numerous metabolic actions. At the onset of puberty in men, testosterone production increases dramatically and its action results in the changes that occur during adolescence. These include enlargement of the male sex organs, increased oiliness of the skin with the development of acne in susceptible individuals, deepening of the voice, the development of axillary and pubic hair, increased growth of body and facial hair, and establishment of beard growth. One of the most dramatic effects of testosterone is a rapid increase in height, often at the rate of 3 to 4 inches per year, which then tapers off until full statural growth is achieved. Along with the increase in height, there is thickening of the skeleton and an increase in muscle mass and strength to adult proportions.

The small amounts of testosterone that are normally present in women have some of the same effects, but to a much lesser degree. They play a role in the adolescent growth spurt and the development of acne in women, and if present in excess amounts may result in the growth of facial hair, deepening of the voice, enlargement of sex organs, abnormalities of the menstrual cycle, and increased muscle mass.

In the normal adult man, testosterone levels are high and the body tissues are already fully stimulated. There is no evidence that the administration of additional hormone will increase the effects further, and in fact some undesirable side effects may occur. The most common one is the retention of salt and water in the body, which may account for some of the gain in weight that is observed.

A large number of substances have been made synthetically that have chemical structures similar to that of testosterone but that do not possess all of its actions to the same degree.[13] The group, called anabolic steroids, has been developed to produce an increase in the growth of body tissues while keeping the effects of sexual development at a minimum. These substances are used in medical treatment to stimulate the production of blood cells, to promote retention of nitrogen in the body, and to aid in the treatment of certain types of cancer. Dosage levels are well standardized and are usually much lower than the amounts that have been used by athletes.

The use of anabolic steroids in an attempt to enhance athletic performance must be condemned for several reasons. First, in the adult man there is no sound scientific evidence that high doses of anabolic steroids have any additional effect on muscle strength above that produced by training and normal levels of testosterone. The weight gain that may occur with their use is largely due to the retention of salt and water and does not represent a true increase in muscle tissue. Because dosage levels commonly far exceed those used in medical practice, little is known about the potential harmful effects on the body of such long-term use.

In women, anabolic steroids do appear to increase muscle size and strength to some extent, but this is not well documented scientifically. Since none of the compounds yet developed are totally free of testosterone-like side effects, women using anabolic steroids will develop certain male sexual characteristics including deepening of the voice, growth of hair on the face and body, increased oiliness of the skin with resulting acne, recession of the scalp hair, enlargement of the clitoris, and menstrual irregularities. Although some of these changes will regress after discontinuation of the steroids, some, such as deepening of the voice, increased hair growth, and enlargement of the clitoris may be permanent.

Under no circumstances should anabolic steroids be used by preadolescent or adolescent boys or girls. Permanent effects on body growth and development may result—a large price to pay for a desired temporary increase in muscle size and strength.

In summary, the use of anabolic steroids among some groups of athletes is widespread in the hope that this, like eating large quantities of meat or taking protein tablets, will increase muscle strength and performance. There is no sound evidence that this is the case and the potential risks of this practice, although not well understood at this time, would appear to far outweigh the supposed benefits. The use of anabolic steroids has no legitimate place in athletics and should be soundly discouraged whenever it is practiced.

CONCLUSION

In general, the best approach to proper nutrition for maximal performance in sports is to eat a well-balanced diet with a total caloric intake adjusted to the demands of the training program. Unusually large amounts of protein or vitamin supplements are of no proven benefit and the use of anabolic steroids should be avoided. For those participating in endurance events lasting longer than 30 minutes, the practice of carbohydrate loading may enhance endurance and provide greater reserve for the final push during competition. A high-carbohydrate meal should be avoided however, during the hour or so before competition since this may decrease the utilization of fat for energy and may decrease endurance. Caffeine ingestion prior to competition may increase fat mobilization and enhance performance. During endurance events, frequent feeding of small amounts of a drink containing glucose and salt will aid in replacing fluid and salt losses and in maintaining a glucose supply for energy production. Ultimate success in sports will depend on the individual's natural abilities and learned skill, his or her training program, and a sensible approach to good nutrition.

REFERENCES

1. Cahill, G.F., Jr. Starvation in man. *N Engl J Med.* 282:668–675, 1970.

2. Felig, P., and Wahren, J. Full homeostasis in exercise. *N Engl J Med.* 293:1078–1084, 1975.

3. Havel, R.J., Naimark, A., and Borchgrevink, C.F. Turnover rate and oxidation of free fatty acids of blood plasma in man during exercise: studies during continuous infusion of Palmitate-1-C^{14}. *J Clin Invest.* 42:1054–1063, 1963.

4. Holloszy, J.O., and Booth, F.W. Biochemical adaptations to endurance exercise in muscle. *Annu Rev Physiol.* 38:273–291, 1976.

5. Christensen, E.H., and Hansen, O., III. Arbeitsfahigkeit und Ernahrung. *Skand Arch Physiol.* 81:160–171, 1939.

6. Bergstrom, J., and Hultman, E. Nutrition for maximal sports performance. *JAMA.* 221: 999–1006, 1972.

7. Bergstrom, J., Hermansen, L., Hultman, E. et al. Diet, muscle glycogen and physical performance. *Acta Physiol Scand.* 17:140–150, 1967.

8. Hickson, R.C., Rennie, M.J., Conlee, R.K. et al. Effects of increased plasma fatty acids on glycogen utilization and endurance. *J Appl Physiol.* 43:829–833, 1977.

9. Ahlborg, G., and Felig, P. Substrate utilization during prolonged exercise preceded by glucose ingestion. *Am J Physiol.* 233:E188–E194, 1977.

10. Foster, C., Costill, D.L., and Fink, W.J. Effects of pre-exercise feedings on endurance performance. *Med Sci Sports.* 11:1–5, 1979.

11. Ivy, J.L., Costill, D.L., Fink, W.J. et al. Influence of caffeine and carbohydrate feedings on endurance performance. *Med Sci Sports.* 11:6–11, 1979.

12. Fordtran, J.S., and Saltin, B. Gastric emptying and intestinal absorption during prolonged severe exercise. *J Appl Physiol.* 23:331–335, 1967.

13. Goodman, L.S., and Gilman, A. *The Pharmacological Basis of Therapeutics.* 5th Ed. New York: MacMillan, 1975.

CHAPTER 22

The Athletic Alchemist: Drugs in Sport

E. C. Percy, MD

With the excellence in performance expected in all areas of competitive athletic endeavor today and with the demands placed on sportspersons involved to attempt to improve upon this performance, it is no wonder that many forms of artificial aids are utilized. The term "ergogenic aids" is generally applied to techniques or substances used to improve athletic performance. This broad classification includes anything which might, through its use, increase work output or performance of the competitor. Generally speaking, these aids can be divided into five broad classifications: physiological, physical, psychological, nutritional and chemical.

In the first category, physiological aids would be included; for example, the use of supplemental oxygen in athletic competition. There appears to be little or no effect upon performance with the ancillary use of oxygen before or following strenuous physical activity. There appears to be evidence, however, to suggest that the use of supplemental O_2 during exercise may improve performance and endurance through increasing VO_2max, reductions in blood lactic acid and the lowering of the ventilatory rate.[1] The encumbrance of carrying a portable O_2 supply would seem to mitigate any such possible advantages. The hypoxia of altitude is physiologically compensated for (over a period of time) by increasing the hemoglobin level. On this basis, ill-advised athletes have attempted to simulate the hypoxia of altitude by breathing air with a lower O_2 content than normal. Blood boosting, blood packing or blood doping is a technique which has also been used in an attempt to improve the O_2 delivery system to the working muscles. Gledhill[2] has shown that the reinfusion of 900 cc of an athlete's blood some two months following its removal did improve VO_2 max in endurance performance as well as raise the hemoglobin level in that individual. The dangers of infection, mismatched transfusions, interference in the clotting mechanism and future blood-typing and the expense would have to be considered before subjecting an athlete to these risks.

In the physical aids category, equipment can be a vital asset to the athlete in improving performance. For example, the fiberglass pole was introduced to the sport of pole vaulting in 1963, and within six months new heights had been reached—increasing the world record by nine inches.[3] In the same vein, the use of synthetic tracks on the running surfaces has probably led to increased performance by reducing running times. Sprinters, for example, apply force to the surface for a short time and perform better on a firm surface. Endurance runners, on the other hand, perform better on a softer track due to less impact stress from the repetitive efforts required.

Psychological aids have long been recognized as an important factor in winning or losing a competitive event. This may vary from a simple pep talk from the coach prior to a game to the actual use of posthypnotic suggestion by members of the coaching staff trained in psychological methods. Medical teams in international competitions now routinely include a number of athletic psychologists. The psychologist can also play a definite role in the management of pain and in the rehabilitation of an injury to the athlete.

Nutritional aids are that group of substances which have been employed as ergogenic aids that date back to the birth of sport. There is probably more quackery in this area than in any other field. Athletes are particularly susceptible to false advertising claims, especially in the vitamin and protein supplement areas. Few, if any, athletes require supplemental substances beyond the Recommended Dietary Allowances (RDA). Indeed, there are dangers inherent in the excessive use of, for example, vitamins. (Megavitamin doses, incidentally, have not been shown to improve performance.) Obviously, nutrition is an important aspect of conditioning and training, and a basic RDA diet is essential to all athletes. Dietary manipulation is not uncommonly used by athletes, but it seems that results of such techniques as far as improving performance are largely psychological. It should be emphasized, however, that most athletes have little or no idea of what is a nutritionally adequate diet.[4]

The use of chemical substances by athletes in an attempt to improve performance has become widespread. Indeed, the abuse of these materials by sports persons has been labeled "chemical warfare,"[5] and those who use these materials in this way have been referred to as "athletic alchemists." No longer is the use of these materials confined to the professional athletic level—their use is now apparently wide spread at the high school and collegiate level. The spectrum of drugs used varies from stimulants to steroids.

The history of sport relates that drug testing was first employed in race horses in 1910. The demand for tests arose because of flagrant misuse and abuse of substances used in attempts to improve the animals' performance. The actual use of chemical substances in humans, however, goes back further; there are references to their use in the early history of the Olympics, which started in 776 BC. A number of deaths have been reported from the abuse of drugs over the past few centuries, and the sudden apparent increase in the use of these materials following World War II led the International Olympic Committee (IOC) to form a medical commission to investigate and attempt to arrest the use of these materials. A list of banned substances was introduced in 1967 and was first used in the Olympic movement in 1968 during the games in Mexico City.[6] Attempts were made to educate the athletes but the warning seemingly fell on deaf ears and although the drugs were prohibited, they were still taken prior to international competition and disqualifications resulted. Whereas stimulants were initially the principle drugs that were abused, it soon became apparent that the use of these materials was being overshadowed by that of the anabolic steroids, which were taken to improve strength and power. Tests were then introduced for these substances in the 1976 Olympics in Montreal to determine whether or not the athlete had taken this "forbidden fruit."

It is interesting to note that the original premise of the IOC Medical Commission stressed the negative effects of drug taking. It is now realized that some of these materials and methods do in fact improve performance, but in general the possible advantages gained by their use are far outweighed by the health hazards associated with taking them. For the 1984 Olympics, the Medical Commission of the IOC again stressed the dangers of taking these drugs but also attempted to stress to the athletes that improving performance may be best achieved with far less danger by physiological and biomechanical means rather than chemical means.[7]

Stimulants The most widely used group of drugs has been stimulants. While amphetamines are the most commonly used substances in this group of drugs, even strychnine has been used as a possible ergogenic aid! The amphetamines do have an effect on aerobic performance by decreasing fatigue and probably increasing the work output. Strength may be improved and reaction time decreased. It also seems that in trained athletes there can be improved times for short distance events. That is to say, there is a distinct possibility of improved performance with the use of amphetamines but inherent in their use are the health dangers to the taker. This spectrum can vary from diminishing the normal physiological warning symptoms of fatigue to actual collapse and death. It allows the athlete to "run the red light." The athlete may become more aggressive and, as such, be more apt to injure himself or other competitors. The drugs are a central nervous system (CNS) stimulant and lead to wakefulness, a sense of well-being and euphoria as well as heightened self-confidence. The peripheral effects do lead to increased blood pressure and pulse rate and the redistribution of blood from the skin and splanchnic bed to skeletal muscle, and the brain thus interferes with the bodily heat dispersion mechanisms. There is a possibility of the use of these drugs resulting in a rise in free fatty acids and some carbohydrate sparing.[1]

Their use has been very common in professional sport as evidenced by the number of autobiographies by former athletes that include specific references to the use of drugs. Their use was widespread during World War II in the armed forces. The taker can, of course, become dependent on these materials and often large amounts are taken with a resultant rebound effect when their use is stopped. Occasionally the athlete who has been taking uppers will have to take anti-anxiety agents (downers) following the competition to come down from the high caused by the stimulants.

Another substance which is widely used as a stimulant is caffeine. It also is a powerful general stimulant of the CNS and has been shown to enhance performance, particularly in endurance events. It may have a direct effect on muscle itself by reducing the threshold of motor neurons and allowing larger recruitment of muscle fibers. Apparently it has a similar effect as amphetamines on immobilization of fat and CHO.[8] Caffeine was tested for in the 1984 Summer Olympic Games (a positive test demonstrates a concentration in urine exceeding 15 mg/mL).[9] When one considers the fact that caffeine occurs in so many products which are consumed by athletes (chocolate, some soft drinks, tea and coffee) the findings of a "positive" test will be on somewhat tenuous legal grounds.

Diuretics In an attempt to "make weight," athletes involved in sports where competitors are assigned to different levels according to their body weight, often take diuretics to lose weight through fluid loss. In this manner the athlete can increase muscle bulk by vigorous training and then, by sudden rapid loss of weight, compete in a lower weight category. Athletes have been known to dehydrate and starve themselves 24 to 48 hours prior to competition. Sweat suits and diuretics supplement these techniques. Usually following the competition the athlete can be reinfused with fluids and regain normal weight and fluid distribution in the body. There have been a number of complications associated with this practice, and its use has been condemned by the American College of Sports Medicine.[10,11] The fluid loss is, of course, accompanied by loss of electrolytes, and it has been shown that this practice can result in decreased performance. Athletes will even go to the extremes of voluntary emesis in an attempt to lose weight and have been known to run around with spitting cups!

Alkalinizers Because lactic acid is formed as a result of intensive exercise, it is thought that the use of these substances could result in a higher serum pH level so that the athlete would be able to make more lactic acid before exhaustion and presumably be capable of a greater work output. A recent study by Wilkes et al has shown that the ingestion of $NaHCO_3$ by trained middle-distance runners prior to an 800-m race has an ergogenic benefit.[12]

Pangamic acid This substance is more commonly known as B15 or even as vitamin B_{15}. Historically it is said to have first appeared in the USSR, where apparently it was isolated from the liver in 1950. It was called B15, and at a later date Krebs and his group isolated a crystalline form which they called pangamic acid. It should be realized that there is no definite chemical entity known as pangamic acid. In the United States the Food and Drug Administration (FDA) has called B_{15} a hoax and has attempted to remove it from the market. It has been described by this group as "not an identifiable substance . . . not a vitamin nor a provitamin . . . no accepted scientific evidence established as any nutritional properties of the substance or any deficiency . . . in man or animal . . . no medical, nutritional, or other usefulness for these substances has been established." It has been labeled and sold as DMG.[13] It would appear that there is no sound scientific evidence to lend any credibiltiy to this substance as an ergogenic aid.[14]

Aspartates It has long been felt that the fatigue that accompanies strenuous exertion may in fact be related to the increased rate of ammonia production. A recent study by Maughan and Sadler demonstrated no beneficial effect of oral aspartate administration on work capacity.[15]

Alcohol This substance has frequently been used by competitors in athletic events particularly those involved in cycling, shooting and in the biathalon and pentathalon. It has been used as an ergogenic aid because of its possible tranquilizing effect on steadying the aim. Beer has been used as a readily available source of calories and fluid as well as having a diuretic effect. Other substances which have been used as a tranquilizer include chlordiazepoxide and diazepam. These drugs, along with alcohol, do have the effect of reducing the velocity of saccadic eye movements.[16] These substances do, however, produce a doll's-eye type eye movement, which does impair visual acuity in following moving targets. The American College of Sports Medicine has again taken a firm position against the use of alcohol, and apart from its obvious ill effects systemically and the dangers of dependency, it has not been shown to improve physical performance capacity.[17] Indeed it may lead to decreased performance in many areas. Probably the only benefit an athlete might get from alcohol or tranquilizers is the disinhibiting effect, although this in itself could be dangerous to the participant or fellow competitors.

Beta blockers These materials have been used to diminish anxiety for years by musicians, ballet dancers, public speakers, college professors and even surgeons prior to performing. Their effect in this area is to block the sympathetically mediated effects of stress and to reduce central anxiety. For these reasons, athletes involved in shooting competitions take these substances. A large number of studies, as reported by *Lancet*, have shown that patients with primarily somatic anxiety may be helped with the use of these substances, but those patients whose anxiety is primarily psychic have not been helped.[18] It is of interest to note that in 1982 and 1983 the pharmaceutical product with the largest volume of prescription sales in the United States was Inderal (propranolol).[19]

Because of the cardiovascular effects of this drug, a number of studies have been carried out to see if performance is affected. Wilmore has recently carried out a study in which he has shown that there is a definite decrease in performance in endurance athletes who are on these drugs. He has also shown that these drugs will have no adverse training effect on the untrained athlete during the training period.

These materials are now being used in the recreational field to reduce the anxiety associated with taking cocaine. It is reported anecdotally that they are being used as a new type of "Mickey Finn." In addition, they are said to be used at parties as a recreational drug.

Narcotic analgesics These materials have been taken by athletes in an attempt to improve performance. They do, of course, reduce pain and, as such, would help an injured athlete perform without pain. Unfortunately, over the years they have also been used in an attempt to improve performance. There is no evidence that such substances do improve performance, and they are banned by the medical commission of the IOC.[9] Marijuana has also been used by athletes but a recent study has shown that there is no competitive edge from the use of this material (J.H. Wilmore, personal communication, September 1984).

Anabolic steroids In 1954 while in Vienna during international competition, a physician with the American weightlifting team was first exposed to the concept of the use of anabolic steroids to improve muscle strength in athletics.[21] The concept of the use of these materials was by no means new, having first been used in the 1930s and reported to have been taken by German soldiers during World War II to increase aggressiveness. The substances have long been used in animal sciences to increase "the beef."[22] Initially, both the male and female hormones were used, but the use of diethystilbestrol has now been prohibited in animal husbandry. It is interesting that the male slaughterhouse animal is castrated (to minimize aggressiveness and to limit stud activity to selected bulls) and then given the male hormone to increase beef production. It was not long before the athletic population seized upon this effect on animals destined for the slaughterhouse. Their use by sportspersons (male and female) has grown to staggering proportions. It is now estimated that, for example, almost 100% of body builders take this material to improve muscle development. Initially, the medical profession reacted negatively to the use of this substance because of its serious health effects. It was not felt that these materials improved performance. While the issue of increased strength and performance is still controversial on a scientific basis, there appears to be little doubt among the users that these materials improve their performance.[23] The difficulties associated with producing sound scientific data in this area is based on the dangers associated with taking this material. This difficulty is compounded by vast amounts of this substance taken by athletes. There are few indications medically for the use of this drug, being confined largely today to its use in metastatic carcinoma, renal transplants and kidney failure. The athletes who use this material use up to 50 times the prescribed therapeutic use for this material. Scientific double-blind studies that use this amount of material cannot pass the human subject studies guidelines. Side effects of this material include interrupted growth, early maturation in children, possible birth defects in the unborn, reduced sperm count, and testicular atrophy with reduced blood levels of gonadotropins and testosterone in the adult male. It can result in sludging of the bile with cirrhosis and liver dysfunction. Recently reported in the press was the death of an athlete, who was taking large doses of this material, from liver cancer. The androgenic portion of the drug results in changes in the libido and increased aggressiveness. A case of a Wilms tumor is reported in the literature from an athlete who was taking this material.[24] Gynecomastia may also occur in the male from its use. Testosterone is being used in conjunction with the anabolic steroids and as a substitute for anabolic steroids prior to drug testing, and it unfortunately possesses the undesirable androgenic properties. The possible advantages to be gained from the use of this material are far outweighed by the health hazards. No reputable physician should prescribe this material to athletes. The Arizona State Board of Medical Examiners issued a policy statement on this material and declared that "the prescribing and dispensing of anabolic-androgenic steroids by a duly licensed physician to a normal healthy human being rather than for therapeutic purposes is unprofessional conduct." The American College of Sports Medicine has also taken a strong stand on the use of these materials.[25] (Unhappily, the athletes have not stopped at the use of anabolic steroids and are now resorting to the use of many other hormonal substances produced by the body such as human growth factor.)

It is to be emphasized once again that the IOC will continue to test for anabolic steroids at all international competitions. Universities in the United States are planning to test for this material in their varsity athletes. Random testing for anabolic steroids in training camps has been instituted in Europe. It would appear that the only way in which the medical profession can limit the use of this material is by institution of penalties, as attempts to stifle the use of this material through education is falling on deaf ears and blind eyes.

REFERENCES

1. Williams, M.H.: Ergogenic Aids in Sport. Champaign, Ill: Human Kinetics Publishers, 1983.
2. Gledhill, N.: The ergogenic effect of blood doping. *Phys Sportsmedicine* 1983; 11:87–90.
3. Epstein, SH: World records: Any limit? *Science* 1984;5:84.
4. Wilmore, J.H., and Freund, B.J.: Nutrition abstracts and reviews. *Rev Clin Nutri* 1984; 54(1):1–16.
5. Percy, E.C.: Chemical warfare: Drugs in sports. *West J Med* 133:478–484, 1980.
6. Prokop, L.: *The Problem of Doping*. Lausanne, Switzerland, International Olympic Committee Medical Commission, 1972.
7. Introduction: *Medical Guide*. International Olympic Committee, 1984, p 19.
8. Wilcox, A.R.: The effects of caffeine and exercise on body weight, fat-pad weight, and fat-cell size. *Med Sci Sports Exerc* 14(4):317–321, 1982.
9. *I.O.C. Medical Controls Brochure*. Los Angeles Organizing Committee: Games of the XXIIIrd Olympiad. Los Angeles, 1984.
10. American College of Sports Medicine: Position stand on weight loss in wrestlers. *Med Sci Sports* 8:11–13, 1976.
11. Croyle, P.H., Place, R.A., and Hilgenberg, A.D.: Massive pulmonary embolism in a high school wrestler. *JAMA* 241:827–828, 1979.
12. Wilkes, D., Gledhill, N., and Smyth, R. Effect of acute induced metabolic alkalosis on 800-m racing time. *Med Sci Sports Exerc* 15(4):277–280, 1983.
13. Gray, M.E., and Titlow, L.W.: B_{15}: Myth or miracle? *Physician Sportsmedicine* 10(1):107–112, 1982.
14. Gray, M.E., and Titlow, L.W.: The effect of pangamic acid on maximal treadmill performance. *Med Sci Sports Exerc* 14(6):424–427, 1983.
15. Maughan, R.J., and Sadler, D.J.M.: The effects of oral administration of salts of Aspartic acid on the metabolic response to prolonged exhausting exercise in man. *Int J Sportsmed* 4:119–123, 1983.
16. Wilkinson, I.M.S.: Disorders of eye movement. *Proc R Soc Med* 69:479–480, 1976.
17. American College of Sports Medicine: Position statement on the use of alcohol in sports. *Med Sci Sports* 1982;14:9–11.
18. Editorial: Beta-adrenergic blockade and anxiety. *Lancet* 611–612, 1976.
19. The top 200 prescription drugs of 1983. *American Druggist*, January, 1984, pp 42–43.
20. Steadward, R.D. and Singh, M.: The effect of smoking marijuana on physical performance. *Med Sci Sports* 7:309–311, 1975.
21. Todd, T.: The steroid predicament. *Sports Illustrated*, Aug 1, 1983, pp 62–77.
22. National Research Council Committee Report. Publication No. 1415. Washington, DC, 1966.
23. Lamb, D.R.: Anabolic steroids in athletics: How well do they work and how dangerous are they? *Am J Sports Med* 12(1):31–38, 1984.
24. Prat, J., Gray, G.F., Stolley, P.D., and Coleman, J.W.: Wilms tumor in an adult associated with androgenic abuse. *JAMA* 237(21): 2322–2323, 1977.
25. American College of Sports Medicine: Position statement on the use and abuse of anabolic-androgenic steroids in sports. *Sports Med Bull.* 13(1):1–3, 1978.

CHAPTER 23
Hyperthermia, Hypothermia, and Drowning

John S. Hayward, PhD

We take the stability of our body temperature for granted. Aside from occasional fever, we seldom consider and appreciate the importance of our regulated body temperature and the complex of sophisticated controls necessary to maintain this "homeothermy." Such indifference can be fatal to those participating in many athletic and recreational activities. Above-normal increases in body temperature (hyperthermia) can occur during competitive sports or recreation in warm, humid environments. Significant lowering of body temperature (hypothermia) is the major hazard accompanying being lost, injured, or fatigued during outdoor recreational pursuits in cold or cool-wet weather, and of accidental immersion in cold water. Death is imminent for those whose body temperature rises more than about 5°C or falls about 10°C. It is therefore necessary for those involved in athletic training or direction of outdoor recreational activities, to be fully aware of the problems of hyperthermia and hypothermia, and the preventive measures required to avoid these insidious, neglected killers of otherwise healthy persons. Because drowning has an important relationship to immersion hypothermia, this topic will also be considered here.

HYPERTHERMIA

There are many excellent reviews of the topic of hyperthermia in man. The intent of this presentation is to give a general overview of this problem and to put special emphasis on some of the misunderstandings that have led to tragic fatalities from heat stroke.

Mild hyperthermia is associated with all sustained muscular activities, even in cool weather. A rise of 1° to 2°C in body temperature can be observed while jogging, hiking, playing tennis, basketball, football, and so forth, and has no direct adverse effect. It is readily apparent that a problem with hyperthermia can arise if the extra heat production of vigorous athletic activity is not matched by extra heat loss from the body. It is this failure of adequate heat loss that leads to the higher levels of hyperthermia associated with heat exhaustion and heat stroke. Heat stroke is frequently lethal. It is accompanied by collapse and coma, and convulsions are common. These are the observable symptoms of dying cells, particularly brain cells (hence the term "stroke"). With inadequate blood flow to the brain and the direct effect of high temperature, enzymes are destroyed and cell membranes are disrupted, leading to fluid shifts (eg, brain edema) and electrolyte and excitability changes. Persistence of such conditions is rapidly irreversible, making resuscitation difficult.

The main emphasis of any treatment of this condition must be to explain the factors that contribute to inadequate heat loss from the body and how these must be recognized and avoided.

The "Will to Die" from Hyperthermia

Despite deliberate efforts to avoid it, a person can die from hyperthermia while producing minimum body heat if the environment is warmer than the body temperature, and evaporative cooling is limited by body dehydration (desert situation), or high ambient humidity (situation in moist tropics). However, to die from hyperthermia when the ambient temperature is significantly below body temperature requires a "will to die."

To reach a fatal level of hyperthermia when there is still some significant cooling capacity of the environment (by conduction, convection, and radiation, as well as evaporation), requires the body heat production to be maintained at an elevated level. Normally, this will be avoided by the condition of heat exhaustion, which is characterized by significant motor and mental impairment and tendency to collapse at a body temperature perhaps only 2° to 3°C above normal. By definition, therefore, such exhaustion would tend to stop the vigorous activity and its associated elevation of heat production at a lower, sublethal level of hyperthermia. Unfortunately, it is possible for a person to force himself mentally to continue activity beyond the safeguard of heat exhaustion. Such an inadvertent will to die is an understandable feature of competitive sports where coach, colleagues, and self-respect discourage "quitters," even if quitting is caused by a severe physiologic limitation. This phenomenon of heat death because of high motivation to continue activity despite physiologic rebellion has also been observed in military maneuvers in warm weather, and in industrial or mining activity in hot conditions. Recently, a young man died from hyperthermia while hiking in British Columbia (ambient temperatures about 30°C, bright sunshine, humidity unknown). The symptoms of heat exhaustion in the victim were misinterpreted as lack of motivation combined with the usual fatigue. His fellow hikers encouraged him so strongly to continue climbing that he willed himself onward to death.

This emphasizes the dilemma of those demanding high performance of themselves or others in situations where heat stress is likely. Pushing hard is desirable. Pushing too hard can be fatal. One must be aware of this common denominator of all types of exercise-induced heat death.

There are many circumstances where potentially lethal heat stress is encountered in athletic and recreational activities. The major considerations relate to adequacy of heat loss mechanisms of the body.

Factors Influencing Heat Loss

Ambient temperature and humidity Increased temperature and humidity of the environment, especially when combined with exposure to the sun and low wind speed, are obvious factors that will be most important in limiting heat loss. Even at fairly moderate temperatures of about 20°C, hyperthermia death can occur because of limitation of evaporative cooling if the humidity is high. At higher temperatures such as 30°C, heat deaths occur at lower relative humidities (eg, 50%) because of limitation of the conduction, convection, and radiation routes of heat loss. Surveys of heat stroke deaths in athletic activities such as American football, can be used to derive a graph (Figure 23-1) that provides guidelines as to the environmental conditions under which significant heat stress and heat stroke are potentiated for persons exercising vigorously. It is obvious that this graph must be adapted to other particular circumstances. For example, extra caution is required if the participants will be in full sunshine and if there is little wind to aid evaporative cooling.

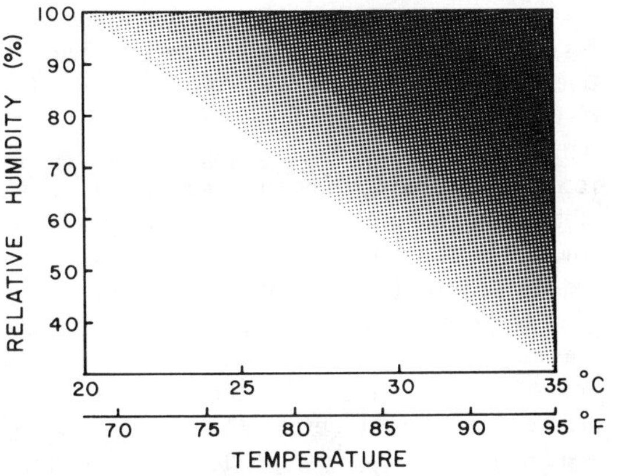

Figure 23-1 Approximate temperature-humidity relationship that potentiates serious hyperthermia during exercise. The shaded zone is that in which heat stroke fatalities have occurred in athletic activities. The darker the shading, the more likely that cases of heat exhaustion and heat stroke will occur.

It is also important to realize that it takes time to reach heat stroke levels of hyperthermia. Brief workouts at 30°C and 80% relative humidity can be safe. It is prolonged activity under these conditions that leads to fatalities. It is difficult to provide concise guidelines as to this third dimension (exercise duration) because of the large variation of exercise thermogenesis associated with different types of activities. It is sufficient to say that great caution should be applied to exercise under the temperature and humidity conditions that potentiate heat stroke. Keep workouts short and watch for the early signs of heat exhaustion in the most susceptible individuals (see later section). As many recommend, a sling psychrometer for obtaining temperature and humidity at the time and site of the vigorous physical activity is cheap insurance against the tragedy of hyperthermia.

Clothing Everyone understands that the major route of heat loss of exercising man is through the skin. Obviously, clothing impedes such heat loss by reducing radiation and convection from the skin, and by creating a microclimate of higher humidity near the skin, leading to less evaporative cooling and wasted sweating. Clothing that becomes saturated with sweat is relatively ineffective in providing heat loss, as is sweat that drops off the skin. Although the foregoing seems painfully obvious, it is surprising the number of recreationists and athletes who wear inappropriate clothing (tight-fitting, low permeability to air) without realizing the extent to which these can reduce the effectiveness of sweating. In awareness of this problem, many teams that must have players wear shirts over the important sweat loss area of the trunk, now make sure that these shirts are well ventilated and provide little barrier to outward diffusion of water vapor (eg, use of fish net fabric).

Other barriers to heat loss are various types of protective equipment (helmets, pads, etc) that must be worn by athletes. Football players working out in the warm, humid weather of the southern United States have been particularly susceptible to death from hyperthermia. Ice hockey players who wear similar gear and need to lose much body heat can thank the heat sink they skate on for sparing them deaths from heat stroke.

Individual differences in heat loss capacity This category of the factors that relate to probability of heat stroke is the least appreciated. It must be carefully emphasized that under similar environmental and work load conditions, some individuals in a team or group are significantly more likely to suffer heat exhaustion and proceed to heat stroke than are others. The three features of individuals that are most important in this respect are: body size and build, level of physical fitness (aerobic fitness), and level of acclimatization to exercise in the heat. Before analyzing the reason for these personal determinants of susceptibility, it is necessary briefly and simply to review the physiologic mechanisms of losing the extra heat that is produced during exercise.

The extra heat produced in working skeletal muscles and their back-up tissues such as heart, liver, and respiratory muscles must get to the skin for loss to the environment. Two methods interact: conduction outward through tissues along a gradient of temperature to the cooler skin (dependent on ambient temperature being below body temperature and/or evaporative cooling of the skin); and convection outward to the skin by blood circulation. With this understanding, the role of individual differences can be explained.

Effect of body size and build The farther heat is from the skin, the slower its rate of transport outward through tissues will be. The larger a person is, and the more bulky his trunk and limbs are, the greater the problem with heat loss. Consequently, under similar circumstances of temperature, clothing, and exercise, adults are more likely to become hyperthermic than children, and mesomorphs (well-muscled, stocky body build) and endomorphs (fat persons) are more susceptible to hyperthermia than equivalent body weight ectomorphs (tall, thin, lanky body build). The principle (exaggerated) is simple: large spheres cool more slowly than small rods. Actual evidence to support this factor as being important in potentiating heat stroke is the fact that among football players, death from heat stroke is restricted almost exclusively to interior linemen. These are typically large mesomorphs who lose their body heat less readily than the fleet pass receivers. A secondary consideration is that more heat is produced in moving a heavier body across a field or up a mountain.

Effect of physical fitness This factor relates mainly to the convection of heat to the skin via the circulatory system. Exercise in heat makes great demands on the circulatory system. The working muscles require a large increase in blood volume and flow rate. At the same time, blood flow to the skin must be greatly increased to convect the extra heat produced to the site for loss to the environment. This competition for blood volume and circulation rate between muscles and skin can easily require maximum circulatory capacity of individuals (eg, heart rates over 160 beats/min are common in heat exhaustion). An essential feature of physical fitness is that working muscles can better extract oxygen from the blood perfusing them, thereby necessitating a lower volume flow of blood and a lower heart rate than in the case of a less fit person. Therefore, the fit person has more circulatory capacity for convection of blood to the skin cooling site. Lower levels of fitness lead to inadequate circulation to both muscles and skin, the consequences of which are the fatigue and dizziness of heat exhaustion as well as higher levels of body temperature. Mesomorphs, for reasons previously explained, have to rely more on circulatory cooling then do ectomorphs. If mesomorphs are unfit as well, they are at high risk for hyperthermia.

Dehydration also has a role in generation of heat exhaustion and heat stroke. If the considerable amount of water that is lost in sweating is not adequately replaced by drinking, fluid compartments of the body will be reduced. This includes the blood volume. Obviously, this is a further insult to a circulatory system that is already near or over functional capacity. It is essential to maintain water balance during exercise in hot conditions so that blood volume and sweating capacity can be maintained. Unfortunately, it has been shown that the level of drinking by persons exercising in the heat does not match water loss, and there is a significant voluntary dehydration of the body (about 2% to 4% of the body weight) that accentuates circulatory strain. Therefore, during hyperthermic stress, persons should force themselves to drink somewhat more than seems to satisfy them. During prolonged exercise, this provides an opportunity to replace salts lost in sweat by adding small amounts of salt to the water. This avoids the heat cramp problem that occasionally is seen in conjunction with hyperthermia. Most are aware of the specially formulated drinks available for maintaining salt and water balance of athletes during exercise. Taking salt in tablets alone is not recommended. Heavier salting of food before and during exercise in the heat will usually suffice to avoid heat cramps. It should be mentioned here that there is one good aspect to heat cramps: such cramps will probably stop a person exercising, and thereby cancel the main heat source for hyperthermia. As emphasized earlier, it is possible in the absence of this disorder to keep exercising despite heat exhaustion symptoms, and slowly continue progress to fatal heat stroke.

Acclimatization to exercise in the heat After a period of approximately five days of exposure to hot environments, during which there are daily periods (2 to 4 hours) of work or exercise, an individual demonstrates significant increase in ability to lose body heat, and thereby reduce the chance of serious hyperthermia. Aside from some fitness benefit of this program, the major change involves increased sweating efficiency. During heat stress, sweating is initiated sooner, is better proportioned to the actual need for heat loss, and the sweat is more dilute (avoiding excessive salt loss). Also, control over the distribution of blood in the body is changed so that less blood is sent to the abdominal viscera during exercise in the heat, thereby easing the strain on circulation to muscles and skin.

In summary, it must be recognized that certain individuals are more susceptible to hyperthermia than others. Coaches and leaders of recreational activities must be aware of this fact and adjust their activities in hot conditions to the predicted weakest link in their group. Otherwise, they must be prepared to pay very careful attention to heat stress symptoms of individuals, especially those that combine any two of the three predisposing factors explained here. A tragic example will help to emphasize this point. Earlier in this chapter, the case of heat stroke death of a young man hiking on a mountain in British Columbia was mentioned. He was one of about ten hikers. After the incident, the question arose as to why this particular individual in the group should reach a fatal level of hyperthermia. None of the participants had significant acclimatization to the heat that was encountered on that warm day in early summer. However, the victim exhibited more than any other person in the group the combination of large body build (well-muscled, weight 90 kg, favorite sport was football) and low level of aerobic fitness (based on very poor performance in morning jogs on two days before the hike).

Other factors that can predispose to hyperthermia problems are: illness, especially fever or gastrointestinal disorders; lack of sleep (fatigue); alcohol intoxication; use of certain drugs (amphetamine); and old age (lower circulatory capacity).

Symptoms and Treatment of Serious Hyperthermia

The previous coverage has been on prevention of serious levels of hyperthermia in sports and recreation. It is necessary to give some information on symptoms and treatment of hyperthermic disorders in the event that precautions have failed. There are many references that document the behavioral symptoms of heat exhaustion. These include many ways of describing impaired motor performance and mental acuity. General symptoms are extreme fatigue, dizziness, and lethargy. Obviously, a leader who is aware beforehand of the possibility of hyperthermia will interpret such symptoms as those of the circulatory crisis of significant hyperthermia. Insistence on prolonged rest out of the heat is the simple therapy for this exhaustion phase of hyperthermia. Others may easily make the mistake of deciding these symptoms are those indicating fatigue per se and inadequate motivation, and implore the victim to try harder to carry on. At this stage, the body temperature is often near 39°C (about 102°F), and a rise of another 2 to 3 degrees is all that separates the average person from potential heat stroke. There is no need to make decisions based on guesswork. If in doubt, an oral thermometer will verify whether the symptoms really are those of hyperthermia. If the victim is at all irrational or violent, so that it is difficult to take oral temperature, rectal temperature may be safer, especially if an electronic thermometer is used. Unless dealing with highly trained athletes such as marathon runners, who are acclimatized to hyperthermia, a temperature over 39°C should prompt immediate rest and cooling of the victim. One other behavioral symptom of hyperthermia that can be useful to help distinguish this type of exhaustion is hyperventilation during rest. It has been shown experimentally that at body temperatures just over 39°C, persons will begin to pant like a dog. Although hyperventilation is a symptom of many stresses, in this situation it is probably driven by an ancestral reflex to increase evaporative heat from the respiratory tract (panting) at a time when normal heat loss by sweating is inadequate.

If exercise, heat production, and exposure to a hot or warm/humid environment continue because of high motivational circumstances as described earlier, then heat stroke is imminent. Body temperature may continue to rise rapidly or slowly. The most famous situation is the rapid rise associated with cessation of sweating due to dehydration and sweat gland fatigue. The skin feels hot and dry. However, it must be realized that total failure of sweat production is not a prerequisite to the heat stroke level of hyperthermia. This level can be reached more slowly while sweating continues if the amount or effectiveness (must evaporate from skin) of that sweating is inadequate to meet the demand for heat loss. In fact, the majority of victims treated for heat stroke in the hospital are still sweating. This point can be further illustrated by the example of the hiking incident described previously. After forcing himself to continue climbing despite symptoms of heat exhaustion (including hyperventilation), and being given some water to drink along with some salt, he sweated continuously until he collapsed into delirium and convulsions about one hour later. The point is, the dry skin symptom is not a reliable criterion to signal a heat stroke situation. One final insight can be gained from this tragic example. During all phases of the hike, the victim took frequent, short rests. It is probably valid that in his case, each rest was long enough to reduce exhaustion or fatigue so that he could climb again, but not long enough to provide anything but brief plateaus in the inexorable rise of his body temperature to the fatal level. The lesson here is to provide longer than usual rest periods during work or exercise in the heat, and to use this time for drinking as much as possible. To help illustrate how the heat stroke level of hyperthermia can be reached either rapidly or slowly, Figure 23-2 presents two hypothetical curves for body temperature change in comparison to that of a person who is able to avoid serious hyperthermia.

Unfortunately, there is no pain associated with core hyperthermia, or any discrete neural information that rises to the conscious level to warn a person of impending heat stroke. One must depend on circumstantial evidence unless a thermometer is available.

Treatment of heat stroke concentrates on increasing heat loss from the body. Heat production is already minimized by the comatose state. Victims must be transferred to a cool, shaded location and all possible means of extra skin-cooling utilized. This includes immersion in cold water or application of ice packs, water, or alcohol to the skin combined with fanning. Give special attention to extra cooling of the head, neck, and chest. Have the victim breathe air that is as cold as possible. Elevation of the arms and legs will help to increase central blood volume. Watch for vomiting so that the airway can be kept clear. Be prepared for cardiopulmonary resuscitation. In all cases of heat stroke, the victim should be taken to the hospital for more intensive care. Unfortunately, it takes time to reverse the trend of increasing body temperature, such that brain damage or death can easily occur. The near-fatal level of hyperthermia is very unforgiving. Irreversible changes are occurring in basic cell function. This is in contrast to near-fatal *hypo*thermia in which tissues are temporarily "refrigerated" and successful resuscitation is facilitated.

In conclusion, hyperthermia can impair performance during athletic and other physical activities, and if not respected, can kill. Due attention to environmental conditions, clothing characteristics, individual differences in susceptibility, and the early symptoms of heat stress should prevent the need ever to have to attempt treatment of the life-threatening stages of hyperthermia.

HYPOTHERMIA

Other than during the warm months of summer, hypothermia is the major life-threatening factor associated with outdoor sporting or recreational activities on land or water. Examples of such activities would include hiking, mountaineering, cross-country and down-hill skiing, snowshoeing, snowmobiling, hunting, sailing, canoeing, kayaking, rowing, and fishing. To avoid death from hypothermia, it is necessary to be familiar with the basic physiology of hypothermia and factors that influence body cooling rate.

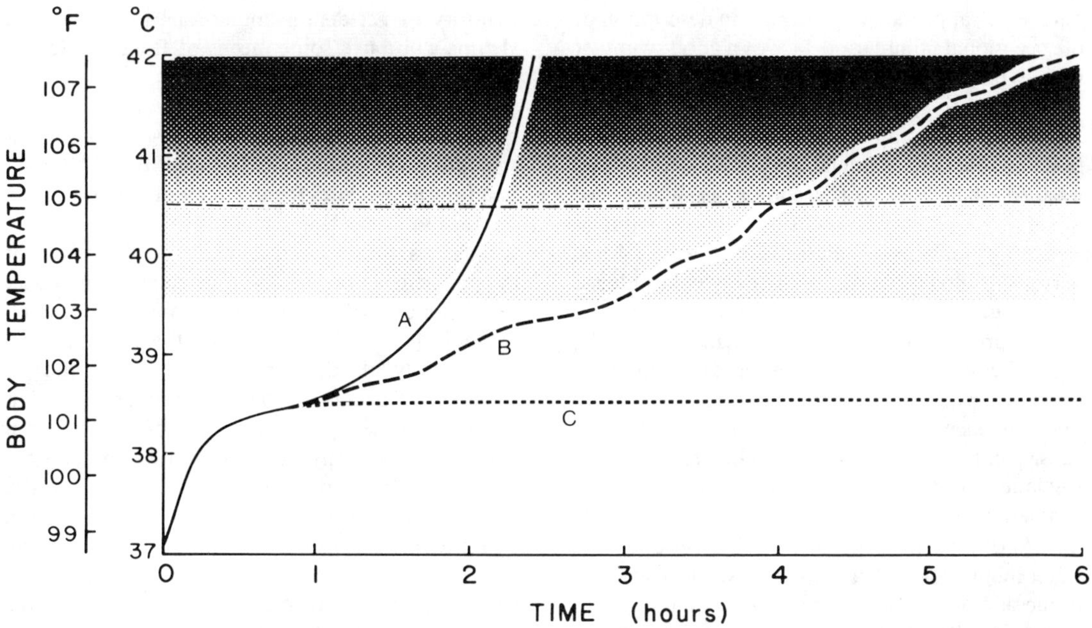

Figure 23-2 Three hypothetical examples of body temperature change during vigorous exercise in a heat stress environment (eg, 30°C, 65% relative humdity). The temperature range of 39.5° to 40.5°C (shaded) potentiates heat exhaustion symptoms. Temperatures beyond about 40.5°C (increasing density of shading) are those which frequently cause heat stroke. Body temperature typically rises 1 to 1.5°C for all individuals early in the exercise period. The longer-term progress of body temperature depends on the effectiveness of heat loss mechanisms. Line A is typical of failure of the sweating mechanism due to dehydration and/or blockage of sweat evaporation by clothing or protective gear. Line B represents the situation where hydration and sweating are maintained, but are inadequate to balance heat production in an unfit mesomorphic person, unacclimatized to work in the heat. Increase in temperature only slows during brief rest periods. Line C represents the temperature profile of a person with good tolerance to work in the heat (hydration and sweating maintained, good aerobic fitness, average body size and fatness, acclimatized to work in the heat).

Hypothermia from Cold Water Immersion

We all have some anxiety or fear of water that is evidenced during dangerous boating excursions. That anxiety is based on childhood warnings related mainly to avoidance of drowning during swimming in warm water. However, when the water is cold (below about 15°C), swimming is not a common activity, but boating is. In this case, drowning is a problem that is easily solved by wearing a personal flotation device (PFD). The diversity of PFDs, boats with mandatory inherent flotation, and the wide teaching of survival swimming techniques (drownproofing) make it inexcusable to drown if one is engaged in boating activities. On the other hand, hypothermia resulting from accidental immersion in cold water is not easily solved, and therefore deserves the careful attention of those at risk.

Cold water can kill in several ways. These can be categorized and explained under the topics of short-term and long-term immersion.

Short-term cold water immersion The sudden and drastic cooling of the skin that accompanies initial immersion in cold water causes certain shock responses involving the respiratory and circulatory systems. Central blood pressure can rise rapidly due to simultaneous peripheral vasoconstriction and alarm-induced increase of heart rate. Those with weak circulatory systems (such as the elderly) are susceptible to heart failure at this time. Another initial response is hyperventilation. The first few seconds of immersion are accompanied by huge gasps, and followed by several minutes of significant increase in ventilation rate. This involuntary response makes it possible that if one plunges totally underwater, or is in rough water with waves breaking over the head (even while wearing a PFD), hyperventilation could lead to unintentional aspiration of water followed by drowning. Some authorities have termed this the "sudden disappearance syndrome" in description of the occasional failure to surface of a good swimmer who is not wearing a PFD after diving into cold water.

A further complication of hyperventilation is that it reduces circulating CO_2 levels and leads to alkalosis. This is accompanied by reduced blood flow to the brain, resulting in fainting and increased probability of aspiration of water. Most persons do not succumb to this early cold-induced drowning, but the problem is so significant that special precautions should be taken. If possible, enter the water gradually. Never dive into cold water even if it is deep. Consciously control breathing as much as possible during entry and the subsequent minute or so. The more clothing and insulation being worn, the less the initial hyperventilation response will be.

Another aspect of the early response to cold water immersion is that the strong vasoconstriction of the skin, arms and legs leads to the establishment of a cold outer shell of the body compared to the warmer core. This is an important means of tissue insulation of the body, but can hasten death in certain circumstances. That is, cooling of muscles and nerves of the limbs and outer trunk produces slower and weaker movements with less coordination. If a person is not wearing a PFD or holding on to some floating object, the ability to swim or tread water is greatly impaired, so that even good swimmers drown more quickly than expected. This tendency increases with the coldness of the water, and instances where swimming failed within ten minutes are common in water below 5°C.

One other way in which cold water increases the likelihood of death during the early phase of accidental immersion is the following. Occasionally, capsized boats, helicopters, airplanes, or submerged automobiles will trap a person inside. Escape may involve a short swim underwater, requiring a modest period of breath-holding. Recent findings have shown that the breath-holding capacity of persons submerged in cold water is greatly reduced compared to that in the warmer water in which one usually swims. In 10°C water, average breath-holding duration is only about 20 seconds, and greatly complicates successful escape.

It should be recognized that these explanations of how cold water can kill in the early phase of an immersion incident do not involve death from hypothermia of the core of the body, but from ventilatory, circulatory, and neuromuscular effects of hypothermia of the periphery.

Long-term cold water immersion In the vast majority of accidental immersions in cold water, victims who have some means of flotation do not die from the short-term problems just outlined. Instead, they are at risk of a slower death. By 10 to 15 minutes of immersion, shivering begins to be conspicuous and continuous. The victim feels "lousy," and fully appreciates the dilemma of cold water immersion in a way that cannot be appreciated while sitting in a warm room reading this discussion of the problem. If the person is rescued at this stage, he or she often feels "I couldn't have lasted much longer." This is a reflection of the fact that one feels nearly dead, and looks nearly dead to observers. This has led to the false assumption that one dies from hypothermia after only minutes in cold water. Actually, it takes 15 to 20 minutes for the core of the body to begin to cool consistently.

Typical experimental results on immersion hypothermia Figure 23-3 provides actual mean data on major responses of ten, nonexercising, seminude, male subjects in 10°C water, followed by rewarming in a bath.

Within 5 to 10 minutes, the skin temperature is down to near water temperature and metabolic rate (heat production) has gone through an elevated shock response and settled down to a level about twice that of preimmersion. After 15 to 20 minutes, core temperatures (as measured at the rectal and tympanic sites) begin to fall consistently. Shivering metabolic rate increases in proportion to the core cooling. When the core temperature reaches 34° to 35°C, maximum levels of shivering are attained that are equivalent to a heat production four to five times that of preimmersion rest. However, all this shivering heat production fails to halt progress into hypothermia. The subject is in a personal "energy crisis." The amount of the body's heat production is suitable to match heat loss in cold air, but not in cold water. Accompanying physiologic changes during cooling that are not shown in Figure 23-3 include elevation of heart rate to as much as 140 to 150 beats/min, high blood levels of noradrenaline, and increase in urine production to about four times normal. Mentally, experimental subjects begin to perceive early stages of impairment of function when cooled to 34° to 35°C. For example, they have lessened ability to maintain a logical sequence of ideas. This effect could account for tales of strange and inappropriate behavior by victims waiting for rescue. The rewarming phase of the data shown in Figure 23-3 is accompanied by cessation of shivering when the skin temperature rises to normal levels despite afterdrop of the core temperatures. Ten to fifteen minutes after entering

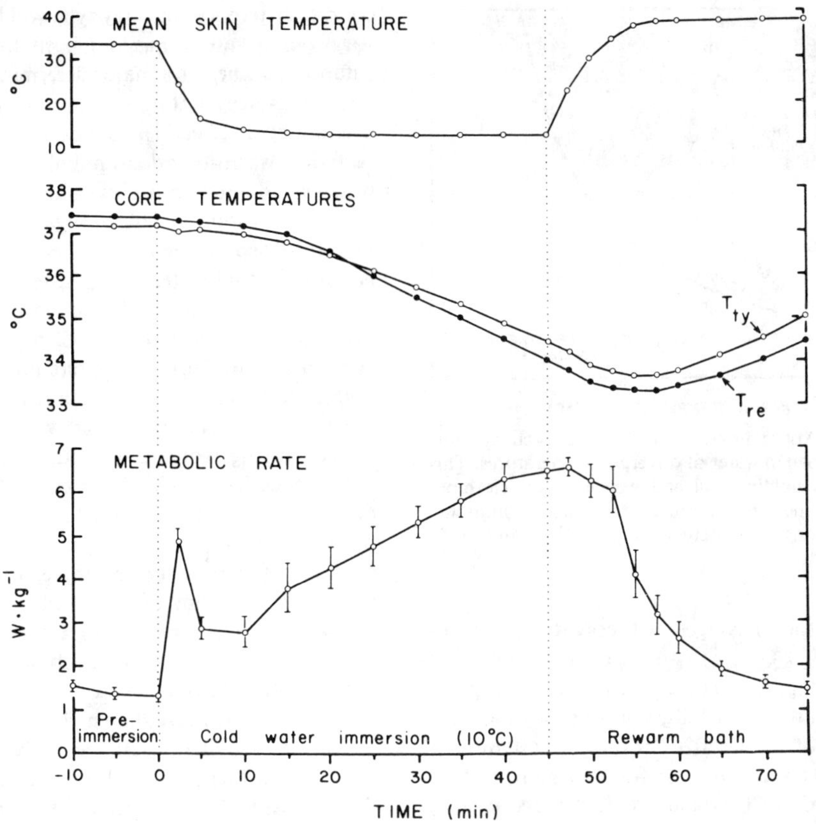

Figure 23-3 Relationship of skin and core temperatures (rectal and tympanic) to metabolic heat production during cooling and rewarming. Subjects were not exercising and wore only bathing trunks. Metabolic rate above rest level is solely from shivering.

the warm bath, the subject feels good, even while having his or her lowest ever core temperature. This illustrates that one can feel a cold skin, but not a cold core. This will have relevance in a later section where it will be shown that how one feels and how one cools can be two different things.

It is interesting to note that hypothermia rarely has any sublethal effects. That is, if one is rewarmed efficiently, there are no residual problems other than fatigue and some muscle soreness from shivering.

Cooling rate and survival time Figure 23-4 provides a generalized scheme for the process of entry into deeper levels of hypothermia. When core temperature falls to near 30°C (severe hypothermia), unconsciousness can occur. It is impossible to give a precise temperature for such a change because there is a great deal of individual variation in this respect according to accident records. At this stage, victims can easily drown due to hypothermia if they cannot keep waves from splashing water into

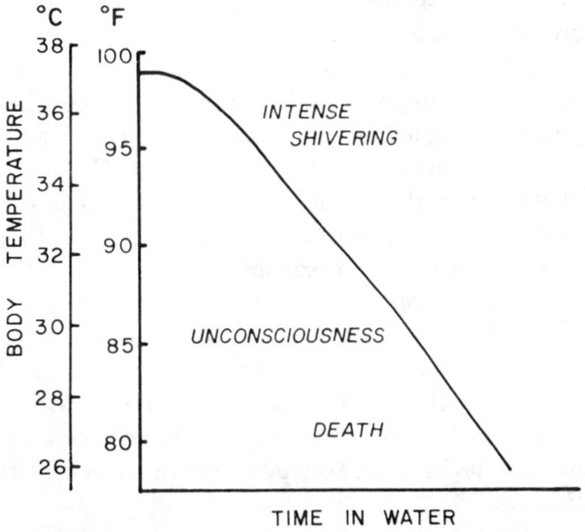

Figure 23-4 Generalized curve for body cooling during hypothermia, showing approximate temperatures of unconsciousness and potential death.

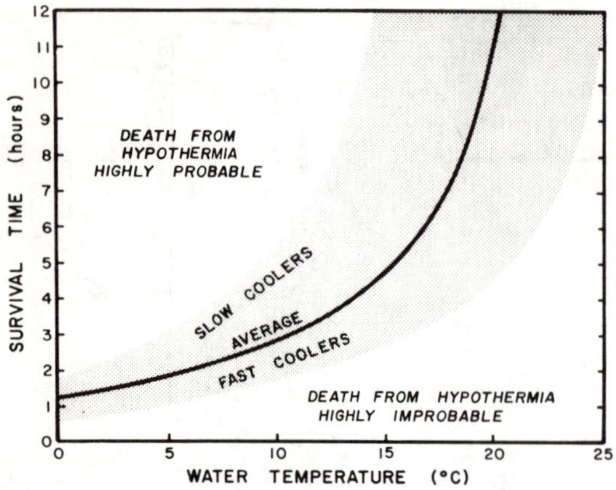

Figure 23-5 Approximate mean curve for predicted survival time of man in water of different temperatures. This is for persons holding still and wearing light clothing. Shaded zones indicate the range of variation commonly seen for persons of different fatness, size, and body build.

their respiratory passages. At core temperatures below about 30°C, the rhythmic contraction of the heart is in jeopardy. There is no precise temperature at which the heart fails, but it usually happens in the range of 25° to 30°C. If one was attempting to calculate a survival time for a person, a core temperature of 30°C would provide an acceptable, conservative estimation of a probable end-point for function of the circulatory system. "Death" of a hypothermia victim is hard to define.

Based on several studies, it is known that cooling rate into severe hypothermia is fairly linear, and is inversely proportional to water temperature. A graph that relates predicted survival time (according to the 30°C core temperature criterion outlined above) to water temperature is shown in Figure 23-5. The graph is for average men and women who are holding still while wearing a standard life jacket and light clothing. The graph shows, for example, that estimated survival time in 10°C water is about two and one-half to three hours. It is not until water temperature is greater than 15°C that there begins to be a reasonable amount of time for search and rescue. Since a great deal of recreational and commercial boating is done on waters at or below this temperature (especially in spring and fall), the risk of hypothermic death is obvious. As a rule of thumb, if you do not see people swimming at the beaches, you are in a hypothermia alert situation.

Individual variation in cooling rate and survival time Figure 23-5 estimates survival times for average or standard adult men and women. Of course, differences in body type will be expected to vary cooling rate. It has long been known that subcutaneous fatness is a major determinant of cooling rate differences among humans. It could be called the "blubber effect" in acknowledgement of the fact that warm-blooded animals (such as whales) who are adapted to life in cold water use this insulative method of defense against hypothermia. For most aspects of human health, extra fat is a liability; in cold water it is an asset. Cooling rate is decreased from the low blood flow to fat, thereby providing more insulative shell to the body. This attribute is an important prerequisite to being a long-distance (eg, English Channel) swimmer. It is largely responsible for the cold water exploits of the Korean diving women. Various studies in Britain and France have yielded the generalization that a doubling of skinfold thickness (the common measure of subcutaneous fatness) doubles predicted survival time. For example, at 10°C, survival time may vary from about one hour for a very lean person with only 4 mm average skinfold thickness, up to about six hours for an obese person with an average skinfold thickness of 20 mm.

It has also been shown that, besides fatness, the size and bulkiness of the body are important variables influencing cooling rate in cold water. The operative factor here is the surface-to-volume ratio. The surface of the body loses heat, and the volume (or mass) produces and stores heat. Therefore, large, heavy-set people cool more slowly than small, thin people, even if their subcutaneous fatness is the same. The feature that was a disadvantage in hyperthermia, becomes an advantage in hypothermia. Based on this knowledge, one can make educated guesses about the cooling rates of different people. Obviously, children will cool most quickly because of their small, thin, low-fat bodies. Women, because they commonly have more fat under their skin than men, would tend to last longer in cold water. However, on the average, this advantage is offset by their significantly smaller body size, so they frequently cool somewhat faster than men.

In summary, it is clear that body size and fatness are important factors. However, we should recognize that these are factors that we can do very little to alter (except degree of fatness).

Influence of alcohol on cooling rate There is ample evidence that consumption of alcoholic beverages is a frequent and pleasant accompaniment to many activities near water (eg, recreational boating). In the majority of instances, the level of intoxication is minimal. Occasionally, persons may reach a legal level of impairment such as 0.08 gm of alcohol per 100 ml of blood. It is important to know what effect, if any, this level of intoxication may have on the rate of progress into hypothermia during prolonged immersion in cold water. It has been known for some time that moderate doses of alcohol, consumed under normal environmental conditions, can cause peripheral dilation of blood vessels and slight lowering of body temperature. However, recent studies from three different laboratories have shown that alcohol intoxication of the moderate level does not significantly effect rate of progress into core hypothermia. There is a slight cooling before entering cold water, but it seems that the stimulus of the cold water overwhelms the mild anesthesia of intoxication to this degree, so that the normal defense mechanisms of peripheral vasoconstriction and muscular shivering are still sufficiently operative. Obviously, some higher level of intoxication, to the point of stupor, would affect these defense mechanisms and result in a faster cooling rate.

It has been shown that the combination of alcohol intoxication and fatigue (caused by vigorous exercise) does increase cooling rate. This latter point is not very relevant to most recreational boating, but could be important for competitive athletic events near cold water, or for many situations where fatigue is a factor facilitating hypothermia in land-based activities.

The failure of alcohol to increase cooling rate in cold water should not be viewed as an endorsement of drinking while boating. It has been noted that about 40% of boating fatalities involve significant alcohol impairment.

We can conclude at this point that the basic, involuntary thermoregulatory controls of the human body are inadequate to meet the unusual challenge of accidental immersion in cold water.

Practical Advice on Cold Water Safety

As is usual for humans faced with a problem, voluntary action can be applied to man's functional incompetence in cold water. Man's success and dominance is related to his ability to innovate behaviors and technologic devices that extend his functional capacities. This familiar axiom also applies to the problem of body-heat loss in cold water. For the situation where man deliberately enters cold water (eg, scuba diving), very excellent technologic devices (wet-suits and dry-suits) have been developed. The last few years have seen the importance of accidental immersion in cold water more widely recognized, with resultant development of behavioral and technologic advances to reduce the severity of this hazard. Therefore, unlike the situation for body-type attributes discussed earlier, this section will concentrate on factors affecting rate of progress into core hypothermia that are subject to decision making, and that permit constructive action to gain a measure of insurance against this form of accidental death.

To swim or not to swim From experience in cold air, we know that the extra heat produced by physical activity helps maintain body temperature. Is this true for cold water immersion? Can we power our way out of the problem through muscular activities that yield heat production several times greater than that of shivering? No. Activity such as swimming (while wearing a PFD) increases cooling rate by approximately 35%. This seems paradoxical, but emphasizes that physical activity increases heat loss more than it increases heat production. This occurs in two ways. Physical activity increases water movement through the clothes, thereby decreasing any insulative effect they may provide. More importantly, activity stimulates blood circulation to the peripheral muscles including those of the arms and legs. This largely destroys the insulation effect of having a cool, vasoconstricted shell of tissues between the warm core and the cold water. Figure 23-6 illustrates this point by use of thermography. These pictures of infrared radiation from the body permit visualization of the relative surface temperatures. The whiter the image is, the warmer the temperature. Black regions are coldest. Using examples concentrating on the upper body, which is the main area of concern (the head is usually out of the water), these thermograms dramatically show the differences in surface temperature (and therefore heat loss) for a) preimmersion, warm conditions, b) after cold water immersion while holding still, and c) swimming. Preimmersion surface has a fairly uniform temperature, warmest in the axillary regions. Holding still in cold water shows much cold surface and therefore underlying cool shell. The highest heat loss areas are lateral chest, groin, neck (probably out of the water), and a portion of the central chest. These are areas with a thin shell to guard against heat loss from the warm core. For example, at the lateral thorax, there is only the thin rib cage with very little fat or vasoconstricted

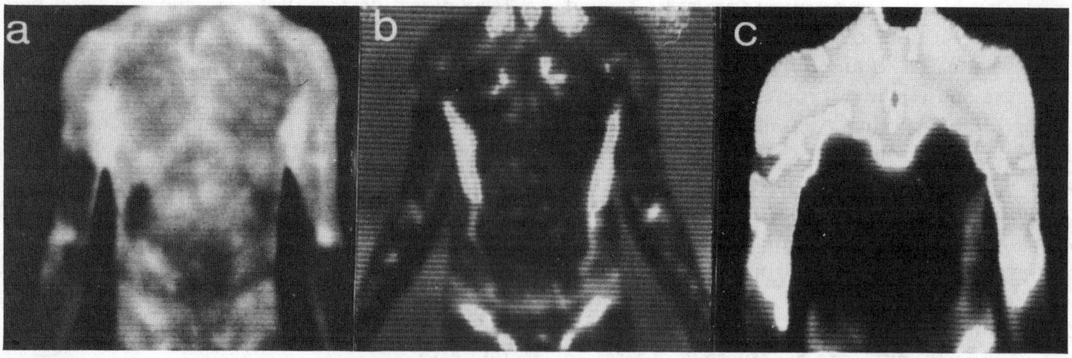

Figure 23-6 Infrared thermograms showing surface temperature distributions of the trunk of male subjects (a) before immersion in water at 7.5°C, (b) after immersion for 15 minutes while holding still, or (c) swimming.

muscle overlying the region. In contrast to this situation, swimming (c), produces much more warm skin over active muscles. Because of more skin that is warm while swimming, one does not feel so cold, but cooling is faster, and death sooner. This is an example that in some cases, how one feels and how one cools can be two different matters.

Advice to avoid prolonged physical activity in cold water must be modified to allow swimming to shore, to a boat, etc, if it is close enough. Should one head for shore or not? The only data available on this question are for eight persons in 9°C water who swam in light clothing while wearing PFDs. They did various strokes to avoid rapid fatigue. Water current and waves were minimal. At the speed they travelled (averaging about 20 m/min), and with the faster rate of cooling of their bodies, it was calculated that they would be incapacitated after a distance just over 1 km. More studies certainly need to be conducted on this issue, involving different water temperatures and conditions, as well as clothing variations. The present data emphasize that being a good swimmer is no insurance against hypothermia, and that the risk of hypothermic death becomes suddenly more compelling once one passes some distance from shore.

Thus it is clear that the means to slow cooling in cold water is not through voluntary methods of extra heat production by the body. Even technologic devices for providing heat are unsuitable because of extremely high cost:benefit ratios that are acceptable only for specialized military use. Consequently, practical advice on cold water survival must concentrate on insulative mechanisms for reduction of heat loss to the cold water.

The dilemma of not wearing a PFD Recent statistics in the United States show that only a small percentage of recreational boaters routinely wear their PFDs while boating. When sudden immersion occurs and no flotation is available, one is forced to adopt antidrowning behaviors (Figure 23-7).

Treading water involves continuous movement of arms and legs in various patterns to keep

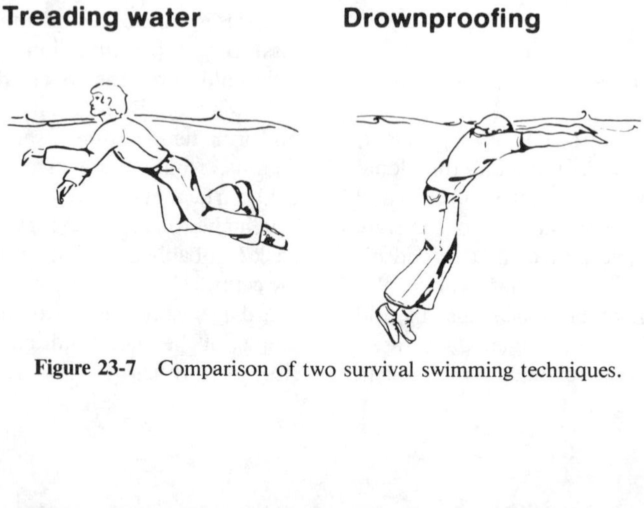

Figure 23-7 Comparison of two survival swimming techniques.

the head out of the water. Test results have shown the average cooling rate of subjects treading water to be about one-third faster than while holding still in a PFD. Besides this faster cooling rate, most people fatigue fairly rapidly while treading water. For this reason, the most effective survival swimming technique (drownproofing) involves restful floating with lungs full of air, interrupted every 10 to 15 seconds for raising the head out of the water to take another breath. By this procedure, even nonswimmers can avoid drowning for many hours in warm water. Unfortunately, this behavior results in a body cooling rate in cold water that is about 80% faster than while holding still in a PFD. This is mostly because of putting another high heat-loss area (the head) into the water along with the rest of the body. Research has shown drownproofing to be the fastest way to die from immersion hypothermia of any behavior studied to date. Therefore, since the best survival swimming technique is so inappropriate for cold water survival, there is a powerful incentive for boaters and others near cold water always to wear a PFD. Drownproofing is a highly valuable technique to include in one's arsenal of water safety methods, but it should be restricted in its use to swimming incidents in warm water.

Strategic behaviors to reduce cooling rate If a person is floating in cold water and waiting for rescue, certain behaviors can be used to reduce heat escape from the body and prolong survival. These involve adopting postures that take advantage of the information previously shown in Figure 23-6B. A Heat Escape Lessening Posture (HELP), as shown in Figure 23-8, can be deliberately adopted. It attempts to reduce the area of exposed body surface, especially of the more critical regions of the lateral chest and the groin. The inner sides of the arms are held in contact with the sides of the chest, and the thighs are pressed together and raised to reduce exposure of the groin area. Experimental results have shown the HELP to provide approximately a 45% increase in predicted survival time over the situation of not curling up in this fetal position. In some types of more wearable PFDs (with less bulky flotation high over the chest and around the neck), raising the thighs can result in flotation instability while doing HELP, in which cases it is best to leave the legs down but held together as much as possible. Some loss of protection to the groin area is not as important as loss of protection around the chest.

Another strategy that may have application in some circumstances is huddling (Figure 23-8). It is obvious that body contact between two or more individuals will reduce the heat loss of each. In experiments where three persons huddled in such a way as to get close apposition of their lateral chest regions, predicted survival time was extended by nearly 50%. In these experiments, the kapok PFDs used had to be tied on backwards in order to expose the chests for contact. Since this is not a recommended general procedure, huddling may only be appropriate if people are not wearing PFDs (unfortunately), and are hanging on to floating wreckage or partially submerged boat. Even with PFDs worn, it may be worthwhile for a group to huddle in some way to attempt reduction of individual cooling rates, especially if a child is present.

It is important to understand that under some particular circumstances of water conditions or types of PFDs, utilization of one or other of these strategies may not be possible. The main purpose of presenting these ideas is to document *principles* regarding behavioral modifications for thermal protection in cold water. With such principles appreciated, immersion victims will be able to max-

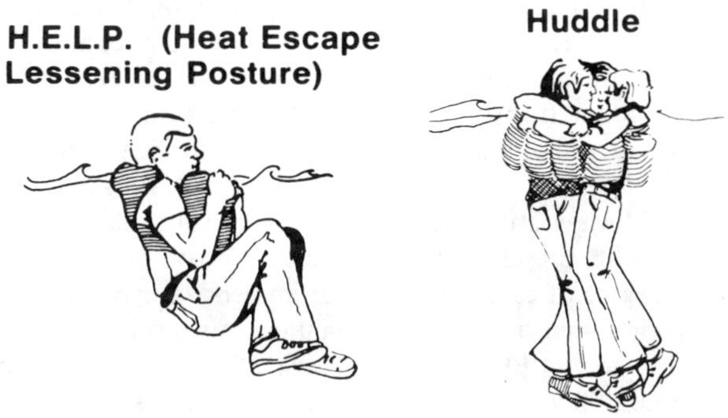

Figure 23-8 Two thermally-protective behaviors during cold water immersion.

imize application of this knowledge to the circumstances of their particular predicament.

The effect of different clothing The fundamental purpose of clothing is insulation in air, not water. The principle is familiar that the more layers of clothing, and air trapped within, the higher the insulation. Clothing reduces convection of air through the materials, while conduction of heat outwards through the air is slight. When a person is immersed in cold water, the benefits of types and arrangements of clothing for cold air are greatly reduced for two reasons. First, due to the high heat capacity of water, even a small amount of convection of water through the clothing can carry away a great deal of body heat. Second, since air spaces among the layers of clothing and fibers of wool will soon be replaced by water, rapid conduction of heat out through the water-filled clothing is impeded very little. For these reasons, experiments that have attempted to quantify the benefit provided by various types of heavy winter clothing show increases in predicted survival time over light clothing that are in the range of only 30% to 40%. This is less than would be desired, but is still worthwhile. Consequently, persons who have the opportunity to foresee the need to abandon ship, and decide there is no use trying to swim to shore, would be well advised to add all the clothes they can if time is available. Wrap towels around the neck, and stuff them inside clothing. Try to reduce access of water at wrists and ankles. Put on any rain gear available. Wrap a blanket around the trunk. In summary, use ingenuity to stabilize water around one as much as possible. The usual habit of taking off shoes and some clothes before entering water is pertinent to *swimming* somewhere. In such a case, clothes and shoes slow one down by their resistance in water. Swimming rapidly is usually not a necessity in cold water immersion accidents. Also, clothes and shoes that feel heavy in air (especially if wet) are not heavy in water.

The only clothing material that can possibly give reasonably effective thermal protection is that which traps air that cannot be displaced by water when submerged. Closed-cell foam (rubber and synthetic) is the most effective material of this type.

Cooling rate in different PFDs It is understandable that in the case of cold water immersion, a PFD cannot really be called a life preserver or a life jacket unless it has some degree of capacity to protect a wearer against hypothermia as well as drowning. The properties of a good PFD are as follows: highly acceptable wearability (storage in the bow of the boat is not acceptable); good flotation characteristics (amount and face-up stability); and preferably some special feature(s) for visibility, but not to the extent that wearability is impaired. To become a life jacket the PFD must provide some heat insulation for the wearer by reducing convective and conductive heat loss to the water. It has been shown that most types of PFDs provide insigificant thermal protection because of high flux of water between it and the wearer. The water comes in neck and arm openings and up from the bottom, despite various ties, belts, and snaps. Vest PFDs that do provide some thermal protection in the water are those that are made of foam, and that can be adjusted to fit snugly to the chest. These usually involve adjustable laces or straps at the side, and a front zipper. With a thickness of closed-cell foam closely applied to parts of the chest, it has been shown that such a PFD can provide about a 40% to 45% increase in predicted survival time.

A further improvement in thermal protection is provided by various flotation jackets or float coats. These are garments that look like ordinary parkas or windbreakers, and are suitable for general wear in cool wet weather. Buoyant and insulative foam extends throughout the body and sleeve portions of the jacket. Therefore, it is like wearing a hidden top of a wet suit except that it is not closely fitted to the body. With sleeves, less water gains access to the trunk of the body, and it has been shown that such jackets yield about a 50% to 75% increase in predicted survival time. Another strong feature of such jackets is that when the water is cold, the air above it is cool as well, so that a jacket has to be worn anyway unless the person is very active. A wearable jacket for cold air that also provides flotation and some thermal protection in the event of sudden accidental immersion is of obvious practical benefit for boating in seasons other than summer. On this account, there has recently been production of specially modified flotation jackets that attempt to improve hypothermia protection features by means of extra foam and convertible features for reducing water access. For two such jackets, it has been shown that thermal protection is improved to the extent that predicted survival time is about two and one-half times that of a person in a noninsulated PFD.

Survival suits for cold water immersion The most effective technologic solution to the problem of immersion hypothermia is the use of survival or antiexposure suits. These are full-body garments, most of which are available only to military and commercial personnel because of high cost and low wearability. Certain types, such as those that look like ordinary coveralls, can be used in sports and recreation, particularly for groups such as offshore sailors. These coverall suits can improve predicted survival time in cold water to four to five times that of an unprotected person. More extensive information of the design concepts and performances of survival suits is available from the author, but is not warranted for inclusion here.

Minimizing the amount of body immersed In all but the most extremely cold, windy conditions, the more of the body out of the water, the lower will be the core cooling rate. For this reason, every opportunity should be taken to exit the water onto some floating object such as a piece of wreckage, log, or protruding bow of the boat. In this respect, new construction regulations for level flotation of boats that are swamped or holed may permit occupants to sit on the partially submerged boat so as to keep their upper bodies well out of the water and thereby significantly retard hypothermia.

Summary

Recreational and sporting activities that occur on or near cold water require that the participants understand that the coldness of the water can kill. Education in the concepts of cold-water safety is necessary as an incentive to learn and obey safe boating practices. Also, when the inevitable accidents do occur, such education will help to minimize the lethality of cold water immersion.

HYPOTHERMIA IN AIR

The problem of cold is frequently encountered in outdoor activities and is familiar to everyone. Many books, articles, manuals, and films warn of the danger of hypothermia in a survival situation. The purpose here is not to repeat these in detail, but to emphasize the principles involved. These can then be adapted to any particular situation in sports or recreation.

The basic thermoregulatory responses of the body to hypothermia in air are similar to those already described for cold water immersion. However, there is one major difference that needs to be emphasized, and that necessitates different strategies for survival. The difference is that the extra heat production that accompanies voluntary physical activity in air can be beneficial in avoiding hypothermia. Whereas in cold water this extra heat production is negated by an even larger increase in heat loss, this is not so in air under most circumstances. The much lower heat capacity and conductivity of air, combined with wearing clothing designed for insulation in air, means that activity thermogenesis results in positive heat balance during cold stress. This generalization, like most others, has limitations, and it is these limitations that cause hypothermic deaths in cold-dry or cool-wet environments.

Failure of Exercise Thermogenesis

Three reasons can be listed as causes of inadequate activity heat production. The most important and commonplace of these is fatigue. Short rest periods are desirable during exercise in the cold, but when fatigue stops activity indefinitely, there can be rapid progress into hypothermia. Not only is the extra heat production obliterated, but there are the further complications that fatigue reduces the ability for shivering thermogenesis and for peripheral vasoconstriction. Fatigued victims also seem less sensitive to the cold, and will often lie passively during the transition to moderate or severe hypothermia. Many stories unfold of how a victim was engaging in strenuous physical activity such as cross-country skiing, was mildly *hyper*thermic and sweating, became exhausted, lay in the snow with hat off and clothes undone; and then in some fairly oblivious mental state, was converted to hypothermia and death. Maintenance of the capacity for thermogenesis (exercise and shivering) is therefore an essential preventive measure against air hypothermia. Consequently, being fit, in the basic, energetic sense of work endurance capacity, is an important safeguard in hypothermia risk situations in air.

Associated with this is the importance of pacing activity to avoid levels producing wasted heat energy and rapid fatigue. Adequate intake of energy food is also an obvious factor in avoidance of fatigue. The carbohydrate reserves of the body should be maximized before any extended period of exercise in the cold, and maintained during the activity. Fit people have the advantage of being better able to use fat reserves as an energy supply for activity and thermogenesis. It is also important to drink adequately to avoid hypohydration of the body. Vigorous exercise in the cold (especially in subfreezing temperatures with low absolute humidity) produces significant dehydration by excess respiratory, skin, and urinary water loss.

Increased viscosity of the blood reduces cardiovascular efficiency and enhances fatigue. One symptom of hypohydration is reduced volume and increased color density of the urine. Use it as a warning. Carrying water in subfreezing conditions is highly recommended (use a thermos bottle) unless a stove is available or a fire can be lit to melt ice or snow. Using body heat to provide the energy to melt ice or snow is only acceptable during the *hyper*thermic phase of activity. Therefore, occasional rest periods should be taken for eating and drinking in order to minimize the risk of fatigue-induced hypothermia.

Two other factors besides fatigue can cause failure of exercise thermogenesis. One is injury. Accidental injury frequently immobilizes, and a relatively minor injury suddenly becomes life-threatening with its potentiation of accidental hypothermia. Second, darkness tends to immobilize. Poor planning and pacing, that leaves one without shelter in the pitch-black of a forest night, is an open invitation to hypothermia. Darkness restricts the extent of gross physical activity possible. Isometrics and shivering are poor substitutes, energetically, if the cold stress becomes severe.

Reduction of Clothing Insulation

Wind, and especially wetness, conspire to potentiate hypothermia by reduction of clothing insulation. Everyone is familiar with the windchill factor that destabilizes air within and over clothing, resulting in increased heat loss. Windproof outerwear and ability to seal openings of the clothing counteract this factor.

Most importantly, if clothing becomes wet from environmental moisture, its insulation is greatly depreciated. Rain or wet snow are the obvious culprits. Rain is the most insidious killer of outdoor recreationists. For example, on what seems a mild spring or autumn day, for which a little exercise and light clothing suffice for thermal comfort, it rains unexpectedly and hypothermia strikes. Rain should never be unexpected. Waterproof outerwear must always be carried if one will be distant from a shelter that guarantees warmth. It is in this wet, cool environment that wool clothing excels because of its ability to maintain air cells even when wet. In colder, dry conditions, other fabrics can be equally effective if they are layered loosely to trap air. In wet situations, this strategy is inadequate unless wool or other air-trapping materials such as closed-cell foam are included. Failure to distinguish between the appropriateness of clothing for intense dry cold, and mild wet cold still leads to many hypothermia deaths despite years of experience. Environmental moisture sometimes comes from other unexpected sources. Hiking through thick bush that is loaded with dew or yesterday's rain soon saturates clothing as one brushes against it. Slipping while crossing a creek easily initiates hypothermia. Drying clothes in the field is very difficult for the unprepared. With clothing that is soaking wet, hypothermia is possible even during exercise thermogenesis, because this tends to mimic immersion hypothermia.

The other major way to decrease clothing insulation is through perspiration. Even in a cold dry situation (eg, below $-10°C$) sensible perspiration (sweating) and insensible perspiration (obligatory water loss through the skin) can significantly impair heat retention properties of the clothing. This is the other reason (beside avoidance of fatigue) why it is necessary to pace the level of physical activity. The extra heat production must not be of a magnitude that leads to significant core hyperthermia and its associated sweating. If the sporting or recreational activity demands a minimum level of heat production that causes sweating, clothing should be removed so that it remains dry, and is available if and when required.

A cardinal rule of good hikers and mountaineers, is "variable clothing." Adjust the type, arrangement, and number of layers of clothing to suit the environmental conditions and level of body heat production of the moment. Do not be too impatient to stop for these important adjustments. Use the occasion to eat, drink, and rest if required. If hypothermia is a risk, carrying a pack is a necessity for clothing adjustment as well as for food, water, and other equipment.

If appropriate attention is given to the modulation of activity thermogenesis and clothing insulation, the problem of hypothermia is minimized. When these measures are inadequate because of accidents causing injury, being lost for extended periods, or extremely cold conditions, other survival methods are necessary. Those with "life insurance" against hypothermia are prepared to provide heat from exogenous sources (fire, stove) and to obtain more shelter and insulation (tent, lean-to, snow cave or igloo, blankets, sleeping bag, insulated ground sheet, etc). Survival blankets or space blankets, as the lightweight, radiation-reflective sheets are called, are useful for trapping air and keeping rain off the clothing when one has stopped. It has been shown, however, that their ability to reflect heat back to the body is minimal when body moisture condenses on the inner surface. Ordinary nylon or plastic sheet (eg, large garbage bags) work equally well when surrounding the body.

When all the clothing and shelter variables are maximized, there can still be a thermal problem with waiting it out while inactive, especially overnight. Then, the following generalizations would apply. Adopting body postures that reduce heat loss (eg, HELP), or huddling with several persons will curtail the chance of hypothermia. In a group, special attention should be paid to individuals predisposed to hypothermia because of small size, lean body build, and low fatness.

In summary of this matter of prevention of hypothermia in air, it is useful to have a simple, quick-reminder system. The "Triple A" is suggested:

Appropriate clothing: relate to activity level and ambient temperature and wetness.
Avoid fatigue: determined by fitness, pace, food, water.
Accessory equipment: carry means for shelter and heat source.

TREATMENT OF HYPOTHERMIA

This is a difficult topic to cover well in a brief presentation. Procedures vary considerably depending on:

1. level of hypothermia
2. treatment site (field or hospital)
3. expertise of the person doing the treatment
4. specialized equipment available.

This presentation will restrict itself to the first-aid, nonhospital situation involving nonmedical personnel, and unavailability of sophisticated equipment for rewarming.

Variation in the amount of shivering, mental and motor impairment, muscular rigidity, and unconsciousness are a typical sequence of events that attend cooling from 37°C to about 30°C. However, these symptoms are extremely variable among individuals and particular circumstances, and are not unique to hypothermia. The importance of knowing approximately how cool a person is relates to the matter that different rewarming strategies apply to different levels of hypothermia. Another type of information that is useful to help assess the level of hypothermia is some knowledge of how fast people cool in air or water. Has there been sufficient time to become significantly hypothermic? For example, those who have read earlier sections know that a 15-minute immersion in 10°C water would only initiate core hypothermia. As with the problem of diagnosing the extent of *hyper*thermia, guesswork is unnecessary. One should use a thermometer. It should be strongly advocated that those in charge of activities in which hypothermia is a possibility, should carry a low-reading clinical thermometer (preferably for rectal measurement).

When a person is suffering from any level of hypothermia, the first requisites are to maximize removal from the cold stress and provision of insulation over all the body. The next step is to determine whether the individual can rewarm with only his or her endogenous heat production. Shivering will usually suffice for people who are mildly or moderately hypothermic (down to about 33° to 34°C) if they are not fatigued or intoxicated, and if insulation is good. With mild hypothermia of a person just removed from cold water immersion, exercise is often effective in providing rapid rewarming as long as the air environment is not too cold. If endogenous heat production of the victim is insufficient for rewarming (as judged by behavioral symptoms, but preferably by thermometer as well), exogenous heat is required. Such a person may be too cool to shiver effectively, be unable to exercise, and have a rectal temperature near or below 32° to 33°C. A victim who is alone, without fire or stove, has poor prospects of recovery.

At this point, it is useful to make a list of some of the main exogenous heat sources that have been used for rewarming in a nonhospital situation. They can be used alone or in combination.

1. Warm shower or bath (even a small tub with arms and legs out of the water). Water temperature near 40°C.
2. Hydraulic Sarong—this is a specially designed wrap placed over the chest that has warm water circulated through integral piping. Some military devices have a whole suit with piped, warm water circulated inside them.
3. Warm objects placed on the body.

Examples include chemical heat packs, water bottles, heated rocks wrapped to avoid burning the victim.

4. Inhalation heat donation. The victim breathes heated (43° to 44°C), water-saturated air or oxygen.
5. Body contact. Warm person(s) donate(s) body heat to the victim.

All these procedures, and others one could innovate, are potentially suitable for donation of exogenous heat to the mildly or moderately hypothermic victim. Warm drinks are useful only if the victim is sufficiently conscious and in control of body function to make sure he does not gag or choke while drinking. Not very much heat can be gained by drinking small amounts of warm fluids. The main benefit is rehydration. As mentioned earlier, a frequent complication of hypothermia in air or water is hypohydration, which also complicates treatment.

A problem arises with severely hypothermic persons (probably unconscious and with a rectal temperature near or below 30°C). An explanation is required. When a hypothermia victim is initially removed from the cold stress, an "afterdrop" of core temperature occurs if the metabolic heat production is very low and insufficient to balance heat loss to the colder peripheral tissues. This may amount to more than 0.5°C even under the most favorable circumstances. It is currently believed that any rewarming method that donates heat to the surface of the whole body (with skin temperature above about 33°C), will soon decrease the peripheral vasoconstriction that is mostly responsible for the large core to shell temperature differential. Circulation of blood to and from the skin, arms, and legs will probably enhance the magnitude of the core afterdrop initially. In a severely hypothermic person, this added cooling could be responsible for extending the hypothermia to the level of cardiac failure (usually 26° to 28°C). Also, venous return from the periphery is believed to contain increased hydrogen ion (because of metabolic acidosis in the ischemic tissues) and electrolyte imbalances (particularly potassium ion) which further insult a hypothermic heart.

Rewarming shock can also occur due to the inability of the hypothermic heart to increase its output in response to decreased peripheral resistance. Therefore, a fundamental principle for field treatment of severely hypothermic persons is to use procedures for core rewarming. Leave the periphery (mainly arms and legs) cold, but insulated. Donate heat to chest, neck, and head. Because of the increased safety of core rewarming, this principle is frequently used in hospitals as well. Peritoneal dialysis—warm saline solutions perfused through the abdominal cavity—is one such technique that has significantly reduced morbidity from hypothermia at the hospital site.

In the field, any of the procedures mentioned should be adapted to the core rewarming principle. For example, body contact rewarming should concentrate on chest-to-chest contact (especially lateral chest) of one or two persons with the victim. Leave the arms and legs alone with their insulation. This has the added social benefit of not having to strip completely. Pants can be left on. Just open the shirt and get as much contact as possible. If any other warm objects are available, place them in the axillary, central chest, neck, and head regions. Also, the warm persons should exhale near the face of the victim to avoid respiratory heat loss of the victim, and perhaps to donate some heat directly to the core by the respiratory system. Of course, insulation (eg, sleeping bag) should surround the group as fully as possible.

In summary, the major principles to understand are:

1. Insulating a hypothermic victim (eg, wrapping in blankets) does not, by itself, rewarm or in many circumstances, even arrest core cooling. Even with perfect insulation around the body, the cool core of a recently rescued, hypothermic person will loose much heat to the cold shell.
2. With any system of heat donation to the victim, concentrate on applying that heat to the most critical core regions (chest, neck, head), especially in the case of severe hypothermia.
3. The primary object of first aid treatment of hypothermia is to arrest further core cooling. The rate of rewarming is of secondary importance.
4. To avoid inducing ventricular fibrillation, handle unconscious hypothermia victims gently.

If the Hypothermia Victim Appears Dead

It should be appreciated that vital signs can be very difficult to detect in the depressed metabolic state of hypothermia. Assuming that careful examination has been made for evidence of breathing and pulse (carotid artery), and that these show no sign of life, it is important to remember that apparently dead hypothermia victims are highly resuscitable. When ventilation and circulation stop because of core cooling, the oxygen demands of critical tissues such as brain and heart, are greatly reduced. Whereas brain damage may be expected in less than five minutes after circulatory arrest of a normothermic person, much longer durations for successful resuscitation apply in hypothermia, even if no cardiopulmonary resuscitation (CPR) was administered after arrest of vital functions. It is hazardous to suggest time limits, because these vary widely with the circumstances, but there are ample case histories to substantiate that the metabolic depression of severe hypothermia can extend resuscitability to about 5 to 10 times that of normothermia. This should not be surprising in view of the common clinical practice to render persons hypothermic during certain surgical procedures that arrest circulation to the heart and brain.

Even with absence of brain electrical activity, hypothermia victims have been fully resuscitated. Every effort should be made in the field to have an apparently dead, hypothermic person transported to hospital for expert treatment. Do not rewarm such a person in the field to over 30 to 32°C unless transport is impossible. Before and during transport, keep the victim cold. CPR should be administered as continuously as possible.

Frostbite

Frostbite is a further risk involved with outdoor activities in very cold weather, and frequently accompanies core hypothermia. Brief mention of prevention and treatment is warranted here.

The physiologic basis of frostbite is peripheral vasoconstriction. In order to try to avoid core hypothermia, blood flow to distal appendages is drastically reduced even in mild cold stress. The body sacrifices the periphery to guard the core. The sacrifice is literal if freezing damage is irreversible. Serious frostbite is almost exclusively limited to distal appendages, especially feet; about 70% of freezing damage involves the toes.

Preventive measures include stimulating heat production of, and blood flow to, the extremities. This is very difficult, especially when not being generally active. The only alternative is good insulation of these regions. Since very little heat gets to them, the insulation has to be good. Mittens are better than gloves for protection of the hands. For the feet, loose fitting, insulated boots, together with dry wool socks are the usual solution. It is very important to give frequent attention to the feet during hiking, mountaineering, and skiing in the extreme cold. Spare socks should be carried and changed frequently to avoid moisture-loading and decrease of insulation.

Loss of skin sensation from the digits is the usual first sign of freezing. Failure of the loose skin over knuckles to move freely is another indicator. Treatment of frostbite, especially when deeper tissues are frozen, involves the following:

1. do not thaw if likely to refreeze
2. do not rub the frozen region
3. thaw rapidly and completely by immersion in warm water (40° to 42°C)
4. protect thawed region, do not break blisters
5. keep whole body warm to avoid peripheral vasoconstriction.

DROWNING

Of the three environmental hazards, hyperthermia, hypothermia, and drowning, drowning is the one that has by far the greatest public awareness and receives attention from specialized organizations such as the Red Cross and Royal Lifesaving Society. It deserves this attention because it is the second most frequent cause of accidental death of persons under 45 years of age. The topic has obvious relevance to athletics and sportsmedicine. Certain key concepts can be extracted from the vast array of information available on this topic.

Most drownings occur in association with swimming activities in warm water. Prevention involves the obvious. Become a better swimmer, especially by learning survival swimming techniques such as drownproofing, which is suitable for warm water. Know one's limitations in water. Do not mix alcohol consumption with swimming recreation, for the statistics that show the high incidence of alcohol impairment in drowned swimmers are alarming; about 40% of drowning victims have significant levels of alcohol in their blood. Another consideration is that there is no significant evidence that swimming right after an ordinary-sized meal increases the incidence of drowning.

One of the important understandings about drowning relates to recognition of the behavioral symptoms at the earliest moments of a victim's plight. This is not as easy as it would seem, for the symptoms can look like play. Nonswimmers display instinctive arm movements early in the drowning process. The arms are partially extended from the sides, and flap up and down in unison. The head goes in and out of the water. Victims cannot yell for help, or wave distress. Recognizing the instinctive arm movements is the key to early rescue, and is of obvious importance to those in charge of water sports and recreations that involve very poor swimmers.

Types of Drowning

There are three types of drowning, all of which eventually kill by hypoxia. Dry drowning involves asphyxia due to intense laryngospasm that blocks detectable amounts of water from entering the lungs (hence dry). This type of drowning occurs in 10% to 20% of lethal instances and is especially prevalent in children. Wet drowning involves significant amounts of water entering the lungs. Secondary drowning refers to delayed death (15 minutes to several days) resulting from long-term effects on lung function of initially sublethal wet drowning. Such effects are progressive edema, atelectasis, and infection.

The amount of water that enters the lungs is obviously one of the two important factors determining whether the victim will be resuscitable. The more water entering, the greater is the dilution of pulmonary surfactant, collapse of alveoli, and pulmonary edema.

Fresh Water vs Salt Water Drowning

Much attention has been given to the differences between fresh and salt water drowning. It was believed that the hemodilution, potential hemolysis, and electrolyte imbalances accompanying fresh water filling of the lung are more likely to cause death than with the opposite osmotic effect of salt water filling. It is now understood that if an amount of water enters the lungs such that the arguments about the differential mechanisms of death between fresh and salt water apply, then the amount of water will probably kill in either case, before expert treatment can be applied. Hemodilution, hemoconcentration, and hemolysis are rarely of clinical significance. Therefore, the fresh vs salt water observations are largely academic.

Cold Water Near-Drowning

A second important factor that determines resuscitability of near-drowning victims is the temperature of the water in which the drowning occurs. With the advent of widespread use of cardiopulmonary resuscitation at the rescue site, and improved techniques for management of near-drowning victims at the hospital, it has been recently realized that those who drown in cold water (below 15° to 20°C) have superior resuscitability to those who drown in warmer water. This effect seems to be stronger in children than adults. The point is, irreversible, hypoxic death of the brain may occur in five minutes for a person drowned in a warm swimming pool, whereas such death is significantly delayed if the drowning occurs for example in 5°C water. Many case histories are now documented of persons being submerged in cold water for 10, 20, and even as many as 40 minutes who have been resuscitated without loss of normal functions. What is the mechanism of this protective effect? Much attention has been given to the mammalian dive reflex (actually the vertebrate dive reflex) in this respect. During face-immersion and breath-holding, strong peripheral vasoconstriction and reflex slowing of the heart (diving bradycardia) occur. This response evolved to save oxygen for the critical tissues (brain and heart) during brief, asphyxic periods. It has been widely believed that the dive reflex is the primary mechanism underlying the spectacular increase in resuscitability of cold water near-drowning victims. However, recent results do not confirm that cold water significantly increases the magnitude of the dive reflex in submerged man.

The much more important mechanism for extending survivability is probably the direct cooling effect of cold water on critical tissues such as the brain. This significantly reduces the oxygen requirement of the unconscious brain, thereby sparing critical hypoxia. Therefore, the colder the water, the faster cooling will occur, and the greater the resuscitability. Furthermore, the smaller the body of the victim, the faster cooling will occur, and this is probably the main reason for high success with resuscitation of children who near-drown in cold water.

This cooling effect on survivability of persons

lacking the common vital signs is the same as that discussed earlier under treatment of hypothermia. Hypothermia victims have the advantage that they are already cool when ventilation and circulation stop, and even longer durations of apparent death, followed by successful resuscitation, can be expected than for cold water near-downing.

Treatment of a cold water near-drowning victim who lacks vital signs is CPR during transport to expert medical care. Do not rewarm the victim in the field. Insulate to maintain the cold temperature of the body.

SUGGESTED READINGS

Belding, H.S. Resistance to heat in man and other homeothermic animals. Edited by A.H. Rose. In *Thermobiology.* New York: Academic Press, 1967.

Buskirk, E.R., and Bass, D.A. Climate and exercise. Edited by W.R. Johnson and E.R. Buskirk. In *Science and Medicine of Exercise and Sport.* 2nd Ed. New York: Harper and Row, 1974.

Hayward, J.S. and Eckerson, J.D. Physiological responses and survival time prediction of humans in ice-water. *Aviat Space Environ Med.* 55:206–211, 1984.

Hayward, J.S., Hay, C., Matthews, B.R., et al. Temperature effect on the human dive response in relation to cold water near-drowning. *J Appl Physiol.* 56:202–206, 1984.

Keatinge, W.R. *Survival in Cold Water.* Oxford: Blackwell, 1969.

MacLean, D., and Emslie-Smith, D. *Accidental Hypothermia.* Oxford: Blackwell, 1977.

Malkinson, T.J., Martin, S., Simper, P., et al. Expired air volumes of males and females during cold water immersion. *Can J Physiol Pharmacol.* 59:843–846, 1981.

Pozos, R.S. and Wittmers, L.E. Jr, (eds). *The Nature and Treatment of Hypothermia.* Minneapolis, University of Minnesota, 1983.

Shepard, J.T., and Webb-Peploe, M.M. Cardiac output and blood flow distribution during work in heat. Edited by J.D. Hardy, A. P. Gagge, and J.A.J. Stolwijk. In *Physiological and Behavioral Temperature Regulation.* Springfield, Ill: Charles C Thomas, 1970, pp. 237–253.

Shibolet, S., Lancaster, M.C., and Danon, Y. Heat stroke: a review. *Aviat Space Env Med.* 47:280–301, 1976.

Wyndham, C.H. The problem of heat intolerance in man. Edited by J.D. Hardy, A.P. Gagge, and J.A.J. Stolwijk. In *Physiological and Behavioral Temperature Regulation.* Springfield, Ill: Charles C Thomas, 1970, pp. 324–341.

Wyndham, C.H. The physiology of exercise under heat stress. *Ann Rev Physiol.* 35:193–220, 1973.

CHAPTER 24
Protection Against Drowning: Training and Equipment

Arnold E. Reif, DSc

Perhaps nothing stimulates one's interest in water safety more than to read stories of water fatalities. Often such accounts help to suggest methods for avoiding future accidents.[1]

The only boating fatality with which I have had close contact is the death of a friend, Lauri Pekkala, while canoeing the Dead River in Maine on an AMC white water trip.[2] I was not there on that weekend in July, 1976, however, I had canoed with him on the same 17-mile class III rapid (the longest continuous set of rapids in New England) on a similar weekend two years earlier. In runs on two successive days, Lauri had negotiated these rapids with ease in an open canoe shared by his son, Keith. Lauri and Keith had also canoed with me on a memorable trip down the Allegash, a 97-mile stretch in Northern Maine that includes 7 miles of gentler rapids.

On the weekend of the accident, Lauri volunteered to lead a group of five open canoes that went down the rapid immediately after a first group of nine boats. Lauri was 56 years old, had had one of his lungs removed long ago, and had emphysema in his remaining lung. Lately, he had to rest after climbing a flight of stairs and fatigued more quickly than he had earlier. The trip leaders were not aware of Lauri's medical problems. On the positive side, Lauri had self-rescued an open canoe after spilling in white water a few weeks earlier, and his physician had told him that he could continue "normal activities."

Despite unusually high water, the early part of the trip went well. However, by the middle of the afternoon, people were getting tired. Lauri mentioned to Keith that he was considering walking Poplar Hill, the last and most turbulent rapid on the river. Starting down a rapid with large standing waves shortly before Poplar Hill, Lauri and Keith went over a 3-ft drop. Lauri, in the bow, said, "Oh, no" and the boat flipped to the left, Lauri's paddle side. Lauri came up gasping short quick breaths behind Keith, on whose shoulders he placed his hands lightly for a few moments; then his hands slipped off. Keith shouted for his father to swim as he drifted off in the heavy water, arms outstretched, head back and gasping. Keith described his own swim in swift water with 2- to 3-ft standing waves as very difficult. Keith left the water after swimming into an eddy, while his father continued around a bend and out of sight. Shortly afterwards, boaters of the first group observed a swamped canoe and what seemed to be a free floating life preserver and hat. One of the boaters quickly reached these objects, and found that they covered an unconscious swimmer floating face up in the water. Despite the fact that mouth-to-mouth resuscitation was begun even before Lauri had been brought to shore, and CPR was then immediately started and continued all the way to a hospital, Lauri did not survive.[2]

What can we learn from this tragedy that will help to save lives in the future? With the clarity granted only by hindsight, we must conclude that Lauri failed to take into account his slowly deteriorating physical condition when matched against long, powerful rapids. Psychologically, though, few decisions are harder than to say one cannot handle a challenge any more that one has met successfully many times in the past. Lauri was wearing a type II "horse-collar" life preserver, which is supposed to float an unconscious person face up (see Equipment). This it did, but the flotation was not sufficient to prevent Lauri from being submerged for considerable periods while floating down a heavy rapid. In retrospect, he should have been wearing a life preserver with more flotation, carefully secured in order not to ride up on the upper body and thereby lose effective flotation. Better yet, he should have passed up a paddle as arduous as the Dead River, or taken out when tired; both are tough decisions damaging to a self-image not yet realistically downgraded to accord with recent medical problems.

Granted, there is inherent danger any time one is around water. However, many more deaths result from boating on flat water than on rapids, for far more pleasure boating is done on gentle streams, on lakes, and in the sea. Still, tragic accidents illustrate disregard for the most important elements in safe water use: modesty in assessing one's own expertise and physical fitness, and caution in assessing the hazards posed by the water.

Thus, it would be unrealistic to downplay the vital role of mental preparedness in avoiding water-related accidents. Certainly, choice of boat and its equipment for the particular conditions of water use is also a vital factor. Preparedness and training usually decide whether or not an upset takes place, while safety equipment plays an important role in survival.

MENTAL PREPARATION

All activities are controlled by the mind. Whether we make what prove to be "good" or "bad" decisions depends on prior experience, and correct evaluation of the match between mental and physical preparedness, physical equipment, and the current conditions of the water.

Following is a brief checklist that water sports enthusiasts could use to evaluate whether a planned trip is really appropriate.

1. A realistic evaluation of the water under the particular conditions of the trip. Items to check include:

a) water temperature

b) waves, or their likelihood

c) current, and possibilities for future changes in current

d) for rivers, gauge readings translated into volume of flow per second

e) for ocean and tidal estuaries, tides and currents.

2. Weather conditions, and the likelihood of changes. Important are:

a) air temperature

b) water temperature

c) wind conditions

d) weather forecast

e) possibility of squalls, rain, thunderstorms, or snow.

3. Location of the water

a) accessibility

b) likelihood of help or rescue in case of trouble

c) maximum distance from land during trip; can it be shortened

d) unusual features of water or surroundings

e) latest conditions for that body of water, if relevant.

4. Distance to be traveled

a) distances look very short on a map, viewed in an armchair at home

b) try to underestimate rather than overestimate distances to be covered in a given time. Much of the fun in most trips on water lies in doing things unconnected with covering distances: swimming, fishing, exploring the land on the banks, taking photographs, watching birds, relaxing.

5. Time available

a) is the time sufficient to cover the planned distance

b) will it be practical to take more time if necessary.

6. Alternative routes and escape plans

a) The safest route is not necessarily the shortest one. For travel on lakes in small boats or canoes, the safe route lies along the shore line, not directly across the lake. This is not necessarily true for larger boats, especially in the sea, where currents and waves may be worse along the shore and may compound the danger of shallow water.

b) can the planned route be shortened if this seems necessary

c) are there escape points at which the trip could be ended, or from which an injured party member could be sent back

d) necessary plans for return from escape points

e) plans for side trips if time permits.

7. Ability of party members

a) how inexperienced is the least experienced member of the party

b) might this pose an additional hazard for that person or for the party as a whole, can this be rectified by prior training

c) if additional training is not feasible, would it be wiser to exclude that person (or persons) from participation.

8. Support by other boats

a) how important is this for the particular conditions and type of water use [the Appalachian Mountain Club (AMC) suggests a minimum party of three boats for white water trips]

b) if support is insufficient, who should be asked to join the trip, or should the trip be postponed until a larger party can be assembled.

9. Equipment preparedness

a) is the boat(s) to be used suitable and safe for the planned trip

b) are spares of whatever equipment is vital for propulsion (oars, paddles, sails, motors) available in case of loss or failure

c) are all necessary items of equipment aboard (a checklist is helpful)

d) is the clothing appropriate for all expected conditions of the weather

e) if an inadvertent swim in cold water may occur, wearing wet suits (with or without gloves and boots, depending on the water temperature) is indicated with an urgency that increases with the likelihood of an upset. For boating in the sea, the presence of survival suits in case of need is increasingly recognized as a vital safety precaution.

f) is a throw line rescue bag (see Equipment) or a 75-ft length of ⅜-inch polyethylene throw rope included

g) are camping and cooking equipment adequate and appropriate

h) are a minimum of tools and duct tape included to make repairs

i) are items that should remain dry all stored in water-tight bags

j) are all equipment and supplies tied into the boat to guard against loss

k) has a sleeping bag been included as protection for a case of hypothermia.

10. Navigational aids

a) on unfamiliar water, it is essential to have maps or charts of appropriately large scale and a compass, and the ability to use both with expertise

b) extended trips on land-locked water require careful planning and use of a map

c) trips on the sea or tidal estuaries require far more detailed charts that include markings of water depth, obstructions, beacons, lighthouses, buoys, plus information on tides and present conditions. Depending upon the type of boat and the conditions of water use, the following equipment may be vital for safety: compass, radio, radio direction finder, ship-to-shore radio, depth finder, and radar.[3]

11. Training in the use of safety equipment

In order to ensure that safety equipment can be used effectively under the highly adverse conditions of real-life emergencies, it is essential to practice with it. Use of all the safety equipment should be practiced at least once a year. Practice should certainly include drills for "man overboard" and for "abandon ship."

For small boat owners, training[4,5] should include:

a) reentering a swamped boat and paddling to shore while awash

b) emptying a swamped boat in deep water (for boats for which this is feasible) and reentering the boat

c) practicing both the above maneuvers in choppy water

d) self-rescue while swimming *behind* a swamped boat in moving water. The swimmer should float downstream on his back, feet-first, legs floating on the surface of the water, so that he can use his feet to ward off impact with rocks and avoid entrapment of his legs against undercut rocks (see section on Skill Training).

For owners and crews of larger boats, rescue drills should include:

a) man overboard rescue under calm water conditions

b) repeat in choppy water with a mannequin-like floating object, to simulate the rescue of a hypothermia victim unable to move his limbs

c) rapidly putting on survival suits

d) abandon boat drill

e) manning and use of flotation equipment and life raft

f) periodic checking of all safety equipment for function and rapid accessibility, and replacement of old batteries or wornout parts.

12. Supplies

a) food, appropriate for length and conditions of trip, with attention to sufficient quantity in case of delays due to weather or rough water, suitability, and ease of preparation under adverse weather conditions

b) gear required to run and moor the boat

c) fuel

d) water

e) contingency and safety supplies

f) supplies for life raft.

While the above list of items is not complete, attention to it will be of great help in insuring safety. However, the most vital items in safety are training and experience. Beyond training in safety equipment, training in skills related to the type of boating and fitness training is essential. Experience is invaluable, and should have been acquired on similar bodies of water and under similar conditions of use. Such experience should provide the confidence necessary to tackle a slightly more difficult trip than has been completed in the past. However, real danger begins when the hazards to be encountered are not expected, understood, or squarely faced, and when the abilities and preparedness of participants and equipment are overestimated. Most important, experience based on past trips is vital in making correct decisions on what constitutes inconsequential risks that are entirely appropriate, and what hazards should and must be avoided. Carelessness, lack of effort in mobilizing people and equipment to the necessary state of readiness, and overconfidence often cost dearly on water.

Certainly, all the above considerations become critical when water activities are undertaken in which one serious mistake can be fatal. This holds true under conditions such as boating in cold water, on large bodies of water, under adverse conditions of waves, currents or weather, or in boating on the sea, in tidal currents, or in rapids. Thus, a single error made while running a violent rapid could cost an expert kayaker his life even though a host of related circumstances might have bearing on the tragic outcome. Even experts can have fatal accidents in water-related sports.[1,2] However, many water-related accidents are the result of insufficient training and experience.

SKILL TRAINING

A large part of the pleasure offered by any sport is the satisfaction of mastering new skills. Through frequent repetition, the complex series of muscular motions required for most sports maneuvers is eventually learned. The brain probably accomplishes this by incorporating into unconscious memory the sequence of neural commands required to activate the muscles that will perform the maneuver. The "feel" of the entire maneuver when correctly executed is also memorized. The expert need only "switch on" that particular program in the brain, and, given the right conditions, the body will then perform the sequence of motions that constitute the maneuver.

Methods for Acquiring Skill

Instruction taken for the specific purpose of acquiring a given skill is the most simple and direct approach. Instruction on water safety is offered by the Red Cross in many areas, and by most clubs that have activities centered on one of the many water sports.

Join a club that concerns itself with water sports. Most of these clubs have active programs in water safety training. This is certainly true of the Appalachian Mountain Club (most active on the east coast) and of the Sierra Club (most active on the west coast). Most sailing clubs also offer such instruction. The US Coast Guard Auxiliary offers a wide variety of courses tailored to the needs of the entire boating public, not just motorboaters. Water safety is best taught in combination with other water sports-related skills.

Continued participation in a water sport while acting as an apprentice to experts, is another excellent way of acquiring the necessary skills and experience. Possibly, learning will proceed more slowly initially than if one joined a club with an active instruction program. In the long run there should be little difference in the acquisition of vital skills.

Watching others is seldom a good substitute for one of the above three methods of acquiring skills. Physically practicing a new maneuver under the eyes of an experienced teacher is a most important part of the learning process.

Learning from a book represents a wonderful way to improve and broaden one's skills, but is a hard way of learning. It is far better to use instruction and participation, supplemented by reading.

Participation without training, or with inadequate training is highly undesirable, especially when this is done alone or with of inexperienced or only partially experienced companions. Sharing ignorance is hardly a substitute for sound instruction.

Skills for Engaging in Water Sports

Swimming ability Tales about ships suggest that many of the old sea-dogs could not swim. If so, this may have contributed to the high death rate that occurred when sailing ships foundered. At any rate, one is unwise to engage in any boating sport if one is not a good swimmer, or has not taken the precaution of wearing appropriate life saving equipment. The natural reluctance of some people who do not swim well to venture onto water, had best be heeded carefully: it may well constitute a valuable defense mechanism against engaging in what constitutes a dangerous activity. Naturally, the degree of expertise in swimming required for safety in a given sport depends on that sport and on the particular conditions. At least in smaller boats, it is wise not to venture out from shore so far that all members of the party cannot easily reach land unaided, following an upset.

A thorough understanding of the cold water hazard is vital to safe boating. Cold water continues to be the major killer in water-related accidents.

Swimming ability fails long before death from hypothermia occurs. A significant percentage of people who fall into cold water experience an uncontrollable respiratory reflex that causes floundering and sudden sinking within a minute or two. In a report by Keatinge et al[6] one of four men swimming in water at 40°F experienced this reflex. In the same study, the three other men were able to swim respectively 8, 10, and 11 minutes before limb movement became too difficult (due to the cooling of muscles and nerves in the limbs) to keep on swimming. In contrast, survival times in water at 40°F vary between 1 and 3 hours, and death is due to core cooling. Both limb and core cooling are retarded roughly in proportion to body fat and body size, but the respiratory reflex seems to be independent of body fat. What is important to understand is the small amount of time one can count on to have available for active swimming in very cold water.

An additional factor to consider is the contrary conditions under which a swim to shore must be made following an upset. Even in water of 50°F, most people wearing a PFD will be able to swim only about 1000 yards under ideal conditions, because of the onset of hypothermia. However, how far one can really swim will depend on factors such as body fat, body size, dress, conditioning, swimming ability, willpower, and the absence of panic. After an upset in rough seas, fighting waves, spray, current, and wind, one might be very lucky to reach shore from more than 200 to 300 yards out in water of 50°F or less.

The above considerations limit the duration of the safe boating season for all types of boats, but especially for small craft. Any time one is boating in a small boat on open water when the water temperature is under 60°F, one is taking major risks in case of an upset. Certainly, it is necessary to wear one's PFD under these conditions. Because PFDs tend to become "elusive" and be swept away under conditions of an accidental upset, PFDs should be worn at all times when boats are under way on open water.

Regarding the decision whether to stay with the boat or swim for shore, the distance one can swim in cold water before being overcome by the respiratory reflex or by hypothermia varies greatly from person to person. Further, distances on water are very deceptive. Last, it is far easier to spot a swamped boat (with people clinging to it) than it is to spot an isolated swimmer. Therefore, the cardinal rule is, *stay with the boat after an upset.* Do not try to swim to shore, unless there is absolutely no chance of rescue and you are absolutely certain that you can make it. If you do swim, use a PFD or some other flotation aid. These are the conclusions of the US Coast Guard, as set out in a pamphlet *Hypothermia and Cold Water Survival* (AUX-202, Rev. 10-77).

While awaiting rescue, it is important to heed the advice in Chapter 23. Tragically, most people have not yet been convinced that "drownproofing" is not helpful in cold water. In fact, because this technique requires putting the head into the water, one cools about 80% faster than if floating with the head out of the water, and survival time is reduced. The best results, virtually a doubling of survival time, is obtained when one wears a PFD and uses the HELP, or the "huddle" posture described in the last chapter. Movement only serves to speed up the cooling process. Obviously, wearing a thermally protective garment greatly reduces the rate of cooling. For this reason, owners of all types of boats for which type III PFDs are legal should purchase the jacket-type PFDs that offer considerable thermal protection in addition to flotation.

An understanding of the hazards of currents, waves and rocks is another vital asset. For those who boat the sea, a knowledge of tides and tidal currents in the area is essential. Swimmers should be aware that one cannot succeed swimming against a current that runs faster than one can swim. Instead, one should try to escape the current by swimming at right angles to it; this is particularly important if caught in a tidal rip.

For white water boaters, the most serious hazard is to have a foot caught underneath a submerged boulder. When that happens, the force of the water is usually sufficient to sweep one downstream, flip one onto one's back and hold one under until drowned.[7] For this reason, rapids should always be swum on one's back, with the legs facing downstream and floating on the surface of the water, ready to fend off rocks.

It is also important to understand the deadly hazard of a "roller."[8-11] As water plunges over an obstruction in the river, such as a dam, it falls down to the bottom of the river bed, then shoots up again to peak above the height of the surface of the water on the downstream side of the dam, thereby forming a "standing" (stationary) wave. Water from the peak of this standing wave runs back into the trough that forms between the wave and the water rushing over the dam. Thus a "roller" is formed, with surface water from the standing wave flowing back towards the dam, while water deep down flows downstream in the normal direction of the current. You can sometimes watch a log caught below a dam as it rolls over and over, at times being sucked under, only to shoot up again where the current emerges and be carried back toward the dam, to repeat the cycle. A boat or swimmer trapped in a roller is often unable to escape unaided. Even a 1-ft dam that has a heavy water flow over it may have a well-formed roller. Larger dams may pull boats in toward the dam from as much as 50 ft downstream. It is therefore standard technique to portage around dams. Holes on the downstream side of ledges or large boulders can also form rollers; these vary in capacity to trap and upset boats, depending upon the volume of water flow, the height of the drop, and the size of the ledge or boulder. One way to negotiate weak rollers is to paddle hard through them, dipping the paddle as deep as possible to reach the deep downstream-flowing current. For a swimmer trapped in a roller from a dam that extends a considerable distance laterally, the method of escape is to take off one's PFD and swim down toward the bottom of the stream, to be flushed away from the dam by the deep downstream-flowing current. If the dam is very narrow or one is trapped near to shore, an attempt to escape laterally into water beyond the fall is worthwhile.

One more hazard, a strainer, should be mentioned, since it concerns flat water boaters as well as white water enthusiasts. A solid obstruction to water flow, such as a protruding rock, produces a pillow of water that bounces off the rock at the point where the water stream hits it. Such pillows are often strong enough to cushion floating objects from a direct contact, as long as these have as little momentum as a canoe or a kayak. In contrast, any object caught against an obstruction that is permeable to water flow, such as the branches of a partially submersed tree, strains out objects unable to pass through the branches. Boats trapped against branches are quickly upset by the current, and then are held against this "strainer" by the force of the current, as are occupants of the boat or swimmers.

For further information on these and additional hazards of white water boating, appropriate books[4,5,8-11] should be consulted.

Skills related to the water sport in question have great value for water safety. They minimize the chances of prolonged exposure to cold water, whatever the type of boat involved. The kayak can be made completely watertight, if the paddler wears a water-proof spray skirt snug around the waist, and stretches the elastic-lined hem of the skirt over the upturned rim of the kayak's cockpit. This allows the paddler to "wear" the boat, which remains dry even if flipped upside down. The boat can then be righted by a brief and fluid sequence of paddle strokes named the Eskimo roll. The ability to roll up again from an unexpected upset is obviously a safety asset. Recently, the white water committee of the AMC has begun to require that anyone who wishes to paddle a kayak or a decked canoe with the club on class III white water must first learn the Eskimo roll.

In a large and active club such as the Appalachian Mountain Club (AMC), skill training occupies much of the time of the leaders. There is a training program run separately for open canoes, and for decked boats such as kayaks. There are programs for paddling on flat water as well as on white water at different levels of difficulty. Well-run sailing and motorboat clubs have analogous training programs for members. Such training programs should become universal at boat clubs. Many clubs (including the AMC) invite the non-member public to participate. The inclusion of safety drills as part of skill training should also be universal.

Certification of skill training provides motivation for submitting to the time and trouble required for training. In the case of the AMC white water program, certification for boating at successively higher levels of difficulty is required. This includes rescue drills.

As an example of the type of safety precautions that need to be taught and practiced, the current safety code of the American White Water Affiliation (a volunteer organization of paddlers and clubs interested in the white water sports) is presented as an appendix to this chapter (see Appendix 1).

For flat water paddlers, many different rescue techniques following an upset can be taught.[4,10] National organizations such as the US Coast Guard Auxiliary and the American Red Cross have available courses in such techniques. However, the most urgent need is for practical instruction, where boaters have a chance to practice the techniques in water. This is best provided by volunteer organizations such as the Appalachian Mountain Club (AMC) in the east, the Sierra Club in the west, and the American Canoe Association nationally. While both the AMC and the Sierra Club have extensive training sessions open to the public, the main focus is on skill rather than on life-saving. This is entirely proper, for these two aspects of boating are inseparably intertwined. Further, more people are likely to attend training sessions when the emphasis is on skills. The great deficiency regarding these programs is the lack of sufficient publicity. The general public cannot benefit from these programs, if they are not widely publicized. Unless announcements are placed in newspapers and aired as public service spots on radio, only a small fraction of those interested will be reached.

For motorboaters, the US Coast Guard Auxiliary offers several courses tailored to meet the needs of the owners of various types of boats and their families.[3] Members of this volunteer organization are active in the "Vessel Examination" program, under which Courtesy Marine Examinations are made on an annual basis, if requested. This purely voluntary action insures that a thorough check is made of a craft and of its equipment.

The Coast Guard Auxiliary's courses "Boating Skills and Seamanship" consist of either 6 or 13 two-hour lessons. They lead up to tests which, if passed, merit a certificate. However, because the Coast Guard does not pay insurance for students taken on board the boats of the volunteer instructors, these courses do not include practical instruction on the water. The same considerations apply to the 6- and 13-lesson courses on "Sailing and Seamanship" that the Coast Guard offers for sailors.

Many local sailing clubs run extensive training programs for certification at different skill levels. A good example is Community Boating in Boston. There, skill training includes instruction of what to do when a sailboat tips over. While the instruction given is adequate for the area in which the boating is done, it is inadequate to prepare a future boat owner for the same predicament when alone in the middle of a lake. Therefore, a stronger emphasis on life saving would seem appropriate at the clubs that do run sailing instruction programs.

For owners of larger sailboats and yachts, it seems high time that the US Yacht Racing Union begin a "Yachtmaster Examination," patterned along the lines of the British model. Beyond testing sailing and navigational skills, such an examination should test performance of man-overboard and abandon-ship drills. As in the case of all other certification programs, more than a single level of skill might be certified, and the question of time interval between renewals would have to be decided. Certainly, examinations for renewal could be abbreviated greatly compared to those for initial certification.

Leadership training is important in certain types of boating such as club-oriented flat water and white water canoeing. In such group activities, the trip leader assumes responsibilities that require specialized training.[9]

In the case of motor boats, sailboats, and yachts, the captain traditionally bears the responsibility for the safety of his crew and guests. Even for amateur boating, the amount of knowledge required to captain a ship proficiently is extensive.[3] Each hand in a boat, whatever the task, needs to acquire competence in it. Still, it is the captain who bears the responsibility for knowledge, training, and experience.

First aid and CPR training are indispensable safety precautions.[12,13] It is highly desirable that at least one person in a small party that takes a water trip should possess such training. Better yet, all boaters should be encouraged to take the necessary training courses, provided free of charge by the American National Red Cross (first aid) and the American Heart Association (CPR). Special attention should be paid in such courses to the restoration of breathing to a person rescued from water, and to the treatment of hypothermia from exposure to cold water.

FITNESS TRAINING

It is important not to confuse physical conditioning with skill training. While physical fitness and good coordination aid learning any sport, it is skill (and not fitness) training that leads to mastery. Still, fitness and skill are complementary. Both types of training are vital for water sports that demand physical exertion.

Boating

Minimum standards of physical fitness for different types of boating are worth considering. However, such standards (or rather recommended guidelines) pose a number of hazards. For example, someone who has passed the minimum swimming requirements test outlined below, may not fully appreciate that this test is valid only for the ideal conditions of warm water, calm surface, and assured safety provided by a swimming pool. An accidental upset in cold and/or choppy waters under stressful conditions far from shore, is certain to reduce a swimmer's performance drastically.

Boaters may feel that, having passed their swimming test, they are now free to boat. They may not fully understand that such fitness achievement does not reduce the need to acquire boating skills. In addition, swimming ability and general physical ability are certain to vary up or down with time, depending on increased or decreased training, and on the general health and age of the boater.

For safe boating in small boats (20 ft or under), participants should feel comfortable in the water. This is achieved when one can swim one-quarter mile in under 15 minutes in a pool, do 50 yards using any type of back stroke in under two minutes, and float on one's back for 90 seconds with minimal (or only languid, occasional) movement of arms or legs. For white water boating or other types of water sports that require increased exertion and the risk of longer swims, these minimum swimming requirements should be doubled, both for distance and time. Each boater would be advised to pass a test for minimum swimming requirements at the start of the boating season each year. If the swimmer passed the test, his certification would be validated for a one-year period.

Special physical conditions, such as youth or old age, recent illness or injury, should be taken into account by individual boaters in assessing their own fitness. A trip leader could use these factors to assess the fitness of trip participants. This would upgrade the requirement for life jacket type (eg, from type III to type II+ or even I), and allow leaders to refuse to accept for their trip people who have problems of any sort.

A warming-up period at the start of each season should be set aside by all boaters to reacquaint themselves with old skills, practice the more demanding maneuvers, test equipment, and get the feel of it once again.

Ice Sports

Natural ice covering bodies of water holds special dangers for the sports enthusiast, whether skater, ice-fisherman, hiker, cross-country skier, or snowmobiler. If one falls into ice-covered water, one has only a short time (approximately 1 to 10 minutes) from the time when water has penetrated through one's clothing, to the point when movement becomes greatly reduced because of hypothermia. The risk of breaking through the ice therefore presents a deadly hazard.

There is much to learn about ice. During the process of freezing, the center of a pond or lake freezes last and is least safe. The reverse is true during thawing: the edges thaw first, while the center remains safe. Further, even slight flow of water greatly thins the ice. Therefore, especially during the freezing or the thawing process, there are places on a lake where the ice may be unsafe: where wind action has whipped up waves that have delayed the freezing process, where there are inlets or outlets or any other sources of moving water such as springs that enter from the floor of the lake, or where side streams or man-laid water pipes enter or exit. There may even be thin ice along the line of slight flow from any incoming water to the lake's exit. During a long cold spell when the rest of the lake may be quite safe, such places may remain open, or (far worse), be covered by a thin layer of ice. For this reason, one is well advised not to venture onto lakes not observed during freeze-up, where the location of hazards is unknown.

Large lakes often have pressure cracks running across the ice. These represent danger spots. Where cracks meet, a chunk of ice may break off. If one falls through such a chunk, getting up onto solid ice should be done as quickly as possible. First, break off jagged ice, so that the chest can face a smooth line of ice. Then, keeping the body floating as much as possible on the surface of the water, stretch out the arms as far forward as possible onto the ice and make circular pulling motions on the ice toward the chest. When the chest is up on the ice, resist the temptation to push the trunk up. Instead, continue to lie flat and pull with the arms, until completely out of the water. Then roll away from the hole. Even when some distance away from the hole, crawling is safer than walking, until firm ice is underfoot. As a last resort, if overweight or unable to extricate oneself from the water and the weather is cold enough, allow outstretched arms to freeze onto the ice before obtaining the necessary purchase to pull yourself out.

Falling through thin ice into deep water when as little as 50 ft from shore can lead to the drowning of even a strong swimmer, unless help arrives quickly. For as one attempts to climb onto the ice, the thin ice keeps breaking off. Soon, one becomes exhausted from repeated unsuccessful attempts, and the deadly cold takes its toll.

In the absence of a rope that can be thrown to a victim, rescuers should knot clothing into as long an imitation rope as is possible, then crawl out onto the ice on their bellies, thereby minimizing weight per unit area. Speed is vital. Throw one end of the rope to the victim, then pull him out when he grasps the rope. Use of a ladder, if available, is much preferable, for it permits closer approach to the victim. If a long tree branch or a dead tree is readily available, it can be used instead of a ladder. A human chain of rescuers[12] should be used only if the ice is safe close to the break-in spot.

A mobile "one man" rescue kit consists of a long rope, an ice piton of the type available in mountaineering shops, and a hammer. The piton can be hammered into safe ice to serve as attachment for the rope. This will insure that the rescuer can haul himself out, should he break through during his attempt to rescue the victim. A long nail cannot be substituted for the piton, since nails shatter ice. This method is useful only if most of the ice is safe, and the victim has fallen through a spot where the ice is locally unsafe. If the ice is unsafe for some distance around the victim, a ladder is the best rescue instrument.

To venture out onto ice covering moving waters, such as a river or tidal inlet, compounds the danger. A multitude of unexpected places may have thin ice covering them: places where water flow is stronger or less even than elsewhere, such as near bridges or other obstructions to water flow (these may be unseen submerged boulders), or where streams or man-made water conduits enter the river. If one should break through thin ice, there is a real danger of being swept under the ice, and no one has enough strength to break ice from underneath.

A different type of danger is posed by warm weather, when even thick ice can become rotten or mushy, so that one can break through. On larger bodies of ice-covered water, a combination of warmer weather and wind can cause startlingly swift ice breakup. This represents utmost danger for someone far out on the ice.

Indications for safe use of ice are when the temperature is below freezing and has been there for some time, one knows the body of water and its own peculiar patterns of ice formation well, one is aware where the inlets, outlets and any springs are, and the ice is at least three inches thick. Even then, there is danger for the unwary. Even on a familiar lake, one should not go out alone. On an unfamiliar lake, individuals in a party should stay apart, and at least one should carry a throw line. WHEN IN DOUBT, DON'T GO OUT.

EQUIPMENT

The choice of all types of safety equipment depends on the type of boat and the use to which it will be put. Relevant factors include the type of boat and its use, water temperature, the type of water to be navigated, the farthest distance from shore during trips, the likelihood of predictable waves or currents, the possibility that sudden changes in weather or tides could cause higher waves or a swifter current, and the protection afforded by the boat once swamped or upset.

Life Preservers

According to the Federal Boat Safety Act of 1971, all boats must have a personal flotation device (PFD) for each person on board. Water skiers towed behind a motorboat are counted as being on board. A wise skipper does not skimp on quality, quantity, or type of PFDs on his boat, and even provides extras for unexpected guests.

Recreational boats less than 16 ft in length, and all canoes and kayaks irrespective of length, must have one PFD aboard for each person; these can be either of type I, II, III, or IV (Figure 24-1 A, B, C, and D). All recreational boats 16 ft in length and over must have one PFD of type I, II, or III for each person, plus one throwable type IV PFD. All PFDs must be readily accessible to all persons on board, and the type IV PFDs must be immediately available for use. Further, for PFDs that come in adult and children's sizes, and for the three sizes of buoyant vests for adults, they must be of an appropriate size for the persons for whom they are intended.

Type I The federal regulations[14] define a type I PFD as any approved device designed to turn most *unconscious* persons from a face downward position in the water to a vertical or slightly backward position, and to have at least 22 pounds of buoyancy for persons who weigh over 90 pounds and at least 11 pounds of buoyancy for persons who weigh less than 90 pounds. This type of life preserver is recommended by the American National Red Cross for offshore cruising.[4] Chapman says, "although the regulations allow a choice of from three or four categories of PFDs, the truly safety-conscious skipper will choose type I. This type provides the maximum buoyancy and will hold a person's face clear of the water so that he can breathe even though unconscious."[3]

Type II According to federal regulations, this is any approved device designed to turn a person from face down position to a face up vertical or slightly backward position and to have at least 15½, 11, or 7 pounds of buoyancy for persons weighing respectively more than 90, 50 to 90, or less than 50 pounds. A type II PFD of the most common horse-collar design failed to provide sufficient flotation to prevent Lauri Pekkala from losing consciousness from successive immersions while floating through the standing waves of a powerful rapid. This life preserver can ride up on the torso, causing loss of support.

Type III Any approved device designed to keep a *conscious* person in a vertical or slightly backward position and to have at least 15½, 11, or 7 pounds of buoyancy for persons weighing respectively more than 90, 50 to 90, or less than 50 pounds. These PFDs are most favored by canoers and kayakers who need to wear them constantly while in their boats, for instance for white water running. They are more comfortable to wear and give more freedom of movement than type II PFDs.

Type IV Any approved device designed to be thrown to a person in the water and *not to be worn,* and to have at least 16½, 18, or 20 pounds of buoyancy depending on whether the material of construction is nonabsorbent or absorbs some water. Either buoyant cushions (Figure 24-1D), ring buoys, or horseshoe life rings (required for offshore races by yacht clubs that participate in the New England ocean racing circuit), fall in this category.

In addition, the federal regulations require that all types of personal flotation devices must bear the USCG (US Coast Guard) approval number and be in serviceable condition. They should therefore not be used as knee pads in canoes, and should be dried out immediately after wetting. If wet in salt water, they should be rinsed in sweet water before drying to prevent corrosion of any metallic parts. (Survival suits are discussed in Chapter 23 on hypothermia.)

The ideal life preserver represents the goal of their manufacturers, of the federal regulatory agency (the US Coast Guard), and of the user. Its properties are:

1. dependent on the intended use
2. dependent on the weight and personal preferences of the wearer
3. comfortable and free-feeling for the intended use
4. worn at the time of mishap
5. rapid to put on or take off
6. adequate for flotation for the intended conditions of use
7. flotation centered above the breast bone, to permit turning an unconscious person face up, and with some flotation around the neck to hold the face above the water
8. adequate for protection against cold water
9. does not ride up on torso even if not tightly secured
10. modest in cost
11. meets USCG requirements for flotation and absence of water logging.

The ideal life preserver of the future will probably be patterned after the type I life preserver manufactured by the Gentex Corporation (Figure 24-1A). This life preserver has sufficient flotation (20 lb or more) for all uses. The bulk of the flotation is on the chest and peaks along the midline of the chest. The modest-size flotation collar protects the back of the head and floats the face out of the water. There are leg straps to prevent the life preserver riding up as it pulls upward on the body. The back of the PFD is stiffened to provide some rigidity. All straps are of rapid-exit type. The width of the preserver can be adjusted through side lacings, and entry is from a zippered side opening. Best of all, the cut-away design above and below the arms allows complete freedom of arm motion. On the debit side are expense (about ten times higher than type II PFDs), the feeling of bulkiness that all type I PFDs seem to possess, and the time required to take it off (about twice that for other life preservers). This could be a disadvantage for white water boaters, whose only recourse if trapped in a wide roller is to take off the preserver and swim downwards below the roller, as near the bottom the current sweeps downstream. Because this life preserver fits snugly, it does offer considerable protection for the upper body against the cold.

A distinction should be made between PFD requirements for active water sports, where manpower propels the craft, and passive water sports, where wind or motor provide propulsion. In active water sports, the extra warmth provided by a jacket

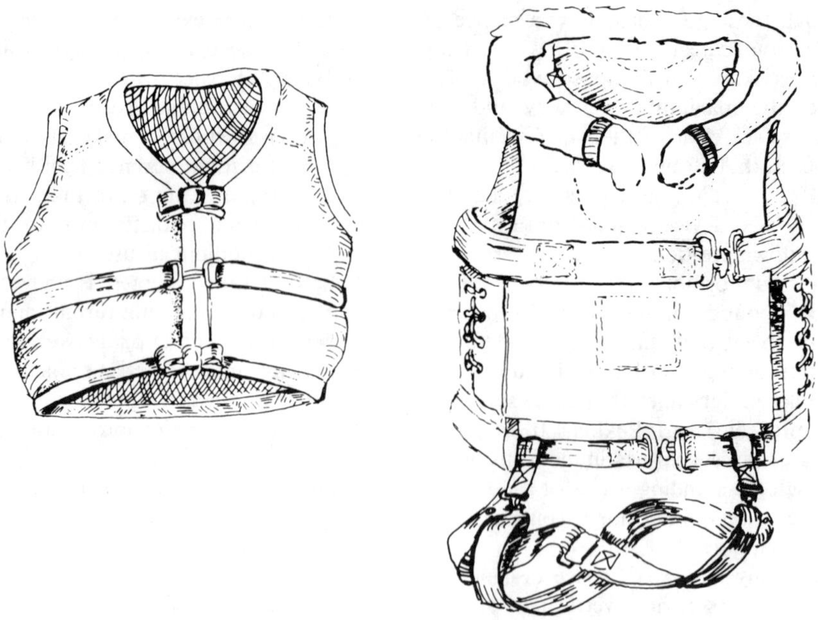

Figure 24-1A PFD life jacket, type I.

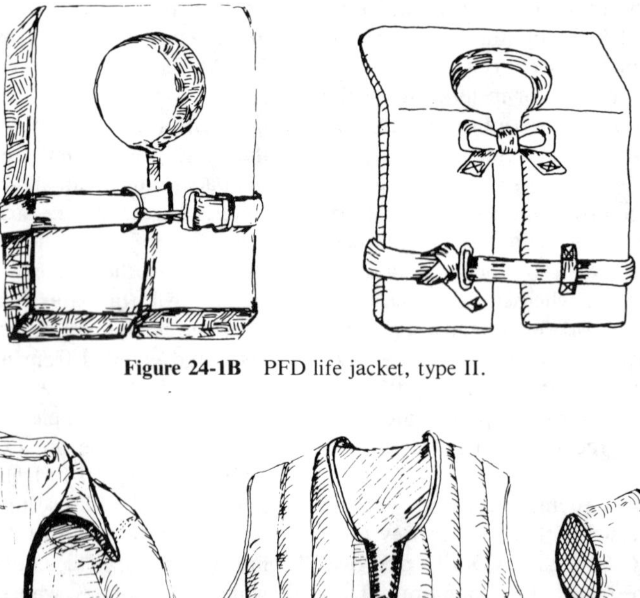

Figure 24-1B PFD life jacket, type II.

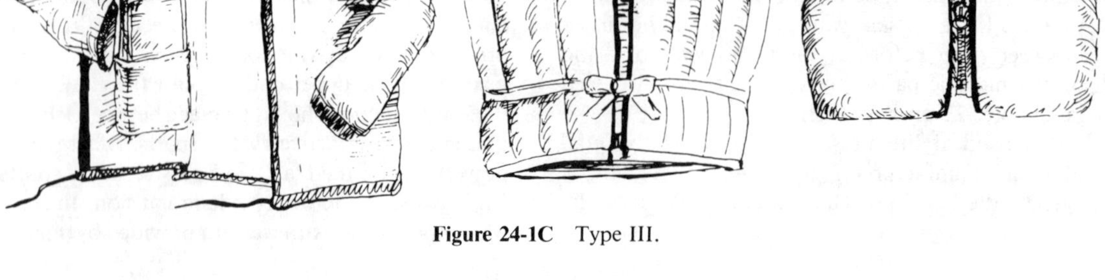

Figure 24-1C Type III.

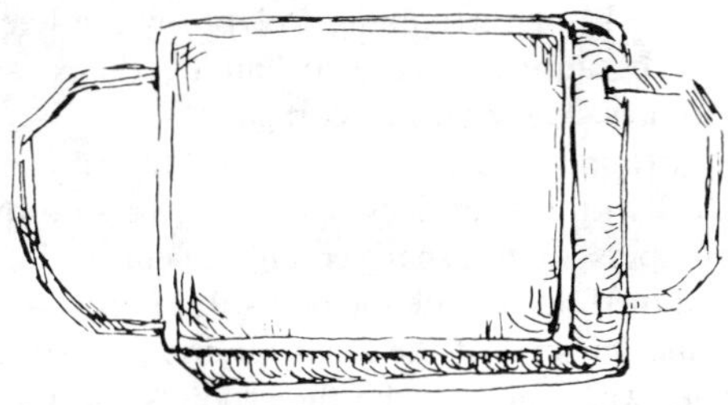

Figure 24-1D Type IV.

(Illustrations by Anne Lemonde)

PFD may not be acceptable because the heat generated by paddling and the restriction of arm movement make it uncomfortable. Even a jacket PFD would not provide sufficient protection against cold water, and a wet suit must be used for this purpose, together with a PFD whose primary function is to provide buoyancy, not protection.

In contrast, in passive water sports there is generally no sustained generation of body heat, or the need for complete freedom of arm movement. Information on the effectiveness of jacket PFDs needs to be more widely appreciated. All jacket preservers need not be type III (Figure 24-1C). Instead, extra flotation could be added above the midline of the breast to convert them to type II or even to type I PFDs, and additional flotation around the neck could be added. Further, warmup pants were almost unknown among skiers ten years ago, yet are worn widely today; there seems no reason why flotation pants could not become equally popular as a complement to flotation jackets. When pants are sealed to the jacket, this greatly reduces heat loss and prevents jacket rideup.

Additional design features include the need to make the life preserver comfortable for its intended use, or it will not be worn. The price must be reasonable, or it will not sell well. Attachment of leg straps to prevent rideup seems highly desirable, and could even be provided as an option at slightly higher price. There seems no reason why all PFDs could not be produced in extra large, large, medium, small, and children's sizes, a trend that the Coast Guard could do much to encourage.

Choice of life preserver for the boater will depend on the user's evaluation of "ideal." The most important point to remember is that a preserver is chosen that will be worn under conditions when it might be needed. A good proportion of drowning fatalities would be avoided through this expedient. Experts and instructors could do much good by setting the example of always wearing PFDs when boats are under way. Life preservers that are not worn become elusive under conditions of a real emergency.

US Coast Guard regulations for the use of PFDs do not at present make allowance for the fact that hypothermia rather than drowning is the underlying cause of most boating fatalities. A complete overhaul of present regulations, with a view to emphasizing thermal protection in addition to flotation, seems overdue as a response to the relatively new data set out in the preceding chapter on hypothermia. Drastic changes in PFD requirements seem warranted, including a change from PFD to PFTPD, to stand for "personal flotation and thermal protection device." Such a change would require a rewriting of such US Coast Guard pamphlets as "Federal Requirements for Recreational Boats" (CG-290), to include the realities of hypothermia that are already well summarized in the Coast Guard pamphlet "Hypothermia and Cold Water Survival" (AUX-202). A good start in this direction would be for the Coast Guard to test and then display ratings of thermal protection provided by survival suits, wet suits and PFDs. These ratings could be on a scale of A (best) to F (worst).

Clothing

Depending on air and water temperature, clothes suitable for boating can vary from a bathing suit to a survival suit. Selection of clothing should be dictated by comfort on board, and safety in case of immersion. For comfort, layers of clothing that permit stepwise adjustments to changes in wind and temperature, rather than use of a single heavy garment, are more suitable. A waterproof shell is a must in case of rain, and also helps to protect against wind chill.

For flat water boating in craft of 18 ft or less, the present considerations suggest use of a PFD that gives thermal as well as buoyancy protection for boating in water between 66° and 54°F. If the water temperature is below 54°F, small craft boating without wearing special garments that afford a high degree of thermal protection is done only at great risk. Owners of small craft who do not possess such garments (wet, dry, and survival suits) would be wise to stop boating when the water temperature is at 54°F or lower. Even owners of larger craft, for which the probability of an upset is far smaller, would be well advised to carry such high-thermal protection garments for all crew members, if they sail more than a very few hundred yards offshore under conditions where the chance for very rapid rescue by other boats is not excellent. Depending on the type, such garments increase the survival time in cold water by a factor of two- to tenfold.

For white water boating in water of any temperature, wearing a wet suit not only adds some buoyancy, but cushions against bruising contacts with rocks. Use of wet suits for thermal protection begins between 70° and 65°F, and becomes urgent at water temperatures between 65° and 60°F, or lower. Below 50°F, neoprene gloves and boots are beneficial. Below 40°F, wearing a Balaklava neoprene head protector is useful. In addition, PFDs are required for buoyancy, but these should leave arm movement unrestricted. For boating in heavy rapids, high buoyancy PFDs (type II+ or type I) are recommended. Additional safety aids, such as helmets, are mandatory for closed (decked) boats, and are recommended for use in open (undecked) boats in white water.[4,5,8-11]

Throw Line Rescue Bag

An excellent way to store rescue line in a form ready for instant delivery to a victim is the throw line rescue bag that the US Navy developed as standard equipment for use in life boats. It consists of a ⅜-inch polyethylene rope about 70 ft long, placed in a nylon stuff bag. A loop, which the thrower keeps hold of, is made at the end of the line that sticks out of the bag. The other end is attached to an Ethafoam disc in the bottom of the bag. The last inches of free line are pushed out through a hole made in the bottom of the bag, and a loop is tied outside. This is the loop that the victim grabs when the bag is thrown to him.

Accessories for Small Boats

Every boat should be equipped with a bailer that should be tied to a thwart to guard against loss. A gallon-size plastic bottle with built-in handle (as used for clothes bleach) can be cut down to make an ideal bailer. Knee pads and foot braces can be permanently installed in canoes to make lake paddling more comfortable. Canoes should be rigged with strong bow and stern lines of one-fourth or three-eighths-inch diameter, about 15 ft long, for use in lining, towing another canoe, rescue work, or cartopping. Polypropylene line is suitable because it is easy to handle, floats, and deteriorates slowly during storage.

Cartopped boats must be carefully and firmly attached with strong lines. One must be sure that the bumpers are not sharp enough to cut the lines. A good method is to tie the bow of the boat to the right and left end of the front bumper, to form a triangle, with knots at the three points of attachment to ensure that the boat cannot move. The stern is then tied down tightly in the same triangular manner to the two ends of the rear bumper. A boat that comes loose while it is being carried on a car becomes a lethal projectile.

Boat Outfitting

The US Coast Guard suggests that home boat builders, or those who would like to equip their boat better to aid survival in case of an upset, acquaint themselves with the safety requirements of its booklet CG-466, *Safety Standards for Backyard Boat Builders,* 1978, which can be obtained free of charge from any Coast Guard District Office. This booklet explains how one should calculate items such as:

a) Safe loading—often, drownings are caused by overloading a boat with people or gear. Owners need to know the maximum load of people their boat can carry as a movable, live load, as well as the fixed load of dead weight that it can carry.

b) Flotation—since August, 1978, the Coast Guard has required that all boats provide "level flotation," meaning that a swamped boat will float essentially level whether upright or upside down. Boats that require flotation but are exempted from the "level" requirement are inboards, sterndrives, and certain other classes. On the other hand, the following types of boats are exempted from all Coast Guard requirements of flotation, safe loading, safe powering, fuel and electrical installations: sailboats (except inboard gasoline-powered auxiliaries), canoes, kayaks, inflatables, submersibles, raceboats, surface effect vessels, and amphibious vehicles. Despite the lack of mandatory flotation requirements for canoes and kayaks, there are very few US canoe manufacturers who do not provide flotation in all canoes. Nor have I encountered a kayaker who fails to use bow and stern flotation bags to float his boat in case of an upset.

c) Survival handles—for boats that have only basic and not level flotation, the Coast Guard recommends installation of survival handles. These should be smooth and large enough, so that they are comfortable for a person in the water to hang on to. Since even boats equipped with level flotation may capsize when swamped and then float upside down, the handles should be installed to be accessible whether the boat floats right side up or upside down after swamping.

Motor Boats and Auxiliaries

The US Coast Guard has available *Rules and Regulations for Recreational Boats* (COMDTINST M16752.2, 1978), which sets out in detail all its requirements for fuel systems, electrical systems, and motor ratings. In addition, it provides more detailed information on safe loading, flotation, and safe powering. This booklet, also, is available free of charge. Many of the safety features discussed, for instance blowers that will remove gas from the engine compartment to avoid an explosion, are vital for safety. Inclusion of bilge pumps as a valuable safety feature should also be considered. Further useful equipment is detailed in the next two sections.

Sailboats and Yachts

The affiliated clubs of the United States Yacht Racing Union all include safety requirements in their instructions for competing yachts. Owners of recreational sailboats and yachts who seldom or never race would be well advised to conform to the same precepts. For instance, some of the requirements specified by the Offshore Racing Council of the New England Ocean Racing Circuit, 1979, include:

a) Owner's responsibility—"The safety of a yacht and her crew is the sole and inescapable responsibility of the owner, who must do his best to ensure that the yacht is fully found, thoroughly sea-worthy and manned by an experienced crew who is physically fit to face bad weather. He must be satisfied as to the soundness of the hull, spars, rigging, sails, and all gear. He must ensure that all safety equipment is properly maintained and stowed, and that the crew know where it is kept and how it is to be used."

b) Basic standards—"Yachts shall be self-righting. They shall be strongly built, watertight and, particularly with regard to hulls, decks and cabin trunks, capable of withstanding solid water and knockdowns. They must be properly rigged and ballasted, be fully seaworthy and must meet the standards set forth herein. All equipment shall function properly, be readily accessible and be of a type, size and capacity suitable and adequate for the intended use and the size of the yacht, and shall meet standards acceptable in the country of registry." Standards for inboard engine installations are also given. A yacht may be inspected at any time for compliance with these regulations, and is liable to disqualification if she does not comply.

c) Structural features—precise specifications are given for construction and seaworthiness of hatches, companion ways, ports, cockpits, cockpit drains, storm coverings for windows, life lines and pulpits, and accommodations such as toilets, bunks, cooking stove, galley, and water tanks.

d) Equipment—minimum requirements for four classes of equipment are specified: general, navigation, emergency, and safety equipment. The *general equipment* includes fire extinguishers, bilge pumps ("at least two, manually operated, one of which must be operable with all cockpit seats and all hatches and companionways closed"), anchors and cables, flashlights, first aid kit and manual, foghorn, radar reflector, set of international code flags and code book, shutoff valves on all fuel tanks. *Navigation equipment* includes compass and spare compass; charts, light lists and piloting equipment; sextant, tables and accurate time piece; radio direction finder; lead line or echo sounder; speedometer or distance measuring instrument; and navigation lights. *Emergency equipment* includes emergency navigation lights and power source, special storm sails, heavy weather jib, two halyards each capable of hoisting a sail, emergency steering equipment, tools and spare parts, yacht's name on buoyant equipment, marine radio transmitter and receiver with a minimum transmitter power of 25 watts, and a radio receiver capable of receiving weather bulletins. *Safety equipment* includes one life jacket for each crew member; whistles attached to life jackets; safety belt (harness type) one for each crew member, life raft(s) capable of carrying the entire crew and meeting carefully designed additional requirements, including items of equipment secured to each raft and provision for emergency water and rations; life rings; at least one horseshoe-type life ring equipped with a drogue and a self-igniting light having a duration of at least 45 minutes within reach of the helmsman and ready for instant use; at least one more horseshoe-type life ring equipped with a whistle, dye marker, drogue, a self-igniting high-intensity water light, and a pole long enough to fly a flag at least 8 ft off the water, attached to the ring with 25 ft of floating line; distress flares (12 parachute type, 8 hand type, 2 smoke signals); and a 50-ft heaving line of floating material.

Accessories for Larger Boats

Some safety devices for larger boats in addition to those listed under Equipment Preparedness are:

a) attachment of strobe lights (in addition to whistles) to all crew members, in case of a fall overboard in the dark

b) survival suits for each crew member on ocean-going vessels

c) use of the latest types of life raft, such as the Givens buoy life raft, which is hydrodynamically stabilized (not ballasted), and has a canopy to protect the occupants.

Unsinkable Boats

If a boat is unsinkable, not only is the chance of total loss greatly reduced, but the boat becomes a safety device for its crew. There are two principal methods for making a boat unsinkable: design it to be self-righting, or add sufficient flotation that it remains afloat when swamped. Both methods have their uses. In addition, self-bailing designs help to prevent swamping.

US Coast Guard rescue boats for use in extremely heavy seas are constructed to be self-righting. So is the Givens life raft, which has a canopy to cover it and a water-filled bag attached to its floor, so that it is self-righting after an upset. Many fixed-keel sail boats and yachts have lead keels that make them self-righting (or very nearly so) if all hatches are intact and secured. To make all larger sailboats fully self-righting would not add heavily to the burden of boat designers.

As we have seen in the section on hypothermia, the best chance for survival after an upset in cold water is generally to follow the rule, "stay with the boat." Obviously, the chances of survival are greatly increased if the boat provides considerable flotation when awash, especially if the flotation is sufficient to lift the stranded sailors out of the water; this is obviously only feasible with larger boats.

Use of closed cell foam, such as polyethylene foam, is an excellent method to keep boats afloat when awash. Certainly, it is far superior to use of air-tight compartments, which may fail through leakage or puncture. The amount of closed cell foam required to float virtually any recreational boat is surprisingly small. Since one cubic foot of water weighs 62 lb, while one cubic foot of polyethylene foam weighs a trifle over 2 lb, each cubic foot of foam provides about 60 lb of flotation, if we assume that it never becomes waterlogged—which may not be entirely correct.

There is, however, yet a third method for floating boats: the flotation bag. All inflatable boats, of course, make use of air for their flotation requirements. Kayaks and some white water canoes use flotation bags. These are often made of heavy duty, 20 ml polyvinyl chloride plastic. Use of flotation bags filled by carbon dioxide cartridge or by compressed air to provide flotation during emergencies has not yet come into general use. However, the Coast Guard has experimented with and used flotation bags for recovery of boats for several years. Indeed, the potentials of this method seem high. The amount of flotation provided by spheres with diameters of 4, 5, and 6 feet, which provide space for respectively 33, 65, and 113 cubic feet of air, are respectively 1, 2, and 3.5 tons. For successful use of built-in flotation bags, factors such as size requirements, material specifications, maintenance, and manner of inflation would have to be investigated in the future. Judging from materials presently available, the chances for success seem high. Use of such inflatable flotation bags for emergencies in sailboats, yachts, raceboats, surface effect vehicles, and amphibious vehicles, which are presently exempted from Coast

Guard flotation requirements, would make exemption unnecessary. Emergency flotation in the form of inflatable bags would have to be carried at all times, and cabin or cockpit design would have to be modified to ensure that the bags could not escape from their designated location once they were inflated when a boat was awash. An average 50-ft yacht might weigh 11 short tons; 5 of which are the keel. Four flotation bags each 6 ft in diameter could keep such a yacht afloat when awash.[15]

There seems to be no good reason why canoes should be exempted from flotation requirements. As mentioned before, most canoe manufacturers provide flotation. As for kayaks, *use* of kayaks (rather than manufacture) without flotation bags could well be prohibited by the Coast Guard, on the same basis as suggested above for larger boats presently exempted from the Coast Guard regulations on flotation. Inflatables might be required to have indestructible flotation; this could easily be accomplished by using closed cell foam for seats and floor boards. Thus, all boats under Coast Guard regulations could be required to possess either permanently installed or emergency flotation, depending on type of boat and intended usage. More stringent regulations in this area might well be welcomed rather than resented, since they would seem to have great potential for saving lives in the future. By making the effective date of any new regulations two or three years in the future, boat builders would have ample time to make adjustments.[16]

Many boaters abhor "regulations".[17] The lifesaving potential from Coast Guard involvement could be achieved instead by legislating a financial "break" for flotation-equipped boats and self-righting sailboats. The repeal of the state purchase tax on all self-righting and unsinkable boats would suffice to persuade many boat builders where their own and the public's interests lay.

For the more distant future, the next stage in the evolution of safe boating designs beyond "level flotation" may be the concept of having boats provide a "dry flotation platform" for occupants even when awash. This would require significant positive flotation plus a canopy for protection. The objective would be to have an awash boat serve as a truly effective liferaft.

Much more needs to be done to make boating safer.[18] A particularly welcome recent advance is the development of community river safety programs.[19] Details of a River Rescue Training Program for fire and rescue personnel are available from the Ohio Department of Natural Resources, Division of Watercraft, Columbus, Ohio. This program provides uniquely useful instruction on the rescue of people caught in the roller below a dam, or involved in other boating accidents.

This chapter is dedicated to my friend Lauri Pekkala, whose tragic death provided the stimulus to attempt to make deeply-loved water sports safer for others. I am greatly indebted to white water boaters Keith Pekkala, T. Walley Williams 3rd, and Warren B. Manhard 2nd, to physiologist Dr. John S. Hayward, to sailor Thomas Sabin, MD, and to Captain K.R. Kellogg and Commander D.W. Kennedy, respectively former and present Chiefs, Boating Safety Division, U.S. Coast Guard, for correcting errors and making most valuable suggestions.

REFERENCES

1. Lesser, R. Those who tempt the river can never rest. *Canoe* 6(5):68–69, 1978.

2. Williams, T.W., III. White water canoeing fatality on the Dead River, Maine. *AMC Appalachia.* 41(3):98–102, 1977.

3. Maloney, E.S. *Chapman Piloting. Seamanship and Small Boat Handling,* 53rd Ed. New York: The Hearst Corporation, 1977.

4. American National Red Cross. *Canoeing.* Garden City, NJ: Doubleday, 1977.

5. Byde, A. *Living Canoeing,* 2nd Ed. London: Adam & Charles Black, 1972.

6. Keatinge, W.E., Prys-Roberts, C., Cooper, K.E. et al. Sudden failure of swimming in cold water. *Br Med J.* 1:480–483, 1969.

7. Walbridge, C. Fatal accident at the icebreaker slalom. *American Whitewater.* 20(6):200–202, 1975.

8. Evans, J., and Anderson, R.R. *Kayaking.* Brattleboro, Vt: Stephen Green Press, 1975.

9. Urban, J.T. *White Water Handbook for Canoe and Kayak.* Boston: Appalachian Mountain Club, 1965.

10. Tejada-Flores, L. *Wildwater.* San Francisco: Sierra Club Books, 1978.

11. Arighi, S., and Arighi, M.S. *Wildwater Touring.* New York: Macmillan, 1974.

12. American National Red Cross. *Standard First Aid and Personal Safety.* Garden City, NJ: Doubleday, 1973.

13. American National Red Cross. *Cardiopulmonary Resuscitation.* Washington: The American National Red Cross, 1974.

14. US Coast Guard. Boats and associated

equipment. Personal flotation devices informational pamphlet and labeling requirement. *Federal Register* 43(47):9766–9772, 1978.

15. Captain Kirk R. Kellogg, Chief, Boating Safety Division, U.S. Coast Guard, made this comment: "As far as vessels having built-in flotation bags, the size requirements, maintenance, manner of inflation, and design constraints would restrict practicality of them to boats of relatively small size." The author believes that the practicality for larger boats will seem better, once experience with their use in smaller boats has been accumulated.

16. Captain Kirk R. Kellogg commented as follows on the exemption of canoes and other boats from flotation requirements: "Generally speaking, the level flotation regulation was aimed at outboard and unpowered boats less than 20 feet in length, not because they tended to sink or because they were unsafe, but simply, because this class of boat led the field in numbers of accidents. They also comprised the largest number of boats those that were commonly operated by more experienced boaters such as canoes and kayaks, or those for which no particular need had been demonstrated. One of the prime considerations for making a regulation under the Federal Boating Safety Act of 1971 is that a need must be established."

17. Reif, A. K-1 deck collapse. *Am Whitewater.* 25(4):27–29, 1980. See also *ibid.* 25(6):30–33, 1980; 25(6):8, 1980; 26(1):5–6, 1981; 26(2):6, 1981; 26(2):22–25, 1981.

18. Bechdel, L., and Ray, S. *River Rescue.* Boston, Appalachian Mountain Club, 1985.

19. Walbridge, C., (ed). *The Best of the River Safety Task Newsletter.* Lorton, Virginia: The American Canoe Association, 1983.

APPENDIX 1

AMERICAN WHITEWATER AFFILIATION SAFETY CODE

Personal Preparedness and Responsibility

1. Be a competent swimmer, with ability to handle yourself underwater.

2. WEAR a lifejacket.

3. Keep your craft under control. Control must be good enough at all times to stop to reach shore before you reach any danger. Do not enter a rapid unless you are reasonably sure you can safely navigate it or swim the entire rapid in event of capsize.

4. BE AWARE OF RIVER HAZARDS AND AVOID THEM. Following are the most frequent **KILLERS.**

High water The river's power and danger and the difficulty of rescue increase tremendously as the flow rate increases. It is often misleading to judge river level at the put-in. Look at a narrow, critical passage. Could a *sudden* rise from sun on a snowpack, rain, or a dam release occur on your trip?

Cold Cold quickly robs one's strength, along with one's will and ability to save oneself. Dress to protect yourself from cold water and weather extremes. When the water temperature is less than 50°F, a diver's wet suit is essential for safety in the event of an upset. Next best is wool clothing under a windproof outer garment such as a splashproof nylon shell; in this case, one should also carry matches and a complete change of clothes in a waterproof package. If, after prolonged exposure, a person experiences uncontrollable shaking or has difficulty talking and moving, he must be warmed immediately by whatever means available.

Strainers Brush, fallen trees, bridge pilings, or anything else which allows river current to sweep through but pins boat and boater against the obstacle. The water pressure on anything trapped this way is overwhelming, and there may be little or no whitewater to warn of danger.

Weirs, reversals, and souse holes The water drops over an obstacle, then curls back on itself in a stationary wave, as is often seen at weirs and dams. The surface water is actually going **upstream,** and this action will trap any floating object between the drop and the wave. Once trapped, a swimmer's only hope is to dive below the surface where current is flowing downstream, or try to swim out the end of the wave.

5. Boating alone is not recommended. The preferred minimum is three craft.

6. Have a frank knowledge of your boating ability. Don't attempt waters beyond this ability. Learn paddling skills and teamwork, if in a multiple-manned craft, to match the river you plan to boat.

7. Be in good physical condition consistent with the difficulties that may be expected.

8. Be practiced in escape from an overturned

craft, in self-rescue, in rescue, and in artificial respiration. Know first aid.

9. The Eskimo roll should be mastered by kayakers and canoers planning to run large rivers and/or rivers with continuous rapids where a swimmer would have trouble reaching shore.

10. Wear a crash helmet where an upset is likely. This is essential in a kayak or covered canoe.

11. Be suitably equipped. Wear shoes that will protect your feet during a bad swim or a walk for help, yet will not interfere with swimming (tennis shoes recommended). Carry a knife and waterproof matches. If you need eyeglasses, tie them on and carry a spare pair. Do not wear bulky clothing that will interfere with your swimming when waterlogged.

Boat and Equipment Preparedness

1. Test new and unfamiliar equipment before relying on it for difficult runs.

2. Be sure craft is in good repair before starting a trip. Eliminate sharp projections that could cause injury during a swim.

3. Inflatable craft should have **multiple air chambers** and should be test-inflated before starting a trip.

4. Have strong, adequately sized paddles or oars for controlling the craft and carry sufficient spares for the length of the trip.

5. Install flotation devices in noninflatable craft, securely fixed and designed to displace as much water from the craft as possible.

6. Be certain there is absolutely nothing to cause entanglement when coming free from an upset craft; ie, a spray skirt that won't release or tangles around legs; lifejacket buckles or clothing that might snag; canoe seats that lock on shoe heels; foot braces that fail or allow feet to jam under them; flexible decks that collapse on boater's legs when a kayak is trapped by water pressure; baggage that dangles in an upset; loose rope in the craft, or badly secured bow/stern lines.

7. Provide ropes to allow you to hold onto your craft in case of upset, and so that it may be rescued. Following are the recommended methods:

Kayaks and covered canoes should have 6-inch-diameter grab loops of ¼-inch rope attached to bow and stern. A stern painter 7 or 8 feet long is optional and may be used if properly secured to prevent entanglement.

Open canoes should have bow and stern lines (painters) securely attached, consisting of 8 to 10 feet of ¼- or ⅜-inch rope. These lines must be *secured* in such a way that they will not come loose accidentally and entangle the boaters during a swim, yet they must be ready for immediate use during an emergency. Attached balls, floats, and knots are *not* recommended.

Rafts and dories should have taut perimeter grab lines threaded through the loops usually provided.

8. Respect rules for craft capacity and know how these capacities should be reduced for whitewater use. (Life raft ratings must generally be halved.)

9. Carry appropriate repair materials: tape (heating duct tape) for short trips, complete repair kit for wilderness trips.

10. Cartop racks must be strong and positively attached to the vehicle, and each boat must be tied to each rack. In addition, each end of each boat should be tied to car bumper. Suction cup racks are poor. The entire arrangement should be able to withstand all but the most violent vehicle accident.

Leader's Preparedness and Responsibility

1. River conditions. Have a reasonable knowledge of the difficult parts of the run, or if an exploratory trip, examine maps to estimate the feasibility of the run. Be aware of possible rapid changes in river level and how these changes can affect the difficulty of the run. If important, determine approximate flow rate or level. If trip involves important tidal currents, secure tide information.

2. Participants. Inform participants of expected river conditions and determine if the prospective boaters are qualified for the trip. All decisions should be based on group safety and comfort. Difficult decisions on the participation of marginal boaters must be based on total group strength.

3. Equipment. Plan so that all necessary group equipment is present on the trip: 50- to 100-foot throwing rope, first aid kit with fresh and adequate supplies, extra paddles, repair materials, and survival equipment if appropriate. Check equipment as necessary at the put-in, especially lifejackets, boat flotation, and any items that could prevent complete escape from the boat in case of an upset.

4. Organization. Remind each member of individual responsibility in keeping group compact and intact between leader and sweep (capable rear boater). If group is too large, divide into smaller groups, each of appropriate boating strength, and designate group leaders and sweeps.

5. Float plan. If trip is into a wilderness area or for an extended period, your plans should be filed with appropriate authorities or left with someone who will contact them after a certain time. Establishment of checkpoints along the way at which civilization could be contacted if necessary should be considered. Knowing location of possible help could speed rescue in any case.

In Case of Upset

1. Evacuate your boat immediately if there is imminent danger of being trapped against log, brush, or any other form of strainer.

2. Recover with an Eskimo roll if possible.

3. If you swim, hold onto your craft. It has much flotation and is easy for rescuers to spot. Get to the upstream end so craft cannot crush you against obstacles.

4. Release your craft if this improves your safety. If rescue is not imminent and water is numbing cold, or if worse rapids follow, then strike out for the nearest shore.

5. Extend your feet downstream when swimming rapids to fend against rocks. **Look ahead.** Avoid possible entrapment situations: rock ledges, fissures, strainers, brush, logs, weirs, reversals, and souse holes. Watch for eddies and slackwater so that you can be ready to use these when you approach. Use every opportunity to work your way toward shore. *[Also, the Red Cross recommends that you should* never *stand up in fast-moving current or in a chute unless the water is too shallow for swimming. Try to get into an eddy or slow-moving water* before *standing up.]*

6. If others spill, **go after the boaters.** Rescue boats and equipment only if this can be done safely.

International Scale of River Difficulty

If rapids on a river generally fit into one of the following classifications but the water temperature is below 50°F, or if the trip is an extended trip in a wilderness area, the river should be considered one class more difficult than normal.

Class I Moving water with a few riffles and small waves. Few or no obstructions.

Class II Easy rapids with waves up to 3 feet, and wide, clear channels that are obvious without scouting. Some maneuvering is required.

Class III Rapids with high, irregular waves often capable of swamping an open canoe. Narrow passages that often require complex maneuvering. May require scouting from shore.

Class IV Long, difficult rapids with constricted passages that often require precise maneuvering in very turbulent waters. Scouting from shore is often necessary, and conditions make rescue difficult. Generally not possible for open canoes. Boaters in covered canoes and kayaks should be able to Eskimo roll.

Class V Extremely difficult, long, and very violent rapids with highly congested routes which nearly always must be scouted from shore. Rescue conditions are difficult, and there is significant hazard to life in event of a mishap. Ability to Eskimo roll is essential for kayaks and canoes.

Class VI Difficulties of Class V carried to the extreme of navigability. Nearly impossible and very dangerous. For teams of experts only, after close study and with all precautions taken.

(Reprinted by permission of the American Whitewater Affiliation, 1977.)

CHAPTER 25

Pediatric Sportsmedicine

John J. Murray, MD

Current statistics on organized youth sports in the United States indicate that over 22 million children under high school age are regularly enrolled in some kind of competitive athletics. Organized interscholastic competition accounts for between three and five million participants. The number of athletes under high school age is staggering—the equivalent of all of the population of the states of New York and Massachusetts combined. This is a stimulating challenge to the skills of those physicians who care for young athletes, for there are very special considerations in the treatment of the developing human organism engaged in strenuous athletic activity. A commitment to physical fitness and general athletic activity the likes of which have never been seen in this country is well under way, children are equally involved with adults. Young athletes are taking part in distance running events, tackle football, weight lifting events, long distance swimming and cross-country skiing. Many things result from their outburst of activity, some are good, some are not good.

In this chapter, we will explore the issues of safety in youth sports—matching by ability, size and maturity, growth, injuries commonly found in young athletes, psychologic and emotional aspects of sports participation for youth, and, most importantly, preparticipation evaluations. We will also look at the issues of young athletes with diabetes mellitus, seizure disorders and other chronic problems influencing levels of athletic activity.

GROWTH AND DEVELOPMENT

The normal growth and development of the human being is a physiologic continuum. Between the age of 8 and 16 (for most children), changes take place which convert the child to a young adult. Interestingly enough, it is from ages 8 to 14 that we find the highest number of participating athletes, critical years indeed. Concomitant with increases in size and strength, maturation of the nervous system takes place, eventually producing the quick reflexes, good balance and muscular control of the healthy adolescent athlete. Although there are many things that are typical of an 8-, 9- or 10-year-old child, there are enough differences so that, for the purpose of this discussion, we will not refer to the "typical" child of any age. Coordination of large muscle groups in particular is extremely variable and must be accounted for when matching children to play any competitive sport. Size and age alone do not suffice for matching young athletes. Any two children of the same age may be greatly different in their levels of coordination. Therefore, some assessment of coordination is essential if young athletes are to be properly matched.

We should not assume that because a young athlete is big, he or she is well coordinated. In fact, children undergoing major changes in height and weight may be exceedingly clumsy, because muscle and skeletal growth have surpassed neurologic maturation. Only time will improve this situation for the young athlete, and this is where coaches and parents must be unfailingly patient. Fortunately, in most of the contact/collision youth sports in this age group, severe collision injuries are rare because the athletes do not have the speed and power of high school and college competitors. Therefore, the poorly coordinated athlete is not as much at risk as he/she would be later on in a higher caliber league.

In addition to the potential injury problem, the uncoordinated child in a clearly impossible competitive situation is likely to become quite discouraged and may feel a failure or quit athletics entirely—not a satisfactory outcome. Competition is good but only under conditions which allow athletes to compete reasonably well with each other; competition is never good when one young athlete or group of them is consistently outclassed by superior performance from their far better coordinated opponents. On the other hand, the smaller child who is well coordinated and the small early-

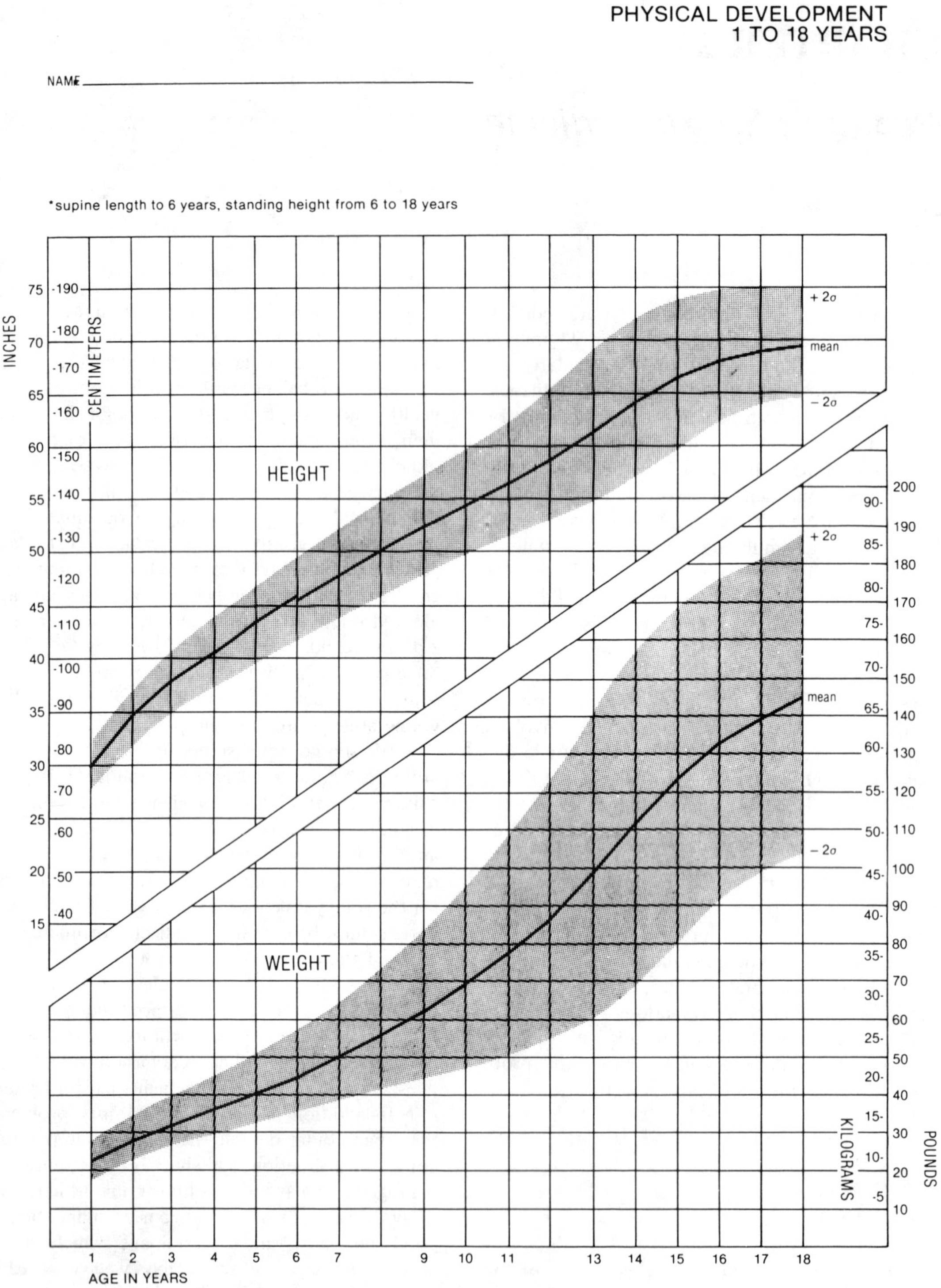

Figure 25-1 Normal physical growth ranges.

Table 25-1
Tanner Classification of Child Development

Genital Development for Boys
Stage 1: Pre-adolescent. Testes, scrotum, and penis are about same size proportion as in early childhood.
Stage 2: Enlargement of scrotum and testes, skin over scrotum reddens and changes in texture. Little or no enlargement of penis at this stage.
Stage 3: Enlargement of penis which occurs at first mainly in length, further growth of testes and scrotum.
Stage 4: Increased size of penis with growth in breadth, and development of glands, enlargement of testes and scrotum, increased darkening of scrotal skin.
Stage 5: Genital adult in size and shape; no further enlargement takes shape.

Breast Development Stages for Girls
Stage 1: Pre-adolescent. Elevation of papilla only.
Stage 2: Breast development, breast bud stage, elevation of breast and papilla a small mound; enlargement of areola diameter.
Stage 3: Further enlargement and elevation of breast and areola with no separation of their contours.
Stage 4: Projection of the areola and papilla to form a secondary mound above the level of the breast.
Stage 5: Mature stage, projection of papilla only due to recession of areola to the general contour of the breast.

Pubic Hair Stages for Boys and Girls
Stage 1: Pre-adolescent. No pubic hair.
Stage 2: Sparse growth of long, slightly pigmented downy hair, straight, only slightly curved, appearing chiefly at the base of the penis or along the labia.
Stage 3: Considerable darkening, coarser and more curly; the hair spreads sparsely over the junction of the pubis. At this stage, it can usually be seen on a black and white photograph.
Stage 4: Hair now resembles adult in type but the area covered by it is still considerably smaller than adult; no spread to thighs.
Stage 5: Adult in quality and type with distribution horizontally and spreading to the thighs in female and extending toward the umbilicus in the male.

Axillary hair usually appears at stage 4. Facial hair in boys usually appears at stage 4, first on the lips and then on the cheeks and midline on the chin. Full facial hair develops at stage 5.

In competitive athletics, stage 1 and 2 development should not compete against stage 4 or 5 development because of the maturity of the body with increase in muscle mass, strength, speed, agility and psychological confidence. This is especially true if it is to be a strenuous contact sport.

maturing athlete who is well coordinated often have a considerable advantage over their large opponents because of agility and quickness. Later, this may cause problems because when the larger athletes have fully developed their coordination, speed and quickness of response, the smaller athlete is then at a disadvantage. Problems in adjustment may occur at that time, and one can easily perceive the difficulties which may arise.

Figure 25-1 shows the range of normal physical growth. For example, an 11-year-old boy has an average weight of about 78 lb. However, the child may vary from 50 to 108 lb and still be within the normal range. Therefore, one child may outweigh another by a factor of more than 2 to 1, but still be in the same age group. This would present an obvious mismatch in many sports, particularly in contact and/or collision sports. Coaches and trainers must keep this in mind continually when they are selecting and matching teams for play in contact sports. In addition, the maturity factor must be considered. The Tanner rating (see Table 25-1) classifies the development of children: 1 = very little puberty changes, 5 = fully developed. Since many athletic skills (muscle power, coordination, oxygen consumption) develop rapidly with hormonal changes of puberty (especially in boys), equal height and weight alone do not imply equal athletic capabilities. Two children of equal height and weight, one pre-pubertal and one post-pubertal, would not be equivalent competitors—the pre-pubertal athlete is at a significant disadvantage. A boy or girl with a Tanner rating of 1 or 2 should not compete with a youth having a rating of 4 or 5.

Proper matching may occasionally call for more changes in certain sports. For example in youth football, running backs may have to be limited to 135 lb or so, as the very large boy who builds up even moderate speed can severely injure a smaller opponent. Large linemen may have to be restricted to a certain area of play in order to prevent injury.

NUTRITION

Coaches and parents often ask questions about nutrition, diets, weight loss and weight gain, the best foods for certain sports, etc. Much nutrition is common sense, yet there are several important points to remember.

In this discussion we will present some basic concepts regarding nutrition in young athletes, look at various food groups and try to show a diet that will be acceptable to the majority of individuals, realizing that the growing child has special needs.

Important points to remember are that children of all ages are undergoing rapid incremental additions to their body weight especially in the immediate prepubertal and pubertal years, but there are changing growth rates at all times. The child begins life in a situation in which the rate of growth is decelerating, for obviously one cannot continue to triple one's weight every year as does the newborn infant in the first year of life. A natural deceleration in the rate of growth takes place from that time to about the age of 6 or 7 when the child reaches what is referred to as the lag stage. Nonetheless, even during the lag stage, there is continuing addition of structures, tissues, muscles, bones, blood, and nervous tissues in a predetermined pattern. If a child is consuming a reasonable, well-balanced diet containing meats, vegetables, milk and dairy products along with fruits and whole grain wheats, this will usually suffice.

This is a time when parents sincerely interested in the welfare of their young athletes may fall into the trap of protein supplements, extra vitamins and irrational high-protein diets. None of this is necessary or even desirable, in fact it may be harmful. Nathan J. Smith states, "There is no place in the diet of a healthy athlete for vitamin, protein, or mineral supplements that are so vigorously promoted to the uninformed, highly motivated, and vulnerable population of athletes."[1] He also goes on to state that there is no necessary increase in the requirement for protein, vitamins, or amino acids that will not be met optimally through the food intake necessary to satisfy the needs of an active young athlete.

Sources of Food

Complex carbohydrates such as those found in pasta, rice, breads and potatoes are preferable sources of fuel. Studies have shown some correlation between high intake of refined sugars and elevated cholesterol and increased coronary disease.[2] As more and more young athletes enter longer and more exhausting endurance events, it has become necessary to look carefully at ways of replenishing glycogen depletion. Coaches will need to pay close attention to weight loss in the conditioned athlete, it may indicate chronic glycogen depletion and will lead to fatigue and poor performance.

Weight Control

A topic of great interest and concern to people involved in health care and athletics in young people is weight control. Obesity has become a definite problem in all age groups, although the recent upsurge in physical fitness may change this in a few years. If there is concern that an athlete may be overweight, determination of body fat percentages will be of great value in assisting the coaches and parents with appropriate diet. There is room for a properly supervised weight control regimen if it is understood by all involved that the purpose is improvement of fitness and performance. The obese child is frequently very unhappy with himself and may have a very low self-image. This image may be developed much more positively if a better physical appearance results. Frequently, actual weight loss does not have to occur. Simply stopping weight gain for a period of time may be sufficient, while increase in height makes the child more congruent in height and weight measurements.

In children, as in adults, the most important single factor seems to be physical exercise. Development of a program of vigorous sustained physical activity, which can be sports-specific coupled with education of athlete and parents about how physical activities burn calories will help prevent experimenting with starvation diets and illogical regimens. The young athlete will need to pursue a lifelong commitment to physical fitness. This in itself will do a great deal to bring obesity under control.

There are problems surfacing in the opposite direction as well. Some athletes become overly motivated toward losing weight and may get into a regimen that resembles that of anorexia nervosa. Some coaches and parents have noted this from time to time. It is a disturbing trend and needs to be looked for very carefully, since the athlete will usually not admit to perverted eating regimens or vomiting. In the past, it has been customary to think of this form of anorexia nervosa occurring only in females; however, it has been noted in males as well and needs to be approached firmly and positively if it is to be controlled.

THE HEALTH EXAMINATION FOR SPORTS

Much confusion exists regarding the advisability of frequent examinations for participation in sports. People who supervise sports programs may be wedded to the idea of the annual physical, or worse, the locker-room physical, as an ideal way in which to determine fitness for sports participation. The so-called regular physical examination will suffice for the child not engaged in strenuous athletics, but the thrust of an examination for sports participation must be in an entirely different direction.

The sports history and physical must concern itself with discovering problems that might rule out the particular sport in question and with the degree of physical fitness of the athlete. It should also make some evaluation of maturation levels, and must discover treatable conditions and organize treatment if necessary.

It has been stated that a more reasonable approach to evaluation of athletes would be a yearly preparticipation health appraisal, during which routine exams would be required only once every three or four years.[3] The appraisal would cover histories of all accidents, injuries, illnesses, or operations that might affect the athlete's performance in a given sport. Examinations for each sport are generally unnecessary and costly. A good quality examination, supported by periodic reappraisal, appears to be the best plan.

High frequency of examination does not and will not guarantee their high quality. Improved quality, less paperwork, and better health in sports can be achieved by directing medical activities specifically to the problems. Certainly the child's pediatrician or family doctor can accomplish this in the office; it can also be done in group fashion utilizing paramedical people, trainers, and assistants.[4]

The health history form as distributed by the American Academy of Pediatrics (Figure 25-2A,B) would be of help in the evaluation process by utilizing a check-off system. The form contains a sheet labeled "Instructions for Physicians," and we have found this very useful for inclusion in the statewide School Health Manual so that people are aware of the conditions and problems that must be found before athletes can begin their respective seasons. The Tanner Stage Maturation Appraisal as seen in Table 25-1 should prove helpful in attempting to match young people for competitive sport.

Flexibility is a very important consideration in determining the total fitness of the young athlete. With few exceptions, most young athletes, male or female, should be able to bend over and touch their toes, or should be able to touch toes while sitting on the floor, knees flat on the floor, feet flat against the wall. A surprisingly large number of young men and women are unable to do this very simple test, and the most common reason for this is excessive hamstring muscle tightness. In addition, strength of the shoulder shrug should be checked. The ability of the head to move well in all directions should be checked, and some assessment of neck muscle strength should be made.

A brief assessment should be made of the athlete while standing. This will reveal many of the problems associated with the extensor malalignment syndrome. This syndrome has accounted for a number of so-called "overuse syndromes" in athletes and consists of the following things:

1. medical patella squinting
2. internal rotation greater than external rotation
3. increased Q angle
4. genu varum
5. patella alta (patella points skyward)
6. external tibial rotation
7. compensatory pronation of the feet.

Sometimes running shoes with a stabilizer, sometimes simple orthotic measures, and almost always advice on distances at which to run and compete will be very helpful to the young athlete in this situation. It is becoming more and more apparent that disorders of and problems with the patellofemoral mechanism are frequent occurrences.[5]

CONDITIONS ALTERING OR EXCLUDING PARTICIPATION IN SPORTS

Parents, coaches, trainers and athletes themselves are always very interested in knowing

EVALUATION FOR COMPETITIVE SPORTS (to be completed by parent and student before student participation in each competitive sport)

You must have had a:

I. Complete physical exam within the last two years

date of exam ______

name of physician ______

positive findings none ______ yes ______

if yes, list ______

II. Do you have now, or have you had

	No	Yes
1) loss of eye, lung, kidney, ovary or testis		
2) loss of vision or hearing		
3) loss of consciousness with head injury		
4) diabetes, seizures, congenital heart disease, rheumatic heart disease, or other serious illness in the last year.		

III. Since last exam have you had any injury to:

	none	yes
head		
neck		
chest		
back		
abdomen		
arms		
legs		
eyes		
kidneys		
genitals		

If yes, please have a physician comlete this section of the form in regard to this injury.

Nature of injury ______

Any disability none ______ yes ______ if so, what ______

Any limitation of physical activities none ______ yes ______ if so, what ______

Comment or Recommendation none ______ yes ______ if so, what ______

Date of exam ______ Signature of M.D. ______

VI. Physical Fitness Test:*

You must be able to successfully complete the following test before you can engage in any competitive sport.

	Boy		Girl	
1)	mile (walk, run) in 8 min.		mile (walk, run) in 10 min.	
2) sit-ups				
	age 10-12	35	age 10 and over	20
	age 13-14	55		
	age 15 and over	60		
3) 50 yd. dash				
	age 10-12	8.5 sec.	age 10 and over	9.0 sec.
	age 13-15	7.6 sec.		
	age 15 and over	7.0 sec.		

*Based on AAJPER Youth Fitness Test Manual and Aerobic by Dr. Cooper.

I agree to the above conditions in order to engage in ______
Name of Sport

Signature of Student ______

Upon completion of the above, I give permission for ______

to compete in ______ Signature of Parent ______

Date: ______

Figure 25-2A Health history form suggested for sports physical examination.

INSTRUCTION TO PHYSICIANS: This young person is going to enter a program of strenuous activity. A general physical exam is important every two years to assess general health, but more importantly, concentrate on the following things in this appraisal to prevent future harm.

I. General:
   A. cardiopulmonary system
   B. abdomen
   C. skeletal system, especially for flexibility of various joints.
   D. secondary sex characteristics
   E. review of medical history questionnaire filled out by parent and student

II. Conditions which may generally act as disqualifiers:
   A. enlargement of the spleen after mononucleosis or of the liver after hepatitis
   B. bleeding disorders
   C. asthma—only during acute episodes or exercise-induced asthma not controlled by medication
   D. acute or chronic strains and sprains of joints
   E. epilepsy if uncontrolled by medication
   F. persistent hypertension not controlled by medication or salt restriction
   G. maturity rating of 1–3 should not be competing with maturity ratings of 4–5 in contact or strenuous sports
   H. acute infection until fever-free
   I. herpes simplex—very contagious among wrestlers and should be disqualifying until all lesions have healed

III. Conditions which disqualify athletes from strenuous sports:
   A. physical signs suggesting mitral or aortic stenosis
   B. coarctation of the aorta, prolapse of the mitral valve, or postinfectious carditis need to be evaluated by a cardiologist
   C. ectopic beats that do not disappear when the pulse rate goes above 140 with exercise need to be evaluated by a cardiologist

IV. Conditions which disqualify athletes from contact/collision sports:
   A. loss of a paired organ—eye, kidney, testicle
   B. concussions—if athlete has one concussion, he should be removed from game; two concussions, disqualified for season, three concussions, disqualify permanently from contact/collision sports
   C. severe strain or sprain or fracture of a limb that has not been evaluated within three months before participating in a contact sport, athlete must prove that limb is back to pre-injury strength.

Tests of musculoskeletal capabilities:

If the candidate cannot do the following 5 tests he should be re-evaluated by an orthopaedist before being allowed to participate in strenuous activity.

A. rotate his head in all directions
B. do a shoulder shrug
C. place both hands together behind head on neck
D. bend and touch toes with knees straight
E. duck walk with buttocks on heels

After reviewing the candidate's history and completing the physical exam based upon the above information, are there any restrictions on participation in physical activities for this athlete?

Any recommendations prior to full activity in this desired sport?

I feel this young person can participate in the sport of his choice based upon the above information providing he can pass the physical fitness requirements set forth by the coach and school in regard to this sport.

Physician's Signature ______________________________

CLASSIFICATION OF SPORTS

Strenuous—contact/collision
- football
- rugby
- ice hockey
- wrestling
- lacrosse (boys)

Strenuous—noncontact
- crew
- swimming
- cross-country
- tennis
- fencing
- track & field
- gymnastics
- water polo
- skiing

Strenuous—limited contact
- basketball
- soccer
- field hockey
- volleyball
- lacrosse (girls)

Moderately strenuous
- badminton
- golf
- baseball (limited contact)
- table tennis
- curling

Nonstrenuous
- archery
- riflery
- bowling

NOTE: *The Diet for Competitive Athletics* is available upon request.

Figure 25-2B

about medical problems that limit or change sports activity. Our perceptions of exclusion or altered participation are also changing as time goes by. With the development of newer and more sophisticated equipment, it is now possible for individuals to be involved in some of the contact/collision sports that were previously prohibited. Moreover, decisions in the courts regarding abrogation of constitutional rights or discrimination have altered what may and may not be forbidden regarding athletic participation. This section will deal with some of the many conditions that can change or alter participation in an attempt to update current thinking and knowledge upon this very vital subject.

Absence of a Paired Internal Organ

Absence of a kidney precludes involvement in collision sports. Currently, people are experimenting with protection from "flack-jackets" for Little League baseball players and also professional football players. Mainly these are directed at protection of the heart and ribs. Research is going on as to what represents effective protection for the kidneys, however, we do not yet appear to have a device on the market which offers total protection during collision sports.

Absence of One Eye

Previously, absence of one eye was thought to deprive an individual of any depth perception whatsoever. This turns out not to be the case. Many people are able to make an adaptation and in some way are able to develop depth perception. Face masks today are very highly sophisticated and it is entirely possible that an individual can play in the contact/collision sports with adequate face protection and be at very little risk for loss of an eye. The face masks and eye protection should be approved by the American Society for Testing and Materials (ASTM) before the athlete is allowed to play. There must be a clear understanding of and sharing of the responsibility involved in allowing someone with one eye to play sports that may damage an eye. It is imperative that the parents, the school authorities and the coaches clearly understand, and, if necessary, put down in writing what the limits of responsibility will be. For people under legal age, this has to be a parental responsibility. There is no question that total blindness is a very high price to pay for playing in a competitive sport, nonetheless, there are children and parents who are willing to take this risk in order to improve the individual's life through athleticism and personal fitness.

Absence of Testicle

This is another situation in which thinking has changed over the last few years. The hard athletic cup again approved by ASTM is the treatment of choice for this situation and will provide appropriate shielding. It is again important that everyone realize the amount of responsibility and the amount of risk involved. The youth must agree to practice with the cup on at all times and most certainly must agree to wear that equipment during competition. As in the preceding conditions, some attempt should probably be made to change the athlete into other sports, which places him at less risk for loss of the remaining paired organ. There is no question that some elements of risk can be reduced when an individual changes from strenuous contact/collision sport to strenuous noncontact/noncollision sports. The basic theme is reduction of the size and scope of risk factors.

Other Considerations

Concussions usually cause a great deal of concern about the athlete's future brain development. By definition a concussion means any period of unconsciousness stemming from a blow or injury to the head. It implies that the brain, regardless of how intensely or actively it may have been functioning, has been reduced to an unconscious state. It also implies that the brain tissue has been injured, and must undergo a variable period of recovery. Needless to say, the brain is rendered more susceptible to injury for the succeeding 24 to 96 hours. Concussions must be treated with respect. The athlete who has sustained a concussion should be removed from the contest immediately and should not return under any circumstances. If games are scheduled within the next three to seven days, he should miss them. Assuming that he has been examined and no residual problems are found, he may return to action in a week. An additional concussion ends his season and bars him from collision/contact sports for one year. A third concussion should end participation in *any* collision/contact sports. The risk of permanent severe brain damage is probably significant after three concussions.

Transient or acute medical conditions often pose problems for coaches and trainers. It is generally agreed that an athlete with high fever and symptoms suggestive of acute respiratory infection should not play in a given contest, but how long he should be restricted is another matter.

In younger athletes, a period of 24 hours without fever or symptoms should elapse before resuming strenuous athletic activity. This would be true in cases of ear infection, streptococcal infections, bronchitis, and sinusitis. Pneumonia would require a longer convalescence.

Mononucleosis presents a special problem. It is a viral infection that saps energy, causes acute tonsillar and lymphoid swelling and frequently affects the liver, producing a form of hepatitis. Because of the swelling of the spleen during mononucleosis, extreme caution must be used, especially in contact sports. Any athlete whose spleen is enlarged should be excluded from contact/collision sports until the spleen is considered to have returned to normal size. This can be tricky under the best circumstances. Additional information such as how the athlete is feeling, how the morning pulse has changed, and how appetite and sleep habits have returned to normal will also be very helpful in determining when the athlete returns to contact sports.

Specific Disease Conditions

Diabetes mellitus, seizure disorders, heart murmurs, and asthma all cause concern to parents, coaches and physicians with regard to how they will affect the young athlete's performance and whether the athletic stress represents a risk to the child with the problem.

Diabetes It is important to remember that the increased physical exercise accompanying practice and/or competition in athletics will result in a decreased demand for insulin, and/or an increased demand for energy sources (food) or both. The overwhelming majority of diabetics can and should indulge in athletics and physical exercise, for both physical and psychological reasons. In all likelihood the child who is wildly out of control with his diabetes will not be reporting for sports activities, simply because his medical problem is so great at the time. There are, however, a good many diabetic children who are physically capable and should be encouraged to become involved in competitive sports.

Coaches may question whether sports participation will make the diabetes worse. It will not. The important point to remember is that if available energy supplies are outstripped by insulin, a hypoglycemic reaction may occur. This is potentially far more dangerous to the child than a mild acidosis, and needs to be dealt with promptly. The symptoms are increased sweating that becomes clammy, complaints of or observation of weakness, irrational or unusual behavior, shaking or trembling, or actual fainting. Treatment is to get some readily absorbing sugar solution into the athlete as soon as possible. This will usually avert serious problems. Following recovery the athlete needs to adjust insulin, diet, or both, but only under medical supervision.

Seizure disorders Seizure disorders cause much alarm and confusion from time to time, mainly due to the dramatic nature of the episodes. The child who is absolutely seizure-free for one year on medication is a reasonably safe candidate for athletic activities. Special head protection would be advisable if the child's seizure disorder stemmed from a traumatic incident in the first place. The most anxiety-provoking aspect of seizure disorders is unpredictability if the control is borderline; for instance, the athlete could be placed in a dangerous situation if a seizure occurred during a time at which maximum strength and alertness are required.

The important point in regard to moderately well-controlled seizure disorders is that the athlete does not engage in those sports which could result in a fatality if a seizure occurred. One example is high rope climbing, another is prolonged under-water swimming, another is swimming itself, unless closely monitored by a responsible water-competent adult. Another consideration would be high-speed cycling in the individual who is not quite well controlled. In short, once again, those sports in which a seizure could cause a potentially fatal outcome should be avoided.

Heart murmurs Heart murmurs in children and their effect on athletic performance is of interest to all parents and coaches. It is safe to say that by eight or nine years of age nearly all of the congenital heart conditions that would preclude or change sports activity have been diagnosed and are being followed medically. This actually involves a relatively small number of all heart murmurs, so there remains a large number of children who have *heart murmurs without heart disease*. It is extremely important to make this distinction. Thirty percent to 50% of all children have heart murmurs at one time or another in their lives, and the overwhelming majority of these are innocent, or nonpathologic, therefore not significant. The characteristics of innocent heart murmurs set them apart from the pathologic ones in that they are usually of short duration, always systolic and may be present or absent from time to time in the same child.

There is absolutely no reason to restrict a child who has a heart murmur that is established as innocent. There is not a shred of evidence to suggest that the nonpathologic innocent murmur ever resulted in physical impairment in any athlete. Moreover, the needless anxiety and frustration over being restricted is ultimately damaging to the child's emotional development and self-image. The old practice of restriction of physical activity because of a heart murmur has no basis in fact. Even patients with certain types of congenital heart disease, such as mild pulmonary stenosis, or mild atrial or ventricular septal defects, all of which produce significant or pathologic heart murmurs, are acceptable candidates for athletics and strenuous events. Obviously, cooperation between coaches, parents, and the child's physician is essential in athletic management.

Another class of heart lesion, the cyanotic congenital heart disease, generally precludes participation in strenuous activity; however, the severity of the condition is obvious. There is one heart lesion that does not produce cyanosis, may not produce any symptoms at all in some patients, but that can result in sudden death. This is aortic stenosis, a narrowing of the valve or the muscle under it. The exact mechanism of the sudden death syndrome is unknown, but it is necessary to be most cautious about patients with aortic stenosis, since the degree of strain of the left ventricle is variable, even in children. These patients should not be involved in endurance events or in events that demand bouts of intense muscular effort. Consultation with a pediatric cardiologist is recommended before these children engage in sports activities.

Any individual who has had a fainting spell during strenuous athletics or exercise should be evaluated for the possibility of abherant left coronary artery syndrome. Although this condition has been associated with sudden death in young persons, there may be no associated abnormalities found on physical examination. It is extremely important that the question must be asked about fainting during exercise.

As mentioned above, aortic stenosis, or, as it is more commonly known, hypertrophic obstructive cardiomyopathy, needs to be considered very carefully. It is the job of the physician who is examining the child or young athlete to make sure that further cardiology evaluation is obtained when there is reason to suspect abnormalities of rhythm or anatomic abnormalities of the heart with or without a murmur.

Asthma Asthmatic children have long posed questions for parents, coaches and physicians regarding their ability to engage in organized sports. Most childhood wheezers can tolerate sustained exercise remarkably well, but attention must be paid to problems associated with particular types of allergies during particular seasons. In general, the child with occasional wheezing who had pollen allergy, if properly premedicated, hydrated and motivated, can and should engage in competitive athletics. Some of the more severe asthmatics who are also seasonally affected can safely engage in competitive sports, even of an endurance nature, during the times when their allergies are least bothersome.

The young athlete who has exercise-induced wheezing may present a very different situation in that the wheezing only occurs as the result of exercise or perhaps exercise in cold environments. The possibility of allergic asthma needs to be ruled out in children like this; however, once the diagnosis is established, there are several different types of medication, both aerosolized and oral, which are very effective in the treatment of exercise-induced wheezing. In general, this will require close follow-up by an interested physician who is familiar with the condition, but most certainly the majority of people afflicted with this problem can and should participate in athletics, including endurance events. Medical evaluation of the severity of wheezing is crucial, again this is done by appropriate medical follow-up.

There are various techniques of exercise which can be used to lessen the effects of exercise-induced wheezing. Additionally, it is now known that asthmatic people who exercise improve exercise tolerance and improve lung ventilatory and physiologic capacity. For all of these reasons, asthmatic children in general should be very carefully screened before they are restricted from a sport, the thrust of the effort should be to keep them as active and as fit as possible.

PSYCHOLOGIC CONSIDERATIONS

The young athlete's attitude about athletic competition is very easily influenced by those who coach him or her. All children need positive input and approval at frequent intervals, sometimes more so in competitive athletics. The player who is yelled at or criticized in public by his coach is not learning anything from the experience, and is probably angry at the end of the episode. Moreover, if this is a frequent phenomenon, the results can be psychologically undesirable over a long period of time. All children "fail" at one time or another and they need to be helped over the obstacle with compassion and understanding. As mentioned before, if "failures" are frequent, then perhaps the organization or the aim of the activity should be reevaluated.

There are some regrettable situations in youth sport wherein parents become part of the game. They may become argumentative with the referees, they may become abusive toward their young athletes who don't succeed on every play, in short they place themselves so much in the picture that one can seriously question for whom the event is scheduled. This is very destructive to the young athlete's image of him or herself. It is very destructive to the aims and ideals of youth sport—namely development of skills in a healthy competitive atmosphere, and it certainly does not improve the coaches' life. All parents need to assess the level of their involvement in youth sport, moreover, they need to assess what is truly motivating them when situations like this occur.

It is our place as parents, coaches, teachers, and trainers to develop in the young athlete an appreciation of the sport itself, as a challenge, a contest, a chance to better oneself. Competition is good, but must be under controlled conditions, and it must be made plain that winning at all costs is not acceptable. The game itself has worth, the contest has some value, and we have to teach, by example and word, that we believe this.

REFERENCES

1. Smith, N.J. Nutrition and the young athlete. *Ped Ann*. 7(10), 1978.

2. Costill, D.L., Dalsky, G.P., and Fink, W.J. Effects of caffeine ingestion on metabolism and exercise performance. *Med Sci Sports*. 10(3): 155–158, 1978.

3. Shaffer, T.E. The health examination for participation in sports. *Ped Ann*. 7(10):27, 1978.

4. Garrick, J.A. Sports medicine. *Ped Clin North Am*. 24(7):737, 1977.

5. Murray, J.J. Chronic knee pain in the athlete. *Ped Ann*. 13(8):613, 1984.

CHAPTER 26
The Psychology of Sports Injuries

Deborah L. Feltz, PhD

Much has been written about sports injuries in terms of their causes, types, and treatments. Most of this information has focused on the physical factors related to injuries. Suggested causes of sports injuries have focused primarily on variables such as equipment used, coaching techniques, and playing conditions. Moreover, the types of injuries and treatments suggested are usually physical in nature. Much less has been written about the psychosocial factors related to sports injuries. These include psychosocial factors that may predispose an athlete to injuries, emotional injuries that may result from sport participation, and the psychological aspects of rehabilitation. For instance, an athlete's emotional stress may enhance his or her chances of receiving an injury, and the emotional trauma of receiving an injury may impede the recovery process. This chapter addresses each of these aspects of psychosocial factors related to sports injuries.

CONTRIBUTIONS OF PSYCHOSOCIAL FACTORS TO SPORTS INJURIES

In spite of the improvements in safety equipment and training and conditioning programs, the number of athletes injured as a result of sports participation has not decreased.[1,2] No doubt this is due, in part, to the increasing number of participants, a greater emphasis on athletics, and an increasing amount of leisure time available. However, MacIntosh[2] postulated that psychological factors might also play a significant role in the occurrence of sports injuries.

Injuries are complex, multifaceted events that occur as the result of a summation of variables that interact with each other.[3,4] These variables include psychosocial as well as physical factors. Taerk[5] has postulated that the genesis of sports injuries involves at least 10 key factors. They include: 1) environment (condition of playing surface, weather conditions, time of day), 2) exposure (playing time accumulated by athlete, position played), 3) physical condition (athlete's health when injury occurs, degree of fatigue, presence or absence of previous disability), 4) amount and quality of protective equipment, 5) rules, 6) experience, 7) quality of coaching, 8) age of the athlete, 9) characteristics of the opponent, and 10) psychosocial factors (personality traits, stressful life events, depression). Rarely, however, have psychosocial factors been considered in the multifactorial process of sports injuries.

A sport participant's personality is one psychological factor thought by some to influence the chances of injury.[6,7] Many medical and psychological reports which deal with psychosomatic illness and injury indicate there is a definite relationship between illness, injury, and personality.[8-10] The few studies that have examined the relationship between personality and injuries in sports, however, have found equivocal results.[4,11-17]

Brown,[11] using the California Personality Inventory, compared personality characteristics of injured and noninjured high school football players and found no significant differences. Other studies, using the Minnesota Multiphasic Personality Inventory[14,15] and the Tennessee Self Concept Scale[17] did not find any significant relationships between personality characteristics and injury rate.

In contrast, both Jackson and his colleagues[4] and Valliant[16] found injured participants to be less tough-minded than noninjured participants on the Cattell 16PF. Though, as Jackson pointed out, these findings should be moderated because athletes in the tender-minded group would probably seek out medical attention more frequently than the tough-minded athletes. Dahlhouser and Thomas[13] found differences between injured and noninjured high school football players on their locus of control. Players who believed they could control their injury-producing behavior (internal locus of control) were less likely to have been injured than players who believed they could not control their injury-producing behavior (external locus of control).

Cohen and Young[12] also found significant differences between injured and noninjured female high school basketball players on self-concept. The differences, however, were opposite of what one might expect. The injured players received more positive scores relative to overall self-esteem, personal self considered apart from relationships with others, and identity. Cohen and Young also suggested that injured players were more apt to take added risks in play, finding themselves in situations which would involve injury.

Much of the research on personality and sports injuries, unfortunately, has been plagued by methodological, interpretive, and conceptual problems. Many investigators have used poor sampling procedures, different definitions of injury, and inappropriate measures of personality. Personality tests have been selected with little or no theoretical basis for their selection, and samples have been chosen on the basis of convenience. Ryan,[18] labeling this the "shotgun" approach to the study of personality and athletics, concluded that it is not surprising that firing into the air at different times and at different places, using different ammunition, should result in different findings. In addition, much of this research has not considered how personality characteristics interact with the many other factors involved in the genesis of sports injuries, including an individual's current subjective stress and transitory life changes.

Life stresses are events that an individual perceives as overwhelming, threatening, unsatisfying, or conflicting. These events may involve a change in job, a move, a death of a spouse or parent, or troubles in job, academic, or athletic performance. In the past 20 years, several investigators[19-22] have found significant relationships between perceived stressors and the onset of physical and psychosomatic illness and accidents. In a study examining the relationship between life changes and auto accidents, those drivers involved in an auto accident in which they were at fault reported seven life changes in the past year, while drivers involved in an auto accident who were not at fault reported only two life changes in the past year.[20]

In the area of sports, the number of life changes an individual experienced has been shown to be a predictor of sports injuries.[3,23] Using the Social and Athletic Readjustment Rating Scale (SARRS), Bramwell and his colleagues[3] found a significant association between the perception of stressful life events and risk of injury. Players suffering major time loss injuries had significantly higher life change scores than noninjured players. In another study,[23] over 55% of high school athletes reporting loss of a parent in the previous 12 months experienced an injury. Only 10% of athletes with no loss were injured.

Life stresses experienced by sport participants may influence the chance of injury by hindering concentration, increasing distractibility, and interfering with one's ability to execute correct performance. As Nideffer[7] suggests, what an athlete attends to and his or her ability to direct concentration in task-relevant ways has a lot to do with injury occurrence. The individual's personality characteristics combined with the pressure imposed by situational and emotional factors interact with performance demands and attentional abilities to increase or decrease the likelihood of injury. Sports participants who are more likely to be stressed in general, to be stressed by certain situational conditions, and to have limited attentional control, are much more likely to be injured.[7]

Social support systems such as friends, counseling centers, or coaches and trainers can help the individual cope with life changes and may have a positive effect in minimizing injury vulnerability.[22] Coddington and Troxell[23] have suggested the provision of some sort of mental health or mental conditioning program aimed at teaching coping skills and providing group support to help injury prevention. Unfortunately, counseling programs have rarely provided services of this type to athletes because they are considered a privileged group and, therefore, are not considered to have special counseling needs.[24]

An additional approach to help sport participants who are experiencing a lot of life stress is to teach them how to exert control over their performance, to reduce distractions, and to improve task-relevant concentration. Nideffer[7] advises identifying those individuals who are likely to be under stress, to be stressed by certain performance situations, and/or identifying those situations which are likely to be stressful (eg, a dangerous skill). These individuals might be identified by administering the SARS and/or an anxiety test. The critical physical and attentional abilities in these specific situations should also be identified. These individuals can then be taught to use cognitive techniques such as mental rehearsal, relaxation, and attention control training to exert that control.

Eliminating individuals from teams on the basis of life stress such as the SARS would be inappropriate and risky. As Bramwell[3] pointed out in his study, some athletes with high life change scores had no injuries. If an instrument such as the SARS is to be used to indentify individuals for counseling purposes, an informed consent procedure should be used to protect the athlete and to deal with the serious ethical issue involved in such screening. Also, any screening and/or counseling provided should be conducted under the direction of a qualified counselor or sport psychologist.

EMOTIONAL INJURIES INCURRED FROM SPORT PARTICIPATION

When one thinks of sports injuries, one usually thinks of injuries to the knees, head, back, ankles, etc. The fact that one could suffer emotional injuries through sports participation doesn't immediately come to mind. The possible emotional injuries that sports participants could suffer may include competitive stress, lowered self-esteem, and depression.

Youth sports is one area of sports participation where there has been much controversy, though little evidence, as to whether or not competitive athletes are too stressful for children. Anecdotal evidence has been mentioned that indicates that some elite young athletes routinely vomit before competition, have had mental breakdowns, develop ulcers, have committed suicide or contemplated committing suicide.[25] Whether their sport participation caused their emotional disturbances cannot be said. There is some research evidence, however, that has indicated the extent to which youth sports is stressful, the antecedents of competitive stress, and the consequences of competitive stress.

The term "stress" has been used interchangeably with tension and anxiety and refers to an unpleasant emotional reaction associated with arousal of the autonomic nervous system as a result of situational demands perceived as threatening. Participation in youth sports has the potential to be stressful to children because of the situational demands imposed on players. Scanlan and Passer,[26,27] in their tests of youth soccer players, found, however, that most children reported rather low levels of stress before and after their soccer matches. Still, about 20% of the children reported high levels of stress before the game, and many reported high levels of stress after games which their teams lost. Also, players who tended to have high competitive anxiety (competitive trait anxious), who had low self-esteem and who had low performance expectations, experienced greater stress than those who were low competitive trait anxious who had high self-esteem, and who had high performance expectancies. Thus, there is evidence that sports can be anxiety-inducing, at least for some children and under some circumstances.

The importance of the game and/or situation within the game has been shown to have an effect on the stress experienced by children.[28-31] For instance, Hanson[28] conducted a study with Little League Baseball players examining within-game variation in children's stress. Stress was measured by continuously monitoring each player's heart rate with a telemeter. Results indicated that players' average heart rate before the game was 95 beats per minute (bpm). The average heart rate rose to 127 bpm when they were in the field, and to 167 bpm when players came to bat. The players responded with the greatest stress at bat when evaluation potential was at its height. This emotional stress was short-lived, however. After the game, the average heart rate dropped to 110 bpm. Other studies have shown that children who find themselves trailing their opponents or losing to them report more anxiety than those who find themselves ahead or winning.[29-31]

Individual sports, which have a higher evaluation potential than team sports have elicited higher stress responses prior to competition.[32] Simon and Martens[32] examined the precompetition anxiety levels of 468 9- to 14-year-old boys in baseball, basketball, football, ice hockey, gymnastics, swimming, and wrestling. They found that wrestling and gymnastics were the two most anxiety-inducing sports. Players in these sports had significantly higher precompetitive levels of anxiety than players in football, hockey, and baseball, which were the least stressful sports.

From the research presented, it appears there are several factors that can influence how much stress children might experience during competition. These include: 1) the evaluation potential, 2) the importance of the game and situation within the game, 3) whether one is ahead of or behind the opposition, and 4) the outcome of the game.[33] These factors correspond to the reasons players provide for their worry.[34,35] Junior elite players have reported that they worry most about performing up to their level of ability, improving on their last performance, participating in championships, not performing well, and losing.[34,35] These sources of stress represent players' fears of failure and social evaluation and feelings of inadequacy.

Although some evidence exists indicating that youth sports are stressful for some participants, evidence also exists that youth sports are no more stressful than other evaluative activities in which children participate.[32,36] Simon and Martens[32] examined the state anxiety levels of boys in band solos, band competitions, an academic test, and physical education class in addition to the sports previously mentioned and found that the anxiety levels of the boys engaged in sports were no greater than the anxiety levels of those engaged in other activities. In fact, band soloists demonstrated higher competitive anxiety levels than the athletes.

Just because some stress is associated with youth sport competition does not imply that competition is necessarily detrimental to children. At times, stress may have no consequences beyond the immediate unpleasantness associated with the child's emotional state. To determine whether competitive stress is psychologically detrimental to children, one must examine the consequences of that stress.

One of the consequences of experiencing too much stress is dropping out of the sport. In our study of young swimming dropouts, we found that, "not liking the pressure," ranked fifth out of 32 possible reasons for discontinuing participation, and 16% rated this reason as very important.[37] Other consequences of stress may be loss of sleep or loss of appetite. Skubic[38] found 11% of the young baseball players she surveyed reported that losing a game decreased their appetite and 60% reported occasional or frequent sleep disruptions the night before or after competition. In addition, the State of Michigan Youth Sports Study[39] found that 21% of 1118 youth sport participants sampled indicated that there were times when they lost sleep because of their involvement in sports. Of the participants experiencing sleep loss, 46% indicated worrying about performance as a contributing factor and 25% reported that being upset after losing was a reason. However, another sample of children in the same study who engaged in recreational activities other than youth sports reported an even higher incidence (36%) of sleep loss, and 50% of these children indicated concern about performing well as the cause of sleep loss. Therefore, athletic competition appears to affect children's sleeping patterns no more than other activities.

Although the studies reviewed in this section do not reveal whether youth sports are too stressful for children, they do provide needed information about the factors that create stress, the types of children for whom competitive stress will be greatest, and the consequences of competitive stress. Children with low self-esteem and high competitive trait anxiety who are placed in highly evaluative situations will probably be the most vulnerable to emotional injury.

To guard against possible emotional injuries in youth sports, Smith and Smoll[40] have developed some prevention techniques. These techniques can be organized into three general categories: 1) modifying certain features of the athletic environment, 2) training coaches to relate more effectively to their players, and 3) providing individual counseling in stress management. Although individual counseling might be needed in some cases of high competitive stress, most stress-related concerns in youth sports can be handled by modifying the environment and training coaches.

The competitive setting can be modified to reduce stress in a number of ways. For instance, rules could be changed to allow for a greater degree of success. Game scores, league standings, or individual performance statistics could be eliminated to reduce the fear of evaluation and take the emphasis off winning. Training coaches to provide a supportive rather than punitive environment can also minimize players' stress by reducing their fear of failure. Likewise, parents can also reduce fears of failure by being encouraging and supportive of their children.

Other preventative and treatment techniques for emotional injuries provide children with stress-coping skills.[40] These may involve relaxation, altering irrational beliefs, and replacing self-preoccupational thoughts with specific cognitions designed to reduce stress.

PSYCHOLOGICAL ASPECTS OF REHABILITATION

A physical injury has several psychological effects on a sports participant. These include the emotional trauma of experiencing an injury, the psychological factors that influence the recovery process, and the psychological impact of an injury on the individual's future performance.

It is a devastating, emotional blow to receive an injury in sports, especially one that sidelines the individual for a week or more. The emotional stress involved does not come from the injury itself, but rather from the interruption of participation. For some sports participants, an injury causes a severe disruption in their overall lifestyle, and for a few, ends their athletic career.

Rotella[41] has described the sequence of psychological reactions that an athlete typically undergoes after an injury. These steps involve: 1) disbelief, denial, and isolation; 2) anger; 3) bargaining; 4) depression; and 5) acceptance and resignation while continuing to remain hopeful. Before the physical rehabilitation process begins, it is important that the injured player learn to accept or cope with the injury while still remaining positive and enthusiastic about the prospect for recovery. The more serious the injury, the more difficult this will be, especially if it ends an athletic career.

One of the difficulties that may interfere with accepting the injury is the development of emotional and irrational thinking.[41] The athlete may become preoccupied with self-defeating thoughts that interfere with recovery. For instance, the athlete might exaggerate the seriousness of the injury, decide he or she is injury-prone, believe the coach will eliminate him or her, or believe he or she will never be able to catch up with the competition.

To help the athlete learn to cope with an injury, the personnel involved with his or her rehabilitation need to be supportive and reassuring, and, at the same time, encourage the athlete to view the injury in a rational, self-enhancing way. The athlete should understand that it is appropriate to feel irritated, frustrated, and sad, but unreasonable to feel the situation is hopeless.[41]

Another factor that may interfere with the athlete's ability to cope with the injury is the failure of rehabilitation personnel to provide honest and accurate information and eliminate uncertainties or misconceptions.[41-43] Steadman,[42] chair of the US Alpine Ski Team Medical Group, recommends explaining fully the nature of the injury and what the progression will be. It is also important to encourage the athlete to have realistic expectations about the prescribed treatment, with honest estimates of the time involved.[43]

Once the injured player has accepted and learned to cope with the injury, the rehabilitation process will be easier because the player will be more cooperative in pursuing the prescribed treatment. To maintain the athlete's interest in the rehabilitation process, Steadman[42] recommends that he or she be kept active. For instance, if a player is recovering from surgery on the left knee, exercise for the right leg and upper extremities is prescribed. Setting realistic short-term goals in rehabilitation is also recommended to give the athlete something immediate for which to aim. Injured players should also be encouraged to take an active part in their rehabilitation, with interplay between them and health-care personnel about what seems to be working well. As Steadman noted, athletes may come up with rehabilitation techniques that are more effective than what the physician suggests.

Another suggestion to help keep the injured player active and interested in the rehabilitation process is to use visuo-motor behavior rehearsal (VMBR) training.[44] The period of inactivity caused by a sports injury can subject the individual to growing doubts about the strength of the injured part and the loss of coordination and timing from lack of practice. VMBR allows the athlete to practice the skills mentally that he or she is unable to do physically. This type of mental practice can help to alleviate the growing fears the athlete may have concerning loss of ability.

VMBR, a technique developed by Suinn,[44] involves training in deep muscle relaxation followed by training in imagery. The relaxation procedure is used to enhance the ability to use imagery. According to Suinn, VMBR imagery is more realistic than just mental practice because it also includes using all muscle groups involved in the skill. However, much of the evidence in support of the effectiveness of VMBR has been anecdotal in nature, and no controlled studies to date have assessed its effectiveness in helping athletes recover from injury.

Body rehearsal[41] is a similar mental rehearsal technique but with a different purpose. More than just keeping the injured player active during rehabilitation, body rehearsal is thought to actually aid in the healing process. The injured player is first given a detailed explanation of the injury accompanied with colored pictures to help him or her develop a mental picture of the injury. Next, the healing process and purpose of the rehabilitation techniques are explained so the individual can visualize what is happening internally to the injured part during the rehabilitation process. The individual is then asked to visualize the healing process during treatments and at intervals throughout the day.

Much of the evidence for the effectiveness of this technique as an aid to healing has been anecdotal and in the treatment of cancer.[45] The technique typically involved picturing the destruction of cancerous material by the body's immunological system and disposing it through the circulatory system. Systematic, controlled studies that are causal in design are presently being conducted in this area. However, the issue of causality is not necessary to justify the use of this technique in conjunction with physical rehabilitation as it is a noninvasive technique.

Biofeedback is another technique that can aid in the healing process of certain injuries. Through the use of electromyography (EMG), athletes can learn to reduce the strain that excessive muscle tension places on the injury.[7] However, biofeedback is an expensive procedure that may not be used frequently enough to warrant its purchase.

Some of the physical therapies used in rehabilitation can be somewhat painful (ie, icing). There are a number of techniques that athletes can use to control or eliminate pain. The injured individual can try to dissociate with the pain by using attention diversion techniques such as doing mental arithmetic, daydreaming, playing music in his or her mind, etc. Relaxation, biofeedback, and hypnosis have also been used effectively to gain control over pain.[45-47] Athletes using these techniques must be careful, however, not to completely block out pain signals which could otherwise warn them of danger.

If surgery is involved in the rehabilitation process, it may cause additional anxiety or fear on the part of the athlete. To help alleviate some of the anxiety in preparation for surgery, a technique called mastery rehearsal or positive self-talk can be used. With this technique, athletes rehearse positive self-statements that prepare them for the surgery, control negative thoughts, psych themselves up, and help themselves cope with the feelings of being overwhelmed.

An example of the type of positive statements used in this technique is given in the following example by Rottella[41] in an athlete's preparation for knee surgery:

> I'm looking forward to surgery and feel great about the upcoming operation and rehabilitation. I'm glad I'll no longer be bothered by my knee. I have a well-qualified surgeon who'll do a successful operation. I'll begin rehabilitation shortly afterwards with a caring and talented athletic trainer. Rehabilitation will be short and successful. Each day, I'll make progress. In a few weeks, I'll be training again. I'll feel good and be excited. I know I'll be successful.

These types of statements should be rehearsed whenever the athlete starts to become anxious or worried about the surgery.

Although a player may have recovered from an injury physically, he or she may not have recovered emotionally enough to be an effective competitor. The athlete may have some anxiety about returning to competition, lack confidence in his or her ability, have irrational thoughts, which lead to an inability to concentrate on performance, or fear future injury. For instance, a basketball player who gets a severe ankle injury from playing underneath the boards may try to avoid that area of the court when he or she returns to competition. A baseball player who has been hit in the head by a pitched ball may back away from every ball that is pitched after returning to play. Or a football player who has been out of competition for a long time with a knee injury may have severe doubts about his ability to perform up to his previous performance level, which causes anxiety and in turn poor performance. This self-doubt–anxiety-poor performance cycle just spirals to the point where he can no longer manage his performance anxiety.

When the trainer, physician, or sport psychologist suspects the athlete has a fear of reinjury or anxiety over performance capabilities, techniques such as desensitization, hypnosis, VMBR, stress inoculation, or other stress management techniques may be used. These techniques should be timed so that psychological rehabilitation is completed when the athlete is physically ready to return to practice. The technique employed should be based on the type of anxiety response displayed by the athlete. Desensitization, hypnosis, and VMBR are generally used when the athlete has a specific fear. Stress inoculation and other stress management techniques are more frequently used when treating anxiety concerning performance incompetence.

Desensitization, as described by Wolpe,[49] basically involves three parts: training in deep-muscle relaxation, construction of anxiety hierarchies, and relaxation paired with imagined anxiety-evoking stimuli from the hierarchies. For example, a gymnast who is fearful of a front aerial dismount off the beam because of an ankle sprain she suffered as the result of a previous attempt may first be taught deep-muscle relaxation. Then progressively threatening tasks leading up to the dismount can be constructed by the sport psychologist in cooperation with the gymnast. Tasks might include simple routines on the beam without a dismount, simple dismounts, and the front aerial dismount with spotting. The gymnast would then relax and imagine first the least anxiety-provoking scene. While being relaxed, the mild anxiety that might arise is inhibited by the deep relaxation. Then progressively more anxiety-provoking situations are imagined until the gymnast has worked through the hierarchy. When the gymnast actually returns to practice, she can work through the hierarchy physically with her coach.

Suinn[50] has used VMBR successfully to help a recreational skier return to skiing after sustaining a knee injury. The woman in this example fell while skiing and had to have a knee operation. After going through a physical rehabilitation program, she was still unable to return to skiing because of the anxiety she felt about falling again. VMBR was used to enable her to use the imagery to face all of the stimulus conditions leading up to and associated with the fall, but without the anticipation of having a fall, and allow her to re-experience skiing to the point of the fall, but continue on with the correct responses of making the right turn without falling and continuing down the hill.

When an athlete's self-doubts about his or her playing ability become overwhelming, the stress involved can have a severe effect on the individual and performance. Stress inoculation is one procedure that can be useful not only in the treatment of this type of anxiety response, but also in its prevention.[51] As its name suggests, stress inoculation is based on an immunization model that allows the individual the opportunity to cope with small, manageable units of stress.

The procedure involves three phases. The first phase is the educational phase that provides the individual with an explanation for how stress occurs. It also involves helping the athlete break down the stress response into its component phases. The goal here is to have the individual see the stress as a series of phases rather than one overwhelming experience.

In the second phase, the sport psychologist provides the individual with coping skills to be rehearsed. The goal in this phase is to enable the individual to replace maladaptive thoughts with adaptive ones. Some form of physical relaxation is usually employed as a strategy to counteract physical tension. The coping skills to be rehearsed are positive self-statements which typically involve preparing for the stress, confronting the stress, coping with being overwhelmed, and reinforcement for carrying out the procedure as prescribed.

The third phase (the application phase) simply consists of actual practice of the previously outlined steps. Stressful situations are introduced in a graduated fashion, often proceeding from imaginary to real-life situations. The goal in this phase is to get the individual to start using skills he or she has learned in naturally occurring stress situations.

The techniques that have been discussed for the psychological rehabilitation of the injured sports participant are considered clinical techniques and should be conducted under the direction of a qualified counselor or sport psychologist. Furthermore, the sport psychologist or sport counselor must maintain close contact with and supervision by a physician and/or trainer when using these techniques. Cooperation among the sport psychologist, physician, trainer, and coach is essential in athletic injury situations. If the sport psychologist is unsure of the ethical standards for service provision in this area, I suggest the following book: *The Ethics And Practice of Applied Sport Psychology* by Robert Nideffer.

The psychological state of an athlete can influence the chances of a sports injury as well as influence the rehabilitation process once an injury has occurred. If sports medicine professionals pay as much attention to the psychological aspects of sports injuries as to the physical aspects, injury occurrence might be reduced and recovery might be faster.

REFERENCES

1. Garrick, J.G. Requa, R.K. Injuries in high school sports. *Pediatrics* 61:465–469, 1978.
2. MacIntosh, D.K., Skrien, T., Shephard, R.J. Physical activity and injury: A study of sports injuries at the University of Toronto. *J Sports Med Physical Fitness* 12:224–237, 1972.
3. Bramwell, S.T., Masuda, M., Wagner, N.N., et al. Psychological factors in athletic injuries: Development and application of the social and athletic readjustment rating scale (SARRS). *J Human Stress* 2:6–20, 1975.
4. Jackson, D.W., Jarret, H., Bailey, D., et al. Injury prediction in the young athlete: A preliminary report. *Am J Sports Med* 6:6–14, 1978.
5. Taerk, G.S. The injury-prone athlete: A psychosocial approach. *J Sports Med* 17:187–194, 1977.
6. Hayes, D. Risk factors in sport. *Human Factors* 16:454–458, 1974.
7. Nideffer, R.M. *The Ethics and Practice of Applied Sport Psychology.* Ithaca, New York, Mouvement Publications, 1981.
8. Dunbar, F. *Mind and Body: Psychosomatic Medicine.* New York, Random House, 1955.
9. Kunce, J., et al. Psychological factors in high school accidents. *Personnel Guidance J* 45:140, 1966.
10. Tiffin, J., Parker, B.T., Haberstat, R.W.

Visual performance and accident frequency. *J Applied Psychol* 33:499, 1949.

11. Brown, R.B. Personality characteristics related to injuries in football. *Res Quart* 42: 133–138, 1971.

12. Cohen, D.A., Young, M.L. Self-concept and injuries among female high school basketball players. *J Sports Med Phys Fitness* 21:55–61, 1981.

13. Dahlhouser, M., Thomas, M.B. Visual disembedding and locus of control as variables associated with high school football injuries. *Perceptual Motor Skills* 49:254, 1979.

14. Goven, J.W., Koppenhauer, R. Attempt to predict athletic injuries. *Med Times* 93:421–422, 1965.

15. Kraus, J.F., Gullen, W.H. An epidemiological investigation of predictor variables associated with intramural touch football injuries. *Am J Public Health* 59:2144–2156, 1969.

16. Valliant, P.M. Personality and injury in competitive runners. *Perceptual Motor Skills* 53: 251–253, 1981.

17. Young, M.L., Cohen, D.A. Self-concept and injuries. *Am Corrective Therapy J* 33:133–142, 1979.

18. Ryan, E.D. Reaction to sport and personality dynamics. In *Proceedings of the National College Physical Education Association for Men.* 70–75, 1968.

19. Holmes, T.H., Rahe, R.H. The social readjustment rating scale. *J Psychosomatic Res* 11: 213–218, 1967.

20. Holt, P.L. Stressful life events preceding road traffic accidents. *Injury* 13:111–115, 1981.

21. Rahe, R.H., Meyer, M., Smith, M., et al. Social stress and illness onset. *J Psychosomatic Res* 8:35–44, 1964.

22. Sheehan, D.E., O'Donnell, J., Fitzgerald, A., et al. Psychosocial predictors of accidents-error rates in nursing students: A prospective study. *International J Psychiatry Med* 11:125–137, 1981–82.

23. Coddington, R.D., Troxell, J.R. The effect of emotional factors on football injury rates — A pilot study. *J Human Stress* 6:3–5, 1980.

24. Lanning, W. The privileged few: Special counseling needs of athletes. *J Sport Psychol* 4:19–23, 1982.

25. McDermott, B. The glitter has gone. *Sports Illustrated* 57(20):83–96, 1982.

26. Scanlan, T.K., Passer, M.W. Factors related to competitive stress among male youth sport participants. *Med Science Sports* 10:103–108, 1978.

27. Scanlan, T.K., Passer, M.W. Factors influencing the competitive performance expectancies of young female athletes. *J Sport Psychol* 1:151–159, 1979.

28. Hanson, D.L. Cardiac response to participation in Little League baseball competition as determined by telemetry. *Res Quart* 38:384–388, 1967.

29. Corbin, C.B., Nix, C. Sex-typing of physical activities and success predictions of children before and after cross-sex competition. *J Sport Psychol* 1:43–52, 1979.

30. Gill, D.L., Martens, R. The role of task type and success-failure in group competition. *International J Sport Psychol* 8:160–177, 1977.

31. Martens, R., Gill, D.L. State anxiety among successful and unsuccessful competitors who differ in competitive trait anxiety. *Res Quart* 47:698–708, 1976.

32. Simon, J.A., Martens, R. Children's anxiety in sport and nonsport evaluative activities. *J Sport Psychol* 1:160–169, 1979.

33. Passer, M.W. Psychological stress in youth sports. Edited by R.A. Magil, M.J. Ash, F.L. Smoll. In *Children in Sport.* Champaign, IL, Human Kinetics, 1982, pp 153–177.

34. Gould, D., Horn, T., Spreeman, J. Sources of stress in junior elite wrestlers. *J Sport Psychol* 5:159–171, 1983.

35. Feltz, D.L., Albrecht, R.R. Psychological implications of competitive running in elite young distance runners. Edited by M. Weiss, D. Gould. In *Competitive Sport for Children and Youth/Proceedings of the 1984 Olympic Scientific Congress.* Champaign, IL, Human Kinetics, in press.

36. Skubic, E. Emotional responses of boys to Little League and Middle League competitive baseball. *Res Quart* 26:342–352, 1955.

37. Gould, D., Feltz, D. Horn, T., et al. Reasons for attrition in competitive youth in swimming. *J Sport Behavior* 5:155–165, 1982.

38. Skubic, E. Studies of Little League and Middle League competitive baseball. *Res Quart* 27: 97–110, 1956.

39. State of Michigan: Joint Legislative *Study on Youth Sports Programs: Phase II, Agency Sponsored Sports.* East Lansing, MI: Author, 1978.

40. Smith, R.E., Smoll, F.L. Psychological stress: A conceptual model and some intervention strategies in youth sports. Edited by R.A. Magill, M.J. Ash, F.L. Smoll. In *Children in Sport.* Champaign, IL, Human Kinetics, 1982, pp 153–177.

41. Rotella, R.J. Psychological care of the injured athlete. Edited by D.N. Kulund. In *The*

Injured Athlete. Philadelphia, J.B. Lippincott, 1982.

42. Ferstle, J. The medical side of the Sarajevo games. *Physician Sportsmed* 12:180–183, 186, 1984.

43. Watson, G. Some psycho-social aspects of athletic injury. *Sports Coach* 3:23–25, 1979.

44. Suinn, R. Removing emotional obstacles to learning and performance by visuomotor behavior rehearsal. *Behav Therapy* 3:308–310, 1972.

45. Pelletier, K.R. *Mind as Healer, Mind as Slayer.* New York, Dell, 1977.

46. Evans, M., Paul, G. Effects of hypnotically suggested analgesia on physiological and subjective responses to cold stress. *J Consulting Clin Psychol* 35:362–371, 1970.

47. Reeves, J. EMG-biofeedback reduction of tension headache: A cognitive skills training approach. *Biofeedback and Self-Regulation* 1:217–225, 1976.

48. Johnson, R. Suggestions for pain reduction and response to cold-induced pain. *Psychol Rep* 18:79–85, 1966.

49. Wolpe, J. *The Practice of Behavior Therapy.* New York, Maxwell House, 1974.

50. Suinn, R.M. *Behavior Modification For Athletic Injury.* Fort Collins, Colorado: Colorado State University, 1975.

51. Harrison, R.P., Feltz, D.L. Stress inoculation for athletes: Description and case example. *Motor Skills: Theory into Practice* 5:53–61, 1981.

CHAPTER 27
Psychological Aspects in the Care and Treatment of Athletic Injuries

Steven J. Danish, PhD

> I've always been concerned about health. But when you start getting good, achievement becomes the #1 thing in your life. If you are a person like me who lives for now, achieving #1 is the most important thing.
>
> *Beverly Francis, Women's World Record Holder in Power Lifting*

Statements such as these have become all too common among elite athletes. Many of these athletes judge their total worth as a person by their athletic performance. Their self-esteem and self-respect depend on the outcome of competition and all their energies become directed at winning. It almost seems as if some athletes will go to any end to achieve this goal.

Whether this attitude is right or wrong has been debated ad nauseam by philosophers, psychologists, and sociologists of sport.[1,2] Regardless of the reader's opinion about this attitude, it exists and has significant implications for athletes' behavior and health. For example, it is probably a major impetus for the decision by some athletes to use steroids and other so-called performance enhancing drugs. However, more importantly for this chapter, it has profound implications on the incidence of athletic injuries and the recovery process. When an athlete adopts a "winning is everything" philosophy, there is a greater likelihood that more injuries will occur because the athlete takes more risks during competition. A "go for it regardless of the costs" attitude develops. Moreover, the athlete is more likely to play with pain. Admitting to pain may mean that the athlete will be withdrawn from competition and lose the chance to attain all the self-esteem associated with winning. If the injury does require that the athlete not participate, the impatience about recovery is often so overwhelming that it may inhibit the rehabilitation process. This impediment exists despite the willingness of the athlete to work hard.

In the previous chapter, Feltz looked at the psychology of sport injuries from three perspectives: the psychosocial factors predisposing athletes to injuries (such as the attitude held by Beverly Francis); the emotional injuries which result from sport participation; and the psychological aspects of rehabilitation. In this chapter, the emphasis will be almost entirely on the latter, the psychological aspects associated with the care and treatment of athletic injuries. The purpose of the chapter will not be to review the relevant literature since Feltz has done an admirable job examining the literature on the psychology of sports injuries. Instead, a framework for working with injured athletes will be developed.

A FRAMEWORK FOR UNDERSTANDING THE PSYCHOLOGICAL REACTIONS TO ATHLETIC INJURIES

Because the treatment of sport injuries primarily involves physical interventions, the psychological impact of the injury is often overlooked. When the injury is treated as if it is not related to the person having the injury, the rehabilitation process is affected. It is the person, not his or her knee or shoulder, which must be treated. For this reason, it may be useful to understand individuals from a general systems theory perspective.[3-5] For example, Miller, in his book *The Living System*,[5] applies the general system theory to living systems. He contends that information is organized at seven levels—the cellular, organ, organism, group, organization, societal, and supranational. While treating sport injuries may not require attention to all levels, a comprehensive rehabilitation program must consider many of these levels.

Stresses of Athletic Injury

Being injured and undergoing treatment and rehabilitation can be highly stressful, especially to someone whose body and physical activity are the main source of self-esteem. As Gruen[6] has noted:

> When a person is incapacitated . . . he is not only severely debilitated by physiological imbalance, but his whole psychological adjustment is in severe turmoil. He is faced with the sudden termination of his customary life-style, which has abruptly passed out of his control. He suffers pain, strange symptoms, and a frightening disruption of physiological processes that were once either automatic or taken for granted. . . . He must leave his immediate future up to the 'experts,' most of whom he has never met before. He is concerned about the disruption in his family, friends, and work circles and its consequences; and he worries about his capacity to reenter these circles. He faces an uncertain future in which resumption of normal activity is questionable for him.

In sum, the athlete's life becomes uncertain; the sense of control over oneself, so necessary for outstanding performance, is gone. He/she questions the reasons for the injury and how to prevent a recurrence. Being injured threatens not only an athlete's physical well-being, but acts as a threat to the athlete's self-concept, belief system, social and occupational functioning, values, commitments, and emotional equilibrium. In Table 27-1 some of these threats are categorized and considered in more detail. Thus, dealing with the injury exclusively without an understanding of how the injury may impact on the athlete's self-concept, future plans, and social roles may have a negative impact on the morale of the athlete and the rehabilitation process.

Table 27-1
The Potential Psychological Effects of Injuries and Athletes

1. Threats to bodily integrity and comfort (from the injury, the diagnostic procedures, or the medical treatment itself)
   - Bodily injury or disability
   - Permanent physical changes
   - Physical pain, discomfort, and other negative symptoms of the injury or treatment
   - Incapacitation
2. Threats to one's self-concept and future plans
   - Necessity to alter one's self-image or belief systems
   - Uncertainty about the course of the injury and about one's future
   - Endangering of life goals and values
   - Loss of autonomy and control
3. Threats to one's emotional equilibrium, that is, the necessity to deal with feelings of anxiety, anger, and other emotions that come about as a result of other stresses described
4. Threats to the fulfillment of customary social roles and activities
   - Separation from family, friends, and other social supports
   - Loss of important social roles
   - Necessity to depend on others
5. Threats involving the need to adjust to a new physical or social environment
   - Adjustment to the hospital setting
   - Problems in understanding medical terminology and customs
   - Necessity for decision-making in stressful and unfamiliar settings

Adapted from Cohen and Lazarus.[7]

Coping with Stresses of Injury

There is considerable clinical evidence that athletes with similar injuries recover at different rates of speed. Some of these differences can be attributed to the athlete's coping strategies. Coping is defined as one's efforts, both action-oriented an intrapsychic, to master environmental and internal demands that exceed a person's resources.[8]

The coping process starts, and is greatly influenced by, the appraisal made of the situation. Appraisals consist of an evaluation of the significance of the event (injury) on the individual's well-being, and on an assessment of the resources available for coping. For example, when an athlete is injured and cannot compete, the significance of the injury is greater than when an attorney is injured and is unable to compete athletically but can continue his or her legal activities.

The extent of one's psychosocial resources also becomes a factor. Obviously, the more resources one has, the better one is able to cope. The appraisal determines whether one views the event (injury) as deleterious, essentially non-intrusive, or as an opportunity for growth.[9-11]

Once the appraisal is complete, the individual begins to implement the coping strategies. Several coping processes or modes can be identified: taking direct action, using intrapsychic mechanisms, and seeking social support.[7,11] Taking direct action involves the use of intrapersonal skills such as setting goals, seeking relevant information, rehearsing alternative outcomes, and learning specific injury-related procedures.

Taking action is often the result of what Janis[12] has called the "work of worry." Experiencing a *moderate* amount of anticipatory fear about the treatment and rehabilitation process may promote a positive coping response. Coping through direct actions often facilitates rehabilitation by making the athlete self-directed, aggressive, and unwilling to accept the dependent patient role. By taking some control of the situation, the athlete feels more responsible for the treatment process.

Kubler-Ross[13] identified a sequence of psychological reactions followed by a patient facing death. These are disbelief, denial, and isolation; anger; bargaining; depression; and acceptance and resignation. Rotella[14] has suggested that these intrapsychic processes apply to athletes facing injuries as well. While the defense mechanisms experienced by injured athletes may differ somewhat from those identified by Kubler-Ross, such intrapsychic processes do occur. Further, in certain situations, such as when the athlete is feeling helpless, this coping process may be of real value. However, as with the use of defense mechanisms in general, too much reliance on them may hinder the rehabilitation process.

The final mode of coping is seeking social support from others. Supportive networks such as family, friends, and teammates often serve as a buffer to the experience of stress. Consequently, the treatment and recovery process is often enhanced by social support.[15]

An individual may use one or more of these methods of coping. Essentially one will try anything that works. If the coping strategies are successful, the individual will reduce the harmful effects of the injury and enhance the prospects of recovery, be able to adjust to or tolerate the events being encountered, maintain a positive self-image and emotional equilibrium, and continue satisfying relationships with others.

The purpose of this section has been to develop a framework for understanding the psychological effects of an athletic injury on the athlete's likely reaction.[5] If the health care professional understands what the athlete is experiencing *and* can respond to the athlete in a manner which communicates this understanding, the athlete is more likely to feel that the health care professionals can be helpful. The development of this rapport is crucial to the success of a rehabilitation program. As will be seen in the next section, rapport between the health care professional and athlete is a necessary component for increasing the level of compliance to the treatment.

FROM THEORY TO PRACTICE: A PROGRAM TO INCREASE COMPLIANCE

Compliance or adherence to medical regimens is notoriously poor. Based on a large body of research, it has been estimated that one-third to one-half of all patients fail to follow the treatment prescribed for them.[16–18] Noncompliance has been described as the least understood health behavior.[16] Numerous variables have been tested in an effort to explain and predict the phenomenon. These variables fall into four main categories: patient characteristics, characteristics of the illness, quality of the interaction between the expert and the patient, and the characteristics of the prescribed regimen. The patient's age, sex, religion, education, socioeconomic status, and personality have been found to be unrelated to adherence, as have the characteristics of the illness.[19] On the other hand, both the quality of the interaction between the health care professional and patient and the nature of the regimen have been found to influence compliance.

When patients do not feel understood, do not find the health care professional warm and friendly, and are intimidated by the technical terminology, noncompliance is likely. Furthermore, when the regimen is complex, requires considerable change in the patients' life-style, and is given to them without any of their input, adherence levels decrease. Rosenstock[20] developed the Health Beliefs model to explain under what circumstances health measures would be followed. The elements identified were: belief that the nature of the threat is sufficiently severe to constitute a danger to well-being, belief that a specific action has benefits which will protect against the threat, and belief that the costs in taking action outweighed the threat. Costs might include financial costs, pain, and inconvenience. In sum, then, the keys to reducing compliance according to Rosenstock and his colleagues are the perceived susceptibility, the perceived seriousness, the perceived benefits of taking action, and the perceived barriers to taking action. *Readiness is determined from the individual's perspective, not the professional's perspective.* For a change to take place it must be based on a want or need, not an ought to, should, or have to.

The term "ought to" is synonymous with *compliance.* As delineated by Kelman,[21] compliance is one of the three levels of motivation individuals may choose when reacting to injuries and illnesses. Compliance occurs when an individual's motivation is to gain external rewards, avoid punishment, or do something because they are supposed to. The performance of the behavior is seen as required, and maintenance is not likely to occur. When an athlete follows a regimen without an understanding of why and without a commitment to it, it is compliance. Motivation to continue the program will be low.

A higher level of motivation is *identification*. Patients follow the regimen in an effort to please the health care professional or to be part of the group. Satisfaction is derived from conforming. Problems occur with maintenance and transfer of these behaviors because the patient will not likely follow the regimen in the natural setting. In other words, the injured athletes may work at rehabilitation only in the training room where they can impress the health care professional and be part of the group rehabilitating an injury.

The highest level of motivation is *internalization*. Internalization occurs when the behaviors are performed because they are meaningful to the patient as well as the health care professional. The athlete, then, is working for him or herself and not for the health care professional. The treatment is seen as intrinsically rewarding because it is perceived as being effective.

Given the definition of compliance and the lack of inherent rewards in certain activities, it is understandable that athletes often do not follow treatment regimens. Developing intrinsic motivation to rehabilitate is difficult. It may be that injured athletes go through all three levels of motivation in successful treatment programs.

Reducing Delay in Initial Treatment

Understanding the Health Beliefs model, the reasons for noncompliance, and the stresses experienced by injured athletes helps explain why they may delay coming for help. They fear losing playing time. They are frightened that the rehabilitation may be worse than the injury itself. Equally as important, they often don't feel understood. They feel as if they are being treated as a lateral meniscus or an osteochondral fracture, and not as individuals. Consequently, if they can, they often minimize the injury and continue playing. Perhaps they seek advice from "knowledgeable" friends. Unless the injury is serious, you may be the last to know.

The first step in reducing the delay is having the athlete recognize that you understand the consequences of injuries to athletes and are concerned about him or her as a person. The development of such rapport probably begins before the injury occurs. You must have conveyed caring and concern previously. This caring is communicated through your nonverbal behavior (eye contact, posture, head and facial movements), verbal behavior, and your ability to understand the athlete as a person. Developing this rapport is a skill-learning process similar to the skills required for implementing some of the treatment modalities. Just as reading about how to do an arthroscopy will not produce a skilled surgeon, reading about developing rapport or being empathic will not produce a skilled communicator. Learning skills, any skills, entails *describing*, *demonstrating*, and *practicing*[22] each facet or component of the skill. In the same way that courses and training programs exist for new surgical procedures, they exist for developing communication skills.

It is impossible to present a complete program as part of this chapter, however, some strategies for understanding and communicating with patients will be considered. Some of the material is based on a training program entitled *Helping Skills: A Basic Training Program*.[23]

Strategies for Understanding and Communicating with the Athlete

The following questions and considerations should help you determine what the athlete is experiencing and how to begin the communication process.

1. If you are with the athlete when the injury occurs or detect anxiety when you see the athlete, focus your initial attention on the athlete as a person, not the injury. Attempt to quiet and calm down the person. Watching the reactions of the athlete to the injury should provide important information about the athlete's initial physical and emotional state.

2. If you have had contact with the athlete previously, questions such as how well you get along and what kind of person he or she is are crucial to consider. Having had previous contact with athletes may provide an indication of how they will relate to you. Are you trusted; are you seen as being supportive and understanding? If so, your changes for making an impact are heightened. Also, previous contact with the athlete may enable you to predict how he or she will react to the injury. For example, some athletes will focus on physical pain, others on the impact of the injury on other

aspects of their lives, and still others may feel relief because they can now avoid practice and the pressures of competition for a period of time. Previous contact will also give you some information about the athlete's tolerance for pain.

3. After the athlete has had time to react to the psychological ramifications of the injury, which threat listed in Table 27-1 do you think the athlete considers paramount? Some of the threats may be seen as more pressing than others given the nature of the injury and the situation. It is necessary to consider the threats from the athlete's perspective. It is not helpful, and in fact may be harmful, to speculate on how you would react to the injury or on how you believe the athlete should react. In other words, try to separate your own reactions from the athlete's and understand how the athlete is experiencing the injury.

4. How do you think the athlete feels about the injury and its consequence? Once you can understand the athlete's beliefs and thoughts, it is helpful to identify his or her feelings. Feelings refer to the emotions being experienced, eg, frustration, shock, anger, relief, cheated, disappointment, upset, etc. They are usually something experienced in the heart and/or stomach as opposed to the head. For example, one can *feel* shattered or empty, but one *believes* the injury to be unfair.

5. Communicate to the athlete your understanding of the situation and his or her feelings. Understanding and communicating this understanding are two different processes. When an understanding has been developed, communication becomes the key. It is helpful to summarize your understanding of how the athlete is experiencing the injury and the feelings associated with the perceived threat. Such a statement might be: "From what you've said, it seems that you are concerned that the injury may affect your future plans and that makes you feel disjointed. Right now the pain almost seems secondary. You also wonder how your teammates will treat you if you're not playing . . ."

In making your response, avoid asking questions, especially closed-ended ones. Closed-ended questions are ones which actually limit conversation by calling for a yes or no, or a one- or two-word answer. By summarizing and reflecting, you are communicating your understanding and encouraging a response.

6. Next consider the different coping modes. What way is the athlete likely to cope or what way is the athlete presently coping with injury? As you consider the coping modes, it is useful to consider whether the athlete has the resources to cope. It may be important to point out certain resources to the athlete. It also may be possible to facilitate the coping process. For example, you may know of another athlete rehabilitating from a similar injury who could serve as a model or source of support.

7. Finally, as you have previously learned, it is valuable to communicate your understanding of the athlete's coping mode to him or her. Demonstrating your understanding of how the athlete is or will be coping is a means of making a transition between the "understanding and rapport building phase" and the "rehabilitation program" phase. You might say: "You're not sure how best to deal with the injury. Sometimes you blame yourself for trying to do more than you should but when you really sort out your feelings it seems that all you want to do is find out what is involved in rehabilitation and get started. Both feelings are reasonable at different times. It is easier sometimes to wish it didn't happen. However, when you're ready, I'm ready to get started designing a rehabilitation program with you."

Strategies for Developing Treatment Plans

For rehabilitation to succeed, the patient must be considered the agent for guiding his or her own program. The way in which the patient construes the injury then becomes crucial to effective self-management. Therefore, the choice of treatment must be, in part, mediated by the closeness of fit of the treatment to the patient's understanding of the problem and how it can be treated.[24]

Patients, in general, tend to be concerned about a number of kinds of information: 1) information about the nature of the injury or about the medical reasons for initiating particular treatments, 2) information about the goals of the treatment, 3) information describing in detail the medical procedures to be carried out, 4) information about particular sensations or side effects to be expected, and 5) information about coping strategies the person can use in adjusting to the upcoming threat.[7] Involving the patient in the planning and implementation will provide the patient with the information they seek.

The initial step of planning is goal setting. It is likely that you and the athlete may have different goals. Your ultimate goal should be to return the athlete to participation as quickly and as safely as possible at a level of competence in terms of the athlete's physical, mental, and emotional state equal to or better than the pre-injury level. While the athlete may agree with this goal in general, the specifics may differ. Athletes often focuses on how quickly they can return. In addition they may want to be assured no effect of the injury will remain. Discussion between you and the athlete about the general goals of rehabilitation are going to be important. Explaining your goals and providing information about the *possible* consequences of the injury is the first part of goal setting.

How the ultimate rehabilitation goal is to be achieved is the second step. Once the initial pain of the injury has subsided, the restoration and maintenance of motion, strength, endurance, and power begins.[25] This stage is difficult and often trying for the athlete. Without strong motivation and "teamwork" between you and the athlete, progress may be slow and frustrating. It is here that having the athlete set specific goals becomes most valuable.

While it may be sufficient to have the athlete involved in every level of decision with regard to rehabilitation, having the athlete determine specific goals with your participation makes the rehabilitation process a more collaborative venture. Moreover, the responsibility for success becomes, in great part, the athlete's. The process of setting goals is difficult. While the energy involved in attaining the goal is considerable, if the goal is not identified clearly and in a form which makes achievement possible, all the energy expended is useless.

Goal setting begins then with goal assessment. Goal assessment involves three parts: goal identification, goal importance, and delineating the barriers to achieving the goal.[11] Goal identification involves the specification of a positive, behavioral goal. A positive goal is emphasized because goals which include negatives involve a large expenditure of attention and energy on a behavior to avoid rather than a behavior an athlete wants to achieve. Encouraging athletes to state goals in a behavioral way provides a clear endpoint for evaluating whether or not the goal was reached. Using these criteria, goals such as "I don't want my ankle to hurt" and "I want to be back to normal" would be inappropriate. The first goal is behavioral, but negative. The second goal is positive, but not behavioral. An example of a positive behavioral goal is "I want to develop range of motion in my ankle by March 1. To do this I must practice range of motion exercises, three sets of 10 every day, with at least one of the sets being done in the whirlpool." When such specificity is determined, you can provide reality testing by determining how possible such a goal is. If, in your opinion, the goal is based on wishful thinking or overly demanding expectations, you should discuss your impressions with the athlete and see if the goal can be altered somewhat. However, it is probably better to allow athletes to maintain their "unrealistic" goals if they want to and fail rather than to "force more reasonable" goals on them. The most important aspect of goal identification is that the determination of positive, behavioral goals provides an opportunity for athletes to initiate and then evaluate their actions.

In addition to setting positive and behaviorally-stated goals, the importance of the goal must be assessed. Goals which are more important to significant others, such as coaches, parents, or friends, are less likely to be attained than goals which are important to the athlete. Achieving goals takes energy, and if athletes are setting goals to please another person, maintenance of the rehabilitation program over a long period of time is unlikely.

Once the goal has been set and its importance determined, it is necessary to recognize what barriers and roadblocks exist to goal achievement. In other words, what will or is likely to prevent the athlete from achieving the goal? Four roadblocks have been identified which may interfere with goal achievement: a lack of knowledge, a lack of skill, an inability to assess the risks involved in reaching the goal, and a lack of social support. A lack of knowledge refers to not having information or facts which prevents goal achievement. For example, the athlete may not know what is wrong with him or her or what rehabilitation processes are necessary. Lack of knowledge would, therefore, be the roadblock interfering with goal achievement. You will probably be the main source of this kind of information for the athletes. When athletes lack skills they may know what to do, but not how to do it. Skills can be either physical or mental. For example, the athlete may not know how to do a certain exercise or may not have the necessary self-control to work toward a goal. When the athlete lacks skills you may become a teacher of skills, even mental ones. Some athletes know what to do and how to achieve their goals but are afraid to initiate the necessary actions because of the risks involved. Risks are the benefits of an action minus the costs. When the costs outweigh the benefits, the risk is too great and actions are rarely taken. Thus, athletes may want to rehabilitate and may know how but are afraid that if they try, they may not be able to play effectively again or will re-injure themselves, and therefore, do not want to take the risk. You may want to help the athlete carefully evaluate

Table 27-2
Rehabilitation Goal Setting Guide

I. *Goal Assessment*

A. Describe your rehabilitation goal in positive, behavioral terms.
____
____

B. To whom is the goal most important?
____ me
____ friends
____ family
____ coach
____ someone else; if so, whom? ____________

C. Is the goal based on:
____ realistic expectations
____ wishful thinking
____ Other factors; describe: ____________
____

D. How will attaining this goal affect your life?
____
____

E. Do you think you can achieve this goal?
____ yes
____ no

F. What are the realistic problems you will face in trying to achieve the goal?
____
____

G. Goal Roadblock Analysis What is your understanding of the barriers you must overcome to achieve the goal?
____ Knowledge roadblock. Describe. ________
____
What do you need to know? ________
____
____ Skill roadblock. Describe. ________
____
What skills do you need? ________
____
____ Risk-taking roadblock. Describe. ________
____
What risks do you have to take? ________
____
____ Social support roadblock. Describe. ________
____
What social supports do you need? ________
____
____ Some combination of knowledge, skills, risk-taking, and social support. Describe. ________
____

II. *Goal Attainment*

A. Identify the rehabilitation steps using the Goal Ladder. Are the steps small and manageable? If not, divide the most complex step. More than ten steps is possible.

GOAL LADDER

GOAL ______________________
____

Steps	Time Frame (in # of weeks or by date)
10	
9	
8	
7	
6	
5	
4	
3	
2	
1	

B. With what step(s), if any, are you likely to have trouble? ________
What kind of help will assist you to overcome this trouble? ________
____
Who can offer this assistance? ________

Adapted from Danish.[30]

the benefits and costs. The final roadblock has to do with the lack of social support. Even when athletes know how and are willing to rehabilitate, the lack of support from important people in their lives may inhibit action. You may be one of these important people. Therefore, being positive and supportive during both the good times and the bad times will be essential. Social support is especially crucial in maintaining new behaviors.

It is very possible that more than one roadblock can interfere with goal achievement. It is the health care professional's job to know what the roadblocks are and to help the athlete devise strategies to overcome them so rehabilitation goals can be achieved.

The focus on roadblocks adds a new dimension to understanding why some athletes may not follow treatment regimens. Usually the assumption is made that the athlete is not sufficiently motivated. While this may be true, two other possible reasons for noncompliance should be examined—lack of mental skills and inability to take the risk. For example, failure to maintain a regimen may be due to the athlete's lack of mental skills such as self-control or time management. We can all remember important things that we don't get done because we cannot organize our lives effectively. Assuming it is a lack of motivation is too often a simplistic explanation. Another possible explanation involves risk taking. Rehabilitation often involves pain without a clear indication that the pain will result in full recovery. Athletes unaccustomed to injury may be afraid of undergoing the pain, especially if the outcome is in doubt. The fear of re-injury when the athlete is once again able to compete may also hinder the athlete from full participation in the rehabilitation regimen.

Once a workable rehabilitation goal has been identified, the process of goal attainment can begin. Setting and attaining goals are two distinct steps. While the process of goal setting influences how easily goals can be attained, the real work for the athlete occurs after the goal is set—during the actual rehabilitation period.

Because the rehabilitation process is often very lengthy and time-consuming, athletes may be prone to give up or get easily discouraged. For this reason, the process of attaining the goal must be divided into small manageable steps so the athlete can see the progress being made and the route that must be taken. When breaking the goal down into steps it is essential that the first steps be especially small and manageable so that a successful experience is developed. There is no predetermined series of steps or time sequence for a particular injury. Injuries are different and athletes rehabilitate at different rates. However, constructing a treatment ladder with the athlete which includes projected dates often proves to be a motivating force.

Several authors[25,26] have provided general treatment programs for various injuries. For example, Scott[25] describes a general regimen involving restoration and maintenance of motion, strength and endurance, and the refinement of motor skills. Roy and Ervin[26] present a specific five-stage rehabilitation program for ankle injuries. Programs such as these, combined with some of the mental training approaches,[14,27-30] may serve as the basis for the rehabilitation ladder. In Table 27-2 a guide, including a rehabilitation ladder, is presented to assist the athlete in designing a goal-oriented regimen.

In this section we have focused on techniques and strategies for developing and implementing a rehabilitation program for athletes. We have identified two major components of a comprehensive program; developing rapport and understanding between the athlete and the health care professional; and developing a goal-oriented approach to treating and restoring the injury. When these techniques and strategies are used within the framework presented in the chapter, the health care professional works with a more motivated athlete and the rehabilitation process is enhanced.

ACKNOWLEDGMENT

The author would like to thank Angela Carlson and Linda Tardiff for their comments and suggestions and Joseph Smey, David Tiberio, and Michael Zito for providing the opportunity to develop a better understanding of the rehabilitation process.

REFERENCES

1. White, S.W. (Ed.). Sports in America. *National Forum* 2-42, 1982.

2. Ogilvie, B., Tutko, T. Sport: If you want to build character, try something else. *Psychology Today* 5:61-63, 1971.

3. von Bertalanffy, L. *General Systems Theory*. New York: Braziller, 1968.

4. Schwartz G.E. The brain as a health care system. Edited by G.C. Stone, F. Cohen, N.E. Adler, and Associates. In *Health Psychology—A Handbook*. San Francisco: Jossey-Bass, 1979, pp 549-573.

5. Miller, J.G. *Living Systems*. New York: McGraw-Hill, 1978.

6. Gruen, W. Effects of brief psychotherapy during the hospitalization period on the recovery process in heart attacks. *J Clin Consult Psychol* 43:223-233, 1975.

7. Cohen, F., Lazarus, R.S. Coping with the stresses of illness. Edited by G.C. Stone, F. Cohen, N.E. Adler and Associates. In *Health Psychology—A Handbook*. San Francisco: Jossey-Bass, 1979, pp 217-255.

8. Lazarus, R.S., Laurier, R. Stress-related transactions between person and environment. Edited by L.A. Pervin, M. Lewis. In *Perspectives in International Psychology*. New York: Plenum Press, 1978.

9. Danish, S.J., Smyer, M.S., Nowak, C.A. Developmental intervention: Enhancing life-event processes. Edited by P.B. Baltes, O.G. Brim, Jr. In *Life-span Development and Behavior* (vol. 3). New York: Academic Press, 1981, pp 339-366.

10. Danish, S.J. Musing about personal competence: The contributions of sport, health, and fitness. *Am J Community Psychol* 11:221-240, 1983.

11. Danish, S.J., D'Augelli, A.R. *Helping Skills II: Life Development Intervention*. New York: Human Sciences Press, 1983.

12. Janis, I.L. *Psychological Stress: Psycho-*

analytic and Behavioral Studies of Surgical Patients. New York: Wiley, 1958.

13. Kubler-Ross E. *On Death and Dying.* New York: Macmillan, 1969.

14. Rotella, R.J. Psychological care of the injured athlete. Edited by D.N. Kulund. *The Injured Athlete.* Philadelphia: J. B. Lippincott, 1982, pp 213–224.

15. Wallston, B.S., Alagna, S.W., DeVellis, B.E., et al. Social support and physical health. *Health Psychol* 2:367–392, 1983.

16. Becker, M.H., Maiman, L.A. Sociobehavioral determinants of compliance with health care and medical care recommendations. *Med Care* 13:10–24, 1975.

17. Sackett, D.L. The magnitude of compliance and noncompliance. Edited by D.L. Sackett, R.B. Hayes. *Compliance with Therapeutic Regimens.* Baltimore: Johns Hopkins University Press, 1976.

18. Stone, G.C. Patient compliance and the role of the expert. *J Soc Issues* 35:34–55, 1979.

19. Haynes, R.B. A critical review of the 'determinants' of patient compliance with therapeutic regimens. Edited by D.L. Sackett, R.B. Hayes. *Compliance with Therapeutic Regimens.* Baltimore: Johns Hopkins University Press, 1976.

20. Rosenstock, I.M. Why people use health services. *Millbank Memorial Fund Quarterly* 44: 94–127, 1966.

21. Kelman, H.S. Compliance, identification, and internalization: Three processes of opinion exchange. *J Conflict Resolution* 2:51–60, 1958.

22. Danish, S.J., Galambos, N.L., Laquatra, I. Life development intervention: Skill training for personal competence. Edited by R.D. Felner, L.A. Jason, J. Moritsugu, et al. *Preventive Psychology: Theory, Research, and Practice.* Elmsford, New York: Pergamon Press, 1983, pp 49–66.

23. Danish, S.J., D'Augelli, A.R., Hauer, A.L. *Helping Skills: A Basic Training Program* (2nd). New York: Human Sciences Press, 1980.

24. Turk, D.C., Meichenbaum, D., Genest, M. *Pain and Behavioral Medicine: A Cognitive-Behavioral Perspective.* New York: Guilford Press, 1983.

25. Scott, S.G. Current concepts in the rehabilitation of the injured athlete. *Mayo Clinical Proceedings* 59:83–90, 1984.

26. Roy, S., Irwin, R. *Sports Medicine: Prevention, Evaluation, Management, and Rehabilitation.* Englewood Cliffs, New Jersey: Prentice-Hall, 1983.

27. Danish, S.J., Krimmel, R.S. Mental imagery: The swimmer's edge. *Penn J Health, Phys Ed, Recreation Drama* 54:2–3, 1984.

28. Danish, S.J. You play the way you talk to yourself. *NAGWS Bowling/Golf Guide* 85:131–135, 1983.

29. Danish, S.J., Hale, B.D. Sport psychology: Teaching skills to athletes and coaches. *J Phys Ed, Recreation and Dance* 73:11–13, 80–81, 1983.

30. Danish, S.J. Goal setting for athletic excellence. Manuscript submitted for publication.

CHAPTER 28
The Role of the Trainer

Steven T. Gaunya, RPT
Earl F. Hoerner, MD

The trainer assists the athlete by preparing him for maximum performance in competitive athletics, shielding him from possibly damaging sequelae, and restoring him to maximum performance should injury occur.

Medical care is concerned with preparation of the athlete for competition, protection of the athlete from injuries by way of specific conditioning regimens, and rehabilitation of the athlete following injury. These principles apply to both the novice athlete and the champion.

Our knowledge of the training of athletes is derived from three sources: 1) traditional beliefs and practices, 2) writings of historians, and 3) scientific investigation.

TRADITIONAL BELIEFS AND PRACTICES

Much of man's information concerning the training of athletes and care of athletic injuries is thousands of years old. Many of our traditional beliefs and practices stem from our ancestors' efforts for survival. The hunter's urgent need to continue providing impelled him to search for methods of promoting more rapid healing of his injuries. The medicine man was considered a member of the learned profession of medicine and he utilized herbs and heat to treat his patients and to speed up the healing process.

WRITINGS OF HISTORIANS

Much of Cretan culture spread across the Mediterranean Sea to ancient Hellas, the site of the first written records of training regimens. The Olympian games were first held in some time prior to 776 BC, probably in honor of the dead. Competitors were expected to spend ten months in hard training. A training schedule was provided and an upper age limit of 35 was established. Women were banned both as participants and as spectators.

Spartans viewed athletics as part of military training and as a means of developing beauty and harmony of body and spirit. Socrates (470 to 399 BC), himself a distinguished warrior, spoke of body training as a priority goal for health and strength.

The first team physician with specialized knowledge of the treatment of athletic injuries appears to have been Galen (131 to 201 AD) who tended the gladiators. He said that exercise: 1) produced strength by hardening the organs, 2) increased the respiration and intrinsic body warmth, 3) produced improved nutrition, 4) produced better metabolism, and 5) stimulated better elimination of waste materials. Galen stated that all men should regulate their exercise, food, and sleep by one word: moderation.

However, athletes preparing for competition practiced immoderately, sometimes all day at their objective. The athlete required the services of a trainer to teach him the necessary motor skills and a physician to advise him what to do to produce a desired effect in the body.

Following the fall of Rome and with the ascendance of Christian doctrine, the body was considered worthy only of contempt and humiliation. The church emphasized intellectual learning and neglected the development of the body. Athletic training during the Dark Ages was used primarily for training the fighting men.

The wars of the 18th century aroused an interest in the role of athletics as means of increasing the fitness and patriotism of youth. From this movement arose Ling's system of medical gymnastics in Sweden. This system of formal exercise was introduced into the United States and certain of Ling's calisthenic exercises are used in athletics today as warm-up and conditioning routines.

The American youth has long insisted that his physical training be achieved through competitive sports. This thinking leaves much to be desired, as a period of formal, specific exercise training is required to achieve athletic success.

Rowing was the first competitive sport in American colleges with established training routines prior to competition. At the time of the first intercollegiate football game in the United States in 1869 the athletic trainer was generally a masseur or an expugilist without technical preparation or professional education. The field has progressed until today it is highly specialized and professional.

PROCEDURAL MANUALS

Health care is one of the fastest moving sectors of today's society. Athletic training is a component of that sector in which the trainer acts as the administrator, managing personnel and material resources.

Concern with budgetary expenditures for supplies and equipment, capital costs, and personnel, plus a growing demand for services through the development of women's sports have further pressured the trainer into an administrative role. Establishment of a policy and procedural manual can be a valuable tool in the trainer's effectiveness.

The procedural and policy manual is a document that evolved from requests by regulatory agencies (Joint Commission on Accreditation of Hospitals, insurance companies, etc) for formal rules and regulations to standardize trainers' modes of operation and to assure delivery of quality health care.

Policy serves as a criterion on what is to be done. Procedure complements policy as defining how things are to be done. The manual should be written by the athletic trainer in consultation with the athletic director, team or institutional physician, and any other medical or administrative person directly involved with the athletic training program. To insure medicolegal correctness, the document should be reviewed by an attorney.

The manual can be divided into four parts:

1. statement of purpose or function,
2. personnel policies,
3. operational procedures, and
4. fiscal policies.

The introductory statement of purpose or function is the definition of philosophy from which an athletic training program operates. As a measure of justifying the program's presence, the statement defines its role within the context of the institution's athletic commitment. A training program's objectives must be compatible with those of the athletic department and the institution.

In formulating the statement of purpose the following points are to be considered:

1. Purpose of the program—defines the degree and measures of involvement in care and prevention of injuries to participants in the program. It specifies if care is extended to the athlete during the off-season, and if so, the mechanism of referral and treatment.
2. Intrainstitutional status—clarifies involvement of the training program with regard to treating students, staff, and faculty, and the manner of referral and medical direction during treatment. If the athletic training program serves as a clinical setting for an athletic training curriculum or any other educational program, it should specify the criteria for supervision and evaluation of students' level of involvement in the management of athletic injuries.
3. Community relationship—often an established athletic training program is requested to make available its resources to individuals from outside the institution. High school, amateur, and recreational athletes, are in areas that often lack accessibility to a formal sportsmedicine program and approach the athletic trainer for health care. To prevent abuses of the training room facility, there should be stipulated the extent outside parties are allowed to use the services of the room and staff.
4. Educational activities—as in any health care profession, athletic trainers should be aware of the opportunity to educate those associated with athletics to the aims and objectives of athletic training. This form of public relations can be achieved through many forums: clinics, workshops, articles, and media presentations.

Personnel Policies

Concise description of personnel policies is essential through recognized guidelines such as job descriptions and qualifications, salary and benefits,

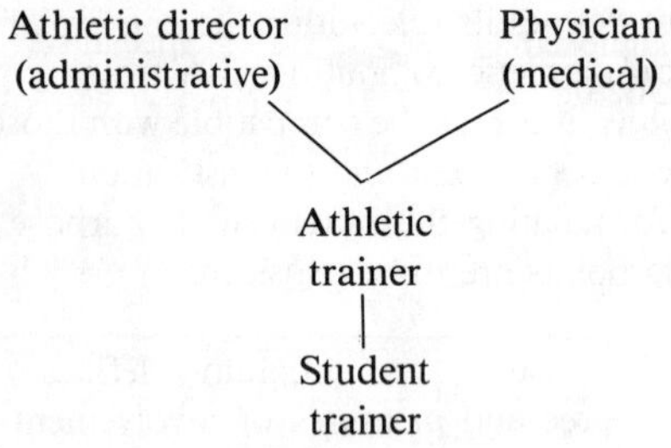

Figure 28-1 Personnel organizational chart.

and hiring mechanisms. Other areas are standards for evaluation and promotion of staff. Figure 28-1 is a line chart depicting an organizational and reporting system. For example, the student athletic trainer reports to the athletic trainer on medical and administrative problems. In turn, the athletic trainer reports to the athletic director on administrative matters but to the team or referring physician on medical problems and situations.

The job description informs the individual on qualifications and responsibilities assigned to the position. It should be detailed to prevent any misunderstanding encountered about the job. An athletic trainer, for example, could have the following job description:

1. educational and professional requirements, level or degree, licensure, or certification
2. level of experience
3. expertise in a specific area (exercise physiology, curriculum development).

Duties would include:

1. administer first aid and therapy
2. direct and supervise rehabilitation programs
3. direct daily training room operations
4. advise on equipment purchase and supervise equipment fitting
5. inspect playing facilities for safety factors
6. assist with medical examinations and physical fitness screening
7. training coverage of athletic events, home and away.

A similar job description should be used for the team physician, dentist, or other medical personnel employed by the athletic department. It should detail educational and professional qualifications, such as board certification in a medical specialty for a physician. The responsibility section should indicate coverage requirements and define medical duties:

1. determination of the medical criteria for participants
2. diagnosis and treatment of injuries and medical problems
3. supervision of training room operations
4. overall direction of health and medical aspects of sports.

Operational Section

The operational section is the most extensive part of a procedural manual. It defines the daily workings of the training room in handling athletic injuries and health problems. This section can be separated into the following areas:

1. Procedure for the care of injuries and health problems—specifies the methods and steps taken from initial complaint or evaluation and rendering first aid through referral to team doctor or dentist and ensuing medical care and treatment (Figure 28-2). To define and insure proper medicolegal channels, it may be appropriate to institute formal standing orders from the physician to the athletic trainer defining the amount and type of care that may be given with or without a physician's involvement. For example, if an athlete sprained an ankle, standing orders would indicate the manner of first aid and follow-up treatment to be used by the athletic trainer. Such a measure could place the athletic trainer into a position of serving as an agent of the physician in management of the injury. However, athletic trainers must check into the legality of using standing orders before implementing them, as in most cases legal statutes vary from state to state.

Also under this section should be the procedure for referring the athlete to specialists or, if requested by the athlete, to a physician not associated with the athletic program. This is important as many insurance policies stipulate that the athlete must be seen initially by the team or institutional physician before going elsewhere or the insurance company will not pay for medical costs incurred. Since the athlete's health is important at all times, mechanisms for an emergency medical

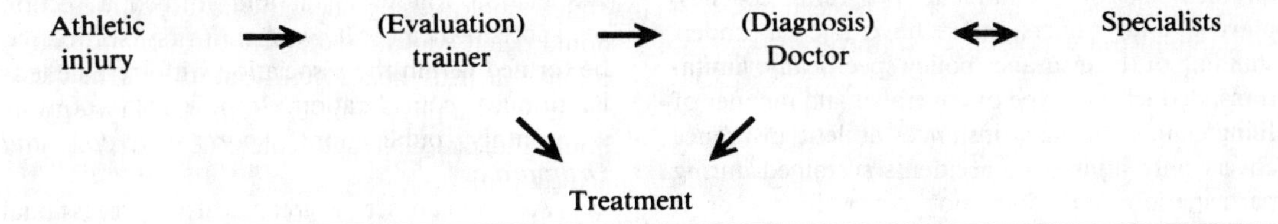

Figure 28-2 Steps of caring for an injured athlete.

referral system should be arranged to assure the availability of health care especially when the athletic trainer or team physician is unavailable.

2. Policy on injury information—this applies not only to the media, but also to the way in which the coach is appraised of an injured athlete's status. In dealing with the public, proper respect and confidentiality of the athlete should be observed. Designation of how, where, and by whom information is given to the press should be set forth, indicating approval of the athlete, coaching, and administrative staffs. Authorization releases should be employed in transfer of information and records to interested parties, such as recruiting colleges, and professional teams scouting for player draft. A daily injury status form may be used in notifying the coaching staff of the status of an injured athlete and the degree to which he may be able to participate during practice.

3. Training room management—covers the day-to-day operation of the training room and coverage of services to the athletic program. Among the components of this section are:

1. manner and availability of dispensing medication,
2. manner and method of record keeping,
3. coverage assignments by professional and student staff, what events are covered by whom and hours of operation that the training room is open,
4. specification on maintenance of facility and equipment,
5. procedure for obtaining emergency vehicle and medical assistance,
6. stocking supplies in the training room and medical kits,
7. specification as to athletes' conduct in the training room (loitering, attire, using equipment, requesting supplies).

In some instances to prevent misuse of equipment, standardized procedures for operating the various treatment modalities are also specified. This may be of value in programs where equipment is operated by more than one individual.

Fiscal Policies

An understanding of the financial funding of an athletic training program is essential in operating this service. Knowing the source of funds assists the trainer in establishing budgets and determing priorities in purchasing supplies and equipment.

Each institution or athletic program has a different manner of funding. This varies primarily between private or public status. In private or major university programs, funding may be derived from the resources of the intercollegiate athletic program, an entity in itself, and separate from the academic area of an institution. In such places, there may exist greater freedom with less administrative control of purchasing. Public institutions, on the other hand, must deal with a bureaucratic channel that proceeds through a maze of levels gathering approval for buying supplies or equipment. In many instances, bidding procedures are required by law for items purchased over a specified dollar amount. The following points should be included under fiscal policies:

1. position or person authorized to order and purchase supplies and equipment,
2. procedure for purchasing items,
3. source and manner of paying for items not included in budget,
4. inventory procedure and manner of issuing supplies,
5. timetable to be used in preparing a budget and ordering supplies.

The complexities and problems incurred in dealing with athletic insurance demand that information on this matter also be included in the procedural manual. Athletic insurance coverage varies according to the size, scope, and structure of the program. As a deterrent to any budding problem, all members of the athletic program: coaches, players, and trainers, must have a clear understanding of the insurance policy specifically: limitations, deductions, type of coverage, and manner of filing claims. In many instances athletic insurance covers only injuries or accidents sustained during participation and does not cover illness or a medical condition. Therefore, the athlete must be made aware of this situation and advised to have the necessary health insurance to supplement and cover for any medical costs incurred in such health problems. A special account or the use of a catastrophe insurance policy is usually established by athletic departments for extensive medical costs not covered by the normal policy or by a budgeted item.

Conclusion

Periodic revisal of the procedural manual is essential if the document is to be operational and in compliance with current standards of health care.

With time and research, a procedural manual can be formulated, streamlining the administrative function of an athletic training program. For the most part, this information is available, and all that is needed is for the athletic trainer to gather and organize the material.

SCIENTIFIC INVESTIGATION

The introduction of modern methods of scientific investigation into the fields of biology and medicine has resulted in a more accurate understanding of the body's functions and its response to injuries.

Athletic trainers in the United States formed the National Athletic Trainers Association in 1950 for the purpose of raising their professional standards and exchanging information. This organization publishes a quarterly journal and sponsors an annual athletic training clinic in the United States. Physicians and others interested in sportsmedicine organized the American College of Sports Medicine in 1954.

In 1962, the American Academy of Orthopedic Surgeons voted to form a specialized section on sportsmedicine to advance the knowledge and education of those physicians treating athletes. This was a significant step in the medical treatment and consideration of athletic injuries.

In 1974, the American Physical Therapy Association followed suit and formed a section of sportsmedicine. It was the first section to be formed within the association with treatment as its primary consideration. It now also sponsors a monthly publication: *Sports Therapy and Orthopedics*.

As one can see, a great deal of professional effort is being conducted and launched on the topic of injuries to athletes and their treatment. Many and varied health specialists are joining forces and sharing knowledge to improve the health and welfare of the competitive athlete in our society.

KINESIOLOGIC FACTORS IN COMPETITIVE ATHLETICS

Athletic performance is in large part a dynamic expression of the design of the human body.

The belief that an individual's morphology is related to his capacity for athletic achievement appeared early in written history. The Greek coaches classified their Olympic prospects as bear-, lion-, and eagle-athletes. Thus there are three general groups of athletes, ie, round, muscular, and slender.

Sheldon and Carter have classified athletes morphologically and correlated them with athletic performance. His method, termed somatotyping, was based upon the relative predominance of the particular embryonic layer from which the various body tissues are derived: endoderm, mesoderm, and ectoderm.

1. Endomorphy: roundness and softness of body; small bones, large head, short neck; central concentration of mass; short limbs and comparatively weak extremities; hypoplastic genitalia.
2. Mesomorphy: large, heavy bone; massive musculature, slender waist and board hips; genitalia nearly always well-developed.
3. Ectomorphy: thin bones; slight muscles and long thorax; usually hypertrophic genitalia.

Endomorphs are stronger than ectomorphs, but ectomorphs possess more speed, agility, and endurance.

Excess weight is a handicap to endomorphs and insufficient strength is a handicap to ectomorphs in performing physical tests. The physical performance of extreme somatotypes in motor and strength tests was studied by Sills and Everett.[1] In addition to the above, they also found that mesomorphs are stronger, more agile, and are superior in speed and endurance. However, mesomorphs had little or no relation to weight and taller individuals tend to have a less mesomorphic component. Thus, the combination in one individual of extreme height and the rugged characteristics of the mesomorph, which would constitute an ideal build for many sports, is seldom found.

Willgoose and Rogers[2] administered the Physical Fitness Index Test to 153 male college students. An average score of 100 points has been established on national norms in this test. They reported that extreme endomorphs scored 68.4 points, extreme mesomorphs scored 112.8 points, and extreme ectomorphs scored 102 points.

Obviously, all individuals are not extremes of any somatotype, but rather each individual possesses some degree of each of the three components. Each component exists in an individual and Sheldon suggests a numerical value on a scale of 1 (minimum) to 7 (maximum) for each of the three components.

Selection by morphologic means is an instrument in the coaches' armamentarium in the development of successful athletes. Although other factors, such as motivation and diligence in training, may override morphologic constituents, the athlete's chance for success is enhanced if he engages in sports well suited to his specific physical characteristics. These findings are well documented in the literature and are a part of recorded history.

PHYSIOLOGIC/PSYCHOLOGIC INTERACTION

The process of conditioning for athletics is a specific and absolutely deliberate one. Through repeated exposures graded in intensity and adhering to the physiologic principle of overload, the organism responds in two different ways:

1. by an improvement in the organization of the neurophysiologic mechanisms, represented and demonstrated quite dramatically by increases in agility and body quickness, and
2. by adaptive alterations in body tissues,[3] demonstrated by increases in strength, power, flexibility, and cardiovascular endurance.

The conditioning process is a stressful one in the terms of psychologic as well as physiologic tolerance levels. These levels are individual and what is stressful and painful to one may not be of sufficient stress to another to produce desirable physiologic change. This physiologic change in the organism is the goal of all well-planned and implemented physical conditioning regimens.[4]

Since the conditioning process is stressful, and at times seemingly unbearable (psychologic stress), the athlete should be educated as to the reasons for and direction of his program. He will be better prepared psychologically to endure the pain of fatigue, the daily dull aches of muscular effort, and the burning of laborious breathing. As training continues he will hurt less because he has an increased tolerance, arising from a gradually lessened sensitivity to the acid metabolites of muscular work and the irritating dryness of excessive ventilation.

Education and knowledge can best be presented by those specializing in exercise physiology. The minimal time required to present scientific data supporting strenuous and specific exercise regimens is of unmeasurable value to the competitive athlete. With tolerance to specific exercises improved by knowledge of conditioning principles, the athlete will be motivated to pay the price.

Learning to endure the pain of fatigue is necessarily an uncomfortable one. Aside from the lowering of sensitivity thresholds, certain homeostatic adjustments are taking place in the athlete's body as it becomes accustomed to increased metabolic demands. The blood circulates more freely, owing to more effective adjustments by the vasomotor system, which goes into action even before the activity is commenced and shifts the blood to the working muscles in just the right amounts as the work continues. Pulmonary ventilation keeps pace with the requirements for gaseous exchange rather than overresponding to the excitement of exercise, producing giddiness from chemical imbalance resulting from hyperventilation. The athlete no longer fights for air with a continually expanded chest, but permits a full excursion of his thoracodiaphragmatic bellows to provide efficient ventilation of his lungs.

The phenomenon termed second wind is a sensation that signals attainment of homeostatic adjustments during hard muscular steady-state exercise. Early in the work, before second wind occurs, there is a piling up of lactic acid and other metabolic acids. There is a lag in production of sweat, and peripheral dilation, and a lag in the vasomotor shifting of blood from splanchnic pools to the working musculature. As a result, the work is performed with difficulty and pain, the body becomes overheated, and the athlete feels sluggish. At the onset of second wind, the athlete experiences a sensation of sudden relief because of the homeostatic adjustments, in which energy production is facilitated and is balanced by the mechanisms of heat dissipation. The organism is now functioning adequately to support the intensity of the work underway.

In addition to the improvements of the organization of the neurophysiologic mechanisms previously described, training makes imprints upon the organism that are marked enough to differentiate the athletes from nonathletes.[5] There is a power-giving hypertrophy of muscles, heart, and skeletal musculature. The heart beats at a slower rhythm, delivering a greater volume at each stroke. Previously dormant alveolar capsules on the lungs' surface provide for the passage of gases between the lungs and the oxygen-hungry bloodstream. Through the blood flow induced by vigorous exercise, aged and fragile blood corpuscles are replaced by young and vigorous ones. Increased chemical buffers in the blood can handle larger amounts of the waste acids of metabolism. The working muscles receive improved irrigation and nourishment through the abundant capillary system which has been opened in response to the physical demands of a strenuous exercise regimen.

Nothing but vigorous exercise will bring about these physiologic changes. The rewards of training are not the gifts of any age, sex, or race; they are the hard-earned rewards of exhausting effort and are attainable by those willing to pay the price.

THE QUADRATIC TRAINING CYCLE or A Trainer's Approach to Decreasing Football Injuries

Preparing an athlete for maximum physical performance in competitive athletics is a major objective of any training and/or conditioning regimen. Training must be thought of principally in terms of prevention of injury. Coaches and medical staff alike now recognize that a lack of physical fitness is one of the prime causes of athletic injury.

Muscular imbalance, improper timing due to poor neuromuscular coordination, a lack of ligamentous or tendinous strength, lack of flexibility, and inadequate muscle bulk, are among the causes of injury directly attributable to insufficient or improper physical conditioning. Conditioning and proper medical rehabilitation rank among the most vital factors in the ultimate success of the individual athlete, and show a direct correlation to total team effort and objectives. The athlete's contribution to the success of the team will be directly related to his physiologic and psychologic readiness and ability to participate to his maximum potential.

The Quadratic Training Cycle, is designed to develop the athlete to his maximum potential. At the present time, there are no pharmacologic ergogenic aids that can be safely used to promote the fitness quality necessary for success in professional football. A hard contest demands a hard training regimen. The objectives of the Quadratic Training Cycle are to promote maximum individual fitness and motor performance based on principles of exercise training.

Injuries are of major importance in determining a team's chance for success or failure. A summary of current findings by many researchers follows.

1. Medical questionnaires are vital to isolate and identify the players entire history of injury, from high school to professional level, to prevent development of permanent disability and/or ineffectiveness.
2. The law of natural selection can be used to weed injury-prone people out of football programs from high school to the first two to three years of professional activity.
3. Professional football has traditionally shown a penny-wise, pound-foolish approach to the whole problem of prevention of injuries and rehabilitation for key personnel. The players' association, insurance payments, compensation laws, and the pro football image have all contributed to this problem.
4. A three-year collection of statistics in Seattle showed no appreciable difference in injury rate between natural and artificial surfaces.
5. Tight-jointed athletes will tend to suffer muscle pulls and/or bone breaks, while loose-jointed athletes will suffer ligamentous injuries.

6. One out of four athletes will require some kind of surgery during his professional career.
7. The biggest single factor contributing to injury is momentum.
   a) The safest position in football is offensive center, because the area is congested and momentum is low.
   b) Offense is safer than defense because the player is aware of the hit or contact before it comes.
   c) Special teams are the least safe positions, with chances of being injured three times greater than those of an offensive or defensive regular.
   d) After special teams most danger is to the running backs, followed by the wide receivers, defensive ends, and line backers. Offensive linemen and defensive tackles are relatively safe from injury.
8. Proper and specific physical conditioning is imperative in the prevention and/or minimization of athletic injuries. Thus, development of the Quadratic Training Cycle. Professional athletes traditionally have looked for an easy answer to fatigue. The athlete by nature tends to be a prima donna of sorts, and does not want to pay the price of strenuous physical conditioning. It is this conditioning process which is vital to his decreased susceptibility to injury and to his ultimate success and contribution to team objectives. The easy road the athlete seeks often leads to a trail of drug abuse. Medical research leads to the scientific approach as a means of arresting the problems related to fatigue and resultant athletic injury. The scientific method and available research data direct us to the specificity of exercise training for competitive athletes.

The Quadratic Training Cycle strives to promote and develop necessary fitness levels for maximum athletic performance. Injury prevention is a primary objective. The ultimate goal to be achieved by training is decrease in time lost from practice and competition, within specific and recognizable medical guidelines. There are four specific training periods: postseason (February to May), off-season (May to July), preseason (July to September), and in-season (September to January). Each period is designed to meet specific objectives and is preceded by a series of programmed kinetic tests and measurements. The results of these tests are computer-programmed and remain as a permanent profile of each player. The results of the test battery are utilized to evaluate and prescribe appropriate training regimens for each individual. The postseason training cycle is medical and oriented to rehabilitation. The time period correlates with the termination of the season and/or postseason play. It will most probably occur in early February. The major objectives of this phase are to reevaluate in-season injuries and medical rehabilitation achievements such as:

1. Review specific injuries.
2. Discuss possible surgical corrections as indicated vs continued nonsurgical therapy.
3. Perform medical evaluations of prospective trade personnel and/or possible draft selections. These evaluations must be detailed and include history of injuries and medical care rendered to date.
4. Perform specific tests to measure physiologic status of each athlete. These tests are to include the following:
   a) strength, flexibility, and agility
   b) motor fitness and reaction time
   c) movement time
   d) lean body mass as determined by underwater densiometry or adipose tissue measurement
   e) exercise stress test and oxygen consumption determination—maximal performance treadmill stress test.

Note: Period from February to April is free time for uninjured veterans, and conditioning is voluntary. Veterans are tested in May.

The postseason cycle is mandatory for injured players. It is a time for maximal rehabilitation and affords the players an early start toward their rehabilitation objectives.

The off-season training cycle is for conditioning and oriented to injury prevention. This time period correlates with free-agent and rookie camp, most likely to occur in early May. The major objectives of the off-season cycle are to evaluate the physiologic status of all returning veterans, and to establish individual training programs to ready the squad for preseason camp. This cycle is very important and serves to set the tempo for the coming season. It is a cycle where physiologic readiness is the major objective. Others are to:

1. Review any old injuries.
2. Evaluate progress made by those individuals who have partcipated in the postseason cycle.
3. Make medical evaluations of trades and draft selections consummated during the winter.
4. Perform battery of tests for all to determine their physiologic readiness. Tests and measurements are identical to those given during postseason cycle.

Note: Period from May to July is concerned with strenuous physical conditioning in preparation for preseason training camp.

The preseason cycle correlates with the start of training camp. The major objective of this phase is to evaluate the results of the postseason and off-season cycles. At that time it is necessary to:

1. Review rehabilitation progress of injured players.
2. Review progress of all personnel tested in February and May.
3. Discuss player contracts accordingly.
4. Outline specific training objectives to be achieved in summer camp.

Note: Installation of circuit training program to maintain and/or improve fitness levels—aerobic in nature.

The in-season phase of the cycle is designed to review the status of injuries and is oriented to treatment. However, there is a constant review and upgrading of conditioning methods to negate the always present problems of deconditioning. For example, it was demonstrated that the physiologic condition of the University of Pittsburgh varsity football team was lower in the late November than it was in mid-August.

The in-season cycle must be strenuous and adhere to the scientific principle of progressive overload. This is imperative and should show a significant correlation to decreased injury and loss of valuable playing time.

In summary, the Quadratic Training Cycle was developed to insure maximum quality of performance by professional football players. It is based upon sound scientific, anatomic, physiologic, and kinesiologic principles, and should serve to promote a keen awareness of the value of specific exercise training in competitive athletics.

The program must be implemented by the all-out effort of a coaching and medical team. Education of playing personnel as to the reasons for such an aggressive and strenuous program is mandatory and ultimately essential for maximum benefit and performance.

REHABILITATION OF THE INJURED ATHLETE

The injured athlete presents a different and unique problem to the physician and paramedical staff. The problems are different because the periods of rest necessary for healing to occur are shortened for the injured athlete, whose career in competition is relatively short. Every day lost from practice represents a deterioration in his physical condition that he trained long and hard to acquire. In addition, time lost from practice represents a loss in his opportunity to develop motor skills so vital to success in all competitive athletics. Add these factors to the psychologic stresses of losing one's position to a fellow competitor and/or teammate, and the physician finds that he is dealing with a highly impatient individual—one who insists on returning to competition as early as possible, even at the risk of permanent disability.

Obviously, a sportsmedicine philosophy of medical care must be shared by team members, parents, physicians, trainers, and coaches if the objectives of the sports program are to be achieved at their highest level. Working together, the team physicians, athletic trainers, and physical therapists have developed methods of effective and active medical rehabilitation for the injured athlete. The philosophy we strive to adhere to is best exemplified by an ounce of prevention being worth a pound of cure.

However, once injury does occur, rehabilitation of the injured athlete must begin immediately. We must decrease lost time from practice and competition, within specific medical guidelines. The player's contribution to the team objectives will be directly related to his physiologic readiness and physical ability to participate to his maximum potential. Immediate rehabilitation enables him to attain this state of readiness at its earliest possible moment. Some of the principles of immediate rehabilitation are as follows:

1. Early recognition, evaluation, and medical care of athletic injuries. The training of the medical staff in sports-medicine is a major factor in achieving this.
2. Effective treatment of the injured athlete, beginning with immediate and proper first aid including:
   a) immediate application of cold and pressure, and elevation of the injured part to inhibit and decrease edema
   b) splinting where indicated
   c) immediate physical therapy to maintain and restore joint, range of motion, muscle flexibility, and muscular strength, as well as circulation to the injured area or part.
3. Effective reconditioning once proper and adequate healing has taken place.
4. Effective strapping (taping) of the injury until the athlete can be weaned from this support.
5. Medical decision on return to action.

An example of a physical restoration program is the program *How to Strengthen a Weak Leg* using an isotonic mode.

HOW TO STRENGTHEN A WEAK LEG

Sport scientists recommend strengthening exercises for patients with a weak leg or unstable knee. It is important for the doctor to know whether the leg will respond to such strengthening exercises because further evaluation may be needed if he does not. The same exercise may be used to strengthen the leg regardless of whether the weakness is due to old knee trouble, recent injury, disc trouble, or other causes. Hence, different patients with different conditions will do the same exercise. Increasing overall leg strength to peak levels is a key factor in regaining proper function of the leg.

EQUIPMENT

Weights are used for the strengthening exercises and there are different types which can be used:

1. They can be in the form of scale weights, sand bags, stones, bricks, lead shot, coins, etc. They should be small enough to fit into a small airline bag, a large handbag, or a traveling bag. Weights can also be placed inside a piece of stockinette, nylon hose, or knee socks. Weights should be in assorted sizes up to 25 lb to start.
2. Velcro wraparound weights.
3. Weight boot.

EXERCISES AND GOAL-SETTING PROCEDURES

The Progressive Resistive Exercise (PRE) Program consists of eight exercises. For each exercise, determine the maximum weight the leg can lift for one repetition and record it. This is the SLM, single lift maximum. The maximum weight will vary with each exercise. Do the same thing for the opposite leg, even if it is not involved. Record the difference so that you know how great it is and how much you will have to work.

The single lift maximum (SLM) is used to determine maximum weight. This is the maximum amount of weight you can lift for one repetition from an amount of flexion (30° to 90°) to 0° or full extension (without pain or discomfort). SLM is determined by trial and error.

After determining the maximum weight you are able to lift one time, calculate 70% of this weight. This is the amount of weight you will use for the PRE program. Do 6 repetitions of the exercise using this amount of weight (70% of maximum weight). Hold for 5 seconds. Progress to 10 repetitions as you are able. It is not necessary to do more than 10 repetitions. When you are able to do 10 repetitions, redetermine your maximum weight and repeat exercise procedure.

EXAMPLE: Knee Extension (Exercise 1).

You have determined the maximum weight you are able to lift one time for knee extension is 20 lb. Seventy percent of 20 lb equals 14 lb. Using 14 lb do 6 repetitions of knee extension. Continue using 14 lb until you are able to do 10 repetitions of knee extension. This will usually take two to five days. Once you are able to lift 14 lb for 10 repetitions and hold 5 seconds each time, you will redetermine your maximum weight. You find the maximum weight you are now able to lift one time is 25 lb. Seventy percent of 25 lb equals 17½ lb.

Weight Program Progress Record

Name: Date Started:	Weight Amount (lbs) Side Lift		Weight Amount (lbs) Hip Flex.		Weight Amount (lbs) Leg Rotation		Weight Amount (lbs) Knee Ext.	
	Left	Right	Left	Right	Left	Right	Left	Right
Initial Maximum Ability Tests: Record the largest amount of weight that you can lift 25 times in a row. (Use these as the amounts to start lifting at.)								

PROGRESS RECORD Week Number	Week of: (date)	Use the spaces provided below to record the amount of weight you have been lifting.							
1									
2									
3									
4									
5									
6									
7									
8									
9									
10									
11									
12									

Comments:

Record each treatment session

Figure 28-3 Patient progress report.

Using 17½ lb do 6 repetitions of the exercise. Build to 10 repetitions of the exercise. Redetermine your maximum weight and repeat the procedure.

Remember that the amount of weight used will vary with each exercise. In this regard a daily record should be kept of the amount of weight lifted (Figure 28-3). An important point to remember when doing these exercises is that excessive pain during exercise is detrimental to your progress. If this should occur, either lessen the amount of weight being lifted in that exercise to a tolerable level, or discontinue that exercise with the doctor's advice.

NOTE: If you have a back condition then you must always do the PRE program with the back supported or braced.

Exercise 1
Knee Extensions
(Quadriceps Muscle)

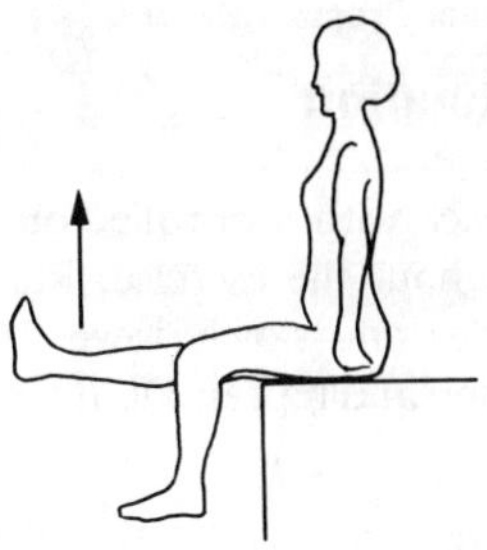

Sit on a high desk or table with the legs hanging over the edge at a 90° angle. Place a rolled towel under the knee. Straighten the knee completely and hold 5 seconds. Slowly lower, and return to starting position.

Exercise 2
Hip Flexion

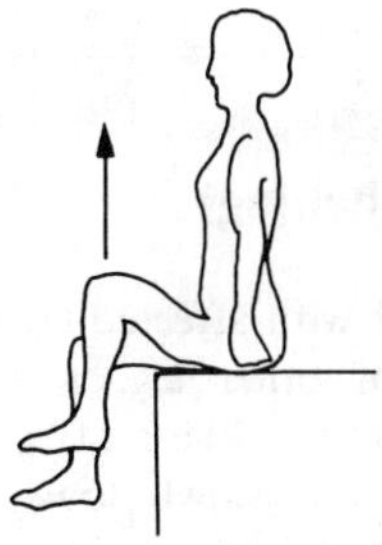

Sit on a high desk or table with the legs hanging over the edge at a 90° angle. Grasp the edge of the table with both hands; do not lean back. Keep the knee bent, and raise it up towards the shoulder. Hold for 5 seconds. Slowly lower.

Exercise 3
Side Leg Lifts—
Upper Leg (Hip
Abductor Muscle)

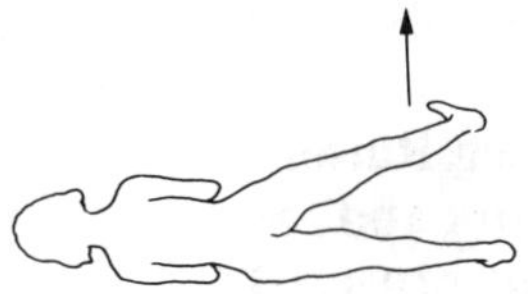

Lie on your side with upper leg and back straight. Raise top leg up. Keep the leg in a straight line with the trunk and do not bend at the hip or knee. Hold for 5 seconds. Slowly lower. Do not exceed SLM.

Exercise 4
Side Leg Lifts—
Lower Leg

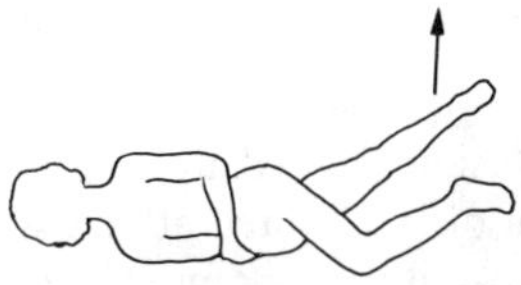

Lie on side with top leg flexed at hip and knee. Keep bottom leg in a straight line with the trunk and do not bend at the hip or knee. The top leg should lie in front of the bottom leg. Raise bottom leg up. Hold for 5 seconds. Do not exceed 12 lb of SLM.

Exercise 5
Knee Flexion Prone
(Hamstring Muscles)

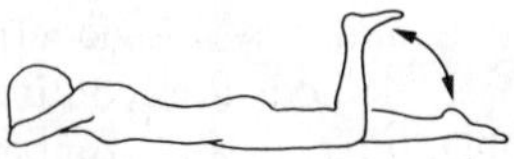

Lie on stomach with arms folded under head and legs out straight. Place a small rolled towel under the leg above the knee cap. Bend knee as far as possible. Slowly return to straight position.

Exercise 6
External Rotation

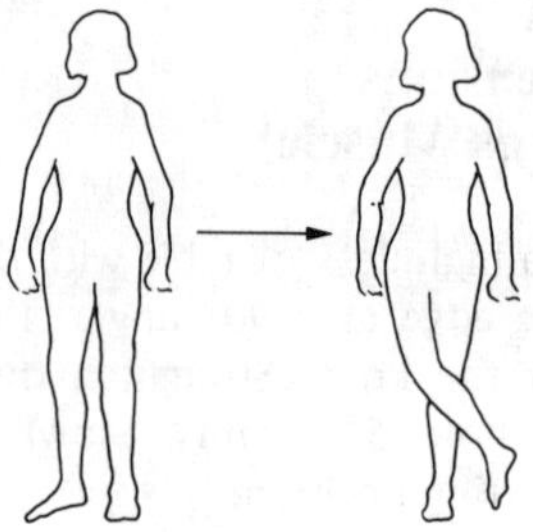

Lie on back with foot rolled out. Keep leg extended throughout the exercise. Raise leg up and across other leg and slowly lower. Bring back to starting position and repeat. Do not exceed 20 lb of SLM.

Exercise 7
Crossover (Inside Knee Strengthening)

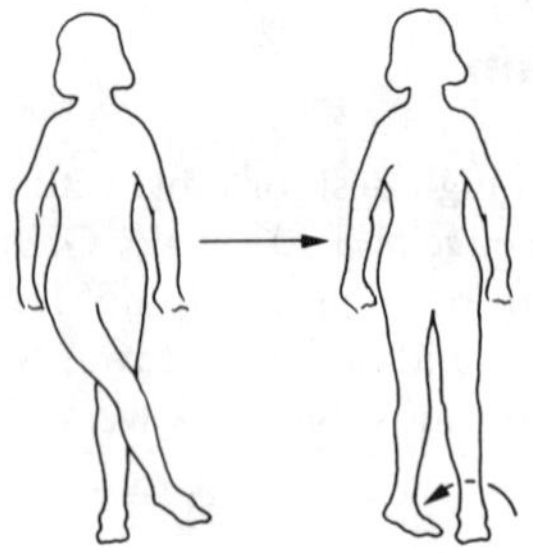

Lie on back with affected leg rolled in and on opposite side of other leg. Keep leg rolled in throughout exercise. Raise affected leg up and across other leg and slowly lower. Move back to starting position and repeat. Do not exceed 20 lb of SLM.

Exercise 8
Straight Leg Raises (Hip Flexors and Quadriceps Muscles)

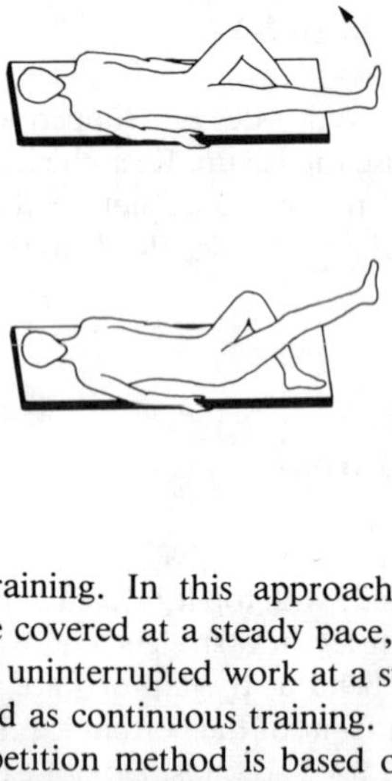

Lie on back with the leg to be exercised in full extension. Bend the opposite leg and keep foot planted on table. Keeping the leg straight, raise 12 inches and hold for 5 seconds. Lower to starting position and repeat.

In conclusion, immediate and proper care and rehabilitation of the injured athlete are vital to the success of most athletic programs. It is imperative that the coach and medical staff be well educated in the field of sportsmedicine.

CLASSIFICATION OF TRAINING METHODS

There are five training methods that have different structural and physiologic effects on the organism. These methods are: continuous, repetition, changeable, interval, and competition.

The continuous method is based on a relatively long duration of uninterrupted work at a constant intensity. It is extremely popular in marathon training. In this approach, very long distances are covered at a steady pace, but shorter durations of uninterrupted work at a steady rate is also classified as continuous training.

The repetition method is based on repeating the same activity a number of times. Recoveries between repetitions are kept sufficiently long to assure an optimal readiness of the organism for the next phase of work. Accumulation of oxygen debt and fatigue are avoided.

The changeable method is based on uninterrupted work, relatively long in duration, but not at constant intensity. The characteristics of work are changed without recoveries. The Swedish training process is a typical example of this method as changes can be made not only in the intensity of the activity, but also by using variations in conditions (running up or down hill, running on sandy or firm surfaces, etc).

Interval method has a format somewhere in between the changeable and repetition methods. Certain set work, similar to repetition work, is performed a number of times, but not with full recoveries. The work, executed at relatively high intensity, is adjusted so that each new repetition is started with some oxygen debt. The oxygen debt and fatigue symptoms continue to accumulate as work progresses.

Recoveries can be performed by changing to milder types of work, such as jogging or walking. However, the types and the lengths of recoveries are strictly regimented.

The competition method is based on performing at maximum intensity in a competitive atmosphere. It must include some training partners to assure real competitive conditions. Performing alone against the stopwatch, as in an individual time trial, is not satisfactory because it does not create sufficient emotional stress.

Continuous Method

The main factor in the continuous method is the duration of work, to adapt the organism to a prolonged load by an economical exploitation of energy reserves over an extended time period. This results in:

1. development of energy potential of the organism
2. a more economic use of energy reserves
3. development of functional stability
4. development of aerobic work capacity.

Some studies have found contradicting results to this approach, with no stress signs noted when recoveries have been restricted to pulse rates in the range of 130 to 150 per minute. This suggests that interval training can be divided into extensive and intensive categories. The extensive interval training should be used in the preparation phase of training, and the intensive category before the start of the competitive season or important competitions.

It should be kept in mind when choosing recoveries that the pulse rate drops faster when the athlete is lying down. However, this position is not favorable to eliminate lactic acid concentrations. That is best achieved when the work phase is followed by muscular activity of a lower intensity. An intensity of about 40% of maximum oxygen uptake capacity may serve as the most efficient for the active recovery interval.

Interval sprints, in which short distances (about 30 meters) are repeated at full speed and followed by jogging or walking recoveries, represent a variation of the interval method. It is based on the theory that 20- to 40-second recoveries after 10 seconds of intensive work do not increase the lactic acid level in the blood. It appears that, because short bursts at maximum or near maximum speed are produced by utilizing the enzyme and metabolic actions of creatin phosphate and creatinine phosphate kinase, no oxygen debt is created. Creatin phosphate acids are resynthesized in 20 to 30 seconds, justifying the use of interval sprints in the development of speed.

Changeable Method

Physiologically, the changeable method is something between the continuous and interval types of training. It can be adjusted toward one or the other by regulating the intensity and duration of the work. Several phases of submaximal or maximal efforts can bring it closer to interval training. Relatively small changes in intensity will produce results similar to the continuous method.

Repetition Method

Repetition training has an important place in learning new skills, developing skills already acquired, and improving speed, strength, and agility. It is closely related to the functions of the central nervous system with the number of repetitions of a particular activity. To increase the number of repetitions without undue fatigue in the central nervous system, requires sufficient recovery intervals between phases of work.

Fox and Matthews[6] have shown that the stimulus to the central nervous system following physical work, makes a wavy pattern. The response of the central nervous system to stimulus drops considerably at the end of heavy and prolonged work, before it reaches a new, improved level. However, it remains on a high level immediately following short and intensive activities before dropping to a low level of response. Optimal stimulus is reached on the crest of the waves, indicating that recoveries should be adjusted to begin the next work phase at the optimal moment.

According to Fox and Matthews,[6] systemic,

prolonged loads lead to increased glycogen reserves in the muscles and liver and improve the activity of oxidative processes, allowing for more economic muscular work. Prolonged work is also responsible for an increase in the tone of parasympathetic nerves that play an important role in the functioning of several organs, particularly the economic functioning of the heart. It is reflected in a lower pulse rate of well-trained athletes.

Continuous training develops the ability of the organism to function at a relatively high level over long time periods because of more efficient oxygen transport and uptake. Improved oxygen uptake and capillarization are the main factors in development of aerobic work capacity.

Development of the functional capacity of the heart in continuous training depends on the intensity of work performed. It is claimed that such training requires the heart to work over a prolonged time at a maximum stroke volume, achieved at a pulse rate of not less than 130 beats a minute. This means that the intensity of continuous running must exceed a pulse rate of 130 but not reach a level at which anaerobic processes become involved. That would accumulate oxygen debt and reduce the time in action. It is generally accepted that anaerobic metabolism is approached at a heart rate of about 160 a minute; continuous running should therefore be performed with the pulse rate maintained at 130 to 160 beats a minute.

Interval Method

From the physiologic standpoint, the interval method is based on work performed under conditions of oxygen debt to develop anaerobic work capacity of the organism. Oxygen debt is accumulated rapidly by performing several repetitions of an exercise at submaximal intensity. To avoid reaching the tolerance limit of oxygen debt, the work is performed in several phases with recovery intervals. The recoveries are kept short so that the next working phase is started before the oxygen debt has been eliminated. This results in:

1. allowing the organism to work under oxygen debt conditions over a longer time
2. performing with a continually increasing oxygen debt
3. allowing the oxygen debt to reach a level higher than is possible by single submaximal or very intensive performance of an exercise.

It has been suggested that interval training should be adjusted according to heart rates. Pulse rates exceeding 180 or even 200 beats a minute may be a sign of overloading in the working phase, in which case the intensity should be dropped or the recoveries extended. Recoveries should be adjusted so that the pulse rate can drop to 120 to 130 beats a minute, allowing a great deal of the oxygen debt to be eliminated before the next working phase begins.

There are different opinions on the loads to be used in repetition training to develop strength. Some claim that no development takes place if the resistance in isometric exercises is below 20% to 30% of maximum strength, and it has been demonstrated that the limit in dynamic exercises is 20%. Optimal results may be achieved through the use of isometric exercises with a resistance of about two-thirds of maximum. It has been shown that maximum loads reduce the number of repetitions and the total time of stimulus, and that there are biomechanical problems in using close-to-maximum loads.

CATASTROPHIC SPORTS INJURIES AND EARLY INDICATIONS FOR CARE

HEAD AND FACIAL INJURIES

Concussion

Mild concussion *Signs and symptoms* Transient losses of consciousness lasting less than 15 seconds.

Emergency treatment Keep athlete out of game. Ask questions concerning events immediate to injury. Assess level of consciousness frequently. If athlete loses consciousness for more than 15 seconds, transfer him to the hospital immediately.

Moderate concussion *Signs and symptoms* Loss of consciousness, mental confusion, retrograde amnesia, dizziness, unsteadiness.

Emergency treatment Keep athlete out of game. Ask questions about events immediate to injury. Assess level of consciousness frequently. Transfer athlete to hospital for further evaluations.

Severe concussion *Subdural hematoma*

Signs and symptoms Headache, intermittent drowsiness, lack of concentration, mild confusion, a gradual loss of consciousness. Seizures are possible.

Emergency treatment Transport athlete to hospital immediately. Elevate head slightly during transport. If seizures occur, protect the airway and tongue. This injury is life threatening.

Epidural hematoma Signs and symptoms Initially athlete usually appears well and oriented. Loss of consciousness and motor problems appear 10 to 20 minutes after blow to head. Seizures are possible.

Emergency treatment Transport athlete to hospital immediately. Elevate head slightly during transport. If seizures occur, protect the airway and tongue. This injury is life threatening.

For further information on concussion, see Chapter 10.

Skull Fracture

Basilar skull fracture *Signs and symptoms* Possible loss of consciousness, unequal pupils, bleeding or fluid from ears or nose, blurred vision, headache, nausea and vomiting, dizziness, changes in personality, "raccoon" eyes, respiratory distress, or seizures.

Emergency treatment Transport athlete to hospital immediately. Elevate head slightly and support it carefully. Be prepared to protect tongue and airway in the event of seizure. In the event of respiratory arrest, provide artificial ventilation.

Depressed skull fracture *Signs and symptoms* Possible loss of consciousness, unequal pupils, bleeding or fluid from nose or ears, amnesia, decreased motor strength, seizures, or respiratory distress.

Emergency treatment Transport athlete to hospital immediately. Elevate head and support neck. Do not remove helmet. Be prepared to protect tongue and airway in the event of seizure. Provide respiratory assistance as necessary.

For further information on skull fracture, see Chapter 11.

Facial Fractures

Signs and symptoms Bloody nose, swelling and ecchymosis of face.

Emergency treatment Apply ice, gentle pressure, elevate head and transport athlete to hospital. This injury could be catastrophic if airway becomes obstructed with blood. Be prepared to aspirate blood from pharynx as necessary.

For further information on facial fracture, see Chapter 11.

SPINAL CORD INJURIES

Cervical Sprain

Signs and symptoms Pain and muscle spasms after 2 or more hours following injury.

Emergency treatment Apply ice to affected area. Cervical collar may be necessary. Apply heat 24 to 48 hours after injury. This injury could be catastrophic if a cervical fracture goes unnoticed. Have neck radiographs performed.

Cervical Fracture

Undisplaced cervical fracture *Signs and symptoms* Possible neck pain and weakness in arms and legs. Respiratory distress may also occur.

Emergency treatment Maintain airway as necessary. Transport athlete to hospital immediately. Transport should be done using a backboard and sandbags to stabilize the head and neck. Do not remove helmet.

Displaced cervical fracture *Signs and symptoms* Paralysis of legs, arms, or both may occur immediately after injury. Respiratory distress or arrest are also possible.

Emergency treatment Maintain airway and provide artificial ventilation as necessary. Transport athlete to hospital immediately. Transport should be done using a backboard and sandbags to stabilize the head and neck. Do not remove helmet.

Lumbar Fractures

Signs and symptoms Pain in lower back that may radiate down the legs and to the abdomen and chest. Paresis, numbness, tingling, and decreased sensation in the legs are possible when the underlying spinal cord has been damaged.

Emergency treatment Place the athlete on a backboard and transport to the hospital immediately.

For further information on spinal cord and back injuries see Chapters 10 and 17.

INJURIES TO THE UPPER EXTREMITY

Complete Shoulder Dislocation

Signs and symptoms Any movement of the shoulder will be painful, and muscle spasms may be present. Athlete may hold the arm in a protective fashion.

Emergency treatment Apply ice, immobilize shoulder with a Figure-8 bandage/splint, and place arm in a sling.

Fractures

Signs and symptoms Any fracture that compromises circulation and nerve function can be catastrophic. Severe pain, weakness, swelling, and deformity may be present. Compound fractures will pierce the adjacent skin.

Emergency treatment Splint, apply ice, and transport athlete to the hospital immediately. In compound fractures bleeding must be controlled and the puncture site cleaned of obvious dirt.

Severed Finger

Signs and symptoms Obvious deformity accompanied by severe bleeding. Athlete may show signs of shock: pallor, sweating, shortness of breath, and fainting.

Emergency treatment Apply bandage to injured site. Attempt to control bleeding. Locate the severed portion of the finger, and place on ice. Severed fingers can often be reattached surgically if promptly and adequately treated. Transport athlete to hospital immediately.

For further information about injuries to the upper extremity see Chapter 18.

INJURIES TO THE LOWER EXTREMITY

Hip Dislocation

Signs and symptoms Pain, swelling, malalignment of the leg, and inability to bear weight are often seen. The athlete will usually lie with hip flexed and adducted.

Emergency treatment Apply ice and immobilize hip. Transport athlete to hospital immediately.

Knee Injuries

Locked knee *Signs and symptoms* Athlete may be unable to straighten knee. Pain, swelling, and difficulty in bearing weight are often seen.

Emergency treatment Apply ice and immobilize knee. Transport athlete to hospital.

Lateral collateral ligament injury *Signs and symptoms* Pain, tenderness on the lateral aspect of the knee, and swelling are usually seen. Adduction test is positive when the leg is flexed 30°.

Emergency treatment Apply ice and compression and elevate leg. Transport athlete to the hospital.

Anterior cruciate ligament injury *Signs and symptoms* Athlete may feel a pop or giving way of the ligament. Pain, swelling, instability, and a positive drawer test often accompany this injury.

Emergency treatment Apply ice and compression and elevate leg. Transport athlete to the hospital.

Fractures

Signs and symptoms Severe pain, swelling, and inability to bear weight. In femoral shaft fractures the athlete may show signs of shock: pallor, perspiration, cold, clammy skin, and tachycardia. In compound fractures the fracture bone is seen piercing the overlying skin. Bleeding can be profuse.

Emergency treatment Make sure pulses are present and circulation is adequate. Splint extremity by applying gentle traction. Also apply ice and compression and elevate leg. In compound fractures clean the injured site of obvious dirt and debris. Apply a dressing and attempt to control bleeding. Transport athlete to hospital immediately.

For further information about injuries to the lower extremity see Chapter 19.

DEEP LACERATIONS

Signs and symptoms Bleeding may be moderate to severe and pulsating. Open wound is usually obvious.

Emergency treatment Gently clean wound of dirt and debris, and apply compression dressing. If the bleeding is profuse or involves a major vessel, apply direct pressure to the bleeding site. Transport athlete to the hospital.

INJURIES TO ABDOMINAL ORGANS

Injury to the Spleen

Signs and symptoms History of a severe blow to the left upper abdominal quadrant or lower left portion of rib cage. Tenderness in this area and signs of shock are possible.

Emergency treatment Transfer athlete to the hospital immediately.

Injury to the Liver

Signs and symptoms History of a severe blow to the right upper abdominal quadrant or lower right rib cage. Tenderness in this area and signs of shock are possible.

Emergency treatment Transport athlete to the hospital immediately.

Injury to the Small Bowel

Signs and symptoms History of severe blow to the abdomen. Early signs may be mild or lacking.

Emergency treatment Transport athlete to hospital if injury is suspected.

Injury to the Kidneys

Signs and symptoms History of direct trauma to the flank or lower posterior rib cage. Pain and tenderness in this area is usually seen. An expanding flank mass indicates severe hemorrhage. Shock is possible.

Emergency treatment Transport athlete to the hospital immediately.

Injury to the Bladder

Signs and symptoms History of trauma to the lower abdomen. Rupture of bladder is possible when lower abdominal pain, tenderness, and swelling are present.

Emergency treatment Transport athlete to the hospital immediately. For further information on abdominal injuries see Chapter 15.

INJURIES TO THE CHEST

Fractured Ribs

Signs and symptoms History of blow to rib cage. Pain, tenderness, and difficulty in deep breathing may be seen.

Emergency treatment Observe athlete for shortness of breath or other respiratory distress. Transport to hospital.

Pneumothorax

Signs and symptoms History of blow to rib cage or penetrating wound to the chest. Shortness of breath and shift of mediastinum away from the collapsed lung are usually seen.

Emergency treatment If the chest wall has been penetrated, cover the site with sterile gauze. Observe the athlete for signs of shock, respiratory and cardiac arrest. Give oxygen if it is available. Transfer the athlete to the hospital immediately.

LARYNGOTRACHEAL INJURY

Signs and symptoms History of blow to the neck. Shortness of breath, hoarseness, loss of voice, and coughing up of blood may be seen.

Emergency treatment If the injury is severe enough, airway obstruction can occur. Complete airway obstruction must be treated with cricothyrotomy or emergency tracheostomy. Oxygen should be given if available. Be prepared to give CPR. Transport athlete to the hospital immediately. For further information on laryngotracheal injury see Chapter 11.

AIRWAY OBSTRUCTION

Signs and symptoms Inspirations may be stridorous and labored. Breathing may stop. Lips and fingernail beds may become cyanotic. The victim may loss consciousness. Pupils may enlarge.

Emergency treatment If victim is coughing, do not interfere, except to encourage slow deep breathing. If victim becomes unconscious and stops breathing, roll him onto his side and strike between his shoulder blades and remove any foreign debris (vomitus, gum, tooth, or mouthpiece) from the mouth. Place victim on his back and maintain airway by elevating jaw forward. Give mouth-to-mouth resuscitation if victim is not breathing. If air does not pass through the airway causing the chest to rise, the airway may still be obstructed. Use the Heimlich Maneuever. If repeated attempts to clear the airway fail, cricothyrotomy with a large bore needle or emergency tracheotomy may be necessary.

RESPIRATORY ARREST

Signs and symptoms No visible movement of the chest and loss of consciousness are seen. Tongue, lips, and fingernails will turn bluish.

Emergency treatment Begin mouth-to-mouth resuscitation immediately. Put the victim on his back. Place one hand under the victim's neck and tilt the head back making sure that the tongue is not obstructing the airway. Pinch the nostrils with one hand, open your mouth and take a deep breath. Place your mouth tightly over the victim's mouth and blow into his mouth making sure that the victim's chest rises as you blow. Repeat this maneuver 12 times per minute. Transport athlete to the hospital and continue mouth-to-mouth resuscitation while en route.

CARDIAC ARREST

Signs and symptoms Before the heart stops the victim may experience chest or left arm pain, shortness of breath, cyanosis, pallor, perspiration, and shock. When the heart stops, consciousness is lost, breathing stops, no carotid pulse will be felt.

Emergency treatment Begin CPR. (Only those trained in CPR should do so.) Transport athlete to the hospital immediately continuing CPR while en route.

THERMIC INJURIES

Hyperthermia

Heat stroke *Signs and symptoms* Skin is flushed, hot, and dry. Heart rate will be increased. Body temperature is elevated, and the athlete may be unconscious.

Emergency treatment Undress the athlete and bathe body surfaces with cool water or alcohol. Do not use ice. Transport the athlete to the hospital immediately.

Heat exhaustion *Signs and symptoms* Skin is usually pale, cool, and clammy. Body temperature is usually normal. Athlete may feel faint or complain of dizziness, weakness, or nausea.

Emergency treatment Have athlete lie down with feet elevated and take small sips of water. Loosen tight clothing and apply cool wet compresses to exposed skin. Transport to hospital immediately.

Hypothermia

Signs and symptoms Athlete will usually be shivering and complain of numbness in extremities. Drowsiness, weakness, and confusion may also be present.

Emergency treatment Watch for signs of shock, irregular heart rate, respiratory distress. Remove wet or constricting clothing. Keep warm. Administer warm liquids if the athlete is conscious. Do not give alcohol.

For more information on thermic injuries see Chapter 23.

SUGGESTED READINGS

Fox, E.L., and Matthews, D.K. *Interval Training. Conditioning for Sports and General Fitness.* Philadelphia: W.B. Saunders, 1974.

Morehouse, L.E., and Miller, A.T. *Physiology of Exercise,* 2nd Ed. St. Louis: C.V. Mosby, 1963.

Rasch, P.J., and Morehouse, L.E. The effect of static and dynamic exercise on muscular strength and hypertrophy. *J Appl Physiol.* 11:29–34, 1957.

Sills, F.D., and Everett, P.W. The relationship of extreme somatotypes to performance in motor and strength tests. *Res Q.* 24:223–228, 1953.

Willgoose, C.E., and Rogers, M.L. Relationship of somatotype to physical fitness. *J Ed Res.* 42:704–712, 1949.

APPENDIX

Contents of the Sportsmedicine Bag

Paul F. Vinger, MD
Earl F. Hoerner, MD

First aid is the fundamental aspect of all injury control. As stated by Oswals of the American National Red Cross, first aid training is comparable with a need to plan for accident prevention. There is no doubt that there is a significant effect of properly applied first aid on sports injuries. Individuals who have applied first aid develop a sensitivity to the after-effects of injuries and often strive to prevent them.

Factors that are of value in planning and preparing for appropriate early care and first aid include:

A. In-Service Training

- Cardiopulmonary resuscitation
- Emergency care and transportation
- Analysis of injury and accident causes
- Effectiveness of early care
- Principles of follow-up medical treatment

B. Role of Environment and Playing Surface

C. Participant Responsibility

D. Leadership Responsibility:

Athletic director

Coach	Fireman	Physician
Trainer	Policeman	Nurse

Emergency medical technician

E. Emergency Planning

- Defined plan in writing
- Procedural manual
- Appropriate support systems
- Plan ahead for away games

F. First Aid Supplies[1]

1. To establish airway
   - Bolt cutter for removal of face masks
   - Oral airways – small, medium, and large
   - Nasal airways – medium and large
   - Endotrachial tubes – cuffed, small, medium, and large
   - Laryngoscope
   - Ambu bag with face mask and adapter for endotrachial tubes
   - Syringe, 50 ml, and large catheter for suction
   - Mouth screw to open mouth
   - Tracheostomy kit and tubes for use on field as absolute last resort
   - Padded tongue blade
   - Towel clip
2. To maintain blood pressure
   - Tourniquet for use if direct pressure fails
   - Cardiopulmonary resuscitation medications
     - Epinephrine – 1:10,000 in 2-ml syringe to be given if chest massage unsuccessful
     - Epinephrine – 1:1000 for direct instillation through endotrachial tube
     - Lidocaine hydrochloride (Xylocaine) – 100 mg vial for prevention or treatment of arrhythmia
     - Lactated Ringer solution – 500 ml with sterile tubing and needles
   - Supplies
     - Backboard with strap restraints
     - Stethoscope
     - Aneroid manometer
3. To prevent and treat hypothermia and hyperthermia
   - Thermometer – oral and rectal
   - Thermometer to measure air and water temperatures
   - Sling psychrometer with tables to determine heat stress index
   - Blankets, wool (hypothermia)
   - Source of shade, ice, cool water (hyperthermia)
4. To protect the brain and spinal cord
   - Neck precautions should be known by all
   - Stretcher (Penn State)[2]
   - Sandbags – 5-pound
     - Medications
       - Diazepam (Valium) – 10-mg ampule for injection to control severe convulsion
       - Dexamethasone (Decadron) – 4 ml in preloaded syringe for spinal cord injury

5. To treat severe allergic reactions
    Anaphylaxis kit
    Medicated inhaler for asthmatic attack
6. Eye injuries
    Vision card
    Penlight
    Hard metal or plastic protective eye shield
    Eye patches, sterile
    Tape, transparent or micropore
    Irrigating solution, sterile
    Sterile cotton swabs
    Fluorescein strips (sterile)
    Erythromycin eye ointment
    Proparacaine—0.5% dropperette
    Sterile adhesive strips
    Magnifying glass
7. Lacerations (only minor lacerations should be sutured outside the hospital)
    Suture kit, sterile, with suture material
    Sterile gloves
    Disposable sterile towels
    Lidocaine
    Syringes with needles
    Scissors, heavy duty
    Tape adherent, can
    Dressings, sterile, 2 × 2, 4 × 4, nonstick
    Bandage, roller, sterile, 1 inch, 2 inch
    Band-Aids
    Povidone-iodine solution
    Liquid soap
8. Bone, joint, muscle injuries
    Slings, for upper extremity—have safety pins available
    Crutches, adjustable lengths, underarm
    Ice packs, chemical or in plastic bags from ice-making machine
    Screwdriver and pliers
    Ace bandages, 2-, 3-, 4- and 6-inch widths
    Foam rubber and felt padding, ⅜ inch
    splints, air or cardboard for upper and lower extremities
    Splints, aluminum finger, foam-covered
    Cotton, absorbent
    Tape, assorted sizes, white, surgical plastic, elastoplast
    Spray, ethyl chloride
    Plaster bandages, 3- and 6-inch
    Cotton web roll 4-inch
9. Miscellaneous
    Notebook and pen—records of treatment are essential.
    Ophthalmoscope/otoscope (optional)
    Aspirin/acetaminophen
    Petrolatum jelly
    Antacids
    Ammonia capsules—not recommended as sudden head jerk could aggravate neck injury.
    Tongue blades
    Swiss army knife

G. First aid practices to be posted with first aid equipment:

Specific procedures to be followed for common injuries and emergencies.

To summarize, all the components as outlined must be available with the basic ingredients being leadership and availability of first aid equipment and supplies. After first aid, get the severely injured player or spectator to a hospital for definitive care:

Phone: should be at site with emergency telephone numbers immediately available

Vehicle should be on site to transport victim, on a stretcher, to the hospital if the ambulance is detained.

The frequency and severity of injuries and illness from physical activity and sport participation, and the peculiar problems created by the variety of environmental conditions, place a great need for a high degree of first aid competence on sport leaders and participants.

REFERENCES

1. Mayne, B.R. If sports medicine is your bag—equip it well. *Physician and Sportsmedicine.* 3:67–69, 1975.

2. Loomis, J.L., Johnson, D.A., Hochberg, W.J. et al. Equipment update: Penn State's foldable rigid stretcher. *Physician and Sportsmedicine.* 7:135–136, 1979.

SECTION IV

Protective Devices and Rules

EDITORIAL COMMENT

Protective Equipment: Its Value, Capabilities, and Limitations

Earl F. Hoerner, MD
Paul F. Vinger, MD

Although catastropic injury in sports, recreational activities, and leisure-time pursuits are facts of life, use of suitable fitted protective equipment can do an excellent job in decreasing this at-risk factor.

The designer of protective equipment for any sporting activity must consider such factors as the economic position of the buyer, fit, weight, restriction of motion, limitation of visual or auditory input, usefulness, comfort, durability, and user acceptability of the product. A designer must also carefully consider trade-off. Every piece of protective equipment has certain advantages and disadvantages. By designing to eliminate one danger, the manufacturer may create another. Or by selecting or using a material for one purpose, the manufacturer may create a problem in its combination or use with another material.

An example is seen in the manufacture of mats for wrestling and gymnastics. The designer and manufacturer are required to have a balance between a mat that will absorb kinetic energy and thereby prevent injuries, and yet one that will be firm enough not to restrict freedom of movement. A mat that truly meets the first criterion would be soft and thick, but motion and movement would be restricted and decreased, thereby modifying the sport.

Designers and manufacturers of eye guards for hockey, racquetball, and squash face litagation in which users of the protective equipment claim that injury occurred to the eye despite wearing of the eye guard. In reality, the only way to guarantee total safety under these circumstances would be to cover the eyes totally and thereby remove all eye exposure. However, by such over-designing, the manufacturer could entirely eliminate the use of the protective equipment. In hockey, reducing the size of the eye openings on goalies' and other players' face masks increases safety, but there is a point where impairment of vision could occur and become a safety factor.

The manufacturers of football, hockey, and baseball helmets have an interest in attempting to consider all of these factors and trade-offs involved in the design and the future use of this equipment. From the standpoint of sizing alone, the range of players in age and growth is from eight years of age to the fully grown adult. Helmets must be capable of absorbing kinetic energy in a range of high mass (weight of the player or participant) and low velocity (speed of moving of the player), to low mass (hockey puck, baseball), and high velocity (speed of the moving object). The equipment should protect against each extreme of these different energy levels without impairing absorption of energy at the average levels of these two energy-absorbing situations. These helmets will be worn on the participants' heads for two or more hours per day, five or six days per week, over a period of at least three to six months. They will be used in temperature extremes of freezing cold and blistering heat. Hockey helmets are used at extremes of $-20°F$ environmental temperature, while inside the helmets the temperature approaches that of the human body. Conditions vary from humid and dry to rain and snow. Baseball and football helmets are exposed to mud, dust, grass, artificial surfaces, and even, at times, macadam or concrete. The helmet must be light enough not to inhibit the wearer in using his or her skill of the activity, but strong enough to resist impacts, provide coverage to as much of the head and neck as possible, and yet not restrict the vision, hearing, or movement of the wearer.

Over the years, designers have learned to apply trade-offs involved in the manufacture and use of helmets to meet these criteria. The strap suspension system within the helmet has been adopted as an excellent protective concept in that it aids the head and its contents to move away from an external blow. However, how does the manufacturer provide suspension systems that in order to be effective, fit tightly and fit all shapes of skulls? This last criterion must be realized through a padding system that can be modified for sizing, fitting, and various skull shapes. Padded systems, however, have air circulation limitations within the helmet, and are hotter, heavier, and do not move the head away from the impacted blow. The ideal helmet is one which combines both the suspension system and padding within the same helmet.

Also to be taken into consideration is the ongoing aging and molecular change of the material used, whether during manufacture or during product use. In time, plastics, leather, and foams thus become modified and lose their energy-absorbing effectiveness. The level of energy absorption provided by any helmet is dependent on its exposure to weather, temperature, humidity, and most of all, the number of impacts delivered to the helmet, especially in rapid succession. All of the adverse factors are superimposed on usual life of materials used in production.

At this time, with the state of the art and taking into consideration the factors of trade-offs, the protection given by many helmets today is similar, regardless of the protective system, padding, or suspension system within the shell. However, as materials improve, and as more is learned of the interface between the equipment and the wearer, better head protection will be available. For proper selection of a helmet, a player, participant, coach, or athletic director must decide which is the most practical and what trade-offs are involved.

In addition, if a participant uses padding that completely encircles the head and allows no space for the flow of air, the wearer must remove the helmet frequently so that the head can cool and body heat or sweating around the head can be reduced.

Continued work in the laboratory and on the playing field is being performed in an effort to determine the level of tolerance of human beings to injury. Much is known, but more needs to be defined, and documented results must be correlated for practical use and application. It is not known precisely at what level of energy concussion or other damage occurs to the brain; nor can it be determined precisely how much energy was involved in a blow that caused a particular injury. Do human factors such as shape of the head, thickness of the skull, length of the neck, age of the participant, or previous injury to an anatomic area have a positive or negative value in any individual's level of tolerance?

Designers, manufacturers, clinicians, and researchers are continuing efforts in an attempt to find, and thus use, ideal materials for application in helmets to bring the energy of a blow to a stop before it reaches the skull and head. This is necessary because once the body is in motion, it possesses kinetic energy which must be expended. As the energy comes to a stop, it creates force, the magnitude of which is governed by the time and distance over which the body stops moving.

One concept for the absorption of energy has been the use of an energy-absorbing material in the helmet consisting of polystyrene beads, enclosed in a Styrofoam pad. This type of protective equipment is used in vehicular crash helmets, and is of value in motorcycle and automobile race drivers' head protection. However, unfortunately in low-level energy absorption, it has been demonstrated that the degree and incidence of cerebral concussion has been increased.

Another concept advocates the employment of a soft outer shell for athletic and recreational activities where participants may collide with one another in the course of their activity. This occurs in contact sports such as hockey, soccer, lacrosse, field hockey, basketball, and football. This soft shell has been primarily advanced as a means for protecting the players and participants from blows administered by the helmet wearer to another player. As of this time, no field or laboratory studies have been performed to determine the effects to the neck and head of the wearer of this proposed modification. There must also be taken into consideration the possible changing of the game due to such equipment changes.

Another concern in equipment design and manufacture is that rims or edges of the helmet can impose a force upon the neck in a manner similar to a bending edge of a mallet in a steel bending mill. The situation could exist when the helmeted head is rapidly extended posteriorly—the rim of the helmet strikes the neck with excessive force because of the increased leverage caused by the use of the helmet itself.

From a biomechanical principle this does, in fact, appear possible. However, radiographic motion pictures with volunteers wearing helmets and involving hyperextension of the cervical area within the experimental laboratory, have demonstrated that when the head is extended backwards the rear rim of the helmet moves down and away from the neck area, rather than contacting it. Further studies have shown that contact in the use of football helmets usually occurs at the seventh cervical vertebrae, while in hockey helmets such contact occurs at the sixth cervical vertebrae. The reason for the difference in location of this anatomic distribution could relate to the wearing of a helmet for different sporting activities. The problem is compounded by the fact that the elevation of the back rim in football and hockey helmets also exposes the occipital area and the upper cervical region to energy absorption on impact, and now these become more vulnerable sites of possible injuries.

It is evident that a situation could arise where the forces on the athlete are so extreme that effective protection is impossible. In these cases, the sport itself must be modified to make participation safer.

CHAPTER 29
Sports Equipment Standards

William F. Hulse

Standards are essential and all-pervasive elements of modern society; yet most people, from the man in the street to the highest officers of the community, understand little about what standards are, what they do, who develops them, and why.

The process of standards-writing is being discussed in many new and significant circles. There are daily comments about standards in newspaper consumer columns. The federal government has established a new and powerful commission whose responsibility is to upgrade the safety of consumer products through standards.

There are several different kinds of standards in use and being developed in the United States. Company standards are written by employees of corporations, principally within such departments as design, development, production, and purchasing. Industry standards are written by representatives of companies under the aegis of a given industry trade association. Professional standards are written by committees of individual members of the professions, eg, the American Society of Mechanical Engineers. Government standards are written by the employees of a governmental agency or department. However, these are sometimes written by one person. Finally a full consensus standard, as written by an American Society for Testing and Materials (ASTM) technical committee, achieves agreement by all the several elements of the community that have an interest in their development and/or use. In ASTM these elements include producers, users, ultimate consumers, and those representing the general public interest.

A standard, the document, rather than a standard thing, is a result of a standardization effort under an agreed-upon set of regulations. It consists of common language to promote the flow of goods between buyer and seller and also perhaps to promote the safety of a thing, in this case, sport equipment.

Many people think that the word standard is synonymous with the word specification. Just as all football players are athletes but all athletes are not football players, a specification is only one of five distinctly different types of standards. In ASTM, the word standard is used predominantly as an adjective to describe the following: 1) standard definitions, 2) standard practices, 3) standard test methods, 4) standard classifications, and 5) standard specifications.

A brief description of each type will enable the reader to distinguish them. A standard definition creates a common language of terms for the given area of knowledge. Standard definitions have been developed for sports injuries so that, for example, a sprain and a strain can be distinguished. A standard practice is a procedure or guideline, and is a document stating how to do something such as selecting, preparing, installing, or inspecting. A standard test method is a concise description of an orderly procedure for determining a property or constituent of a material. It generally contains the essential details so that the method is accurate and the precision is high when the same or different operators in different laboratories conduct the test.

A standard classification defines systematic arrangements or divisions into groups based on similar characteristics, such as origin, composition, properties, or use.

Finally, a standard specification is a concise statement of requirements to be satisfied by a product, material, or system, indicating the procedures by means of which it may be determined whether the requirements given are satisfied. It is desirable that the requirements be expressed numerically in terms of appropriate units together with their limits. Specifications can describe a product, or the performance requirements for a product or system. The five types of ASTM standards are called voluntary consensus standards. They are developed and used voluntarily. Their use becomes mandatory only when government action makes it so.

ASTM is a management system for the development of voluntary full consensus standards. It provides a legal, administrative, and publications forum within which producers, users, ultimate consumers, and those representing a general interest can meet on a common ground to write standards that will best meet the needs of all concerned.

ASTM defines a consensus standard as "a standard produced by a body selected, organized, and conducted in accordance with the procedures of due process." The consensus is achieved when substantial agreement is reached by concerned interests according to the judgment of a duly appointed review authority.

ASTM believes consensus implies much more than the concept of simple majority but not necessarily unanimity, which often can be achieved only by compromises that reduce the quality of the standard. The present regulations make it mandatory for a minimum of 90% affirmative votes to achieve final approval by the duly appointed review body which is the Committee On Standards (nine members appointed from the ASTM membership-at-large of 30,000 and who serve a three-year term).

What does ASTM mean by due process? Eight points have to be followed.

1. Timely and adequate notice of a proposed standard undertaking to all persons likely to be materially affected by it,
2. Opportunity of all affected interests to participate in the deliberations, discussions, and decisions concerned both with procedural and substantive matters,
3. Maintnenace of adequate records of discussions and decisions.
4. Timely publication and distribution of minutes of meetings of main and subcommittees,
5. Adequate notice of proposed actions.
6. Meticulously maintained records of drafts of a proposed standard, proposed amendments, action on amendments, and final promulgation of the standard,
7. Timely and full reports on results of balloting,
8. Careful attention to minority opinions throughout the process.

It is now important to look at how standards are created by ASTM technical committees. There are at present over 140 such committees, with over five new ones formed each year when various organizations, groups, and even individuals express a need and the need is verified by a planning meeting of interested knowledgeable people. This meeting is followed by an organizational meeting and all parties that might have an interest are invited. Over five thousand invitations were sent out by the ASTM staff for one broad-based technical committee. Committee F-8 on Sports Equipment and Facilities was formed that way in 1969.

Standards-writing committees are groups of experts who volunteer their time for standards draft development sessions. They are seeking the mutual benefit of all concerned through consensus. ASTM takes precautions to see that the development of standards under its preview reflects full consensus as defined by the regulations for committee operations.

If the committee's scope concerns products and systems having a commercial bearing then, 1) the number of producer voting members must not exceed the number of nonproducer members, 2) the chairman of the main committee must be a nonproducer, 3) membership must be open to all knowledgeable individuals, 4) all negative votes on letter ballots must be considered, usually in discussion, thereby giving minority opinions a full hearing, 5) all committee meetings considering technical matters relating to standards must be open to visitors, 6) validated test data must be a part of standards action where applicable, this gives the standard a sound technologic base, 7) all standards actions must be equitable, meaning every organization, large or small, and every individual member is given a vote (size is not a factor), one interest equals one vote.

In ASTM there is the main committee as a whole, subcommittees covering a particular area, and task groups who are the workers of the subcommittee who write the first draft or conduct an interlaboratory testing program to validate the precision and accuracy of their new test method.

Together those groups function like this: when a task group prepares a draft document, it is reviewed by its parent subcommittee through a balloting procedure. If the document is approved by two-thirds of those returning ballots (a minimum of 60% of the voting interests must return the ballots) the document proceeds to a main committee ballot. Here 90% of those returning ballots (again a 60% return is required), must approve the document. It then goes to a Society ballot, which means that each of ASTM's 30,000 members has an opportunity to comment on the proposed standard.

All negative ballots must be considered by the originating subcommittee before a document can be published as a standard.

To be valid, a negative vote must be accompanied by a written explanation of what the member considers improper technical or procedural consideration.

Once the document has received approval by the Society ballot, it is submitted to ASTM's Committee on Standards, which checks for compliance with procedual requirements and serves as a body to which the disposition of negative comments can be appealed. On approval by the Committee on Standards, the document is published as an official ASTM standard.

The heart of a standard, of course, is its technical credibility, but it must also rest on sound legal foundations if it is to stand for very long.

In the United States, there are four legal principles that standards must consider: due process, restraint of trade, authority and responsibility, and liability. Standards that are technically sound and consider these principles will most likely be upheld by the courts if they are challenged in litigation. On the other hand, a standard may be technically excellent, but if it fails to consider any one of these principles—especially due process or restraint of trade—it is likely to be struck down and may even jeopardize the organization responsible for its development.

For the sports world the most important principle is liability. However, we are not talking about product liability, but the liability of ASTM and its members.

In Pennsylvania, where ASTM is chartered, the nonprofit corporation law flatly states that the members of a nonprofit corporation shall not be personally liable for the debts, liabilities, or obligations of the corporation. Thus ASTM members, its officers, and staff are free from personal liability should litigation occur.

Liability could be imposed upon the corporation, however, because it is the corporation that holds itself out as the expert on standards and publishes them for use by the public. Thus, if a suit were instituted for negligent misrepresentation (and that is the essence of legal liability), the corporation and not the individual would be the primary target.

It is necessary to understand the background of standards and standardization, including the legal foundations, to realize what a powerful tool a standard is and how it can be used in the protection of an athlete.

Specifically, ASTM Committee F-8 on Sports Equipment and Facilities, is a duly constituted committee approved by the ASTM Board of Directors. It has been operating for 15 years and has regularly held two- to three-day meetings twice a year. As with most ASTM committees, the meetings are held in various hotels around the country.

The committee had its original impetus from football injuries and the original subcommittees were entitled Head and Neck, and Body and Extremities. Head and neck injuries were the main focus and football helmet tests were the first to be addressed.

In 1971, a new subcommittee on Skiing Safety was formed to address the problems of ski bindings. An early subcommittee on gymnastics equipment had its roots in investigating the injuries from trampolines. The first ASTM consumer safety specification was on the trampoline and its use. A wrestling subcommittee was formed and attention given to wrestling mats and the measurement of shock attenuation.

After four to five years of operation, the executive committee found it more difficult to put the various sports into categories dealing with parts of the human anatomy. The committee was restructured into subcommittees dealing with the sport, whose job it was to write performance or product standards on the protective equipment being sold. Resource subcommittees with members having engineering, medical, and biomechanical expertise, were set up to furnish test methods or practices for the specification writing subcommittees. Thus, the existing committees on headgear, footwear, medical aspects, biomechanics, and statistics, were formed.

New sports and activities came in, such as a small group on fencing, and a large group on ice hockey. Subcommittees on padding and playing surfaces were formed to bring together a wide variety of experts who could furnish the expertise and research that is necessary before a standard can be written.

One of the more recent subcommittees is one on the female athlete. As women's sports accelerated it was noted that there were no standards for equipment, and most equipment was modified men's equipment. Women's sports shoes were built on men's lasts and gave poor fits on women's generally narrow feet. At the time of this writing there is a group on jogging and running footwear, which is a task force under the main subcommittee on footwear. Skiing has also started a group on cross-country skis. Previous work dealt with alpine skiing.

It is important to note that the primary work deals with the protective equipment worn by the athlete or the surface upon which he performs.

Thus there is no activity with basketball, which is supposed to be a minimum contact sport, but whose injuries run very high when compared to all sports. Baseball, with its batting helmet that has been satisfactory for preventing disabling injury, has not had an active role in the committee.

The sports community responds to the statistics of injuries as reported by the National Athletic Injury/Illness Reporting System (NAIRS) and Consumer Product Safety Commission's National Eelectronic Injury Surveillance System (NEISS).

Thus far, sports such as track and field, soccer, volleyball, tennis, and golf have not had enough equipment-related injuries to cause concern for standards. There has been minor interest in lacrosse helmets, and shin guards for field hockey players. Future activity may occur for protective devices for the female athlete for protection of the breasts and pelvic area.

The current status of existing standards and draft standards can be categorized by looking at each piece of protective equipment or device.

In football helmets, ASTM has published since 1974 a test method for Shock Attenuation Characteristics of Protective Headgear for Football. This test method is backed up by interlaboratory test data from seven laboratories, none of which is a football helmet manufacturer.

A performance standard was established with limits that football helmets should meet.

An ice hockey helmet specification is also in draft form. The test methods to determine the force of blows to the head are incorporated to minimize injury from the puck, a stick, a goal upright, other players, and the penetration of a skate blade.

A specification has been published to afford eye and face protection by specifying the characteristics of a clear plastic face shield or a wire cage, both of which are attached to a helmet.

Supplemental to both hockey and football, and available for other sports, is a draft specification and a standard practice for use of mouth guards.

In the padding area, task forces have been active for football shoulder, knee, and hip padding, using an existing test method that measures the shock-absorbing properties of the pad material or pad itself.

In footwear, the committee has published a practice for fitting, as it has been adequately demonstrated that the proper fit of equipment to an athlete's anatomy lessens the injury or protects better.

The group on running and jogging shoes is looking at test methods that will measure the impact of the foot in the shoe on the running surface. Recommendations may allow shoe designers to develop a product that can lessen the occurrence of stress fractures which the medical researchers are just beginning to understand.

The knee and ankle injuries associated with long cleats in football shoes have been lessened by the shoe designers going to a smaller soccer-type shoe cleat that reduces the locking of the shoe to the natural or synthetic turf. There has been no need expressed for a shoe or cleat specification at this time.

The playing surface subcommittee developed, and has revised, a test method that can measure shock absorption properties. This test has been used for wrestling mats and trampoline padding criteria.

The release of ski bindings to prevent leg injuries is one of the more complicated problems that has involved the skiing subcommittee for over five years. A test method has been published which enables the moments of force to be measured. Further work on adjusting binding release settings is underway. The mounting of the binding plate to the ski has occupied one group of experts and there are methods published on screw strength retention characteristics, using a specified test screw.

An eye protection specification is being balloted and attention is being given to ski poles and ski brakes.

One small group has been looking into fencing equipment such as vests, masks, and the blade or foil metal characteristics.

Finally the gymnastics group has published a specification on trampolines that includes instructions on labeling and use. It has been reported that trampoline injuries dropped when manufacturers and users followed the voluntary standard. Work is under way for performance standards on the balance beam, vaulting horse, parallel bars, and rings.

A good case history of a standard development project that has had a definite effect on minimizing face and eye injuries, can be found with the ice hockey subcommittee and its standard specification on face protection. The subcommittee chairman was the technical director of the Amateur Hockey Association of the United States (AHAUS), which controls over 200,000 youths playing ice hockey.

Development of the standard specification, which took over two years, was coupled with a certification program that depended on an independent testing laboratory testing face shields and guards and certifying that they met the criteria in the specification. A certification seal was awarded each product that passed, and the rules committee of AHAUS then set forth a rule that mandated use of certified equipment.

There has been no damage of eyes with loss of sight since this program was implemented. The program is self-sustaining and will serve as a model for the ice hockey helmet and other equipment.

Since all youth hockey is not under AHAUS control, it is hoped that the high school federation and the NCAA will adopt the same or a similar program. The possibility of large product liability suits may cause all ice hockey jurisdictions to follow the lead of AHAUS.

The conclusion can now be drawn that when there is a national standard, albeit voluntary, with the legal credibility backed by an independent testing program that involves a visible certification logo, coupled with the power of sports rules that are mandatory, injuries will be minimized and approach zero.

Everyone benefits, with the possible exception of plaintiffs' attorneys. The manufacturer is free from product liabilty suits; his insurance premiums are reasonable; the testing laboratory earns a profit while carrying out a public service; parents and children, the ultimate beneficiaries, can participate in a contact sport with reasonable assurance that a severe injury can be avoided.

Thus the quadruple effect of standard, testing, certification, and mandatory rule make youth ice hockey a safer sport.

The problem has been partially solved in the recreational skier area in a different way. All these risk sports, where injury does occur, can minimize injury on a volunteer basis where a consensus standard has been developed. The manufacturers who took part in the effort now voluntarily follow the standard by changing their product to conform. The recreational skier does not have rules which mandate his skiing, so an educational program needs to be developed.

The two major ski magazines both have talented, safety-conscious skiers on the ASTM committee. The readers of their magazines know about the work of the committee and now more ski retailers, ski rental shops, and ski area operators are attempting to educate their customers by educational precepts.

A new study is under way in the ski subcommittee to gather injury statistics for the next three years. With this data base it will be easy to demonstrate the effect of standards as well as the other effects that will make skiing a safer sport yet still retain the element of risk which gives the thrill and excitement a lot of Americans want in their recreational and school and college sports.

To summarize, this chapter has pointed out that a viable system is available for the development of voluntary consensus standards. The system is working and has produced standards in many varied sports areas. Injury statistics show a trend to fewer injuries when a standard is in place and adhered to. Related beneficial social and economic effects occur when standards are developed and used by participants, manufacturers, and sports administrators. Where there is a low-injury, economically viable risk sport there is generally a standard covering the protective equipment and devices.

CHAPTER 30
National Governing Bodies

Carl S. Blyth, PhD
Voigt R. Hodgson, PhD

The National Operating Committee on Standards for Athletic Equipment (NOCSAE) was organized in 1969 with the purpose of reducing injuries by formulating standards to which athletic equipment must conform. Head injury in football was given the highest priority because of the numbers of serious injuries and the potential for improvement. The Department of Neurosurgery at Wayne State University was selected to develop a football helmet standard and research began in 1971. Fatal head injury incidence has declined by 64% since NOCSAE helmet research began due also, no doubt, to many other factors.

FOOTBALL HELMET IMPACT STANDARD

There are a number of considerations that must be made in setting a standard. Some of the more important ones are as follows:

Types and incidence of injuries In football, as far as closed head injuries are concerned, the two main injuries to be prevented are concussion and cerebrovascular injuries. Something is known about concussions, which are the most numerous. Not too much is known about cerebrovascular injuries, the most common of which are subdural hematomas. These are the head injuries that result in fatalities and paralyzing conditions. One must consider what a standard might do to other injuries in terms of the neck of the player wearing the helmet and in terms of injuries to other players. The tolerance levels of these internal injuries and setting the standard in relation to them must be considered.

Available materials The state of the art of materials and the methods of fabrication must be considered because one cannot just arbitrarily set the standard too high, so that it is impossible to meet the criteria.

Impact environment One has to think of the impact environment; at what velocities are these heads traveling and what are the stopping distances involved? What kinds of surfaces are the players running into? What is the effect of temperature?

Head model If a standard is developed, it should be based on a realistic head model, something to which human tolerance standards can be applied and something that will not cause unrealistic damage to a helmet.

Performance The level of performance standard, or the performance criterion of a helmet, is also important. To what level should a helmet attenuate accelerations of the head? This is very critical. This can be set at various points because it is related to the state of the art.

Failure criteria What, in addition to the accelerations above the maximum tolerable gravity level, should be used as failure criteria? In other words, should failed rivets, cracked shells, damaged liners, be considered as failures?

The test method How comprehensive should a test method be? How many locations should be struck? How many times? What environmental conditions should be simulated?

Size How many sizes should be tested to make sure all sizes in the manufacturers' ranges are as safe as they can be.

Equipment The test equipment used must not be so sensitive that it can only be used in the laboratory where there are people who have worked with it. It must be rugged, withstand repeated tests and be accurate.

Duration Duration of certification of helmets—how long should it be? A year? Ten years? Nobody is certain but it is a question that must be answered.

The cost Is a standard going to put some schools out of the football business? This must be a consideration, since some helmets are already costing $100.00 apiece.

Recertification Is it possible to help schools keep their costs down by recertifying helmets after they have been once certified?

Enforcement The best standard in the world is not going to work unless some kind of a system is developed whereby it can be assured that the helmets turned out by the manufacturers are going to maintain the same quality at which they were originally certified. Furthermore, helmets on the field must be maintained by the equipment people and reconditioning.

INJURY INCIDENCE AND HUMAN TOLERANCE

One study of high school football injuries[1] showed that the most frequently injured parts of the body were: the knee (19.3%); ankle (15.3%); head and neck (8.8% – head 6.2%, and neck 2.6%); shoulder (7.3%); upper leg (5.4%); back (4.7%); and injury to other parts of the body trailing off at lower percentages. While not the most numerous, head and neck injuries are obviously the most serious injuries incurred in football. The most common head injury in this study was a cerebral concussion, projecting across the nation to be 75,000 annually in high school play.

A football fatality study[2] conducted since 1931, shows that of the average deaths that occur annually for all levels of play, head and neck injuries accounted for 80%. The fatal incidence has fluctuated between 1 and 2 per 100,000 participants, with cerebral hemorrhage being the most common cause. From this evidence it can be concluded that either concussions and the rare cerebrovascular injuries occur from different mechanisms, or that it is a matter of force intensity, with concussions usually occurring at the lowest levels among individuals. Occasionally acute cerebral hemorrhagic injuries occur without posttraumatic unconsciousness associated with concussions.

It has been shown[3] that among men of football-playing age in the United States, cerebrovasculardisease incidence is between 1 and 2 per 100,000, about 70% of which are hemorrhagic. Even granting that active young men drawn into football may be atypical of the population, it is doubtful that any practical protective headgear can completely eliminate cerebrovascular injuries in football.

The only tolerable design limit available relates the likelihood of cerebral concussion and the amount of linear acceleration experienced by the head. Furthermore, it is the only limit for which practical instrumentation is available with which to assess the hazard of an impact to a head model wearing a helmet. Based upon the evidence of Gadd,[4] a severity index (SI) of 1500 was chosen as the performance limit which should not be exceeded by the head model in a standard impact test. The SI is defined as follows: $SI = \int_o^t A^{2.5}\,dt \leq 1500$,

where A = linear acceleration in gravity
2.5 = weighting factor
dt = a time interval
t = pulse duration, $0.0025 < t < 0.050$ sec

It is assumed the design to minimize the SI will provide a protective umbrella for all types of internal injury. See discussion and references regarding risk of serious head injury vs SI, Chapter 9.

HEAD MODEL

Since the 1500 SI performance standard is related to clinical studies, human cadaver drops, and volunteer air bag impacts, it is essential that it be used on a head model which is as realistic as possible. Several years of prototypes led to the present head models sizes 6⅝, 7¼, and 7⅝, which are in use evaluating the impact attenuation characteristic of football helmets. The head models have 50th percentile dimensions in each of these three sizes derived from US Army head anthropometry data. These are the critical head sizes (smallest stand-off from the shell) in each of the three shell sizes used by most manufacturers. The head models also have weight/mass distribution and impact response characteristics simiar to the human head as determined from comparison with cadaver impacts. The response of the head model is determined by a triaxial accelerometer mounted at the center of gravity of the head. There are now 51 such test devices in use in this country, including six by manufacturers, 41 by reconditioners, and four by institutions.

Effect of the Standard

As shown in Table 30-1, the effect of the standard has been to produce certified helmets capable of reducing the SI well below prestandard helmet performance. To achieve this change, manufacturers have resorted to size adjustments,

Table 30-1
Comparison of Certified and Precertified Helmets
Severity index performance for the standard second 60-inch right frontal boss drop.

Average of certified models		Precertified helmets tested as received by reconditioner						
Severity index*	866	Below 1199	1200-1499	1450-1999	2000-2499	2500-2900	Total
Number	63	58	80	411	274	26	849
Precentage	–	6.8	9.4	48.4	32.3	3.1	100
				----------83.8%----------			

*Severity index must not exceed 1500 on second drop from 60-inch for certification.

ie, moving sizes in which the head was too close to the shell into larger shells, or eliminating some larger sizes, and making materials and design changes. Most models had to sacrifice some range of fit and comfort, because stopping the head model from a velocity of 17.9 ft/sec in less than an inch means that more of the space between head and shell must be taken up by higher density, stiffer liners. A few models had to increase shell thickness to prevent cracking around rivet holes due to excessive flexure and provide more support for the liner. This also leads to increased shell weight and stiffness, thus creating a more dangerous situation for opponents.

There has been a 64% decline in fatal head injury incidence, comparing the pre-NOCSAE 1964–1970 period to the 1971–1983 NOCSAE period of influence on helmets worn by high school players.[2]

Expense

To date the cost of research leading to the standard has been trivial and there has been no cost for enforcement. Slight increases in cost are to be expected, eg, higher density energy-absorbing foam is more expensive than low-density comfort foams. It has been hoped that, whatever new helmet purchase and maintenance increases were incurred because of the standard, would be offset by lower incidence of injury, litigation, and insurance costs. Unfortunately, litigation and insurance costs have been largely responsible for pushing many helmet model prices to the $100.00 mark, even though head and neck injury incidences are below half of what they were at the inception of the NOCSAE standard.

Length of Certification

It is uncertain how long a helmet will remain certified because of variations in durability among models and differences in numbers and intensities of hits as a result of use. As a direct result of the NOCSAE standard, the National Athletic Equipment Reconditioners Association (NAERA) was formed and all the NAERA members have NOCSAE test equipment for quality control purposes. The NAERA members do a partial nondestructive test on a small sample of each school's helmets coming for reconditioning after the season. Information from the sample test is carried over to all other helmets being processed. The tests are done on all models and primarily in the known critical locations for each model, but with occasional changes to other impact locations. On the basis of results of these tests and visual inspection, the NAERA members recertify previously certified helmets in obviously good condition and work in cooperation with the manufacturers in restoring damaged certified helmets. How long the helmets will stay in recertifiable condition depends primarily on the type of shell and care with which face masks are installed, because a cracked shell will eliminate a helmet from recertification under present conditions. Many recertified helmets are now entering their tenth season with performance either undiminished or in recertified condition with parts replacement.

Neck Injury

Paralyzing neck injuries have been reduced by about 50% from the 21.2 annual average during

1971–1976 seasons for high school and college, apparently resulting from the 1976 rules change prohibiting initial head contact in blocking and tackling. For a more thorough discussion, refer to Chapter 9.

BASEBALL HELMET STANDARDS

NOCSAE devised a baseball batter's helmet standard in 1982 which becomes effective for high schools and colleges for the 1985 season.

OTHER SPORTS EQUIPMENT

Because of limitations in time and numbers of personnel, NOCSAE, rather than spread itself too thin, has concentrated on the development of standards to reduce the most serious injuries in sports, those of the head and neck. It has as its goal, however, establishment of voluntary standards for all sports equipment according to priorities in terms of numbers and seriousness of injuries.

CONCLUSIONS

1. The impact attenuation performances of most NOCSAE-certified football helmets on the market have been greatly improved relative to linear head acceleration concussion tolerance levels, and have significantly helped to reduce the numbers of fatal head injuries.

2. It is felt that the approximate 50% reduction in paralyzing neck injury which has occurred in football is primarily due to 1976 rules changes that research in helmet standards helped to recommend.

3. NOCSAE has devised impact standards for other sports such as baseball, and faceguard and padding standards are in preliminary stages.

4. NOCSAE has devised impact standards for other sports such as baseball, and faceguard and padding standards are in preliminary stages.

REFERENCES

1. Blyth, C.S., and Mueller, F.O. *An Epidemiologic Study of High School Football Injuries in North Carolina.* 1968–1972, Final Report. Washington, DC: US Government Printing Office, 1974.

2. Blyth, C.S., and Arnold, D.C. Thirty-seventh annual survey of football fatalities 1931–1968. In *Proceedings of the Forty-Sixth Annual Meeting.* Hanover, NH: American Football Coaches Association, 1969.

3. Ryan, A.J. *Medical Care of the Athlete.* New York: McGraw-Hill, 1962.

4. Gadd, C.W. Tolerable severity index in whole-head, non-mechanical impact. In *Proceedings of the Fifth Stapp Car Crash Conference.* New York: SAE, Inc, 1971.

CHAPTER 31
Equipment Certification Councils

Earl F. Hoerner, MD

Safety is the responsibility of everyone concerned with an activity. This includes the participant in the realm of sports, whether recreational, leisure, or athletic. The spectrum of interest includes the disciplines of sociology, psychology, medicine, education, law, politics, economics, manufacturing, and commerce.

A monitoring body to collate, review, and analyze data that are available is needed. In the United States, this is the responsibility of the governmental agency known as the Consumer Product Safety Commission (CPSC). The CPSC has the final responsibility to ensure that consumer products are safe.

To implement the findings and recommendations of the Consumer Product Commission, safety codes and standards are developed through the process known as voluntary consensus. These codes and standards include test methods, performance, use, definitions, recommended practices, classification, and specifications. In this country several of the open membership organizations that develop these codes or standards are the American Society for Testing and Materials (ASTM), the American National Standards Institute (ANSI), and the National Operating Committee on Standards for Athletic Equipment (NOCSAE).

The purpose of a Certification Council is to seek out and select such codes and standards as appropriate for any product available that the public, would purchase and use. The Council also assumes the responsibility of establishing the method, criteria, and procedures for the final product or equipment certification. A Certification Council is composed of three major groups—users (consumers), producers (manufacturers and dealers), and general interest (administrators, educators, professionals). These Councils have long been present in the business and industrial sectors, including manufacturing and services areas. Examples are those of the construction, automotive, and electrical industries. These Councils assure that appliances, products, apparatus, or equipment conform to well-identified codes and standards of construction, fabrication, manufacture, and use.

The Equipment Certification Council as known in the sector of sports is composed of coaches, participants, scientists, physicians, manufacturers, and administrators. Its purpose is to seek out and select codes and standards, including test methods and procedures for equipment used in an athletic, sporting, recreational, and leisure time activity. In addition it has as its function the responsibility of identifying and publishing any and all factors associated with safety, whether it be playing surfaces, rules, attitudes, officiating, training, conditioning, and even administration.

Such a system has been designed for ice hockey to ensure that participants, regardless of whether they play on an organized team, in competition, or recreationally, will have available, and hopefully use, equipment and protective paddings that will aid in ensuring safety.

This establishment and implementation of the Hockey Equipment Certification Council (HECC) by its voluntary and independent nature is unique in the sports world. This 15-member council, composed of representatives from all areas involved with the game, was organized and created through the leadership of the national governing body of ice hockey, the Amateur Hockey Association of the United States (AHAUS). The AHAUS was the first of 33 national governing bodies in the United States to establish tested safety standards for sport equipment that met the criteria of the Consumer Product Safety Commission. In addition, within this democratic system, voluntary consensus must be upheld, and in the establishment of this council, thorough steps were taken to weigh and reweigh all recommendations and objections to ensure this.

By this action, precedent has been established. Other national governing bodies have been working in this direction of safety codes and standards for many years. In today's society, the requirement that there be a voluntary process is now being pursued by leaders and suppliers in many other sports.

How did this Hockey Equipment Certification Council come into actuality? In 1977 with increasing public concern and subsequent pressure on the sport through players, coaches, administrators, parents, and spectators, the AHAUS in its role as the national governing body called a nation-wide meeting in Detroit, Michigan in conjunction with the National Collegiate Athletic Association national ice hockey playoffs. As a result, in attendance were leaders from all sectors of ice hockey, as well as representatives of the Consumer Product Safety Commission and the voluntary consensus standard writing organizations. All of the necessary ingredients were present for a combined action toward the establishment of the Equipment Certification Council. From the interest and active participation of the varied people at this organizational meeting, task forces were established to identify the principles and subsequent structure and function of the Council.

The task forces identified needs as:

1. membership
2. charter
3. nominating officers
4. finances
5. validator
6. logo-seal
7. standard-codes certification
8. insurance.

The task forces through their chairman met again in December of 1977. As a result of their activity and recommendations the Hockey Equipment Certification Council became active for the Fiscal year of 1978, and thereafter.

Through the constant motivating leadership of the task forces, an active organization involving all spheres of hockey, including youth, high school, college, semi-professional, and recreational was implemented. Foreign manufacturers as well as United States suppliers were included. A validator was identified, and a logo-seal approved.

Membership classification and participating organizations are:

Users:
- Amateur Hockey Association of the United States
- National Association of Intercollegiate Athletics
- National Collegiate Athletic Association
- National Federation of High Schools
- National Junior College Athletic Association
- National Parks and Recreation Association
- American Hockey Coaches Association

Producers:
- National Sporting Goods Association
- Insurance Underwriters Association
- Sporting Goods Manufacturers Association
- Canadian Sporting Goods Association

General Interest:
- National Safety Council
- American College of Sports Medicine
- National Athletic Trainers Association
- National Operating Committee on Safety for Athletic Equipment.

The Ice Skating Institute of America has been extended an invitation to join the Council as of June 1979.

The Officers of the Council making up the Executive Committee responsible for the administration of the Council include the President—elected from the membership of the User or General Interest category; Vice president—from the membership of the Producer category; Secretary—from the User or General Interest category; and Treasurer from the General Membership.

The secretary of the Council also functions as the Chairman of the Certification Committee, which is responsible for recommendation to the membership of the Council and the Executive Committee the on-going process of reviewing, revising, and modifying codes and standards, as well as suggesting new areas of concern within the sport of ice hockey. This Certification Committee includes two members from the Producer category and one from the User or General Interest group.

The usefulness of these councils is attested to by the following. In 1976 and 1977, sources indicated that over 50% of all hockey injuries were to the face. In March 1979, after one year's experience with face masks produced to standards, Paul Vinger reported an incidence rate of less than 1% injury to the face in protected players.

This experience should stimulate other National Governing Bodies to follow this demonstrated value.

CHAPTER 32
Difficulties of Interfacing People and Materials

Marlene J. Adrian, DPE

Inherent in the setting of standards for safe equipment is the determination of physical dimensions of the protective item, and specification of nontoxic materials in its construction. If these specifications are too general or nonexistent, protective equipment may not meet the needs of the participant because of difficulties of interfacing the sports participant with the protective device. The ultimate goal of interfacing is to obtain the "perfect fit." The fit must be more precise than the fit of ordinary clothing. For example, shoes may be used for walking, going to and from an automobile, and some tolerance in fit could be accepted without causing much discomfort. That same tolerance with athletic shoes would produce blisters and other discomfort, possibly contributing to an injury during high rates of acceleration or changing directions. The following discussion will consider the "ideal" interfacing, or perfect linking, of protective equipment and the athlete.

ANTHROPOMETRY

Athletes and sports participants are of many sizes and shapes. Figures 32-1, 32-2, and 32-3, and Table 32-1, strikingly depict this wide range of characteristics.

These data illustrate the need for a wide range of sizes and shapes for protective equipment; one size does not fit all. No longer do small, medium, large, and extra large fit all sports participants.

At the highly skilled level of competition there has been and still is a tendency toward homogeneity of anthropometric characteristics. This is not true at the recreation, high school, and college levels. With the increased numbers of sports participants, the jogging emphasis, the greater opportunity for competitive sports for girls and women, and the greater concern for safety in sports, the heterogeneity of body shapes and sizes has become evident, and the interfacing problem a critical issue.

Assessment of protective equipment from an anthropometric aspect consists of identifying the anatomy of the body to be protected, thereby covered, and determining if adequate coverage has been achieved. Dynamic fit is more important than static fit. If one merely measured the human body to determine the material required to cover the areas as the person sat or stood, the equipment might not be satisfactory when the person moved. The equipment might move with the body parts and expose other body parts that are to be protected, and therefore, prove to be an unsatisfactory fit. For example, chest protectors must be designed for the sport, the person, and for the movements most often performed.

Questions such as the following need to be asked before fabricating the equipment for best fit. Where are the ball and bat most likely to strike the torso of the catcher? What must be done to protect the groin and collarbone-neck regions when the catcher squats? The same principle for improving all protective equipment in all sports holds true.

CONSIDERATIONS FOR EQUIPMENT

Heat Dissipation and Sweating

Because protective devices add bulk and weight to the body, and usually consist of synthetic nonbreathing materials, even the best protective equipment may be less than ideal with respect to heat dissipation. This difficulty in dissipating heat and perspiration normally may be circumvented by evaluating the rest of the wearing apparel. Changes may be made in the uniform to provide for more adequate ventilation and heat dissipation. Uniforms could be fabricated from materials that are moisture-absorbant or have a wicking action, one of lighter weight and color, and loose in fit.

Some of these same changes may be possible also in the piece of protective equipment itself.

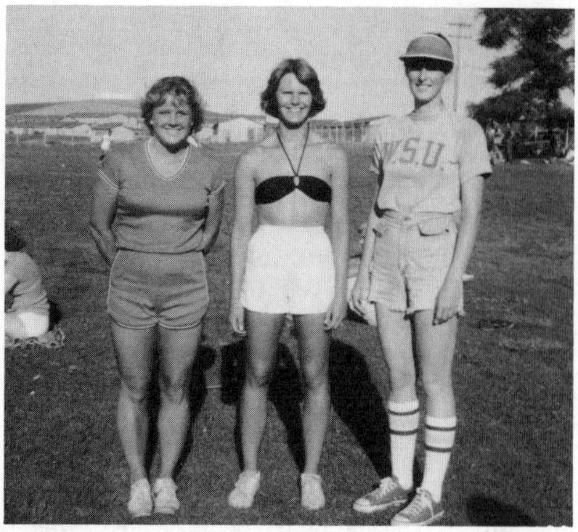

Figure 32-1 College softball players.

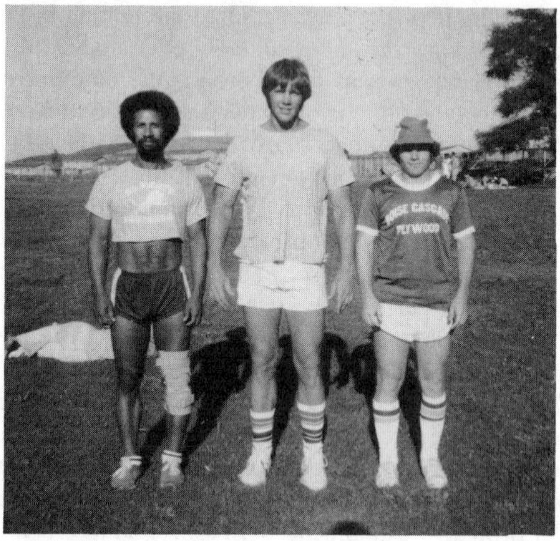

Figure 32-2 College softball players.

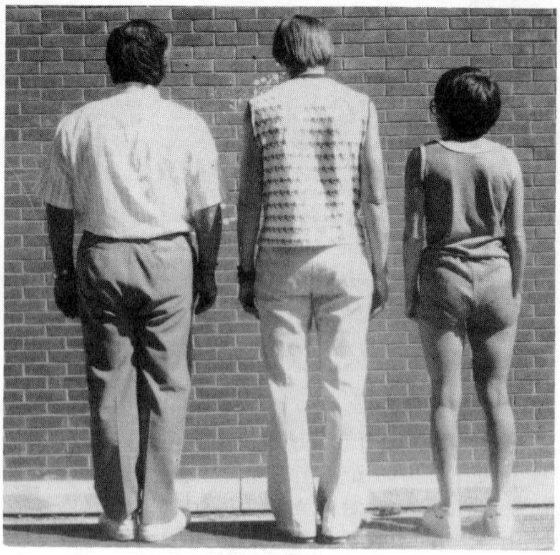

Figure 32-3 Adult sports performers.

Allergies

Another, although minor, problem with protective equipment is selecting materials that are nontoxic and will not cause a physiologic reaction. With ever-changing technology, new materials are created that must be tested against hot perspiring skin. Of particular importance is the appraisal of preservative, water-proofing, or other finishes that are applied to the protective device.

Economics

Ideal fit is not achieved without expense. The more custom-made or individualized the product,

Table 32-1
Anthropometric Characteristics of Sports Performers Depicted in Figures 32-1, 32-2, and 32-3

	Height (Feet and inches)	Weight (lbs)	Girth of upper arm (inches)	Girth of thigh (inches)	Hand length (inches)	Distance between shoulders (inches)
A	5 3	135	11.5	23.0	7.0	18.0
B	5 6	125	10.3	20.1	7.3	17.0
C	5 10	134	9.5	19.8	8.0	16.5
D	5 8	158	12.8	22.0	8.0	18.0
E	6 4	215	14.3	22.3	8.5	20.5
F	5 5	148	12.6	21.6	7.4	19.5
G	5 8	208	12.6	24.4	7.1	20.1
H	5 10	155	11.4	20.9	7.7	16.9
I	5 2	102	8.9	19.7	6.9	15.0

the more expensive it becomes. If the protective equipment is designed specifically for one position in one sport, such as goal-keeper pads in field hockey, the market is reduced considerably. Here also, the popularity of the sport influences the number of participants and therefore, the cost of the item.

The cycle of supply and demand has, in the past, meant inadequate fit or the elimination of sports participants who did not fit the product. This will continue to be a problem, but the trend is toward improved fit with increased cost. Proper interfacing now is one of the major criteria used in the development of protective equipment.

ROLES OF ATHLETE, COACH, AND SPORTSMEDICINE SPECIALIST

Coaches, sportsmedicine specialists, and athletes, must demand improved interfacing of protective equipment with the sports participant.

The coach should assess the fit of equipment for each individual participant. He or she should tabulate the size of the person, the difficulties with fit, and the inadequacies of the equipment. These tabulations need to be summarized and sent to the manufacturers to demand improvement. The ASTM committee could be contacted to determine whether or not safety standards are being violated. If so, the ASTM in cooperation with the National Consumer Product Safety Commission can exert pressure to cause product improvement.

The sportsmedicine specialist, as well as the coach, should tabulate injuries that might be a result of unsatisfactory interfacing of protective equipment with the sports performer. Data should be sent to injury-reporting systems so that their data are compared with many other data, thus identifying more easily interfacing problems. Once again, the manufacturers of the equipment need to be made aware of the problem.

Research by the sportsmedicine specialist, especially the specialist in biomechanics, can provide the necessary information concerning the specific requirements for protection and the anthropometric characteristics of the population using the product. Actual experimental testing of the product will help to produce a change in the state of the art, whether this includes physical fit or nontoxic materials.

The athlete can provide the more subtle identification of lack of fit. He, as well as the recreational sports participant, needs to be educated concerning the questions they could ask: What is an adequate fit? Am I getting an undesirable physiologic reaction to the product? Who should I tell? An educated consumer is vital to the continual improvement of a product and its safety.

State of the Art

Ideal interfacing of protective equipment with the sports participant has not been achieved with such items as shoulder pads used in football, hip and thigh pads used in several sports, or in chest protectors used in several sports and through a wide range of ages. Fit is satisfactory in such equipment as knee and elbow pads and mouth protectors.

Awareness by the public and the people in the sports area has increased in the past decade. This awareness must be enhanced and greater action taken to alleviate the interfacing difficulties.

CHAPTER 33 *Obsolescence in Protective Equipment*

Chauncey A. Morehouse, PhD

The history of the development of protective equipment for sports parallels the establishment of game rules. As individual techniques and game strategies become more complex and sophisticated the risks of injury increase, thus creating a need for more effective protective equipment. As more refined devices become available, older ones become obsolete.

Obsolescence is a gradual process, however, and to a large degree may be considered a matter of personal opinion. Therefore, in order to avoid misunderstandings and misinterpretations it seems essential to introduce this discussion with some basic assumptions and definitions.

ASSUMPTIONS AND DEFINITIONS

There are three basic assumptions that may help to place the subject in proper perspective. First, it must be assumed that sports participation is an educational experience regardless of whether the activity is part of a school program or is sponsored by a nonschool organization. The most important consideration, then, is to provide the best possible protection against injury for all participants. This primary consideration should never be set aside in favor of secondary or tertiary ones such as prestige for individuals or institutions, need to generate financial or community support, and tradition.

Second, it should be realized that despite the use of the best protective equipment presently available, a certain risk of injury remains in all sports competition.

Finally, there is a dearth of objective evidence regarding the direct cause or causes of injuries in sports. Therefore, there is insufficient objective evidence to support many of the statements that follow; however, logical reasoning should lead to similar conclusions.

Protective equipment or practices have been defined in a broad general way. It includes, as well as all personal equipment, all environmental and administrative aspects or objects that assist in protection of sports participants against injury. This definition is offered in contrast to the much more restrictive but usual one of personal equipment designed to attenuate kinetic energy from physical contact or impact between individuals or between an individual and an object within the playing environment. Under the broader definition, a provision for an adequate safety zone around a playing field, or limiting the spectators to the maximum number that can adequately be accommodated would be considered appropriate protective practices.

Obsolescence is defined, by individuals who are knowledgeable in the subject of sport safety or protective equipment, as a piece of personal or environmental equipment or a practice that would not be recommended for use. It must also be recognized that obsolescence is a continuum, and the precise position that a specific article of equipment occupies at a given time on this continuum is very much a matter of personal opinion and subjective judgment.

Use and Fit as Factors Creating Equipment Obsolescence

Usually one thinks of protective equipment as becoming obsolete when it no longer provides adequate protection, cannot be purchased under normal circumstances, or is no longer the newest style. However, there are two other factors that should be mentioned at this point. The first of these is the use of "hand-me-down" equipment, which is a common practice in many school systems. The younger and less skilled players deserve the same protection against injury as the first-string varsity players, yet the newest protective equipment nearly always is purchased for the more highly skilled participants and the younger players must wear the older articles. Often they are not inspected for protective characteristics and are not reconditioned between seasons of play.

A second factor related to obsolescence is the use of ill-fitting equipment. This general practice usually stems from two aspects. First, is the practice of issuing protective equipment without any supervision concerning its fit. Young persons ordinarily do not know how equipment is sized and many do not have sufficient experience to know when it does not fit properly. In fact, some may not even know how to wear it properly. Second, many programs have insufficient quantities of personal protective equipment to provide adequately for the number of candidates who are trying out for a team.

Use of worn out or ill-fitting equipment often is the result of inadequate basic funding for a comprehensive program. In the event that there is insufficient financial support to purchase an adequate amount of suitable protective equipment, the entire program should be evaluated objectively with a view toward replacing some sports with others that require less expense for equipment, limiting the number of participants in certain activities, or curtailing the competitive schedule.

SPECIFIC FACTORS LEADING TO OBSOLESCENCE

There are numerous factors that often make protective equipment obsolete. Each of these is discussed in the following sections and at least one example is given to illustrate the specific point. No attempt will be made to discuss these factors in order of priority, as this would require a value judgment that would be too difficult to make.

Ineffective Injury Prevention

Any piece of protective equipment that fails to provide adequate protection against injury must be considered to be obsolete, for instance, the plastic face guards for football helmets. When hit at certain angles, they may fracture or flex inward and impact the nose or face. The flat shoulder pads are also considered obsolete because much of the force of blows is concentrated on the collar-bone and often results in shoulder injuries. The cantilever pads provide a much safer distribution of forces over a broader area of the shoulder. An example from another sport is the face guard originally used in lacrosse. The openings in many of the masks were so large that a ball could easily pass through and strike a player's eye. Unfortunately, these face guards may still be purchased.

The reed cloth soccer shin guards originally designed for protection against wounds and lacerations, are now thought to be ineffective. They are not capable of attenuating the energy of impact of a direct blow to the shin that is often delivered by the foot of an opponent unskilled in the game.

Most recently, in response to the increasing number of eye injuries occurring in racquet sports, attempts have been made to reduce these injuries, if possible. Investigations of the resistance of eye protective devices to impacts by the balls used in squash and racquetball have come to the same conclusion.[1-3] The results of these investigations indicated that open eyeguards do not effectively protect the eyes from ball impact. The balls deform sufficiently on impact so that they come in contact with the delicate structures of the eye. Easterbrook[4] has verified these results by reported cases of eye injuries during play while wearing open-type guards. Thus, one may conclude that open eyeguards for racquetball and squash are not obsolete. The plano lens type models afford much more effective protection.

Out of Style

For purposes of this discussion, protective equipment is out of style and therefore becomes obsolete when new materials or designs have been developed that provide more effective protection. Perhaps the best example is the extensive use of closed-cell foam rubber for personal and game equipment. Some years ago, foam wrestling mats appeared on the market and soon made the canvas-covered felt mats obsolete for wrestling and tumbling, as protective mats around gymnastic apparatus, and for paddings of walls and posts in gymnasiums. Such padding will retain its shock-attenuation characteristics for longer periods of time. The football side line markers and corner posts (flags) are more recent uses of foam rubber that contribute to greater safety and have made steel and wooden yard line markers obsolete, although many of these older markers are still being used.

New designs in protective equipment have made older models obsolete in a relatively short time. Perhaps there is no better example than the football helmet, many of which now utilize a combination of foam padding and suspension systems. These new designs provide greater protection than either the older full-suspension or completely padded helmets of felt and leather.

Much too frequently athletes, coaches, and administrators follow the lead of more successful teams in purchasing equipment. However, success does not stem primarily from better equipment nor does it ordinarily make good protective equipment obsolete. For instance, there is very little evidence to indicate that performance in basketball or football is improved by changing from high-cut to oxford shoes. The high-top shoes, particularly in football, are rapidly becoming obsolete because of reduced demand for shoes that are laced above the ankle. Athletes may feel they can run faster in low-cut shoes; however, factual evidence to this effect should be gathered before the high shoe becomes completely obsolete, particularly for the young player who may lack the necessary strength to provide adequate stability of the ankle.

Introduction of Additional Hazards

Game strategies and techniques are continually evolving, that tend to make certain items of equipment obsolete. The all-leather football helmet would quickly become soft under the impacts that in today's game, are routinely delivered to the plastic shells. The use of the helmet in blocking and tackling is a newer technique that has made better helmets necessary. Even though the use of the head as an initial point of contact has recently been condemned because of the prevalence of neck injuries, the blows to the head in modern football are much more numerous and of greater magnitude than they were two or three decades ago.

The greater use of the slapshot in hockey in the last few years, and the curved blade of the hockey stick, have created additional hazards for the game's participants. Puck and sticks are more frequently lifted off the ice at head height, creating injuries to the face and head. Therefore, the use of a hockey helmet with a full face guard is recommended. From the standpoint of safety, play without a helmet or with a helmet and no face guard is considered to be an obsolete practice.

Artificial turf, which is being installed in more high school, college, and municipal stadiums each year, has tended to make short knee pads and long cleats in football obsolete. Although there is still some controversy concerning incidence of injuries on artificial turf as compared to natural grass, most objective studies indicate that abrasions occur more frequently while playing on fields with artificial turf. In order to protect participants from these less serious injuries longer knee pads, pads on the elbows, and even knee-length stockings are recommended. If these artificial fields become more popular in the future, the use of the shorter pants with short knee guards may no longer be common in football.

Additional or Unnecessary Weight

If protective equipment adds appreciable weight it may hinder or interfere with player performance. Consequently, players and coaches are continually searching for lighter and more comfortable protective equipment. Such a quest is completely aceptable, if light weight can be achieved without sacrificing protection. The ineffective reed cloth soccer shin guards were originally replaced with fiber ones that were heavier, bulkier, and more difficult to keep in position when running. They have now been replaced with lighter foam-covered guards that conform more closely to the contour of the legs, yet still attenuate the energy of direct kicks quite adequately. The newest models are also fitted with straps at the top and bottom so they are easily held in place.

The fiber football pads are also rapidly being replaced by ones made of foam rubber. These lighter hip and shoulder pads, however, may not give the same degree of protection as provided by the less flexible and heavier fiber ones. All innovative equipment should be thoroughly tested for its protective capabilities before being completely accepted for use. Unfortunately, however, such practice is not often followed.

Some styles of hip and kidney pads are cut quite low, presumably to reduce their overall weight. There is little evidence available at this time to indicate whether protection is being sacrificed for decreased weight. Whether this new style will become popular and thus make the older heavier pads obsolete, remains to be seen.

Bulk as a Deterrent to Performance

Many performances in sport are dependent upon speed of movement, and therefore protective equipment should perform its intended purpose without imposing undue restrictions. The goalie pads and shoes used by women in field hockey are excellent examples of protective equipment that, from the player performance standpoint, should be redesigned. Goalie pads should either be adjustable or be manufactured in different sizes to provide better fit. They should be of lighter material and should conform more closely to the legs so that they do not interfere with movements of running. The shoes could be fitted and also made of lighter material that would enhance movement without sacrificing safety.

Wrestling mats that are thicker then one inch and allow for greater penetration often are a disadvantage to the wrestler who is dependent on his speed of movement. Thicker mats are not necessarily more protective; it is the quality rather than the quantity of material that affords protection to the wrestler or the gymnast. A firm foundation is necessary to provide adequate reaction forces for quick movements. The same firmness is needed for equilibrium in landings in gymnastics.

EFFECTS OF TRADITION ON OBSOLESCENCE

No treatment of obsolescence in protective equipment for sports would be complete without some mention of the effects of tradition. In general, sports are very traditional when it comes to rules and equipment. Changes occur slowly, probably because of the lack of scientific research. The environments in which sports are conducted are complex, and consequently, dependable results of research are not easily obtained. Two major factors that contribute to lack of development of more efficient and better designed equipment, are the concern of only a small number of individuals, and the small commercial market for such equipment.

Specific articles where improvements in design are slow in developing are pants and stockings used in ice hockey, the shoulder and arm guards worn in lacrosse and the headgear and gloves used in boxing. Players, particularly at higher levels of performance, have been slow to accept the baseball batting and ice hockey helmets as standard pieces of protective equipment, probably mainly due to the tradition associated with these sports.

A few research results indicate that the non-cleated shoe may be safer than the cleated shoe on artificial turf surfaces, although performances are not affected significantly. However, cleated shoes have been worn in field sports played on natural grass for almost as long as organized sports have existed. Consequently, it is difficult to accept such innovative ideas as wearing a shoe with a sole similar to that used in basketball or tennis, while playing football or soccer.

FUTURE INNOVATIONS MAY CREATE OBSOLESCENCE

As research develops and becomes more sophisticated, many changes may occur that will make current equipment obsolete. There has been considerable discussion about the possibility of adding a layer of foam rubber to the outsides of plastic helmets in football. Although foam rubber may not be suitable, there are materials that are excellent for shock absorption that are also firm and have a low coefficient of friction. They might well be suitable for use on the outside of football helmets.

Standards and fittings for goals and other field equipment made of shock-absorbing materials may soon make steel or aluminum goals obsolete. Protective equipment in all sports may one day be form-fitting, and provide maximal protection with minimum interference with movement. New protective materials and creative minds may make much of our current protective equipment obsolete.

CONCLUSION

More research concerning sports equipment is desirable. Regardless of the direction of this research, protection and safety must be the first considerations, if sports are to be considered a valuable contribution to the education of young people. Certainly economics must also be considered, but there is no alternative to the best in protective equipment and safety practices. Style, color, and other aesthetic factors should be considered only as last resorts in the purchase and maintenance of protective equipment for sports.

REFERENCES

1. Bishop, J., Kozey, J., and Caldwell, G. Performance of eye protectors for squash and racquetball. *Phys Sportsmed.* 10(3):63–69, 1982.

2. Morehouse, C.A. Preliminary evaluation of

eye protective devices for racquet sports. Unpublished research report submitted to ASTM F-8.57 Subcommittee on Eye Safety, 1983.

3. Feigelman, M.J., et al. Assessment of ocular protection for racquetball. Paper presented at the Annual Meeting of the Association for Research in Vision and Ophthalmology. Sarasota, Florida: 1982.

4. Easterbrook, M. Eye injuries in racket sports: A continuing problem. *Phys Sportsmed.* 9(1):91–101, 1981.

CHAPTER 34
A Manufacturer's Perspective

Dennis Burns, MFA

In order to obtain input for this chapter from some other companies on design, research, and development letters were sent to a number of companies that manufacture protective sports equipment, requesting their comments on such broad topics as:

1. the definition of protection and/or protective equipment;
2. what is the role or responsibility of equipment suppliers regarding protection of the user;
3. what is the procedure for developing a piece of protective equipment;
4. what factor does cost play in designing a product;
5. what is the status of protective equipment today;
6. comment on product liability.

Not one company responded. Some telephone calls were received explaining that for reasons of product liability the manufacturers did not wish to make any written contribution. Thus the perspective of this chapter is from one manufacturer's viewpoint, and that perspective may or may not reflect the views of all manufacturers. However, the perspective of all manufacturers has been drastically affected by the status of product liability. Therefore, they are not entirely to blame for not wanting to go on record; the situation is totally out of hand.

For example, the author was asked a few years ago to relate how a certain product that was designed by his company was developed and manufactured. A lengthy response explained the design development process of this product. Totally by accident, it was discovered that the letter was in the possession of an insurance company dealing in product liability insurance.

A manufacturer jeopardizes himself by making any public or written statement that an attorney may use later. However, the only way to get our society back to reality on this question is to speak out so the consumer has a better understanding of the situation, and the ramifications if the situation is not remedied.

To define protective equipment requires going further than merely consulting a dictionary. It would probably mean one would have to evaluate an individual piece of equipment relative to its intended purpose. But for the sake of discussion, one can define what a piece of protective equipment should do in the broad sense.

First of all, if one were to ask for a definition from ten different players, parents, and coaches, the result would be 30 different answers. Players are primarily interested in improving their efficiency so that they may excel at their game. Consequently they would rather shed more cumbersome, confining equipment in favor of lighter, or even no equipment in some cases, to maximize their performance, even at an increased risk of injury. They are there to play and to win. A parent's definition would probably be slanted in favor of maximizing protection. The coaches, undoubtedly, would take a viewpoint that would stress winning. We cannot or have not identified the "experts," the group that can standardize or supply the official definition of protective equipment, or a list of characteristics that should be found in a particular piece of equipment.

An innovative manufacturer will recognize or determine the need for new articles or the improvement of existing equipment. This is the first and possibly the most important step in the design process. The design process is basically a formula that is the same whether one is designing sports equipment, household goods, cars, billboards, or virtually anything.

Hockey players have been stereotyped as athletes whose faces have so many stitches that they look like road maps crisscrossed with railroad tracks, with puffy eyes, and sometimes even cauliflower ears. The cause of this, of course, is the pucks flying around at speeds sometimes in excess of 100 mph and hockey sticks being swung around like shillelaghs. It is still common in the professional sports for a player to have several hundred stitches on his face alone. Everyone is aware that a good many hockey players are missing teeth, whether they are pro or amateur. There are injuries involving fractures of cheek bones and jaws, and the loss of eyes. These injuries are a common plague to the sport.

This is a classic case of need—the need for a piece of equipment that might bring these injuries under control. Once the element of need is determined, a list of premises or requirements pertaining to the sport must be made. When a possible design solution is arrived at, the list of elements is used as a checklist to evaluate the solution. This is, in effect, defining the goal so it will be recognized once it is reached.

The premises involved in designing a face guard for hockey would include:

1. must have excellent visibility,
2. cannot impair breathing,
3. must be lightweight,
4. must withstand a high velocity/low mass impact (a puck traveling at a high rate of speed), and
5. must attach to helmet for best shock attenuation.

These requirements set up tough problems, however. Hockey is probably the fastest game played, and the players are in continual motion. Therefore they must be able to spot a puck being passed from almost any place in their peripheral plane.

This is unlike a catcher, for instance, who requires vision generally in a frontal direction only. Compared to a hockey player, a catcher is a stationary object, therefore weight is not as important a factor. A football player on the other hand has to have good peripheral vision but since the football is relatively large and the impacts are low velocity/high mass, the bars of the face protector can be larger in scale and also farther apart. Football players can choose between several models or configurations of face guards depending on how much vision and lightness they are willing to compromise in favor of more bars that mean more weight and less visibility, but possibly more protection.

Compromise is the key to design, especially when concerned with protective equipment. The words compromise, or trade-off in reference to a product that is designed to protect, are dangerous when product liability looms from every direction. Compromise in design is a fact and must be discussed. A simple illustration would be to picture on one end of the scale maximum protection, such as a suit of armor, and on the other end maximum performance—no equipment and thus no impairment of performance. The key to good design comes in finding the proper place of protective equipment on that scale. This does not mean a compromise in the quality of the product. It means weighing certain design criteria such as weight vs performance.

Let us assume we could achieve a higher degree of protection if the weight of a particular piece of equipment could be increased 50%, but that increased weight was inversely proportional to decreased performance. The net effect would be that players would not accept it at all and would prefer to go unprotected until a solution was made available. These trade-offs from the players' point of view are usually between protection and performance, but they can involve cost vs protection, appearance vs protection, cost vs appearance, and many others. We must face the important fact that participants in a given sport are there to play and to excel at the game. Therefore, designing equipment that will impair performance is not a solution.

Equipment must reduce the risk of injury without changing the form and appeal of the sport. After all, if football could be made a noncontact sport it would not have the same appeal for the fans or the players. Consequently, it can safely be said that much of the appeal of a given sport can be in the action or inherent danger. In which case, what is the responsibility of a manufacturer? The Consumer Product Safety Council has stated, for instance, that skateboard injuries, which will exceed 200,000 this year, could be greatly reduced if skateboarding was done primarily in parks. But many parks have closed because they cannot buy liability insurance. This means that skateboarding has inherent risks and even under ideal conditions there will be injuries.

The problem from a liability standpoint is that the skateboard park becomes potentially liable for all injuries. Let us say that if all skateboarding were confined to skateboard parks, injuries would be reduced by 65%. The fact that they cannot buy, or cannot afford, the liability insurance premiums clearly illustrates that they are being held responsible for the remaining 35% of the injuries as well.

To correlate this premise more directly to sports equipment manufacturers, whether it is football, skiing, or skateboarding, manufacturers, while trying to reduce injuries are, in effect, being held responsible for all injuries even though they may be inherent to the sport, or born out of actions that are not within the rules or foreseeable risks of the game. The consumer is in effect saying that "the manufacturer will insure me for whatever happens." The responsibility of a manufacturer cannot be to eliminate injuries—he can only reduce risk.

With increased popularity of a sport there are increased numbers of participants. With the increased numbers, a high rate of serious eye injuries is occurring. A manufacturer sets out to design a product that will reduce this high rate of injury. One must work within the parameters of the game in question because the rules, playing surface or court, and equipment (ball, puck, bat, racket) have already been established.

If it were a question of completely putting an end to all of the injuries, it would be necessary either to eliminate the cause of those injuries, ie, the ball, puck, bat, or racket, or cease participation. The assumptions are, however, that: 1) the player wants to play, and therefore 2) certain equipment is required for participation even if it is that very equipment or activity that is causing the injuries. Protective equipment must be designed that will reduce the risk with least impairment to the player and the least change to the form and appeal of the sport.

A piece of equipment that solves an injury problem is not immediately received and applauded. Players, whether professional or amateur, are slow to adopt new equipment especially if there is any danger of it impairing their ability to play. If performance is impaired, they simply will not use the product.

Marketing is essential to introduction of a new piece of protective equipment, especially one that has never been used in the sport before. A new product almost always must be "sold" to a sport before it can take its place with the standard equipment. For instance, it is now the vogue to wear eyeguards in racquetball, but it took years for them to be accepted. Tennis players should wear the same eyeguards but they will not now and may never do so. Eye protection to date has not met the aesthetic or fashion requirements of tennis even though the protective factor may be there. A new product has been developed, however, that will offer both protection and fashion. Sports are traditional, and these traditions must be addressed when one considers introducing a new piece of equipment or changing the appearance or design of traditional equipment.

Another factor that must be addressed, relative to the development of a product, is cost. This is another topic rarely discussed openly but it is a reality. Just as a football helmet cannot weigh 20 lb, it would also be unrealistic to develop a helmet that would cost $900. Even if a product offered the best protection possible, if it weighed 20 lb and/or cost $900, no one would or could buy it.

If the product liability pendulum does not swing back to reality all sports will be on the endangered species list. Because the topic of consumerism is usually mentioned in the context of being pitted against some big corporation in the east or a large oil company, there is a tendency to conjure up an image of a structure that is totally inhuman and monolithic. The fact is that the state of the art of protective equipment in the United States today is on the whole quite good. For instance, football helmets that are being manufactured are excellent products. Yet the manufacturers of these products have lost some expensive law suits. It was not because the product failed or broke, but because the laws are unrealistic.

A company received the threat of a law suit in which an individual described receiving a minor injury while wearing a particular piece of protective equipment. The situation was such that the equipment had actually saved the person from a very serious injury, but nevertheless he was seeking restitution. Another individual described almost identical circumstances except he was commending the product for protecting him from serious injury. At a certain point the costs of defending claims and insurance (assuming they can get it), or the risk of being sued, will outweigh the potential profits. When this happens it will be necessary to cease manufacturing protective equipment. Many companies have been forced out of the market already.

The consumer (player and participant) is responsible for establishing the design criteria for products. Manufacturers must supply what the public wants. If they do not want it, it will not sell, and if it does not sell, it will not exist very long.

This situation has changed since the product liability dilemma arose. This market control is adversely affected by the very small percentage of the consumer market seeking huge damages. Normally a manufacturer would put all efforts into responding to the needs of the market and how that relates to efficient product design. A manufacturer of football face guards, for instance, may find it too risky to offer single- and double-bar models and will offer only full cages, thus taking a choice away from the user. More time, money, and effort are being spent today on addressing the product liability question than are spent on research and development of new products.

In order for us to continue to enjoy sports we must accept the assumption of inherent risk. We can reduce this risk by taking the time to find out and use quality products that are backed with design and engineering technology, rather than those that are imitations produced by copying rather than going through the research development process.

The product liability laws must change. Of course, the consumer must be protected from shoddy products but we cannot continue to sue manufacturers for injuries beyond their control. We must, as participants, assume some risk for the activities we choose to undertake. Toothpaste cannot eliminate all cavities. However, one does not turn around and sue the toothpaste company on discovery of a cavity.

A possible solution would be to eliminate contingency fees to attorneys. Canada does not have product liability problems because contingency fees have not taken hold there.

Product liability laws assume the consumer is absolutely devoid of the ability to make choices and assume some responsibility for them. Therefore, the liability problem that has resulted takes away choices that should belong to the consumer. The manufacturers must offer only products that protect their own behinds, when in fact, they are supposed to be protecting other parts of the anatomy.

CHAPTER 35
Legal Aspects of Sportsmedicine

Joseph M. Healey, Jr, JD

The dramatic increase in the popularity of spectator and participant sports is deeply rooted in the social history of twentieth century America. The rise in affluence, availability of significant leisure time, commercialization of leisure time activities, influence of mass media in reporting sports events and activities, belief that participation in sports enhances one's health—all are factors that have contributed to this increase. No one can seriously doubt the central role that sports play in our social and cultural life.

With the increase in sports activities has come recognition that some participants and observers have been subject to a wide range of injuries resulting from their participation or observation. There are many health problems directly caused or exacerbated by sports activities. Out of this recognition, has developed the field of sportsmedicine.

It is inevitable that the development both of sports and of sportsmedicine would raise substantial legal issues. Sports have become big business, and as such have been subjected to the same legal rules that businesses regularly encounter. Important issues such as the civil rights of players, formation of labor unions, and allegations of antitrust violations have emerged. The process of excessive legalization, so pervasive in our society in general, has clearly affected sports as well.

A particularly vexing series of legal problems arises out of issues of responsibility for the injuries suffered by participants or observers of sporting events. Our inability to resolve them suggests the need for a comprehensive societal policy about liability. These problems are of particular concern because of the absence of clear, appropriate legal answers.

Two questions provide a starting point:

1. Who is liable when a participant or spectator is injured in the normal course of a sporting event?
2. Who is liable when a participant or spectator is injured during a sporting event, by conduct outside the rules and regulations of the sport?

A sample of actual cases suggests the range of contexts in which these questions arise:

Soccer A goal keeper who received a pass and gained possession of the ball in the penalty area was kicked in the head by an opposing forward who ignored the rule prohibiting contact with a goal keeper who has possession of the ball in the penalty area.[1]

Boxing Two boxers were engaged in a scheduled match; one collapsed and died after a blow to his chest. He had been suffering from an unknown heart defect that was aggravated by the punches to the chest.[1]

Golf One golfer who had lost his ball in the woods, waived a second golfer through. While searching in the undergrowth, the golfer was struck on the head and injured by the second golfer's ball.[1]

Baseball A spectator sitting in the grandstand, was struck and injured by a bat accidentally released by the batter during a swing.[1]

Shooting Two individuals were target-shooting when one was seriously injured by a bullet ricocheting off the target.[1]

Ice skating An ice skater slipped and fell on the ice. In turn, several skaters who were skating backwards tripped over her, injuring themselves and aggravating her initial injury.[1]

Basketball During a high school game a player received a blow to his head while pursuing a rebound, and suffered a broken jaw.[1]

Football A high school football player, carrying the ball, realized he was about to be tackled. He put his head down and ran into his tacklers. He had a fracture of a neck vertebra.[2]

Wrestling A wrestler suffered a permanent paralysis of all voluntary functions below his neck as the result of an injury sustained during an interscholastic wrestling match.[2]

Swimming A foreign visitor dove into a swimming pool at a place marked simply "4." She had assumed that the measurement was in meters. It was in feet. She was injured in the shallow water.[3]

Tennis A tennis player went to her right to retrieve a forehand shot. As she did, her foot embedded in a dead spot on the court, resulting in torn cartilage in her knee.[4]

Hockey A teenage hockey player was injured when, after throwing himself down on the ice to block a shot, he was struck in the head by a puck which penetrated the helmet.[5]

These are examples of cases that were presented in legal controversies. They are fairly representative of the complex situations that frequently arise, although many never result in litigation. Nonetheless, it is cases like these that must be confronted and resolved.

The concepts of assault and battery provide protection against harmful or offensive contacts made without the consent of the victim. They represent a commitment to the principle of self-determination and personal integrity. An individual has a legal right to be free from threatening gestures and from physical violence and intimidation. Problems arise in trying to determine what this means in the context of sports that allow bodily contact as part of their rules and their customs. The distinction between contact that is necessary or unnecessary, appropriate or inappropriate, permissible or punishable, is often difficult to draw. The basketball, football, wrestling, and boxing cases all contain aspects that emphasize this difficulty. By engaging in such sports, a participant accepts certain risks and consents to certain contact. But the legal categories of assault and battery do not always permit us to make such distinctions in a fair, consistent manner. As a result, issues of responsibility and liability are cloudy.

The law of negligence is designed to provide protection against harms resulting from the violation of some duty owed to the victim by the perpetrator. If a person acts in an unreasonable way toward a person entitled to reasonable care and those actions cause harm, the perpetrator is responsible for harms that result. Before the advent of no-fault automobile insurance, the system of negligence was used to establish liability for injuries suffered in accidents. The system is still used to determine responsibility in medical malpractice cases. Applying the principles to cases in sportsmedicine is problematic. Determining what constitutes unreasonable behavior is not always possible. It is not often clear what obligation the victim has to avoid unreasonable behavior. In the golf, baseball, shooting, ice skating, and swimming examples, who should be held responsible for the injuries that resulted? These cases suggest how difficult it can be to find answers using the principles of negligence law.

Determining the balance of fault and responsibility between the manufacturer of products used in sporting events and the participants creates further problems. The concepts of strict liability and product liability are designed to provide protection for the consumer against injuries resulting from defectively designed or improperly manufactured products. Under these concepts, a manufacturer could be held liable for injuries resulting from a defective product even if the defect was not caused through his negligence. It is assumed that the manufacturer is in the best position to protect against financial liability by purchasing appropriate insurance. But the cost of such a program is high, and many manufacturers are suggesting that they might withdraw from the manufacture of sporting goods because of the threat of enormous liability. The tennis and hockey cases show the types of situations that arise and are not easily resolved.

In addition to the three chief categories of the civil law, there are several categories of the criminal law that may be called upon to resolve problems in sportsmedicine. The criminal law protects not only the rights of the individual victim, but also society as a whole. As a result, its scope is broad, and includes prohibitions against the unjust taking of life (homicide), assault, battery, reckless disregard of life, and disturbances of public order. The serious nature of some sports injuries could deserve the sanctions of the criminal law. But what circumstances are they? How are such sanctions to be enforced? All are reluctant to use the criminal law because it would seriously detract from the sport events. Yet is it not appropriate in some serious cases?

The frustration encountered in attempting to apply principles of the Anglo-American legal tradition to problems in sportsmedicine should not discourage us from attempting to formulate better social policies. Rather, this frustration should encourage us to seek more intelligent, more comprehensive ones.

The foundations of such a policy should include the following four elements:

1. The law is not the only, and is often not the best, mechanism for resolving some of these difficult issues.

The period of extensive over-regulation we are now experiencing is a result of our excessive reliance on the law as a mechanism for formulating policy and resolving conflicts. We need to develop and to use other mechanisms. Organizational review and establishment of standards for sports equipment is an important example of such a mechanism. Much remains to be done in this area.

2. We must recognize that there are many injuries in sports that can and should be eliminated.

A major contribution of the pioneers in sportsmedicine has been the development and implementation of rehabilitative and preventive strategies designed to reduce and eliminate sports injuries. There needs to be continued work in such areas as equipment, conditioning, training, and performance. Acknowledged leaders in sports and sportsmedicine should provide necessary guidance.

Additional steps are needed. When it can be demonstrated that serious injuries can be prevented by stricter rules, there should be rule changes. Umpires and referees should enforce all rules, especially safety ones, strictly and swiftly. There must be a stern refusal to tolerate reckless conduct that threatens the safety of participants or spectators, whether the conduct is in violation of the rules or not. Finally, injuries that occur to unwilling participants who are forced to engage in sports should be eliminated by allowing the participants (especially children) to choose whether or not to participate, and if so, in which sport.

3. There will remain, however, some risks that may be reduced or minimized, but that regrettably cannot be eliminated. We must learn to live with these risks because they are a part of the fabric of the sports, and even of life itself.

After all reasonable steps have been taken to prevent injuries, there will remain risks that cannot be eliminated. The risk of injury is an inherent part of most sports. This realization should not encourage us to be cavalier about such risks. Rather, it should serve as a reminder that injuries do occur. Part of the ambiguity that results from trying to apply principles of the Anglo-American legal tradition to issues of liability in sportsmedicine occurs because of the desire to find the party at fault. The search for liability can easily become a search for scapegoats with each party denying blame and ascribing blame to another party.

Our efforts should be devoted to finding a way to help the injured victim. We need to develop a comprehensive insurance mechanism supported by manufacturers of sporting goods, owners of sporting facilities, and observers and participants themselves. This mechanism could operate as a no-fault insurance system. Its goal would be appropriate compensation for the victim. There is much work to be done in this area.

4. We should encourage continued research in sportsmedicine and improve the access of participants in sports to knowledge as it becomes available.

Our commitment to research in preventive and rehabilitative strategies in sportsmedicine should increase. It may be possible to discover new strategies. At the very least, current knowledge should be available to all participants. Information clearing houses are needed for all areas of sportsmedicine.

The love of sports unites us in our concern for the injured participant. It is tragic to witness the premature end of an athletic career, or an injury that precludes participation in recreational activities. We must be encouraged to focus attention on injured athletes, on protecting them when possible, and on helping them when necessary. It is our obligation to facilitate development of a wiser, more comprehensive social policy toward sports injuries. Although we need to keep these injuries in proper perspective, they deserve attention. Our failure to act will only result in continued ambiguity.

REFERENCES

1. Barklage, D.K. Torts—participant in athletic competition states cause of action for injuries against other participant. *Missouri Law Review* 42:347, 1977.

2. Korpela, A. Tort liability of public schools and institutions of higher learning for accidents occurring during school athletic events. *American Law Reports,* 3rd series. Vol 35, p. 725, 1978.

3. Stern, J. Swimming pool liability. *Trial Magazine* 14(6):26, 1978.

4. Bortz, B., and Levine, C. Torts on the courts. *Trial Magazine* 14(6):30, 1978.

5. *Everett v. Bucky Warren, Inc. North Eastern Reporter.* 2nd series, Vol 380, p. 683, 1978.

CHAPTER 36
Rules Change: An Example from Ice Hockey

Hal Trumble

The procedure for amending or making new additions to the Playing Rules of Amateur Hockey, which includes those relating to protective equipment, is a very open and democratic process.

Five to six months in advance of the Amateur Hockey Association of the United States (AHAUS) annual meeting, which is held in June, the national office will accept proposals for changes in the playing rules. Any individual who is associated with the organization (AHAUS) may submit a suggested revision or new rule. Everything presented is placed on the agenda for the AHAUS board of directors to review in odd-numbered years. Prior to these items being discussed on the floor of the board of directors, the rules committee will review each proposal and make a recommendation relative to adoption or rejection. A simple majority of the board of directors is required for passage.

Involvement of people from the "grass roots" level across the country is welcome primarily because these people are involved in local programs and are aware of ambiguities that might exist or problem areas that may be solved by a proposed amendment. While playing rules are always written with the idea in mind that there can be no misunderstanding, there is always a possibility that various individuals do not get the same meaning as that which was intended. By having an input from the people in the field, AHAUS can find these items and make the necessary corrections.

The AHAUS is constantly looking for ways to make the game of ice hockey safer, more interesting, and fair for the players who are competing and entertaining for the spectators. A good share of this involves the playing rules. For this reason, each proposal that is submitted is given very careful consideration. The process which brought about the mandatory face mask for all players in the AHAUS program is a good example.

The initial input came from parents who were concerned about their youngsters participating in the game and being subjected to the possibility of the loss of an eye, teeth, or a permanent facial scar. They made these concerns known at the meetings of local organizers, who in turn passed on the information to the National Association, which immediately set up a study project. At the time that this matter was brought to the forefront, there was actually a rule that the face mask could not be worn by a player unless he was already injured. The reasoning was that such a piece of equipment could be harmful to another player who is not wearing a mask. The parents very properly cited that this was protection *after* the fact and that something should be done about preventing the injury from happening in the first place.

The AHAUS safety and protective equipment committee was given the responsibility of studying the situation and presenting a recommendation. Their research was very extensive. They analyzed the questions as to whether the wearing of a face mask would: 1) affect the player's performance because of restricted visibility; 2) encourage rough play; 3) if not properly constructed, be more dangerous to the individual wearing it than not wearing any mask at all; and 4) be the possible cause of some injuries, if not worn by all players.

The result was a unanimous recommendation that face masks be mandatory for all participants at the junior age level and below and was adopted at the 1976 AHAUS annual meeting.

A similar process had taken place years earlier that resulted in the mandatory wearing of helmets and mouthpieces. The safety and protective equipment committee continuously monitors ice hockey games for the purpose of determining what may be needed in the way of changes that are reasonable and practical, in order to reduce the number of injuries to the participants.

Many suggestions for rule changes are directed through the district referees-in-chief who work directly with the approximately 9000 AHAUS registered officials. Many of these ideas come from discussions held on the playing rules at the numerous clinics that are conducted throughout the country at the beginning of each season, where interpretations and applications of the rules are thoroughly analyzed.

Because of the speed of the sport and the continuous action, it is very difficult to write a rule book which covers every situation that could occur. Therefore, the rules are written to: 1) cover the situations which reoccur most frequently, and 2) establish a principle which may be applied to an individual incident.

Application of a principle, as well as the specific rule, is a key factor, particularly at it pertains to preventing injuries. At the lower level of competition, where the participants are just beginning to learn the various skills of skating, stickhandling, shooting, team play, etc, it is most important that the rules are applied by the officials in a very strict manner. As the level of competition increases, and the players become more proficient, more latitude may be applied.

The officials, however, are continuously cautioned to make strict enforcement of those rules that involve situations that might cause an injury.

In addition to the input from those people involved in the AHAUS program throughout the country, the rules committee is constantly aware of rules that are being adopted and that have proven to be successful by other organizations involved in the game of ice hockey (such as at college, professional, and international levels). They are interested in anything that can help improve the game with the thought in mind that the safer it is, the more fun it will be for the participants.

CHAPTER 37
How to Prevent Athletic Injuries: Tackle Football as an Example

Frederick O. Mueller, PhD

In the United States more than 15,000 public and private secondary schools have organized football teams with a total of some 1.2 million young men participating. Another 100,000 young men participate at the college or university level. In addition, it has been estimated that more than 1 million boys participate in competition supported by various community and social agencies. If the many thousands of boys who play in sandlot or semiorganized games were included, the total number playing would probably reach 3 million.

Many physicians feel that as many as half of these participants are victims of at least slight injuries each season. Any health problem that affects over 1.5 million young men and boys annually is significant. Naturally, the problem is recognized by those closest to the game—the coaches, school administrators, team physicians and trainers, physical educators and, of course, parents.

Football injuries have been accepted generally as uncomfortable by-products of participation. In a sport requiring vigorous physical contact, injuries are certain to result. However, every effort should be made to assure that the potential for injury is kept to the absolute minimum. The following suggestions, recommendations, and comments are offered to help everybody involved prevent and ... with tackle football.

...ATION

... evaluation and medical
... at the beginning of each
... s allowed to participate in
... medical history is an im-
... luation and should always
... history and examination
... le with the proper school
... ll be available if needed. It
... physician give written approval to permit a player to participate. In addition, written approval from a physician should be required before a player is allowed to return to practice or competition after injury, especially if the athlete has incurred a head injury. The National Collegiate Athletic Association (NCAA) recommends a thorough medical examination when the athlete first enters the college athletic program and an annual health history update with use of referral exams when warranted. Each state high school association has a set of recommendations for preparticipation medical evaluations, and these should be followed by the coaches of each state. If the physician or coach has any questions about the athlete's readiness to participate, the athlete should not be allowed to play.

A physician should be on the field of play during game and practice sessions. When this is not possible, arrangements must be made in advance to obtain a physician's immediate service if an emergency should arise. Transportation from the game or practice site to a medical facility should also be readily available. Each institution should have a team trainer who is a regular member of the staff and is qualified in treating and preventing injuries.

Every school and institution fielding a football team must subscribe to an athletic injury insurance program. There are several plans available, and the type chosen will depend on the policies of communities and states involved. The National Federation of State High School Associations has an insurance program available on a volunteer basis for all its member schools, and the NCAA will have an insurance plan for catastrophic injuries that will be available to member schools on a volunteer basis in 1985. An excellent source for information on athletic injury insurance is the American Medical Association's Council on Medical Services.

PHYSICAL CONDITIONING

Top performance can only be achieved by the athlete who is in top physical condition; conversely, the athlete in poor physical shape will give a poor performance. More importantly, the poorly conditioned athlete is susceptible to disabling injuries.

A program to aid the athlete in developing a state of physical fitness should be concerned with endurance, speed, flexibility, and strength. Endurance refers to cardiovascular and respiration fitness and is achieved by using an endurance or aerobic program that consists of prolonged continuous work of relatively low intensity. Speed is an asset in all sports and can be improved by following a sprint or anaerobic program. Anaerobic training is accomplished by repeated work of high intensity such as sprints and agility or reaction drills related to the sport. Flexibility involves stretching exercises to give the athlete a more complete range of motion and to prevent possible muscle and ligament injuries. Strength development programs are important in all sports and should be planned to develop both muscle strength and endurance. Strength programs include isometrics, weight resistance machines, and lifting of free weights. It is important to follow strength programs that are planned by experts in the field and are properly supervised. A strength training program for football participation should also include exercises to strengthen the muscles of the neck. This program may not prevent the athlete from sustaining a neck injury, but it will help him keep his head in the proper position when performing the fundamentals of blocking and tackling. This is especially important late in the game when the athlete is fatigued.

It is strongly recommended that the first week of football practice be graded conditioning with particular emphasis on programs that will strengthen the body and reduce susceptibility to fatigue. Considerable effort during the initial conditioning period should be devoted to non-contact activity with emphasis on teaching the fundamental skills.

Preseason Practice

The majority of state high school athletic associations as well as the NCAA require a preseason physical conditioning period of three to seven days for all football athletes before any physical contact between players is permitted. Research has shown that this mandatory conditioning reduces the number and severity of injuries during the early fall practice period. This non-contact period is also excellent for acclimatizing the athletes for hot weather conditions.

When athletes practice and play in hot weather conditions certain precautions should be taken. This is particularly true in football; however, coaches of all sports should be aware of the problems associated with hot weather conditions.

Since 1974 there has been a dramatic reduction in football heat stroke deaths with the exception of 1978, when there were four. All coaches, trainers and physicians should continue their efforts toward eliminating athletic fatalities that result from physical activity in hot weather.

Heat stroke and heat exhaustion are prevented by careful control of various factors in the conditioning program of the athlete. When football is played in hot weather the following suggestions and precautions should be taken:

1. Each athlete should have a complete physical examination with a medical history and an annual health history update. History of previous heat illness and type of training activities before organized practice begins should be included.
2. Acclimatization to heat is a gradual process and is 80% achieved over a seven to ten day period by repeated exercise sessions in the new climate. Full acclimatization will take approximately three weeks and in some cases longer. Graduated practice sessions should be used for the first seven to ten days.
3. Know both the temperature and humidity since, it is more difficult for the body to cool itself in high humidity. Use of a sling psychrometer is recommended to measure the relative humidity, and any time the wet-bulb temperature is over 76° practice should be altered.
4. Adjust activity level and provide frequent rest periods. Rest in cool, shaded areas with some air movement, remove helmets, and loosen or remove jerseys. Rest periods of 15 to 30 minutes should be provided during workouts of one hour.
5. Provide adequate water replacement during practice and games. Water should always be available and in unlimited quantities. Cold water is preferable because it stimulates thirst and is emptied more rapidly from the stomach. Commercial drinks have become popular, but plain water is sufficient.
6. Salt should be replaced daily, and liberal salting of the athlete's food will accomplish this purpose. Coaches should not provide salt tablets to athletes. It should be stressed that plain water and not salt and other electrolytes is needed to restore fluid loss.
7. Athletes should weigh each day before and after practice and weight charts checked in order to treat the athlete who loses excessive weight each day. Generally, a 3% body weight loss through sweating is safe and a 5% loss is in the danger zone.

8. Clothing is important, and a player should avoid the use of long sleeves, long stockings, and any excess clothing. Never use rubberized clothing or sweatsuits.

9. Some athletes are more susceptible to heat injury. These individuals are not accustomed to work in the heat, may be overweight, or may be the eager athlete who constantly competes at his capacity.

10. It is important to observe athletes for signs of heat illness. Some trouble signs are nausea, incoherence, fatigue, weakness, vomiting, cramps, weak rapid pulse, flushed appearance, visual disturbance, and unsteadiness. If heat illness is suspected, seek a physician's immediate service. Emergency procedures are vital.

A sample preseason conditioning program would have the first week of practice limited to noncontact activities with emphasis on conditioning. Shorts, T-shirts, helmets, football shoes and mouth protectors should be worn. During this time the groundwork can be laid for the fundamentals of the game to be stressed.

The second week should include full protective equipment but should be limited to controlled situations carefully supervised by the coach. Practice games and game condition scrimmages should be prohibited until after a minimum of two weeks of practice.

Three weeks of well-planned practice sessions should precede the first regularly scheduled game.

COACHING STAFF

The head football coach is the most important individual in establishing a successful sports program. His attitude and leadership in promoting the safety factor determine whether or not his program will be successful. Much of the responsibility for parts of the program may be delegated to other personnel, but he is the final authority in seeing that all phases are conscientiously carried out.

Securing a competent and experienced coaching staff is one of the most difficult assignments facing the school administration. It has been demonstrated that it is easier to control an athletic program when the coaching staff consists of faculty members. If a school or institution cannot provide a well-trained and professionally prepared coaching staff, consideration should be given to eliminating the sport from the athletic program.

The head coach is responsible for the total program and it is his/her responsibility to seek competent and dedicated assistants. The assistant coach should be a skilled teacher and should have the ability to teach the proper fundamentals of the game. All coaches should take precautions to assure excellence in the physical conditioning of their athletes. Proper conditioning reduces the frequency and severity of injuries and increases morale and desire of the athlete to compete in wholesome physical activity. The coach who does not have the knowledge or expertise in the physical conditioning of the athletes jeopardizes both the health of the students and the total program.

The head coach should be aware of important fundamental changes in the skills of the game and should attend local, state, and national coaching clinics. It is his responsibility to pass this information on to his coaching staff through a series of in-service training sessions.

Participation in football can foster desirable health habits, and the coaching staff should take advantage of teaching situations and inculcate acceptable health practices in their athletes.

RULES AND REGULATIONS

Another method of promoting football safety is to establish and enforce a sound set of rules and regulations. Many unnecessary injuries occur every year because of a poorly defined rule, the lack of a rule, or the improper enforcement of one. It is imperative that each school employ competent officials to officiate at games. Coaches must instruct their athletes within the rules and must not take advantage of them by permitting players to use abusive and hazardous tactics under game or practice conditions. In addition, coaches and school officials must support the game officials in their conduct of the athletic contest.

Athletic governing organizations of colleges and high schools meet each year to promote research to determine the causes of football injuries and vote on rules that enhance safety. The number one criteria for a rules change in football is that the change must be safe for the athletes playing the game. A majority of the rules changes in football over the years have been made to make the game safer. It is important to review the rules each year to make football a safer game and to adjust to the increasing skills, size and speed of the players.

Regulations are extremely important in prevention of injury, but prime importance lies with the officials' responsibility to enforce the rules and the coach's responsibility to coach within them. Coaches should repeatedly warn their players against spearing, piling on, clipping, making initial contact with the helmet while tackling and blocking, and all other illegal tactics.

Football coaches should be thoroughly acquainted with the rules of the game and should be responsible for having the rules taught and interpreted to his players. The coach is responsible for violations of the rules, and both the letter and the spirit of the rules must be adhered to.

EQUIPMENT

It is difficult to suggest that some football protective equipment is safer than others, but the following guidelines should be used to assist the purchaser:

1. The purchaser must deal with reputable sporting goods manufacturers and representatives.
2. The purchaser must buy the best equipment available.
3. Equipment must be properly fitted by someone with the proper expertise.
4. Protective equipment must afford adequate protection against the hazards for which it was designed and not create additional hazards.
5. Old and worn equipment must be renovated properly or discarded. Do not use old, worn out equipment and never hand down this equipment to players of lesser skill or younger teams.
6. Be sure that shoe cleats conform to the standard set forth in the Rule Book.
7. Football helmets should meet the National Operating Committee on Standards in Athletic Equipment (NOCSAE) standard that became mandatory with the 1978 season for colleges and 1980 for secondary schools.

Football protective equipment should be maintained and checked periodically for continued proper fit and absence of acquired defects. Each player should be equipped with a helmet, mouth protector, shoulder pads, hip and thigh pads, knee pads and shoes.

When describing football protective equipment, special consideration should be given to the helmet. Although designed as a protective device, the helmet has been used as a weapon in recent years. An illegal practice referred to as spearing, that is, driving the heat with force into the chest, stomach, or kidney area of an opponent, has developed. When the head is used as a battering ram there is danger of hyperflexion, hyperextension, or compression of the cervical vertebrae, as well as concussion. Head and neck injuries have increased since this tactic was adopted by some teams. Players should be taught to respect the helmet as a protective device and that the helmet should not be used as a weapon. Enforcement of the rules prohibiting spearing, properly fitted helmets, correct methods of blocking and tackling and excellent physical conditioning are factors that will help reduce fatalities and serious head and neck injuries in football.

SUMMARY

Football injuries and fatalities can be eliminated or appreciably reduced if the following recommendations are followed:

1. Mandatory medical examinations and medical history should be taken before allowing an athlete to participate in any football activity.

2. All personnel concerned with training football athletes should emphasize proper, gradual and complete physical conditioning.

3. A physician should be present at all games and practice sessions. If it is impossible for a physician to be present at all practice sessions, emergency measures must be provided.

4. All personnel associated with football participation should be cognizant of the problems and safety measures related to physical activity in hot weather.

5. Each institution should strive to have a team trainer who is a regular member of the staff and is adequately prepared and qualified.

6. There should be strict enforcement of game rules and administrative regulations should be enforced to protect the health of the athlete. Coaches and officials must support the game officials in their conduct of the athletic contest.

7. Only well-trained athletic personnel should be employed and there should be a renewed emphasis on providing excellent facilities and securing the safest and best equipment available.

8. Coaches should continue to teach and emphasize the proper fundamentals of blocking and

tackling to help reduce head and neck fatalities.

9. When a player has experienced or shown signs of head trauma (loss of consciousness, visual disturbances, headache, inability to walk correctly, obvious disorientation, memory loss), he should receive immediate medical attention and should not be allowed to return to practice or game without permission from the proper medical authorities.

10. Finally, there should be continued research concerning the safety factor in football.

CHAPTER 38
Sportsmedicine: An Overview

Daniel F. Hanley, MD

Like Gaul, sportsmedicine may be divided into three parts: trauma, medicine, and research. Unlike Gaul, the dividing lines of sportsmedicine are blurred and indistinct. Also unlike Gaul, each area is expandable, and the very recent development of a sports administration publication may mean a fourth section.

Research of sorts has spilled over into the areas of trauma and medicine. Data collecting and the increasing availability of data retrieval and processing equipment have brought forth a spate of research, much of it inadequate in concept, design, and execution. One of the real threats to the continued development of all of sportsmedicine as an increasingly acceptable specialty branch, is this poor quality of work. The trauma and medicine sections have improved in quality and operation. This improvement in the past 15 years is due largely to the influx of young and well-trained doctors who have brought their techniques and abilities to bear on the care of athletes.

The increasing numbers of individuals involved in exercise and fitness programs, aerobics, yoga, jogging, etc, gives a new meaning to "on the field." In general terms, sportsmedicine deals with the prevention and care of the individual from the inception of the disability through the rehabilitative process, as far as that process can go. It also recognizes that there are times when the disability is not fully rehabilitable. An equally important function is then to convey this information to the injured person at the earliest possible time.

For the most part, patients seen in the medicine section of a sports program are young healthy adults. Their diseases are few, 90% of them minor infections, especially upper respiratory, gastrointestinal, and skin. Infections secondary to trauma are often of a more serious nature. The numbers and ages of participants are expanding so that the chronic and degenerative diseases are showing up more and more. Osteoarthritis, gout, hypertension, diabetes, and cardiovascular diseases, all merit consideration. Of the more serious diseases pneumonia, meningitis, hepatitis, encephalitis, acute iritis, and cholecystitis are usually seen in the older age groups (coaches, managers, spectators). Serious diseases and injuries, although infrequent, must figure prominently in the planning of a good sportsmedicine section.

PLANNING AND PREVENTION

Preseason physical examinations are universally accepted now. These are best done by the regular family doctor and recorded on a form developed by the sports physician in charge of the medical program. Each physical examination form is then reviewed by the sports physician. If medical problems are turned up, he rechecks the patient. Medical forms should be kept available for additions as necessary. The sports physician must survey all the facilities the program will use at home, stadium, field, gymnasium, pool, ice rink. This survey should be done with the objective of removing all hazardous conditions and equipment. It should make certain that the areas have the proper medical equipment and supplies and that transportation is not impeded by locked gates or chains. Hazardous conditions include wooden or steel benches and bleachers too close to the playing field, and wood or metal inflexible yard markers on the football field. On two occasions it was discovered that the white lines on football fields had been marked with unslaked lime, but not before several players suffered chemical burns of the skin. Fortunately, no eyes were involved. Broken wire fence above the boards on a hockey rink, holes in any playing surface, broken glass and rocks on field, and unsanitary water sources are all possible hazards.

Immunizations should be brought up-to-date before the program starts. If the schedule involves foreign travel, a check with the Center for Disease Control in Atlanta, Georgia will determine if additional immunizations (human and animal) are indicated.

SUPPLIES

The physician in charge should develop a list of medical and training supplies and equipment that will be needed for the season. This list must be constantly updated. Some items such as airways, stretchers, cervical collars, air splints, nasal elevators, and slings must be permanently located at each practice and game site.

The usual physician's bag is not enough. The ideal set-up has two additional bags: one containing sterile suture sets, gloves, sterile cloths or towels on which to place the sterile sets, and another set up as a trainer's case for the trainer, coach, etc. For away games an additional medical trunk with all the appropriate permanent equipment mentioned, as well as additional chin straps, cleats, tooth guards, contact lens holders, lamp black, tongue forceps, and sponge pads should accompany the team medical section.

TRAVEL

When the team travels to another city in this country, plans for medical care must be made prior to the trip. A simple call to the opponents' athletic department will determine what facilities, supplies, personnel, and equipment will be available at the game. In addition, the visiting team physician should know what hospital and what specialist he plans to use for serious injuries, and how he will transport an injured player back home.

If the schedule includes foreign travel, more planning is necessary and should start with an area disease survey to include endemic, epidemic, and sporadic human and animal diseases, especially rabies and equine encephalitis. The Center for Disease Control in Atlanta, multinational companies, the United States embassy, and the health department of the foreign city will all be helpful sources of information. In addition to the proper immunizations and checks of water and food sources, availability of medical facilities and medical and dental personnel must be known. Transportation in a foreign city is available but the where and how of transportation for the ill and injured must be documented before leaving home, or at least as soon after arrival as possible.

The same attitude applies to communications. Most foreign cities have an English-speaking operator on call at all times, and someone should know how to reach her.

In foreign travel one also runs into special regulations. The importation of medicines (drugs) and food stuffs is usually forbidden and personal medical instruments, camera, and recording devices should be identified by number and listed prior to departure. Detailed maps of the country and cities to be visited will be extremely helpful and should be studied prior to departure so that alternate bus and subway routes are familiar.

SPORT RESEARCH

Perhaps no more needs to be said on this subject. Some of the work is excellent but it does tend to be repetetive. Sports research has a tendency to follow fads, is often fragmented and uncoordinated, involves statistically invalid (small) numbers of athletes, and often draws conclusions that may be open to question.

Sports administration is a small but growing field and may in time exert a positive, coordinative influence on all phases of sportsmedicine, including research.

Observations of a Competitor

James P. Webb, RN

As I stand in front of a large audience, the music starts. I skate one revolution around the arena and as I elevate into the first jump, I feel what seems to be a piece of rope tearing in two within my calf. I push with my legs, not quite realizing what has happened. The pain is unbearable. "Do I stop skating, do I continue, do I scream? What do I do?" This is a shocking scene that plagues nearly every figure skater during his or her skating career.

Many athletes with whom I have spoken who are involved in athletic competition such as running, diving, crew team racing as well as those competing in my own sport all share a deep concern about avoiding injuries. This concern becomes second nature, a constant battle between feeling the shearing pain of day-to-day training and the pain of an injury. We all have the same feelings about injuries; they are devastating.

To know how an athlete feels about injuries, at least how I, as a figure skater rehearsing for competition regard them, you have to understand how I feel about competition. I feel so strongly, even now 13 years later, that I remember my first major trial.

I drift into the arena not at all conscious of where my legs are or how I am walking. I hear the sounds of something foreign, something new. Yes, a crowd screaming, "go, go, you can do it!" The sounds fade out. The smell of cigarette smoke and exhaust gases fill my sinuses. How hard it seems to breathe. I look to my left and see many long rows of people gazing at the skater on the ice. I look up and see still more smoke and search still higher to the sky, seeing a ceiling higher than I have ever seen before. To my right, I see dozens, what seem like hundreds, of rows of faces examining the ice. I look straight ahead, and see the ice, the only familiar part of these surroundings.

Suddenly I feel my feet, they are cemented to the ground, stuck as if they were welded. I smell a strange acidic odor; I feel my heart pounding, my fingers are throbbing. I look away toward the locker room where I must change into my skates. I try to walk but my feet are still glued to the ground. I see my coach, she gives me a reassuring look as if to say, "you're good, you're very good, you're number one and you're going to do it. You can't lose because you're the best. Let's go, put on your skates." As if my legs suddenly spring into life, I seemingly jump from where I am standing and float toward the locker room.

I hear very faint sounds along the way, "who's he? He's going to beat Ricky Porter. Look, that's him." As I walk inside the locker room, I look around, almost choking on the smell of wet leather, sweat, and salt as it slams against my throat. All eyes are on me, each pair studying the skates I will be putting on. No one makes a sound as I walk over to an empty spot on the bench in the corner to sit and think. Here I am, 11 years old at my first competition, third after the compulsory figures, two places from the top. I have nothing to lose, I am away from home, far away in Pennsylvania. I flew for the first time, how exciting it was. I stop dreaming as my eyes catch sight of Ricky Porter. I listen again to my thoughts. "Ricky's fantastic, he's great, he is good, he has jumps in his program that I don't have." I scrub Ricky out of my mind. I put on my skates, too tight, no—too loose, no—just right, brush off my gray flannel pants, my gray sweater, fix my red tie, and I am ready to go. I am ready to skate, to win; suddenly I feel that I am going to explode from the excitement. I let out a hint of a smile as if to hold the rest inside of me to draw on later.

As I walk back into the arena, a voice so loud that I try to shut it out bellows down at me. "Division One skaters: please take the ice for warm-up." All those thousands of faces are watching me. As I look to my coach, my heart pounds, sweat fills my armpits, and the acid taste in my mouth returns. My coach nods a very reassuring "yes."

Warm-up is over and the burning in my thighs is gone. I feel good. The first skater starts, then finishes. I am to skate third, after Ricky. Ricky takes the ice. I watch as he starts his freestyle program. He attempts his first jump—falls, then tries another—falls again, then executes the rest of his program falling yet a third time. The crowd, as if by direction, signs a sorrowful "Ohh" each time he falls. He has finished his program, my turn is next.

"Will the next skater please take the ice." Wait! Stop! Do I run out onto the ice, skate fast, skate slowly? "Have fun out there!" my coach whispers into my ear, interrupting my thoughts.

I step onto the ice, glide over to where I am to start my routine. I stop, putting my arms out. Why don't they start the music, my arms feel so heavy.

As the music starts, a familiar sound heard each day for the past eight months enters my ears. I execute my routine exactly as I have for the past eight months. As I skate, I see the faces, no bodies, just faces. I hear nothing but the sound of my own breathing. I feel the ice, I see the barriers, and I feel the music. The music is over, they are clapping for me. I did it, I skated flawlessly! A grin springs to my face.

I wait impatiently as the next six skaters finish. I want a chocolate bar. The announcer starts, "Third place," no name that I recognize, did I drop to fourth? "Second place: Richard Porter." As I hear my name being called for first place, I jump into the air shouting, "Yes, I did it!"

One of the hardest aspects of athletic training is being honest with yourself. This is another battle that athletes involved in all sports have in common. Am I running three miles, every step? How fast am I running? Slowly enough so that I won't get that burning pain in my lower back? I push step after step, pounding my knees against the pavement. I want to stop. I don't want the pain in my calves and thighs any longer, but I go on because I know that I must. It's just me against the pain. I am the only one who will know whether I've done it or not. I will be honest with myself—I will go on. I've worked hard all day, just a small nap. No, I must run again. Who will know if I don't? I will know.

Testing myself, me against me. My muscles, bones, lungs, their pain vs my ability to overcome it. I skate day after day, week after week, trying to jump higher each time. Not high enough, try it again, no, still not high enough. My legs ache, my knees feel like rubber, I taste the sweat on my face. One more time, one more exhausting, painful, agonizing time. I try the triple, again I try it, but my knees hurt. "Will I really damage my knees if I try it again? I must do it today, not tomorrow." I leave the ice after practice almost too tired to breathe. As I sit in the locker room with my arms on my knees, I stink and I ache and yet I feel good knowing that I went against myself. I ached and yet I still practiced longer and harder. Those hot, stinky afternoons slither down the drain of a shower stall until the next morning when I do it all over again. It seems like a perpetual grinding 365 days a year, but for what? For that chance to be number one, to be in front of that screaming audience yelling for me.

I feel that my competitors are working as hard as I am so I push harder, grinding my blades into the ice. Deeper and with more vigor, feeling as though I were going to break apart at my joints.

There are many great athletes who seem to win constantly and never falter. Many athletes falter time and time again. Competitive sports are twofold, being divided into practicing and performing. While practice is vital to any sport, the performance is what separates the number one competitor from the rest of the field. Faltering during a performance can be equally as devastating as an injury that keeps an athlete out of competition. The following is a description of how faltering caused my loss and how devastating it can be to the athlete.

It is December 21, 1972, my final exam is over. Rushing home to my dormitory room, I throw my clothes into a suitcase, grab my skates and hurry to a plane heading for Lake Placid, New York for the 1973 United States Eastern Figure Skating Championships. For the next six weeks I will do nothing but skate, eat, and sleep until competition is over. No exams to concern me, nothing to think about but skating. I arrive in New York at 2 AM; everything is cold and white. I am shown to a small room that will be my home for the next six weeks. My head has no sooner hit the pillow than I hear a screaming bell blasting into my ears. It is 5 AM, I have to be on the ice in 30 minutes.

The air outside feels like ice, my limbs like cement. I hurry to the rink following my breath as I walk. There is no sound other than the crunch of snow under my boots. Finally inside the rink, the air feels still colder. I put on my skates barely feeling my toes. I am the only one on the ice.

I skate the school figures until 7 AM, then glide off the ice to look at the work I have done, what a lot I have done. How much I must still do. The ice machine springs into life erasing all. I skate onto the ice to do it over again until 9 AM. Now to practice freestyle.

I push, glide, push, glide, pushing the molasses out of my legs every step of the way. As I stop by the barriers, I put one of my outstretched legs on the boards, how painful my calves feel. Head to knee, keeping my legs straight. The burning in my thighs gets worse. I feel really stiff. The other leg, same thing. "Loosen up, come on, loosen up." I skate along the ice pushing it away from me with every step. By now it is 11:00 in the morning, six hours have gone by in a flash. With so few people on the ice, I skate along feeling that I am the only one. I am off at noon to go home for lunch, so hungry that I could eat a side of beef. Back to the ice at 2 PM to work more until 4:00. Jumping, spinning, gliding, more jumping, working harder. It feels good, I am getting stronger. "I wonder how I did on my final exams."

This goes on for five weeks, no drinking on New Year's, no staying up late at night, always keeping my thoughts on that one day of competition.

A week before the event, I feel as if I am the rink, the rink is me. I know every crack, every crevice, high spot and low. My competitors start arriving one by one. Six days until competition. Many "Hi, how are you's" are exchanged, none of them with much feeling. The tension can already be sliced with a knife.

The evening before the event, as I stroll around the town of Lake Placid, I think about the work I have done, my thoughts quickly turning to my freestyle program with its jumps and spins. "If I can only land all the jumps in the program . . . I can make it, I'll make it to the United States National Championships in Long Beach, California. I know I can, I feel I can."

The day of the event, I enter the arena, atmosphere so thick that I swim through it rather than walk. With my skates on I am ready to go. I have been competing for nine years now. My turn to skate, wow—what a crowd. They are screaming for me—what a great feeling.

The music starts and I execute the first jump higher than I ever have before. Four minutes left in the program, I feel good. I feel and skate with the music. What a great feeling to be performing in front of an audience. To be skating, having practiced so hard, and to be performing so well. Athletic competition—there is nothing like it. As I approach the hardest jump in my program, I trip as I take off and fall. I missed the jump. The one jump I needed to get to the United States Championships. My world seems to have come crashing down on me, how empty I feel.

I continue skating, still trying hard, yet knowing in the back of my mind that my chances for the Nationals are over. As I finish my program I stand there wishing it had not happened, trying to think of something that will change my position. It is over. How lost I feel. A jump that I have been executing for years. I missed it. "How can I go on?" Then a voice starts from my thoughts. "Keep your head up, smile, thank everyone with a bow, and skate off."

INDEX